A Primer of Drug Action

A Primer of
DRUG ACTION

A Concise, Nontechnical
Guide to the Actions,
Uses, and Side Effects
of Psychoactive Drugs

Eighth Edition

Robert M. Julien M.D., Ph.D.
St. Vincent Hospital and Medical Center
Portland, Oregon

W. H. Freeman and Company
New York

Text and cover designer: Blake Logan
Cover illustration: Janet Hamlin

Library of Congress Cataloging-in-Publication Data

Julien, Robert M.
       A primer of drug action : a concise, nontechnical guide to the actions, uses,
and side effects of psychoactive drugs / Robert M. Julien. — 8th ed.
              p.   cm.
       Includes bibliographical references and index.
       ISBN 0-7167-3112-6 (alk. paper). — ISBN 0-7167-3113-4 (pbk. : alk. paper)
       1. Psychotropic drugs. 2. Psychopharmacology. I. Title.
RM315.J75 1997
615'.78—dc21   97-17171
                                                                            CIP

Printed in the United States of America

First printing 1997

Contents

Preface

Psychoactive drugs are defined as substances that act to alter mood, thought processes, or behavior or that are used to manage neuropsychological illness. In the 23 years since the publication of the first edition of *A Primer of Drug Action*, there has been an explosion of knowledge about these drugs and the underlying disorders for which they are used. This knowledge explosion is accelerating, and remarkable advances are occurring in the late 1990s. The three-year period 1994–1997 alone witnessed the introduction of totally new classes of drugs for treating schizophrenia and depression, the recognition of the chronic and disabling nature of persistent anxiety and dysthymia, an increase in the psychopharmacologic treatment of psychological disorders of children and adolescents, new understanding of the biochemical abnormalities in behavioral disorders, new understanding about the usefulness of certain antiepileptic drugs in the treatment of bipolar, conduct, and personality disorders, and increasing interest in the pharmacologic treatment of both attention deficit hyperactivity disorder (ADHD) and obesity. I hope this book reflects that growth and advancement and conveys the excitement of ongoing discovery.

A Primer of Drug Action discusses the general principles of each class of psychoactive drugs and provides specific information about each drug. It also addresses the mechanisms of action of each drug and drug class, current theories about the etiology of major psychological disorders and rationales for drug treatment, and uses and limitations of psychopharmacology in the overall management of the patient.

Drugs of compulsive abuse are again addressed, with new discussions of anabolic steroids, marijuana, the hallucinogens, inhalants, behavioral stimulants (cocaine and the amphetamines), alcohol and other sedatives, and the opioid narcotics. As in the seventh edition, theories of drug-induced behavioral reinforcement, comorbidity of substance abuse with other psychological disorders, and the treatment of substance abuse are emphasized.

In essence, the major changes that have occurred since the publication of the seventh edition in 1995 necessitated a complete revision of the book. Citations are increased, and almost all are from the 1990s, with 40 percent from 1996 and 1997. Up-to-date citations and rewriting are consistent with the effort to make each edition of *A Primer of Drug Action* the most current, objective, readable, and useful introduction to the pharmacology of drugs that affect the mind and behavior.

The goal of the first edition of this book, published in 1975, was to provide pharmacological information that was concise, accurate, and timely. The discussion was presented in clear language, as free as possible of technical jargon, so that it could be easily understood by readers with minimal background in the biological sciences. This philosophy continues in the eighth edition. The pharmacological and psychotherapeutic treatments of psychological disorders are integrated, and the interface between psychopharmacotherapy and the various professions of counseling, psychology, and psychotherapy is addressed. People entering these and related professions now must be knowledgeable about and conversant in the pharmacology of the drugs their clients or patients may be taking, increasingly important since the publication of clinical practice guidelines for the treatment of major psychological disorders. To this end, each chapter contains a brief discussion of the clinical pharmacologic/psychological interface, and Chapter 15, cowritten with a clinical psychologist, is totally devoted to this topic.

Features of the Eighth Edition

In its first two decades of publication, *A Primer of Drug Action* helped shape courses in psychopharmacology, drug abuse, and drug education. Now in its third decade of publication, the book is completely revised and updated with the aim of continuing its history as the most current and most understandable introduction to psychopharmacology. All fifteen chapters and the four appendixes have been rewritten to update each topic of discussion. The literature citations are updated, and most are from 1995 through 1997. Included are not only the newly available drugs but discussions of both current and future directions in drug research (including new drugs that are on the horizon but not yet available for clinical use). New drugs included in this edition include

- The "new-generation" antipsychotics, including clozapine (Clozaril), risperidone (Risperdol), olanzapine (Zyprexa), and sertindole (Serlect)

- New, "dual-action" antidepressants, including nefazodone (Serzone) and mirtazapine (Remeron) and a reversible MAO inhibitor, mo-clobemide (Aurorix)
- New opioid agonists and antagonists, including remifentanyl (Ultiva), tramadol (Ultram), and nalmefene (Revex)
- New psychedelics, including hoasca and ibogaine, the latter being studied as an "anticraving" agent
- New agents for treating obesity, including fenfluramine/phento-lamine ("fen-phen"), dexfenfluramine (Redux), and sibutramine (Meridia)

Also included in the eighth edition:

- Critical review of the various agents used to treat ADHD and obesity
- Discussion of the limitations to lithium therapy and its pharmaco-logic alternatives
- Discussion of clinical practice guidelines for treating psychological disorders
- Discussion of the seven classes of antidepressant drugs
- Four new appendixes, on nonopioid analgesics, oral contraceptives and other pharmacologic means to modulate female fertility, drugs used to treat Parkinsonism, and an introduction to the brain, the neuron, and synaptic transmission
- Discussion of the use of antidepressants to treat depression, panic disorder, OCD, ADHD, PTSD, and other behavioral disorders
- A new chapter devoted to the topic of anabolic steroids and their abuse

As did the previous editions, the eighth edition will, I hope, serve the needs of all those who want a concise, clearly presented introduction to the fields of psychopharmacology, drug education, and psychophar-macotherapy.

Acknowledgments

I would like to sincerely thank Dr. Donald Lange (clinical psychologist, Portland, Oregon) for his generous assistance with Chapter 15. I also offer my thanks to Vina Spiehler, Ph.D., DABFT (forensic toxicology consultant), for her excellent and appreciated review of the manuscript. Finally, I would like to offer my condolences to the family of Dr. John T. Elder (former Professor of Pharmacology, Creighton University School of Medicine, Omaha, Nebraska), who died on November 3, 1995. Dr. Elder graciously assisted with the editing and professional review of the first seven editions.

Dedication

I dedicate the eighth edition to my wife, Judi, who not only has supported the many years of effort on the first seven editions but has recently completed her doctoral training in clinical psychology. Her encouragement and input are invaluable.

Chapter 1

PRINCIPLES OF DRUG ACTION

When we have a headache, we take for granted that after taking some aspirin our headache will probably disappear within 15 to 30 minutes. We also take for granted that, unless we take more aspirin later, the headache may recur within a few hours.

This familiar scenario reveals the four primary events of pain relief. The first is the administration and absorption of the drug into the body; the second is the distribution of the drug throughout the body; the third is the interaction of the drug with its "receptors" in the body, which are responsible for the drug's actions; and the fourth is the elimination of the drug from the body. These factors, coupled with dosage, determine the concentration of a drug at its sites of action and, hence, the *intensity* of drug effect on the receptor as a function of time.[1]

Pharmacodynamics is a term that refers to the study of these drug-receptor interactions and will be discussed later in this chapter. First, however, we will discuss *pharmacokinetics*—the study of how drugs move through and affect the body.

PHARMACOKINETICS: HOW DRUGS MOVE THROUGH THE BODY

Pharmacokinetics, in its simplest form, describes the time course of a particular drug's actions—the time to onset and the duration of a drug's effects. Usually, the time course simply reflects the amount of time required for the rise and fall of the drug's concentration at the target site. Simple though this may sound, the process of transporting a drug from outside the body to its ultimate site of action inside the body is complex (a detailed picture of the process is given in Figure 1.1).

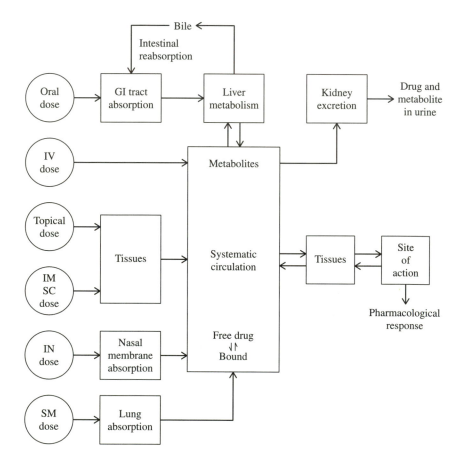

FIGURE 1.1   Schematic representation of the fate of a drug in the body. IM = intramuscular; IV = intravenous; IN = intranasal; SC = subcutaneous; SM = smoked. [Modified from C. N. Chiang and R. L. Hawks, "Implications of Drug Levels in Body Fluids: Basic Concepts," in R. L. Hawks and C. N. Chiang, eds., *Urine Testing for Drugs of Abuse,* NIDA Research Monograph No. 73 (Rockville, Md.: National Institute on Drug Abuse, 1986), p. 63.]

Drug Absorption

The phrase "drug absorption" refers to mechanisms by which drugs pass from the point of entry into the bloodstream. When administering any drug, one must select a route of administration, a dose of the drug, and a dosage form (liquid, tablet, capsule, or injection) that will both place the drug at its site of action in a pharmacologically effective concentration and maintain the concentration for an adequate period of time.

Drugs are most commonly administered in one of six ways: orally (through the mouth), rectally (into the rectum), parenterally (by injection), by inhalation through the lungs, and by absorption through the skin or absorption through the mucous membranes.

Oral Administration

Drugs are most commonly taken by mouth and swallowed. To be effective when administered orally, the drug must be soluble and stable in stomach fluid, enter the intestine, penetrate the lining of the intestine, and pass into the bloodstream.

Because they are already in solution, drugs that are administered in liquid form tend to be absorbed more rapidly than those given in tablet or capsule form. Alcohol, for example, is taken in liquid form. As a result, about one-fourth to one-third of the alcohol that is ingested is absorbed directly from the stomach into the bloodstream (the rest is absorbed from the upper intestine). Thus, absorption is rapid and the effects of the alcohol can be felt rapidly, especially if no food is present in the stomach. When a drug is taken in solid form, both the rate at which it dissolves and its chemistry limit its rate of absorption.

After a drug dissolves in the stomach, it is carried into the upper intestine where it is absorbed across the intestinal mucosa by a process of passive diffusion. This process occurs against a developing concentration gradient of drug at a rate that is determined by the ratio of water solubility to lipid solubility of the drug molecules. Indeed, once they are in the body, drugs exist as a mixture of two interchangeable forms: one that is water soluble (the ionized, or electrically charged, form) and one that is lipid soluble (the nonionized, or uncharged, form). When the drug molecule is in the water-soluble form, it does not readily cross lipid membranes; in the lipid-soluble form, it can freely permeate the membrane. All psychoactive drugs—the topic of this text—are quite lipid soluble and readily cross all cell membranes.

Although oral administration of drugs is common, it does have disadvantages. First, it may lead to occasional vomiting and stomach distress. Second, although the amount of a drug that is put into a tablet or capsule can be calculated, how much of it will be absorbed into the bloodstream cannot always be accurately predicted because of unexplained differences between individuals and differences in the manufacturing of the drugs. Third, some drugs, such as the local anesthetics and insulin, when administered orally, are destroyed by the acid in the stomach before they are absorbed. To be effective, such drugs must be administered by injection.

Despite the disadvantages, about 75 percent of an orally administered drug is absorbed by the body within about one to three hours. This figure can vary widely, however, because of such factors as particle size, formulation, and blood flow to the stomach.

Rectal Administration

Although the primary route of drug administration is oral, some drugs are administered rectally (usually in suppository form) if the patient is vomiting, unconscious, or unable to swallow. However, absorption is often irregular, unpredictable, and incomplete, and many drugs irritate the membranes that line the rectum.

Inhalation

Inhalation is an increasingly popular method of drug administration, because it avoids the unpredictability of administration through the gastrointestinal tract. Drugs that are administered as gases or aerosols penetrate the cell linings of the respiratory tract easily and rapidly. For example, anesthetic gases (such as nitrous oxide or halothane) consist of small, highly lipid-soluble molecules that are absorbed across the membranes of the lungs into the bloodstream nearly as fast as they are inhaled. They are absorbed promptly because of the close contact between the blood and the membranes of the lung.

In a novel variation of pulmonary absorption, some drugs that act directly on lung tissue can be formulated so that they are only minimally absorbed into the bloodstream from lung tissue after inhalation, thereby eliminating or at least minimizing side effects.[2,3] For example, patients with asthma often require cortisone-like, anti-inflammatory steroids to control their attacks of asthma. Steroids (including glucocorticoids) produce undesirable side effects on the body when taken orally in the doses necessary to control asthma. However, by formulating the steroid as large, poorly soluble, and poorly absorbed particles suspended in a carrier gas, the drug can be inhaled through the mouth (on a metered dose of carrier gas) and carried into the trachea and lungs with a deeply inspired breath. The particles sit on the lung tissue and exert their action. Any particles remaining in the mouth are swallowed but not absorbed because of their large size and poor solubility (see Figure 1.2).

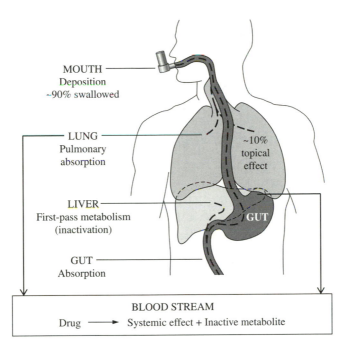

MOUTH
Deposition
~90% swallowed

LUNG
Pulmonary
absorption

~10%
topical
effect

LIVER
First-pass metabolism
(inactivation)

GUT

GUT
Absorption

BLOOD STREAM
Drug ⟶ Systemic effect + Inactive metabolite

FIGURE 1.2 Schematic representation of the disposition of inhaled drugs. [Modified from Talburet and Schmit (1994).[2]]

Less is known about the pulmonary absorption of drugs of abuse, including nicotine, cocaine, marijuana, methamphetamine, and heroin. The pharmacokinetics and pharmacological effects of these drugs are discussed in later chapters.

It is well known that inhalation of substances that are not volatile, such as tars, which are abundant in inhaled cigarette smoke, can injure the sensitive tissues of the lung. Lung cancer, which can be induced by long-term inhalation of cigarette smoke, is thought to be fatal in more than 90 percent of cases and is estimated to result in more than 75,000 deaths a year in the United States.

Administration through the Mucous Membranes

Occasionally, drugs are administered through the mucous membranes of the mouth or nose. A heart patient taking nitroglycerin, for example, places the tablet under the tongue, where the drug is absorbed into the bloodstream directly from the mouth. Cocaine powder, when sniffed, adheres to the membranes on the inside of the nose and is absorbed directly into the bloodstream. Nasal decongestants are sprayed directly onto mucous membranes. Nicotine in either snuff or chewing-gum formulations (see Chapter 6) is absorbed by the buccal membranes directly into the bloodstream. For use before and after surgery in children, the opioid narcotic fentanyl (see Chapter 10) has recently become available as a "lollipop," so this pain-relieving drug can be provided without the necessity of subjecting the child to a painful injection.

Administration through the Skin

Recently, several prescribed medications have been incorporated into patches that adhere to the skin; the pharmacologically active ingredient is slowly absorbed into the bloodstream at the area of contact. Examples include nicotine (used to deter smoking), fentanyl (used to treat chronic, unrelenting pain), nitroglycerin (used to prevent the symptoms of angina pectoris in patients with coronary artery disease), clonidine (used to treat hypertension), and estrogen (used to replace hormones in postmenopausal women). In each case, the drug is slowly released from the liquid in the patch and absorbed into the systemic circulation over a period of days, allowing the levels of drug in the plasma to remain relatively constant.

Injection

Administration of drugs by injection can be *intravenous* (directly into a vein), *intramuscular* (directly into a muscle), or *subcutaneous* (just under the skin). Each of these routes of administration has its advantages and disadvantages (see Table 1.1), but some features are shared by all. In general, administration by injection produces a more prompt response than does oral administration because absorption is faster. Also, injection permits a more accurate dose because the unpredictable processes of absorption through the stomach and intestine are bypassed.

Administration of drugs by injection, however, has several drawbacks. First, the rapid rate of absorption leaves little time to respond to an unexpected drug reaction or accidental overdose. Second, administration by injection requires the use of sterile techniques. Hepatitis and AIDS are examples of disease transmission as drastic consequences of unsterile injection techniques. Third, once a drug is administered by injection, it cannot be recalled.

Intravenous Administration. In an intravenous injection, a drug is introduced directly into the bloodstream. This technique avoids all the variables related to oral absorption. The injection can be made slowly, and it can be stopped instantaneously if untoward effects develop. In addition, the dosage amount can be extremely precise, and the practitioner can dilute and administer in large volumes drugs that at higher concentrations would be irritants to the muscles or blood vessels.

The intravenous route has several important drawbacks, however. First, it is the most dangerous of all routes of administration, because it has the fastest speed of onset of pharmacological action. Second, a normally safe dose may be given too rapidly, causing catastrophic, life-threatening reactions (such as collapse of respiration or of heart function). Third, allergic reactions to a drug administered orally may be mild, but they may be extremely severe when the same drug is administered intravenously. Fourth, drugs that are not soluble in the blood or

TABLE 1.1 Some characteristics of drug administration by injection

Route	Absorption pattern	Special utility	Limitations and precautions
Intravenous	Absorption circumvented Potentially immediate effects	Valuable for emergency use Permits titration of dosage Can administer large volumes and irritating substances when diluted	Increased risk of adverse effects Must inject solutions slowly as a rule Not suitable for oily solutions or insoluble substances
Intramuscular	Prompt action from aqueous solution Slow and sustained action from repository preparations	Suitable for moderate volumes, oily vehicles, and some irritating substances	Precluded during anticoagulant medicine May interfere with interpretation of certain diagnostic tests (e.g., creatine phosphokinase)
Subcutaneous	Prompt action from aqueous solution Slow and sustained action from repository preparations	Suitable for some insoluble suspensions and for implantation of solid pallets	Not suitable for large volumes Possible pain or necrosis from irritating substances

Modified from L. Z. Benet, J. R. Mitchell, and L. B. Sheiner (1996),[1] p. 6.

drugs that are dissolved in oily liquids cannot be given intravenously because of the danger of blood clots forming. Fifth, infection by bacterial contaminants is a danger, and infectious diseases can be transmitted or abscesses induced when sterile techniques are not employed.

Intramuscular Administration. Drugs that are injected into skeletal muscle (usually in the arm, thigh, or buttock) are generally absorbed fairly rapidly. Absorption of a drug from muscle is more rapid than absorption of the same drug from the stomach but slower than absorption of the drug administered intravenously. The absolute rate of absorption of a drug from muscle varies, depending on the rate of blood flow to the muscle, the solubility of the drug, the volume of the injection, and even the vehicle through which the drug is injected.

In general, most of the precautions that apply to intravenous administration also apply to intramuscular injection, but, as a rule, drugs that are intended for intramuscular administration should not be given intravenously. Consequently, one must be careful to avoid hitting a blood vessel when inserting a needle into muscle.

Subcutaneous Administration. Absorption of drugs that have been injected under the skin (subcutaneously) is rapid. The exact rate depends mainly on the ease of blood vessel penetration and the rate of blood flow through the skin. Irritating drugs should not be injected subcutaneously, because they may cause severe pain and damage to local tissue. The usual precautions to maintain sterility apply.

Self-administration of any drug by injection is to be discouraged except when oral administration is not effective or when the drug is being taken therapeutically under the direction of a physician (injection of insulin by a diabetic is a prominent example). The risks associated with injection of a drug (infection, overdose, allergic responses, and transmission of the AIDS virus) are far greater than those associated with oral administration of the same drug.

Drug Distribution

The total amount of a drug in the body (1) governs the movements of that drug through the tissues and its ultimate elimination, (2) determines both the duration and the intensity of the drug's effect, and (3) underlies many of the drug's side effects. Once absorbed, a drug is distributed throughout the body by the circulating blood, passing across various barriers to reach its site of action (its receptors). At any given time, only a very small portion of the total amount of a drug that is in the body is in contact with its receptors. Most of the administered drug is found in areas of the body that are remote from the drug's site of action. For example, in the case of a psychoactive drug—a drug that alters mood or behavior as a result of its effect on the central nervous system (CNS)—most of the drug circulates outside the brain and therefore does not contribute directly to its pharmacological effect. Indeed, this wide distribution often accounts for many of the *side effects* of a drug. Side effects are results that are different from the primary, or therapeutic, effect for which a drug is taken.

Action of the Bloodstream

In the average-size adult, the heart pumps every minute a volume of blood that is roughly equal to the total amount of blood within the circulatory system. Thus, the entire blood volume circulates in the body about once every minute. Therefore, once a drug is absorbed into the bloodstream, it is rapidly (usually within this one-minute circulation time) distributed throughout the circulatory system.

A schematic diagram of the circulatory system is presented in Figure 1.3. Blood returning to the heart through the veins is first pumped into the pulmonary (lung) circulation system, where carbon dioxide is removed and replaced by oxygen. The oxygenated blood then returns to the heart and is pumped into the great artery (the aorta). From there blood flows into the smaller arteries and finally into the capillaries, where nutrients (and drugs) are exchanged between the blood and the cells of the body.

To perform this exchange, the body has an estimated 10 billion capillaries, which have a total surface area of more than 200 square meters. Probably no single functioning cell of the body is more than 20 to 30 micrometers away from a capillary (1 micrometer = 0.0004 inch). After the blood passes through the capillaries, it is collected by the veins and returned to the heart to circulate again. Psychoactive drugs quite quickly become evenly distributed throughout the bloodstream, diluted not only by blood but also by the total amount of water contained in the body.

In addition to solubility, another factor often limits drug distribution—the reversible binding of drugs to proteins present in the blood plasma. A protein-bound drug exists in equilibrium with a free (unbound) drug, as shown in Figure 1.1. Because plasma proteins (albumin, for example) are quite large, they are unable to leave the bloodstream. Thus, the amount of drug that is bound to plasma proteins remains confined within the blood vessels, markedly affecting drug distribution.

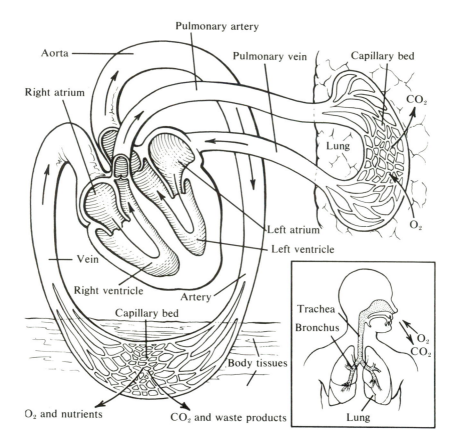

FIGURE 1.3 Heart and circulatory system. Blood returning from the body tissues to the heart via the veins passes through the right atrium into the right ventricle and, with the contraction of the heart, is pumped into the arteries leading to the lungs. In the lungs, carbon dioxide (CO_2) is lost and replaced by oxygen. This oxygenated blood returns to the heart through the left atrium, is pumped out of the left ventricle into the aorta, and is carried to the body tissues, where oxygen and nutrients are exchanged in the capillary beds. Oxygen and nutrients are supplied to the body tissues through the walls of the capillaries; CO_2 and other waste products are returned to the blood. The CO_2 is eliminated through the lungs, and the other waste products are excreted through the kidneys.

Body Membranes That Affect Drug Distribution

Four types of membranes in the body affect drug distribution: (1) the cell membranes, (2) the walls of the capillary vessels in the circulatory system, (3) the blood-brain barrier, and (4) the placental barrier.

Alpha–helix protein

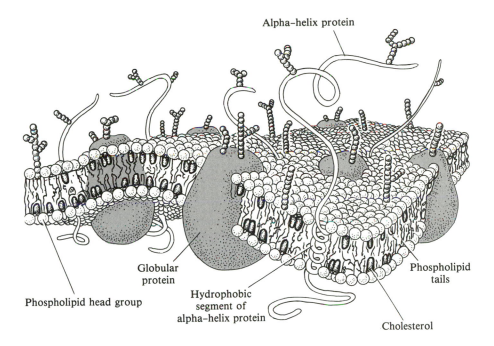

Globular
protein

Phospholipid head group

Hydrophobic
segment of
alpha–helix protein

Phospholipid
tails

Cholesterol

FIGURE 1.4 Diagrammatic representation of the cell membrane, a phospholipid bilayer in which cholesterol and protein molecules are embedded. Both globular and helical kinds of protein traverse the bilayer. Cholesterol molecules tend to keep the tails of the phospholipids relatively fixed and orderly in the regions closest to the hydrophilic phospholipid heads; the parts of the tails closer to the core of the membrane move about freely. [From M. S. Bretscher, "The Molecules of the Cell Membrane," *Scientific American* 253 (1985): 104.]

Cell Membranes. To be absorbed from the intestine or to gain access to the interior of a cell, a drug must penetrate the cell membranes. What, then, is known of the structure and properties of such membranes that determine their permeability to drugs? In Figure 1.4, the two layers of circles represent the water-soluble head groups of complex lipid molecules called *phospholipids*. These phospholipid heads form a rather continuous layer on both the inside and the outside of the cell membrane. The wavy lines that extend from the heads into the membrane are the lipid chains of the phospholipid molecules. Therefore, for our present purposes, the interior of the cell membrane can be considered to consist of a sea of liquid lipid in which large proteins are suspended. This structure has been named the *fluid mosaic model.*

Notice in Figure 1.4 that several large globules and spiral strands appear to be situated on the outer layer of the membrane and extend either into or through the three layers of the membrane, the total thickness of which is about 80 angstroms. (The angstrom is equal to 0.0001 micrometer, or 0.00000004 inch.) These globules and spirals represent protein structures, at least some of which are sites of drug action (i.e., they may represent transmembrane receptor proteins upon which certain psychoactive drugs act).

This membrane, consisting of protein and fat, provides a physical barrier that is permeable to small, lipid-soluble drug molecules but is impermeable to large, lipid-insoluble drug molecules. This is not surprising because the penetration of a drug molecule through the membrane, and thus into a cell, is determined by the solubility of that drug in oil (oil is a fat, and the core of this membrane consists of fat molecules).

These cellular membranes (as barriers to the absorption and distribution of drugs) are important for the passage of drugs (1) from the stomach and intestine into the bloodstream, (2) from the fluid that closely surrounds tissue cells into the interior of cells, (3) from the interior of cells back into the body water, and (4) from the kidneys back into the bloodstream (discussed later).

Capillaries. Within a minute or so of entering the bloodstream, a drug is distributed fairly evenly throughout the entire blood volume. However, most drugs are not confined to the bloodstream because they are exchanged back and forth between blood capillaries and tissues.

Figure 1.5 is a cross-sectional diagram of a capillary. Capillaries are tiny, cylindrical blood vessels with walls that are formed by a thin, single layer of cells packed tightly together. Between the cells are small pores that allow passage of small molecules between blood and the body tissues. The diameter of these pores is between 90 and 150 angstroms, which is larger than most drug molecules. Thus, most drugs freely leave the blood through these pores in the capillary membranes, passing along their concentration gradient until equilibrium is established between the concentrations of drug in the blood and in body tissues and water.

Therefore, the transport of drug molecules out of blood capillaries and into tissues (and, conversely, from tissues back into the blood through the capillaries) is independent of lipid solubility, because the membrane pores are large enough for even fat-insoluble drug molecules to penetrate. However, the pores in the capillary membrane are not large enough to permit the red blood cells and the plasma proteins to leave the bloodstream. Thus, the only drugs that *do not* readily penetrate capillary pores are those rare drugs that are composed of proteins and those that bind to plasma proteins. Therefore, protein-bound drugs essentially become trapped in the bloodstream and do not diffuse into the tissues.

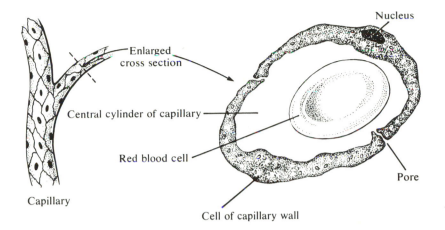

FIGURE 1.5 Cross section of a blood capillary. Within the capillary are the fluids, proteins, and cells of the blood, including the red blood cells. The capillary itself is made up of cells that completely surround and define the central cylinder (or lumen) of the capillary. Water-filled pores form channels, allowing communication between the lumen and the fluid outside the capillary.

The rate at which drug molecules enter specific body tissues depends on two factors: the rate of blood flow through the tissue, and the ease with which drug molecules pass through the capillary membranes. Because blood flow is greatest to the brain and much less to the bones, joints, and fat deposits, drug distribution generally follows a similar pattern. However, some capillaries (such as those in the brain) have special structural properties that can further limit the diffusion of a drug into the brain.

Blood-Brain Barrier. The brain requires a protected environment in which to function normally, and a specialized structural barrier, called the *blood-brain barrier,* plays a key role in maintaining this environment. The blood-brain barrier involves specialized cells in the brain that affect nearly all its blood capillaries (see Figure 1.6). In most of the rest of the body, the capillary membranes have pores; in the brain, however, the capillaries are tightly joined together and covered on the outside by a fatty barrier called the *glial sheath,* which arises from nearby astrocyte cells.

Thus, a drug leaving the capillaries in the brain has to traverse both the wall of the capillary itself (because there are no pores to pass through) and the membranes of the astrocyte cells in order to reach the cells in the brain. Therefore, as a general rule, the rate of passage

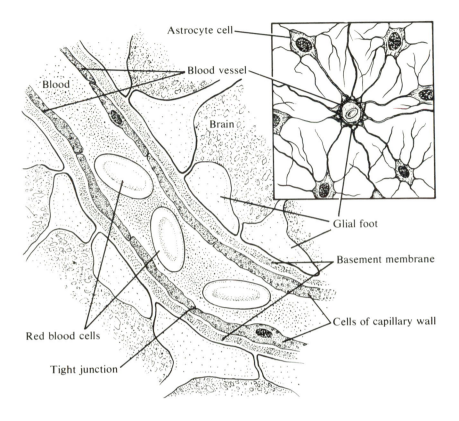

FIGURE 1.6   Blood-brain barrier. Blood and brain are separated both by capillary cells packed tightly together and by a fatty barrier called the *glial sheath,* which is made up of extensions (glial feet) from nearby astrocyte cells (see inset). A drug diffusing from the blood to the brain must move through the cells of the capillary wall because there are tight junctions rather than pores between the cells; the drug must then move through the fatty glial sheath.

of a drug into the brain is determined by the lipid (fat) solubility of the particular drug. Highly ionized drugs (penicillin, for example) penetrate poorly, while fat-soluble drugs penetrate rapidly. Psychoactive drugs (those discussed in this book) are lipid soluble, because they exert their actions only after crossing the blood-brain barrier. Drugs whose therapeutic actions are predominantly exerted outside the CNS are usually more highly ionized (less lipid-soluble) molecules, and, therefore, their CNS actions are usually not of major significance.

Placental Barrier. Among all the membrane systems of the body, the placenta membranes are unique. They separate two distinct human

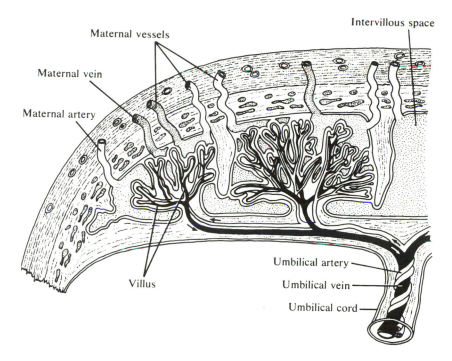

FIGURE 1.7 Placental network separating the blood of mother and fetus.

beings with differing genetic compositions, physiological responses, and sensitivities to drugs. The fetus obtains essential nutrients and eliminates metabolic waste products through the placenta without depending on its own organs, many of which are not yet functioning. This dependence of the fetus upon the mother, however, places the fetus at the mercy of the placenta when foreign substances (such as drugs or toxins) appear in the mother's blood.

A pregnant woman in the United States regularly takes both prescription and nonprescription drugs, and she routinely exposes the fetus to potentially toxic substances in food, cosmetics, household chemicals, and the general environment. The extent to which these substances affect the fetus is not yet known. The consequences of maternal alcohol ingestion, cigarette smoking, and cocaine use on fetal growth and development are now well documented and are discussed in the chapters devoted to these drugs.

A schematic representation of the placental network, which transfers substances between the mother and the fetus, is shown in Figure 1.7.

In general, the mature placenta consists of a network of vessels and pools of maternal blood into which protrude tree-like or finger-like villi (projections) that contain the blood capillaries of the fetus. Oxygen and nutrients travel from the mother's blood to that of the fetus, while carbon dioxide and other waste products travel from the blood of the fetus to the mother's blood.

The membranes that separate fetal blood from maternal blood in the intervillous space resemble, in their general permeability, the cell membranes that are found elsewhere in the body. In other words, drugs cross the placenta primarily by passive diffusion. Fat-soluble substances (including all psychoactive drugs) diffuse readily, rapidly, and without limitation:

> The view that the placenta is a barrier to drugs is inaccurate. A more appropriate approximation is that the fetus is to at least some extent exposed to essentially all drugs taken by the mother.[4]

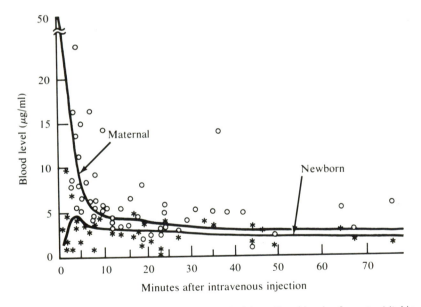

FIGURE 1.8   Effect of barbiturate on mothers in labor. Blood levels of secobarbital in mothers and their newborn infants after intravenous administration of the drug to the mothers. Each point represents one subject (*circles,* mothers; *asterisks,* infants). [From B. Root, E. Eichner, and I. Sunshine, "Blood Secobarbital Levels and Their Clinical Correlation in Mothers and Newborn Infants," *American Journal of Obstetric and Gynecology* 81 (1961): 948.]

The blood levels of a barbiturate (a sedative-hypnotic drug, see Chapter 2) administered intravenously to mothers during labor are plotted in Figure 1.8. The blood concentrations of the drug were determined in both maternal and fetal blood. One can see from this figure that significant amounts of the barbiturate are distributed to the infant and that blood levels in the mother and the newborn baby are almost identical about 10 minutes after injection, illustrating that levels of psychoactive drugs in the fetus usually equal those achieved in the mother.

Termination of Drug Action

Routes through which drugs can leave the body (i.e., be "excreted") include (1) the kidneys, (2) the lungs, (3) the bile, and (4) the skin. Excretion through the lungs occurs only with highly volatile or gaseous agents, such as the general anesthetics and, in small amounts, alcohol ("alcohol breath"). Drugs that are passed through the bile and into the intestine are usually reabsorbed back into the bloodstream from the intestine. Also, drugs can pass through the skin and are excreted in sweat (perhaps 10 to 15 percent of the drug). However, the majority of drugs leave the body in urine. More correctly, *the major route of drug elimination from the body is renal excretion of drug metabolites following the hepatic (liver) biodegradation of the drug into drug metabolites.* These metabolites are more water-soluble, bulkier, less lipid-soluble, and (usually) less biologically active (even inactive) when compared with the parent molecule (the molecule that was originally ingested and absorbed). Thus, in order for a lipid-soluble drug to be eliminated, it must be metabolically transformed (by enzymes located in the liver) into a form that can be excreted rapidly and reliably. Such biotransformation relieves the body of the burden of foreign chemicals and is essential to our survival.

Elimination of Drugs by the Kidneys and Liver

Physiologically, our kidneys perform two major functions. First, they excrete most of the products of body metabolism; second, they closely regulate the levels of most of the substances found in body fluids. The kidneys are a pair of bean-shaped organs (see Figure 1.9), each a little smaller than a fist and weighing about a quarter of a pound. They lie at the rear of the abdominal cavity at the level of the lower ribs.

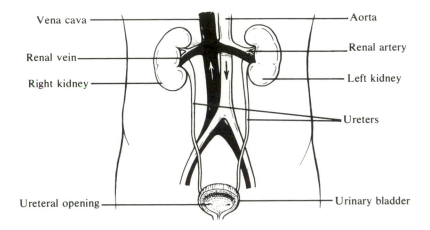

FIGURE 1.9 Architecture of the kidneys.

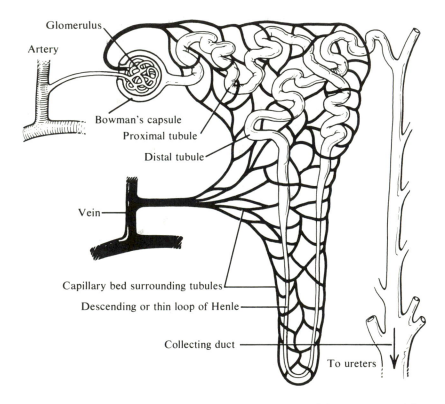

FIGURE 1.10 Nephron within a kidney. Note the complexity of the structure and the intimate relation between the blood supply and the nephron. Each kidney is composed of more than a million such nephrons.

The outer portion of the kidney is made up of more than a million functional units, called *nephrons* (Figure 1.10). Each unit consists of a knot of capillaries (the glomerulus) through which blood flows from the renal artery to the renal vein. The glomerulus is surrounded by the opening of the nephron (Bowman's capsule), into which fluid flows as it filters out of the capillaries. Pressure of the blood in the glomerulus causes fluid to leave the capillaries and flow into Bowman's capsule, from which it flows through the tubules of the nephrons and then into a duct that collects fluid from several nephrons. This fluid from the collecting ducts is eventually passed through the ureters and into the urinary bladder, which is emptied periodically.

In an adult, about one liter of plasma is filtered into the nephrons of the kidneys each minute. Left behind in the bloodstream are blood cells, plasma proteins, and the remaining plasma. As the filtered fluid flows through the nephrons, substances that are not reabsorbed pass into the urinary bladder for excretion later.

Because psychoactive drugs are small, lipid-soluble particles, they are filtered into the kidneys and then easily reabsorbed (by a process of passive diffusion) back into the bloodstream. Reabsorption occurs passively, along a developing concentration gradient—the drug becomes concentrated inside the nephrons (as a result of water reabsorption), and the drugs are themselves reabsorbed into plasma. Thus, the kidneys alone are not capable of eliminating psychoactive drugs from the body, and some other mechanism must overcome this process of passive renal reabsorption of the drug. What occurs is that the drug is enzymatically biotransformed (by enzymes located in the liver) into compounds (metabolites) that are less fat soluble and therefore less capable of being reabsorbed. As the drug is carried to the liver (by blood flowing in the hepatic artery and portal vein), a portion is cleared from the blood by the liver cells and metabolized to by-products (metabolites), which are then returned to the bloodstream (see Figure 1.11). These metabolites are then carried in the bloodstream to the kidneys, filtered into the renal tubules, and are poorly reabsorbed, remaining in the urine for excretion.

Usually, but not always, this process of metabolism decreases the pharmacological activity of the drug. Thus, even though a metabolite might persist in the body for a time, it is usually in a pharmacologically less active (or an inactive) form and does not produce the effects of the parent drug. Sometimes, however, the metabolite is pharmacologically active. In such cases, the metabolite is then further metabolized to an inactive compound, which is excreted (examples of this phenomenon are presented later).

A description of the exact mechanisms by which the liver alters a drug's chemical structure is beyond the scope of our discussion, but

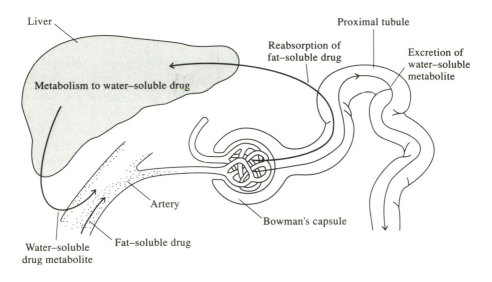

FIGURE 1.11 How the liver and kidneys eliminate drugs from the body. Drugs may be filtered into the kidney, reabsorbed into the bloodstream, and carried to the liver for metabolic transformation to a more water-soluble compound that, having been filtered into the kidney, cannot be reabsorbed and is therefore excreted in urine.

suffice it to state that the reactions are carried out by a special system of enzymes localized in the liver cells.*

Factors Affecting Drug Metabolism

Several different factors can alter the rate at which drugs are metabolized, increasing or decreasing the rate of drug elimination from the body. In general, *genetic, environmental,* and various *physiological factors* are involved. As stated by Benet, Kroetz, and Sheiner (1996)[4]:

> The most important factors are genetically determined polymorphisms in drug oxidation and conjugations, concomitant use of other drugs, exposure to environmental pollutants and industrial chemicals, disease,

*The *cytochrome P450 enzyme family,* physically located in the liver cells, is the major system involved in drug metabolism. Originating more than 3.5 billion years ago, this gene family of enzymes has diversified to accomplish the metabolism (detoxification) of environmental chemicals, food toxins, and drugs. Thus, the cytochrome P450 enzyme system (of which at least 12 different families exist in humans) can detoxify a chemically diverse group of foreign substances.

state, and age. These factors have been thought responsible for decreased efficacy, prolonged pharmacological effects, and increased toxicity.

Many psychoactive drugs have the ability to increase the rate at which enzymes in the liver metabolize drugs, thereby increasing the speed with which the drugs are eliminated. An increased rate of metabolism occurs secondary to an increase in both the enzymatic activity of the cells and the total amount of drug-metabolizing enzymes present in the liver. Thus, tolerance develops, and increasing doses of a drug must be administered to maintain the same level of drug in the plasma and produce the same effect as previously administered smaller doses.

Because drug-metabolizing enzymes in the liver have a low specificity for drugs (that is, one enzyme may metabolize many different types of drugs), an increase in the metabolizing enzymes induced by one drug increases the enzymes' rate of metabolizing not only that particular drug but a variety of others. This process of *cross tolerance* will be elaborated upon later in this chapter.

We have discussed how drugs from the mother are distributed to the fetus through the placenta, and those drugs may be excreted through the umbilical cord back into the mother's bloodstream. The mother can then eliminate the drug through her liver and kidneys. After delivery, however, the newborn baby must get rid of the drug by itself. Unfortunately, the newborn (especially the premature infant) has few drug-metabolizing enzymes in its liver, and its kidneys may not yet be fully functional. Therefore, the infant has difficulty metabolizing and excreting drugs. If it has received a high concentration of depressants (anesthetics, narcotics, and so on) from the mother, the infant may be depressed for a long time after delivery.

Other Routes of Drug Elimination

Other routes for excreting drugs include the lungs, bile, sweat, saliva, and breast milk. Many drugs and drug metabolites may be found in these secretions, but their concentrations are usually low, and these routes are not usually considered primary paths of drug elimination. Occasionally, however, concern arises over the transfer of psychoactive drugs (such as nicotine) from mothers to their breast-fed babies. Similarly, concern has been expressed about the secretion of antibiotics that have been administered to cows into milk that is ultimately consumed by humans. These topics are of obvious importance to the pharmacologist and to the Food and Drug Administration, especially because guidelines for such uses of drugs are needed to minimize danger to the public.

Time Course of Drug Distribution and Elimination

Concept of Drug Half-Life

Knowledge about the relationship between the initial concentration of a drug in the body and the concentration at some time after its administration is essential for (1) predicting the optimal dosages and dose intervals needed to reach a therapeutic effect, (2) maintaining a therapeutic drug level for the desired period of time, and (3) determining the time needed to eliminate the drug. Indeed, it is a fundamental of pharmacology that there is a relationship between the pharmacological response to a drug and its concentration at a readily measurable site in the body (for example, in blood). Furthermore, the therapeutic drug level (as measured in blood) correlates with the level of drug at the "receptor site" (see Figure 1.1).

Figure 1.12 illustrates this time-concentration relationship. Note that after intravenous injection, the drug concentration in plasma peaked immediately, fell rapidly, and then declined more slowly. The rapid fall reflects the distribution of the drug out of the bloodstream (into which it was injected) into body tissues. This process of *redistribution* takes only minutes to spread a drug nearly equally throughout the major tissues of the body. The steeply sloped line in Figure 1.12 (tangent line A) represents this rapid-distribution phase, which is represented by a distribution half-life that indicates the time it takes for redistribution to reduce the initial peak level of the drug by 50 percent (here only 7.9 minutes).

The slower, prolonged decrease in the level of drug in the blood (tangent line B) represents the time required for the body to eliminate the drug through metabolism (by the liver) and excrete the metabolites through the kidneys. The calculated elimination half-life is a measure of this process, and it allows the time course of drug action to be calculated.

Figure 1.12 shows that the peak levels of pain relief produced by the drug fentanyl (a narcotic analgesic) are reached within seconds after intravenous injection. Fentanyl is highly lipid soluble and is rapidly redistributed to muscle and fat, reducing blood concentrations of the drug in the process. The elimination half-life is about 45 minutes.

As shown in Table 1.2, it takes four half-lives for 90 percent of a drug to be eliminated by the body and six half-lives for 98 percent of the drug to be eliminated. At that point, one is, for most practical purposes, drug-free. It is important to remember that even though the blood level is reduced by 75 percent after two half-lives, the drug persists in the body at low levels for six or more half-lives. The so-called "drug hangover" is a result of such calculation.

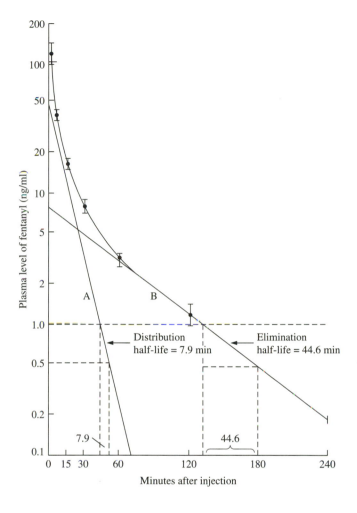

FIGURE 1.12 Plasma levels of a narcotic drug (fentanyl) injected intravenously into a rat in a single bolus dose of 50 micrograms per kilogram body weight. The distribution and elimination half-lives are shown as 7.9 and 44.6 minutes, respectively. The horizontal line drawn at 1 nanogram (billionths of a gram) per milliliter plasma concentration is the level needed for analgesic effect. Thus, analgesia would be lost about 130 minutes after drug injection. [Data from C. C. Hug, Jr., and M. R. Murphy, "Tissue Redistribution of Fentanyl and Termination of Its Effects in Rats," *Anesthesiology* 55 (1981): 369–375.]

TABLE 1.2 Half-life calculations

	Amount of drug in the body	
Number of half-lives	Percent eliminated	Percent remaining
0	0	100
1	50	50
2	75	25
3	87.5	12.5
4	93.8	6.2
5	96.9	3.1
6	98.4	1.6

Throughout this text, drug half-lives will be cited to describe the duration of action of psychoactive drugs in the body. Some drug half-lives can be measured in days, and recovery from the drug may take a week or more. Diazepam (Valium) is an example of a drug that can have a half-life lasting several days, especially in the elderly (discussed further in Chapter 3).

Drug Half-Life, Accumulation, and Steady State

The biological half-life of a drug is not only the time required for the drug concentration in blood to fall by one-half, but it is also the determinant of the length of time necessary to reach a steady state of concentration.[5] If one administers a second full dose of drug before the body has eliminated the first dose, the total amount of drug in the body and the peak level of the drug in the blood will be greater than the total amount and peak level produced by the first dose. For example, if 100 milligrams (mg) of a drug with a four-hour half-life were administered at 12 noon, 50 mg of drug would remain in the body at 4 P.M. If an additional 100 mg of the drug were then taken at 4 P.M., 75 mg of drug would remain in the body at 8 P.M. (25 mg of the first dose and 50 mg of the second). If this administration schedule were continued, the amount of drug in the body would continue to increase until a plateau, or steady state, concentration was reached (Figure 1.13).

In general, the time to reach *steady-state concentration* (the level of drug achieved in blood with repeated, regular-interval dosing) is about six times the drug's elimination half-life and is independent of the actual dosage of the drug. The reason for this is as follows. In one half-life, a drug reaches 50 percent of the concentration that will eventually

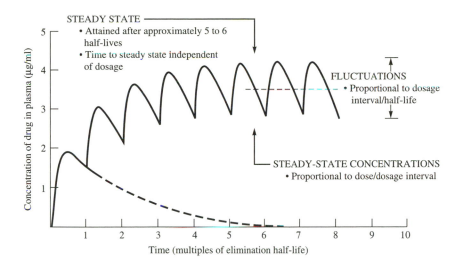

FIGURE 1.13 Plasma drug concentrations during repeated oral administration of a drug at intervals equal to its elimination half-life. The dashed line illustrates the elimination curve if only a single dose is given. Because only 50 percent of each dose is eliminated before the next dose is given, the drug accumulates, reaching steady-state concentration in five to six half-lives. The sinusoidal curve shows the maximal and minimal drug concentrations at the beginning and end of each dosage interval, respectively. The dotted line illustrates the average concentration achieved at steady state.

be achieved. After two half-lives, the drug achieves 75 percent concentration; at three half-lives, the drug achieves the initial 50 percent (of the third dose), the next 25 percent (from the second dose), plus half of the remaining 25 percent (from the first dose). At 98.4 percent (the concentration achieved after six half-lives), the drug concentration is essentially at steady state. This is the rationale behind our general rule. The steady-state concentration is achieved when the amount administered per unit time equals the amount eliminated per unit time. The interdependent variables that determine the ultimate concentration (or steady-state blood level of drug) are the dose (which determines the blood level but not the time to steady state), the dose interval, the half-life of the drug, and other, more complex factors that can affect drug elimination.

In summary, steady, regular-interval dosing leads to a predictable accumulation, with a steady-state concentration reached after about six half-lives; the magnitude of the concentration is proportional to dose and dosage interval. Clinically, these factors guide drug therapy when blood levels of the drug are monitored and correlated with therapeutic results.

Therapeutic Drug Monitoring

Therapeutic drug monitoring (TDM) can aid a clinician in making critical decisions in therapeutic applications. Indeed, in psychopharmacology, TDM can dramatically improve the prognosis of psychological disorders, making previously difficult-to-treat disorders much more treatable.[6]

The basic principle underlying TDM is that a threshold plasma concentration of a drug is needed at the receptor site in order to initiate and maintain a pharmacological response. Critically important is that plasma concentrations of psychoactive drugs correlate well with tissue or receptor concentrations. Therefore, TDM is an indirect, although usually quite accurate, measurement of drug concentration at the receptor site in the tissue of interest (here, the CNS). To make the correlation between TDM, dosage, and therapeutic response, large-scale clinical trials are performed, and blood samples are drawn at multiple time periods during both acute (short-term) and chronic (long-term) therapy. Statistical correlation is made between the level of drug in plasma and the degree of therapeutic response. A dosage regimen can then be designed to achieve the appropriate blood level of a drug. Limiting factors to TDM include imprecision in detecting and quantifying improvement in psychological illness, difficulty in detecting early signs of toxicity, and delays in the onset of therapeutic response.

The goals of TDM are many. One goal is to assess whether a patient is taking medication as prescribed; if plasma levels of the drug are below the therapeutic level (because the patient has not been taking the required medication), therapeutic results will be poor. Another goal is to avoid toxicity; if plasma levels of the drug are above the therapeutic level, the dosage can be lowered, effectiveness maintained, and toxicity minimized. A third goal is to enhance therapeutic response by focusing not on the amount of drug taken, but on the measured amount of drug in the plasma. Other goals include possible reductions in the cost of therapy (since a patient's illness is better controlled) and the substantiation of the need for unusually high doses in patients who require higher-than-normal intake of prescribed medication to maintain a therapeutic blood level of a drug.

Drug Tolerance and Dependence

Drug tolerance may be defined as a state of progressively decreasing responsiveness to a drug. A person who develops tolerance requires a larger dose of the drug to achieve the effect originally obtained by a smaller dose.

TABLE 1.3 Effect of pentobarbital pretreatment on the duration of pentobarbital action

Pretreatment	Sleeping time (min)	Plasma level of pentobarbital on awakening (μg/mL)	Pentobarbital half-life in plasma (min)
None	67 ± 4	9.9 ± 1,4	79 ± 3
Pentobarbital	10 ± 7	7.9 ± 0.6	26 ± 2

Source: H. Remmer, "Drugs as Activators of Drug Enzyme," in B. B. Brodie and E. G. Erdos, eds., *Metabolic Factors Controlling Duration of Drug Action* (Proceedings of the First International Pharmacological Meeting), vol. 6 (New York: Macmillan, 1962), p. 235.
Note: Rabbits were pretreated with three daily doses of pentobarbital (60 mg/kg) subcutaneously, then given a single challenging dose of 60 mg/kg intravenously.

At least three mechanisms are involved in the development of drug tolerance—two are pharmacological mechanisms, and one is a behavioral mechanism. *Metabolic tolerance* is the first of the two classically described types of pharmacological tolerance. Here, as discussed earlier, the presence of a drug in blood perfusing the liver can induce the synthesis of hepatic drug-metabolizing enzymes that are involved in the metabolism of drugs and other chemicals by the liver. Thus, the drug is metabolized at a faster rate, and more drug must be administered to maintain the same level of drug in the body.

An example of enzyme-induction metabolic tolerance is presented in Table 1.3. In this classic experiment, rabbits were pretreated with three daily doses of pentobarbital (a short-acting barbiturate, a class of drugs that when administered are known to result in the development of metabolic tolerance secondary to the induction of hepatic drug-metabolizing enzymes; see Chapter 2). The rabbits were then given a single challenging dose of the same drug. The length of time that the rabbits slept and the blood level of pentobarbital at the time of awakening were measured and compared with the sleeping time and the blood levels of pentobarbital in a control group of rabbits that were not pretreated but were given a single, identical dose of the drug. Although the pretreated animals slept less than half as long as the control rabbits, their blood levels of the drug on awakening were approximately the same. Pretreatment had induced drug tolerance not by affecting any "sleep center" in the brain, but by inducing new drug-metabolizing enzymes in the liver, which caused the drug to be detoxified more rapidly.

A second type of pharmacological tolerance is *cellular-adaptive* or *pharmacodynamic tolerance*. Receptors in the brain adapt to the continued presence of the drug. Neurons adapt either by increasing the number of receptors (thereby requiring more drug to occupy them) or by reducing their sensitivity to the drug (a process called *down regulation*). With either type of pharmacodynamic tolerance, higher levels of drug in plasma are necessary to maintain the same biological effect. Cellular-adaptive tolerance to drugs can be seen in people who develop problems with narcotics, barbiturates, and alcohol (although with the latter two drugs, enzyme induction, through the process of metabolic tolerance, is also involved).

More recently identified is the role of *behavioral conditioning processes* in the development of tolerance. Indeed, simple exposure of drugs to receptors does not account for the substantial degree of tolerance that many people acquire to opioids, barbiturates, ethyl alcohol, and other drugs. Here, tolerance can be demonstrated when a drug is administered in the context of usual predrug cues, but not in the context of alternative cues.[7] Poulos and Cappell (1991)[8] propose a *homeostatic theory* of drug tolerance. They found that, with morphine analgesia, testing in an environment in which tolerance had developed effected the manifestation of tolerance, and an environmental cue could maintain the tolerance. This *contingent tolerance* is pervasive and represents a general process underlying the development of all forms of systemic tolerance.

> The environmental cues routinely paired with drug administration will become conditioned stimuli that elicit a conditioned response that is opposite in direction to, or compensation for, the direct effects of the drug. Over conditioning trials, the compensatory conditioned response grows in magnitude and counteracts the direct drug effects, that is, tolerance develops.9

Physical dependence is an entirely different phenomenon, even though it is associated with drug tolerance in most cases. A person who is physically dependent on a drug needs the drug in order to function "normally" and avoid withdrawal symptoms if the drug is not taken. The state of physical dependence is revealed by withdrawing the drug and noting the occurrence of physical and/or psychological withdrawal symptoms (abstinence syndrome) some time after the drug has been withheld. The symptoms of withdrawal can be terminated by readministering the drug.

PHARMACODYNAMICS: DRUG-RECEPTOR INTERACTIONS

Pharmacodynamics can be defined as the study of the biochemical and physiological effects of drugs and their mechanism of action. The objectives of the analysis of drug action are to delineate the chemical or physical interactions between drug and target cell and to characterize the full sequence and scope of actions of each drug. Such a complete analysis provides the basis for both the rational therapeutic use of a drug and the design of new and superior therapeutic agents.[10]

Before producing any pharmacological effect, a drug must physically interact with one or more constituents of a cell. Indeed, the effects of most drugs result from their binding to, and interacting with, specific components of cells (for psychoactive drugs, such cells are *neurons* within the brain). The cellular component that is directly involved in this interaction with a drug is called the *receptor*. One of the basic concepts in psychopharmacology is that the molecules of a psychoactive drug must attach to specific receptors, which are located either on or within a neuron, and that the occupation of a receptor by a drug leads to a change in the functional properties of that neuron, resulting in the drug's characteristic pharmacological response. Ultimately, the drug-receptor interaction produces a cascade of cellular events involving changes in subcellular components of the target cell, resulting in clinically relevant therapeutic effects and side effects.[10,11]

Figure 1.14 illustrates several important points about drug-receptor interactions. First, receptors are usually located on the surface of or within membrane-spanning proteins. These proteins, in turn, have one or more types of binding sites, usually for one neurotransmitter ("ligand"). Thus, those proteins that serve as drug receptors normally (in the absence of a drug) serve as receptors for naturally occurring endogenous neurotransmitters.

Second, attachment (reversible binding) of the neurotransmitter specific for that receptor activates the receptor, usually by changing the structure of the protein. This change allows a signal to be transmitted through the membrane to the intracellular side of the cell membrane. Thus, the receptor is specialized to respond to one neurotransmitter molecule with great sensitivity and selectivity.

Third, the intensity of the resulting transmembrane signal is determined either by the percentage of the available receptors that are occupied by the molecules of neurotransmitter (or molecules of an agonist

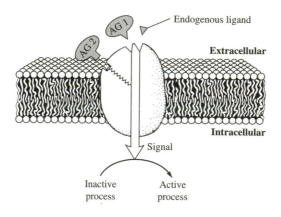

FIGURE 1.14 Diagrammatic representation of classical receptors located on a membrane-spanning protein. A type I agonist (AG 1) fits the receptor site for an endogenous ligand. A type II agonist (AG 2) binds to an adjacent site, thereby influencing (amplifying) signal transmission. Signal transmission activates intracellular processes that are inactive without receptor activation.

drug) or by the rate of reversible binding by either the neurotransmitter or the drug.

Fourth, a drug can either enhance or diminish the generation, transmission, or receipt of the transmembrane signal by binding to the receptor for the endogenous neurotransmitter. Thus, the drug does not create any unique effects; it merely modulates normal neuronal functioning, mimicking or antagonizing the actions of a specific endogenous neurotransmitter. Binding accompanied by drug-induced mimicry of neurotransmitter action is an *agonist* action. Drug occupation of a receptor that is not accompanied by neurotransmitter-like activation blocks the access of the neurotransmitter to the receptor and is an *antagonist* (or inhibitory) action. Agonists and antagonists can bind to the neurotransmitter binding site (to activate or block transduction), to other neighboring sites that influence signal transmission within the membrane, or to intracellular signal reception points (see Figure 1.14).

Drug-Receptor Affinity

A characteristic of the drug receptor is its high (but not absolute) degree of specificity (or affinity) for a particular neurotransmitter and drug molecules. What may appear to be a slight or insignificant variation in the chemical structure of a drug may greatly alter the intensity of a cell's response to it. For example, amphetamine and methamphetamine are both powerful stimulants of the central nervous system. Although their chemical composition is extremely similar, methamphetamine is much more potent and produces much greater behavioral stimulation at the same dosage. Both drugs probably affect the same receptors in the brain, but methamphetamine exerts a much more powerful action on them. The drug molecule with the "best fit" to the receptor elicits the greatest response from the cell. Thus, methamphetamine might fit the receptor better than amphetamine.

Selectivity or specificity of drug action is not due to the selective distribution of drug molecules; rather, it is a function of the selective localization of drug receptors, the specificity of drugs that bind to particular receptors, the strength of the drug's attachment, and the consequences of the interaction between drugs and their receptors.

Current drug research is characterizing in molecular terms the primary sites and mechanisms of drug action. A drug with a seemingly wide variety of actions can frequently be shown to exert such multiplicity of actions via attachment to a specific receptor for a specific neurotransmitter. Side effects result either as a consequence of binding to this specific receptor or as a result of binding to other receptors, with this more nonspecific binding producing unwanted side effects or toxicities.

Following are two examples of the multiplicity of action resulting from a specific action. Aspirin exerts a wide variety of effects (analgesic, anti-inflammatory, and fever reducing), all of which can be explained in terms of inhibition of the action of one or more of the enzymes that are involved in the inflammatory process (see Appendix II). Similarly, the benzodiazepine tranquilizers may exert their sedative, antianxiety, antipanic, and antiepileptic actions by interacting with specific receptor sites in the brain, potentiating the action of an inhibitory neurotransmitter (gamma-aminobutyric acid, or GABA; see Chapter 4).

On the other hand, certain antidepressant drugs (see Chapter 7) exert this action by interacting with serotonin receptors. Some of their side effects (sedation, dry mouth, blurred vision) result from nonspecific binding to histamine and acetylcholine receptors. One goal of this text is to demonstrate, whenever possible, the single actions that may account for the wide variety of effects that a drug produces, as well as the receptor actions responsible for a drug's side effects.

There are three important implications in the fact that drugs act on specific molecular receptors. First, a drug is potentially capable of altering the rate at which any bodily (or brain) function proceeds.

Second, a drug does not create effects but merely modulates ongoing functions. Third, a drug cannot impart new functions to a cell.

The affinity of a drug for its receptor (that is, its ability to bind to a receptor), its intrinsic activity (agonist versus antagonist), and its potency are intimately related to the drug's chemical structure. Indeed, small alterations in chemical structure can result in profound differences in biological action. This presumably follows from the supposition that such structural changes can alter the fit of a drug for its receptor, significantly affecting the drug-induced conformational changes that occur in the three-dimensional structure of a receptor.

It should be noted that receptors themselves are subject to many regulatory, intrinsic, and homeostatic controls, and their sensitivity (and even their absolute numbers) can be modulated (increased or decreased). Such mechanisms appear to be involved in the mechanisms of pharmacodynamic tolerance, genetic variability, and so on.

Dose-Response Relationship

One way of quantifying drug-receptor interactions is to use what are known as *dose-response curves*. In Figure 1.15, two types of dose-response curves are illustrated. In graph A, the dose is plotted against the percentage of persons (from a given population of persons) that exhibit a characteristic effect at a given dosage. In graph B, the dose is plotted against the intensity, or the magnitude, of the response in a single person.

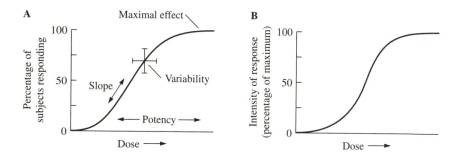

FIGURE 1.15 Two types of dose-response curves. **(A)** Curve obtained by plotting the dose of drug against the percentage of subjects showing a given response at any given dose. **(B)** Curve obtained by plotting the dose of drug against the intensity of response observed in any single individual at a given dose. The intensity of response is plotted as a percentage of the maximum obtainable response.

These curves indicate that a dose exists that is low enough to produce little or no effect; at the opposite extreme, a dose exists beyond which no greater response can be elicited.

All dose-response curves demonstrate important characteristics, three of which are the *potency* (the absolute amount of drug, usually expressed in milligrams, necessary to produce a defined effect), *efficacy* (the maximum effect obtainable), and the *dose* required to produce the maximum effect (Figure 1.15B). One can also use dose-response curves to estimate variability of response and drug safety. (Drug safety and responsiveness are discussed in the next section.)

The location of the dose-response curve along the horizontal axis reflects the potency of the drug. If two drugs produce sedation but one exerts this action at half the dose level of the other, the first drug is considered to be twice as potent as the second drug. Potency, however, is a relatively unimportant characteristic of a drug, because it makes little difference whether the effective dose of a drug is 1.0 milligram or 100 milligrams, as long as the drug is administered in an appropriate dose with no undue toxicity. Thus, the more potent drug is not necessarily the better one. High potency, in fact, can be a disadvantage, because an extremely potent drug may be much more toxic (or dangerous) and require much more careful administration to reach a given therapeutic or behavioral endpoint.

Slope refers to the more or less linear central portion of the dose-response curve. A steep slope on a dose-response curve implies that there is only a small difference between the dose that produces a barely discernible effect and the dose that causes a maximal effect. The steeper the slope, the smaller the increase in dose that is required to go from a minimum response to a maximum effect. This can be good, as it may indicate that there is little biological variation in the response to the drug. Conversely, it may be a disadvantage if it indicates that untoward toxicity occurs with only minimal increases in dose.

The *peak* of the dose-response curve indicates the maximum effect, or efficacy, that can be produced by a drug, regardless of further increases in dose. Not all psychoactive drugs can exert the same level of effect. For example, caffeine, even in massive doses, cannot exert the same intensity of CNS stimulation as amphetamine. Similarly, aspirin can never achieve the maximum analgesic effect of morphine. Thus, the maximum effect is an inherent property of a drug and is one measure of a drug's efficacy. Most psychoactive drugs, however, are not used to the point of their maximum effect, because side effects limit the upper range of dosage. Therefore, the usefulness of a compound is correspondingly limited, even though the drug may be inherently capable of producing a greater effect.

DRUG SAFETY AND EFFECTIVENESS

Variability in Drug Responsiveness

The dose of a drug that produces a specific response varies considerably between individuals. Interpatient variability can result from differences in rates of drug metabolism (discussed earlier), differences in drug absorption, previous experience with drug use, various physical, psychological, and emotional states, and so on. Despite the etiology of the variability, any population of individuals will have a few subjects who are remarkably sensitive to the effects (and side effects) of a drug, while a few will exhibit remarkable drug tolerance, requiring quite large doses to produce therapeutic results. The variability, however, usually follows a predictable pattern, resembling a Gaussian distribution. In a few instances, however, a specific population of individuals (following a genetically predetermined pattern) will skew this distribution by exhibiting a unique pattern of responsiveness, usually due to genetic alterations in drug metabolism.

Although the average dose required to elicit a given response can be calculated easily, some individuals respond at doses that are very much lower than the average and others respond only at doses that are very much higher. Thus, it is extremely important that the dose of all drugs be individualized. Generalizations about "average doses" are risky at best, although we can estimate the dose of a drug that will produce the desired effect in 50 percent of the subjects. This dose is called the ED_{50} for the drug (the effective dose for 50 percent of the subjects). Similarly, we can estimate an LD_{50} (lethal dose for 50 percent of the subjects). The LD_{50} is calculated in exactly the same way as the ED_{50}, except that the dose of the drug is plotted against the number of experimental animals that die after being administered various doses of the compound. Both the ED_{50} and the LD_{50} are determined in multiple species of animals to prevent accidental drug-induced toxicity in humans. The ratio of the LD_{50} to the ED_{50} is used as an index of the relative safety of the drug, called the *therapeutic index*.

To illustrate, two dose-response curves are shown in Figure 1.16. The curve at the left illustrates the dose of drug necessary to induce sleep in a population of mice, and the one at the right illustrates the dose of drug necessary to kill a similar population. In this example, the $LD_{50}:ED_{50}$ ratio is seen to be 100:10, or 10. This may seem like a rather large margin, but note that at a dose of 50 milligrams, 95 percent of the mice sleep while 5 percent of the mice die. This overlap demonstrates both the difficulty in assessing the relative safety of drugs for use in large populations and the biological variation in individual responses

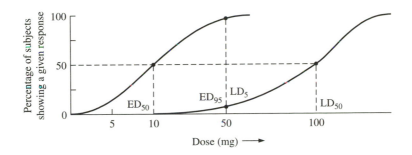

FIGURE 1.16 Two dose-response curves. The curve on the left is the dose of drug required to induce a given response. The curve on the right is the lethal dose of the compound. See text for discussion.

to drugs. With this particular compound, a dose cannot be administered that guarantees that 100 percent of the mice will sleep and none will die. Thus, a more useful indication of the margin of safety is a ratio of the lethal dose for 1 percent of the population to the effective dose for 99 percent of the population (LD_1:ED_{99}). A sedative drug with an LD_1:ED_{99} of 1 would be a safer compound than the drug shown in Figure 1.16. Note that the clinical usefulness of indices obtained from laboratory animals is limited, because these indices do not reflect the occasional unexpected response (from the causes listed earlier) that can seriously harm a patient.

Drug variability is also intimately associated with drug toxicity. Therefore, the side effects that are invariably associated with a drug, as well as its more serious toxicities (including those that can be fatal), must always be considered.

Drug Interactions

The effects of one drug can be modified by the concurrent administration of another drug. This is particularly important in psychopharmacology.[12] For example, alcohol taken after a benzodiazepine tranquilizer (see Chapter 4) has been ingested, or after one has smoked marijuana, increases sedation and loss of coordination. This action may have little consequence if the doses of each drug are low, but higher doses of either or both drugs can be dangerous both to the user and to others. Even though a person may normally be able to ingest a limited amount of alcohol and still drive a car without significant loss of control or coordination, the concurrent tranquilizer or marijuana use may profoundly impair his or her driving performance, endangering the driver, passengers, and other motorists. Logan (1996)[13] studied the interaction between alcohol, marijuana, and methamphetamine on driving performance, noting additive impairments during both methamphetamine intoxication and withdrawal. Drug use was inconsistent with safe driving.

Drug Toxicity

All drugs can produce harmful effects as well as beneficial ones. The nature of these unwanted effects falls into two categories: (1) effects that are related to the principal and predictable pharmacological action of a drug, and (2) effects that are unrelated to this action. It is important to categorize harmful effects of drugs in terms of their severity and to distinguish between those effects that cause a temporary inconvenience or discomfort and those that can lead to organ damage, permanent disability, or even death.

Virtually all drugs exert effects on several different body functions, despite the fact that one is usually interested in obtaining just one (or perhaps a small number) of the drug's many possible effects. The desired effect is usually considered the *main* (or *therapeutic) effect,* while the unwanted effects are labeled *side effects.* To achieve the desired therapeutic effect, some degree of side effects often must be tolerated. This is possible if the side effects are minor, but if they are more serious, they may be a limiting factor in the use of the drug.

The distinction between therapeutic effects and side effects is relative and depends on the purpose for which the drug was taken. Indeed, one person's side effect may be another person's desired therapeutic effect. For example, in one patient the pain-relieving properties of morphine may be sought, while the intestinal constipation that morphine induces becomes an undesirable side effect that must be tolerated. For a second patient, however, morphine may be used to treat diarrhea, in which case the constipation induced is the desired therapeutic effect, and any relief of pain becomes a side effect.

In addition to side effects that are merely irritating, some drugs may cause reactions that are very serious. Such side effects include serious allergies, blood disorders, liver or kidney toxicity, or abnormalities in fetal development. Fortunately, the incidence of these serious toxic effects is quite low.

Allergies to drugs may take many forms, from mild skin rashes to fatal shock. Allergies differ from normal side effects, which can often be eliminated or at least made tolerable by a simple reduction in dosage. However, a reduction in the dose of a drug may have no effect on a drug allergy, because exposure to any amount of the drug can be hazardous and possibly catastrophic for the patient.

Organ damage to the liver and kidneys results from their role in concentrating, metabolizing, and excreting toxic drugs. Examples of drug-induced liver damage include that caused either by alcohol or certain of the inhalants of abuse (see Chapter 3). Certain of the major tranquilizers (the phenothiazines) may induce jaundice by increasing the viscosity of bile in the liver (see Chapter 10).

The toxicity to a fetus of both socially abused and some therapeutic drugs should be mentioned. Data quite clearly show the adverse effects of nicotine (Chapter 6) and ethyl alcohol (Chapter 3) on the fetus. More recently, the effects of cocaine abuse on the fetus (Chapter 5) have received much attention.[14] Indeed, these drugs are thought to be responsible for a majority of preventable fetal toxicities and are three of the major health hazards in the country today.

Placebo Effects

The term *placebo* refers to a pharmacologically inert substance that elicits a significant therapeutic response. Placebos work best on symptoms or diseases that vary (wax and wane) over time. Perhaps the most prominent examples are major depression and chronic pain.[15–18] Because the placebo action is independent of any chemical property of the drug, it arises largely because of what the patient expects or desires. A placebo response may result from a person's mental set or from the entire environmental setting in which the drug is taken. In certain predisposed persons, a placebo may produce extremely strong reactions with far-reaching consequences. Indeed, placebos can therapeutically empower patients to stimulate their psychophysiological self-regulation abilities. Possible mechanisms for the placebo effect include conditioning, expectancy, and self-liberation of endogenous neurotransmitters, including endorphins and adrenaline-like catecholamines.

Remarkably, placebos have been shown to evoke patterns of altered behavior that are similar to, and as long-lasting as, those observed when a pharmacologically active drug is ingested. Thus, in analyzing the pharmacology of a psychoactive agent, we must pay particular attention to the mental set of expectations, the social setting, and the predisposition of the subjects taking the placebo if we are to describe the pharmacological effects of a drug accurately.

The placebo effect is important in understanding the often neglected psychological aspects of therapy. Responses that closely mimic those produced by pharmacologically active drugs can be learned without drugs or placebos. For example, meditation techniques can produce states that closely resemble those produced by drugs, especially altered states of consciousness. Meditation may be used to alter activity in certain centers of the brain in much the same way that a drug would. Certainly, the placebo effect is a powerful element in drug-induced responses.

NOTES

1. L. Z. Benet, "Introduction," in J. G. Hardman, L. E. Limbird, P. B. Molinoff, R. W. Ruddon, and A. G. Gilman, eds., *Goodman and Gilman's The Pharmacological Basis of Therapeutics*, 9th ed. (New York: McGraw-Hill, 1996), 1.

2. A.-M. Talburet and B. Schmit, "Pharmacokinetic Optimization of Asthma Treatment," *Clinical Pharmacokinetics* 26 (1994): 396–418.

3. W. E. Serafin, "Drugs Used in the Treatment of Asthma," in J. G. Hardman, L. E. Limbird, P. B. Molinoff, R. W. Ruddon, and A. G. Gilman, eds., *Goodman and Gilman's The Pharmacological Basis of Therapeutics*, 9th ed. (New York: McGraw-Hill, 1996), 660–664.

4. L. Z. Benet, D. L. Kroetz, and L. B. Sheiner, "Pharmacokinetics: The Dynamics of Drug Absorption, Distribution and Elimination," in J. G. Hardman, L. E. Limbird, P. B. Molinoff, R. W. Ruddon, and A. G. Gilman, eds., *Goodman and Gilman's The Pharmacological Basis of Therapeutics*, 9th ed. (New York: McGraw-Hill, 1996), 11.

5. C. M. Smith and A. M. Reynard, *Textbook of Pharmacology* (Philadelphia: Saunders, 1992), 67–71.

6. S. H. Preskorn, M. J. Burke, and G. A. Fast, "Therapeutic Drug Monitoring: Principles and Practice," *Psychiatric Clinics of North America* 16 (1993): 611–641.

7. S. Siegel, "Drug Anticipation and the Treatment of Dependence," in B. A. Ray, ed., *Learning Factors in Substance Abuse*, NIDA Research Monograph 84 (1988): 1–24.

8. C. X. Poulos and H. Cappell, "Homeostatic Theory of Drug Tolerance: A General Model of Physiological Adaptation," *Psychological Reviews* 98 (1991): 390–408.

9. S. T. Tiffany and P. M. Maude-Griffin, "Tolerance to Morphine in the Rat: Associative and Nonassociative Effects," *Behavioral Neuroscience* 102 (1988): 534–543.

10. E. M. Ross, "Pharmacodynamics: Mechanisms of Drug Action and the Relationship Between Drug Concentration and Effect," in J. G. Hardman, L. E. Limbird, P. B. Molinoff, R. W. Ruddon, and A. G. Gilman, eds., *Goodman and Gilman's The Pharmacological Basis of Therapeutics*, 9th ed. (New York: McGraw-Hill, 1996), 29.

11. L. B. Wingard, T. M. Brody, J. Larner, and A. Schwartz, *Human Pharmacology: Molecular to Clinical* (St. Louis: Mosby Year Book, 1991), 10–17.

12. A. M. Callahan, M. Fava, and J. F. Rosenbaum, "Drug Interactions in Psychopharmacology," *Psychiatric Clinics of North America* 16 (1993): 647–671.

13. B. K. Logan, "Methamphetamine and Driving Impairment," *Journal of Forensic Sciences* 41 (1996): 457–464.

14. R. J. Konkol and G. D. Olsen, eds., *Prenatal Cocaine Exposure* (Boca Raton, Fla.: CRC Press, 1996).

15. R. Rothschild and F. M. Quitkin, "Review of the Use of Pattern Analysis to Differentiate True Drug and Placebo Responses," *Psychotherapy and Psychosomatics* 58 (1992): 170–177.

16. E. D. Peselow, M. P. Sanfilipo, C. Difiglia, and R. R. Fieve, "Melancholic/Endogenous Depression and Response to Somatic Treatment and Placebo," *American Journal of Psychiatry* 149 (1992): 1324–1334.

17. C. Peck and G. Coleman, "Implications of Placebo Theory for Clinical Research and Practice in Pain Management," *Theoretical Medicine* 12 (1991): 247–270.

18. L. White, B. Tursky, and G. E. Schwartz, eds., *Placebo: Theory, Research, and Mechanisms* (New York: Guilford, 1985).

Chapter 2

CENTRAL NERVOUS SYSTEM DEPRESSANTS: TRADITIONAL SEDATIVE-HYPNOTIC DRUGS AND ANTIEPILEPTIC DRUGS

The central nervous system (CNS) depressants are a group of drugs that depress the functioning of the CNS in such a way that calming (*anxiolysis*), drowsiness, and sleep are produced.[1] The older, historically important sedative-hypnotic agents discussed in this chapter produce a dose-related behavioral depression, progressively producing anxiolysis, release from inhibitions, sedation, sleep, unconsciousness, general anesthesia, coma, and, ultimately, death from respiratory and cardiac depression (see Figure 2.1). These relatively nonselective CNS depressants include the barbiturates, a number of sedative-hypnotic agents of diverse chemical structures, alcohols (including ethyl alcohol), the volatile general anesthetics, and the traditional antiepileptic drugs. All except alcohol are covered in this chapter. The unique, nonmedical use of ethyl alcohol in our culture, as well as the widespread abuse of a variety of volatile inhaled substances (the inhalants of abuse) justifies separate discussion (see Chapter 3).

The benzodiazepines (see Chapter 4) have a somewhat lesser capacity to produce deep and potentially fatal CNS depression. Because of this

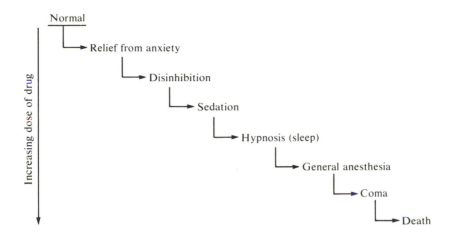

Figure 2.1 Continuum of behavioral sedation. How increasing doses of sedative-hypnotic drugs affects behavior.

improved margin of safety, the benzodiazepines have largely replaced the older agents for the treatment of anxiety and insomnia and are finding use in the treatment of a wide variety of psychological disorders. Even the benzodiazepines, however, are not devoid of potential for toxicity, dependency, or abuse. Therefore, the search continues for hypnotic and anxiolytic drugs with increased efficacy and possibly lower potential for toxicity and abuse. Two such drugs are discussed in Chapter 4—zolpidem and buspirone.

GENERAL CONCEPTS

The terms *sedative, tranquilizer, anxiolytic,* and *hypnotic* can be applied to any of the CNS depressants, because each may diminish environmental awareness, reduce response to sensory stimulation, depress cognitive functioning, decrease spontaneity, and reduce physical activity. Higher doses produce increasing drowsiness, lethargy, amnesia, antiepileptic effects, hypnosis, and anesthesia (see Figure 2.1). The uniformity of action of CNS depressants correctly implies that the effects of any CNS depressant *potentiate* the effects of any other CNS depressant. For example, alcohol exaggerates the depression induced by barbiturates, and barbiturates intensify the impairment of driving ability in a person who has been drinking alcohol.

The depressant effects of sedative drugs are frequently *supra-additive.* Thus, the depression that is observed in a person who has taken more than one drug is greater than would be predicted if the person had taken only one. Such intense depression is often unpredictable and unexpected, and it can lead to dangerous or even fatal consequences. Depressant drugs should not be used in combination without the advice and guidance of a physician, especially if one of the drugs is ethyl alcohol.

Nonspecific antagonism occurs between the CNS depressants and the behavioral stimulants. When a person is profoundly depressed by a sedative drug, the administration of a stimulant, such as caffeine, will not specifically block the action of the depressant and return the patient to normal, although the stimulant may arouse the patient temporarily. In fact, the stimulant may do more harm than good, because when it wears off, the patient will become even more depressed.

Clinically, we have long needed a specific antagonist to CNS depressants—a drug that actually displaces the depressant from its receptors in the brain, thus immediately terminating the action of the depressant. Such a drug would be lifesaving, especially in treating persons who have attempted suicide by ingesting lethal amounts of a drug. The first major step in this area occurred in 1992, when a specific benzodiazepine antagonist, *flumazenil* (see Chapter 4), became available for clinical use. Specific antagonists for the barbiturates and alcohol, however, have not been discovered.

All the CNS sedative-hypnotic agents (from alcohol to the benzodiazepines) carry the risk of inducing physiological dependence, psychological dependence, and tolerance. Physiological dependence is characterized by the occurrence of withdrawal signs and symptoms when the drug is not taken. Signs and symptoms range from sleep disturbances to life-threatening withdrawal convulsions. Psychological dependence follows from the positive reinforcement effects of the drugs. Tolerance occurs as a result of the induction of drug-metabolizing enzymes in the liver and to the adaptation of cells in the brain. In addition, a remarkable degree of *cross tolerance* may occur, in which tolerance to one drug results in a lessened response to another drug. *Cross dependence* also may be exhibited, in which one drug can prevent the withdrawal symptoms that are associated with physical dependence on a different drug. This latter observation underlies the clinical use of benzodiazepines to help moderate the signs and symptoms associated with withdrawal from alcohol.

Historical Background

From time immemorial, human beings have sought ways and means both of achieving release from subjectively distressing and disabling anxiety and of inducing sleep to counteract debilitating insomnia.[2]

Alcohol is certainly the oldest of the sedative-hypnotic agents, having been used since the time of Genesis. It is ingested to ease anxiety, tension, and agitation and to lull the imbiber into a soporific state. The *opium alkaloids* (such as *heroin*) have similarly been used historically to induce a somnolent stupor for relief from anxiety. The addiction potential of the opioids, as well as their lethal potential, have limited their (usually illicit) use as antianxiety agents to relatively small groups of individuals.

In the middle of the nineteenth century, *bromide* and *chloral hydrate* became available as safer, more reliable alternatives to alcohol and opium when used as sedative agents. Then, in 1912, *phenobarbital* was introduced into medicine as a sedative drug, the first of a class of drugs called *barbiturates*. This inaugurated an ongoing search for even safer sedative-anxiolytic agents. Between 1912 and about 1950, hundreds of barbiturates were tested and approximately 50 were marketed commercially. Indeed, "the barbiturates so dominated the stage that less than a dozen other sedative-hypnotics were successfully marketed before 1960."[1]

In 1961 *chlordiazepoxide* (Librium) became the first available *benzodiazepine* tranquilizer (see Chapter 4). As opposed to the older agents, the benzodiazepines exert effects on a specific neurotransmitter receptor that are independent of the nonspecific neuronal depression observed at higher doses. Indeed, the several benzodiazepines that are commercially available display relatively high antianxiety activity relative to generalized depression of CNS function. However, all are sedating to some degree, making them useful as both anxiolytics and hypnotics. Because of a reduced toxicity in overdosage, the benzodiazepines have essentially replaced the barbiturates for these two uses.

In recognition of the limitations to the use of the benzodiazepines (especially the potential to induce dependency), the search continues for equally effective but potentially safer agents. Indeed, in the mid-1990s *buspirone* and *zolpidem* became commercially available, the former as an anxiolytic and the latter as a hypnotic. Both are discussed in Chapter 4. Undoubtedly, the twenty-first century will be accompanied by continued progress in the development of potentially superior anxiolytic and hypnotic agents.

Sites and Mechanisms of Action

The CNS is exquisitely sensitive to the nonselective depressant effects of the barbiturates, the nonbarbiturate sedative-hypnotics, ethyl alcohol, and the general anesthetics.[1] At low and normal doses of these compounds, the polysynaptic, diffuse brain-stem pathways are the first to be depressed. Brain-stem depression continues as dosage increases and accounts for the deep coma and death that can follow barbiturate overdosage. The mechanisms involved in the behavioral depressant action of the barbiturates and related drugs are complex, involving both the depression of "excitatory" synaptic neurotransmitter chemicals and the facilitation of an "inhibitory" neurotransmitter. Each will be addressed.

First, we examine barbiturate-induced depression of excitatory neurotransmission. Recent evidence[3] indicates that pentobarbital (a barbiturate) reduces the synaptic depolarizations produced by glutamate, one of the major excitatory neurotransmitters in the CNS (see Appendix IV). Indeed, it is a specific subtype (the *N-methyl-D-aspartate component*) of the glutamate protein-receptor complex that is blocked.[4,5] Higher doses of pentobarbital (anesthetic levels of the drug) depress ion fluxes through sodium channels, further depressing CNS function.

Second, we examine barbiturate-induced facilitation of inhibitory neurotransmission. To begin, we discuss the GABA receptor; more specifically, we discuss a specific subtype of GABA receptor, the $GABA_A$ receptor, as a site of depressant drug action. The $GABA_A$ receptor is a membrane-spanning ion channel (see Figure 2.2), which is common through the CNS, being particularly prominent in the amygdala and the midbrain. When the neurotransmitter GABA is released from presynaptic terminals, it binds to this receptor, inducing a conformational change that, in turn, opens an ion channel that allows negatively charged chloride ions to pass into the neuron. This hyperpolarizes the nerve membrane, making the neuron less excitable by other transmitters. Located on the outer surface of the $GABA_A$ receptor are specific binding sites for both the benzodiazepines and the barbiturates. Drugs of either class, when bound, affect the structure of the ion channel, making it easier to open or prolonging its opening. This action enhances or potentiates the inhibitory neurotransmitter effect of GABA.

Barbiturates do not bind to the same site on the $GABA_A$ receptor as the benzodiazepines.[6-9] As a consequence of binding, barbiturates increase the affinity of GABA for its receptor and prolong the length of time that chloride channels remain open by a magnitude of fourfold to fivefold. In high doses, barbiturates appear to open chloride channels in the absence of GABA, greatly magnifying CNS depression and potentiating the described inhibition of glutamate receptors, likely contributing to the general anesthetic effects of barbiturates.

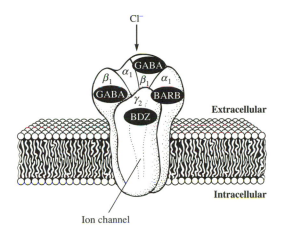

Figure 2.2 Schematic model of the gamma-aminobutyric acid (GABA) chloride ionophore. GABA binding to its receptor (GABA) activates and opens the chloride channel, thus increasing the inward flux of chloride ions. Benzodiazepines bind to specific receptors (BDZ) and increase the effect of GABA on the chloride channel. Barbiturates bind to their receptors (BARB) and prolong the GABA-induced opening of the chloride channel. In high doses, barbiturates may directly open the chloride channel. [Zorumski and Isenberg (1991),[6] p. 168.]

Uses

Use of both the barbiturates and the nonbarbiturate sedatives has declined rapidly in recent years for several reasons:

- They lack selective CNS action.
- They are inherently less safe than the benzodiazepines, being lethal in overdosages.
- They have a narrow therapeutic-to-toxic range.
- They have a high potential for inducing tolerance, dependence, and abuse.
- They interact dangerously with many other drugs.

Despite these disadvantages, the barbiturates are still used as anticonvulsants, as intravenous anesthetics, and, in psychiatry, to sedate (for example, the "amytal interview"). Barbiturates are also used to help protect the brain after severe head injury (by reducing neuronal activity, blood flow to the brain, and intracranial pressure). Some of the older chloral hydrate derivatives are still used as bedtime sedatives for the elderly. Most other nonselective CNS depressants are of such long duration of action that their use for the elderly is restricted, because they impair cognitive function. The decreased availability of barbiturates has tended to limit their illicit use, although instances still occasionally occur.

Certain psychiatric and neurological disorders, such as the dementias, produce characteristic behavioral, intellectual, and cognitive patterns. Sedative-hypnotic drugs can induce a state that closely resembles dementia. One way to diagnose drug-induced dementia (an "organic brain syndrome") is to perform a mental status examination that evaluates 12 areas of mental functioning (Table 2.1).

In instances where a person's neurons are reversibly depressed by alcohol, nonselective depressants, or benzodiazepine tranquilizers, or when a patient's neurons are irreversibly destroyed (as in dementia), 5 of the 12 functions of the mental status examination are particularly altered (sensorium, affect, mental content, intellectual function, and insight and judgment). The person's sensorium becomes clouded, which causes disorientation in time and place; memory becomes impaired, which is evidenced by forgetfulness and loss of short-term

---

TABLE 2.1 Mental status examination: Twelve areas of mental functioning

---

    1. General appearance

*   2. Sensorium

       a. Orientation to time, place, and person

       b. Clear vs. clouded thinking

    3. Behavior and mannerisms

    4. Stream of talk

    5. Cooperativeness

    6. Mood (inner feelings)

*   7. Affect (surface expression of feelings)

    8. Perception

       a. Illusions (misperception of reality)

       b. Hallucinations (not present in reality)

    9. Thought processes: logical vs. strange or bizarre

* 10. Mental content (fund of knowledge)

* 11. Intellectual function (ability to reason and interpret)

* 12. Insight and judgment

---

* Characteristically altered in both organic dementia and reversible, drug-induced dementia.

memory (a "blackout"); the intellect becomes depressed; and judgment is altered. The person's affect becomes shallow and labile, that is, he or she becomes extremely vulnerable to external stimuli and may be sullen and moody at one moment and exhibit mock anger or rage at the next. When such a mental status is seen, it is diagnosed as a "brain syndrome" caused by depressed nerve cell function. In Alzheimer's disease, such dysfunction is irreversible; when caused by a sedative drug, it is called a reversible, drug-induced state of dementia.

Certain persons (such as the elderly) who already have some natural loss of nerve cell function are more likely to be adversely affected by these drugs, experiencing increased disorientation and further clouding of consciousness. Frequently these persons exhibit a state of drug-induced "paradoxical excitement," which is characterized by a labile personality with marked anger, delusions, hallucinations, and confabulations. Treating such a drug-induced dementia requires that administration of the sedative drug be stopped.

SPECIFIC CNS DEPRESSANTS

Barbiturates

The barbiturates were the mainstays in treating anxiety and insomnia for almost 50 years, from 1912 to about 1960. During this period, they were associated with thousands of suicides, deaths from accidental ingestion, wide dependency and abuse, and many serious interactions with other drugs and alcohol. They remain, however, the classic prototype of sedative-hypnotic drugs against which newer drugs are compared.

Pharmacokinetics

Barbiturates are classified according to their pharmacokinetics. As shown in Table 2.2, their half-lives can be quite short (a three-minute redistribution half-life for thiopental), longer (a 24- to 48-hour elimination half-life for amobarbital, pentobarbital, and secobarbital), or very long (an 80- to 100-hour elimination half-life for phenobarbital). The hypnotic action of ultrashort-acting barbiturates (such as thiopental) is terminated by redistribution, while the action of other barbiturates is determined by their rate of hepatic metabolism followed by renal excretion of the metabolites.

Taken orally, barbiturates are rapidly and completely absorbed and are well distributed to most body tissues. The ultrashort-acting

TABLE 2.2 Structures, half-lives, and uses of some barbiturates

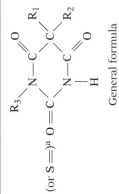

General formula

| Drug name | | | | | Drug name | | Uses | | |
Trade	Generic	R_1	R_2	R_3	Distribution (min)	Elimination (h)	Insomnia	Anesthesia	Epilepsy
Amytal	Amobarbital	Ethyl	Isopentyl	H		10–40	X		
Alurate	Aprobarbital	Allyl	Isopentyl	H		12–34	X		
Butisol	Butabarbital	Athyl	sec-Butyl	H		34–42	X		
Mebaral	Mephobarbital	Ethyl	Phenyl	CH$_3$		50–120			X
Brevital	Methohexital	Allyl	1-Methyl, 2-Pentynyl	CH$_3$		1–2		X	
Nembural	Pentobarbital	Ethyl	Methyl butyl	H		15–50	X		
Luminal	Phenobarbital	Ethyl	Phenyl	H		24–120	X		X
Seconal	Secobarbital	Allyl	Methyl butyl	H		15–40	X		
Lotusate	Talbutal	Allyl	sec-Butyl	H			X		
Surital	Thiamylal	Allyl	Methyl butyl	H				X	
Pentothal	Thiopental	Ethyl	Methyl butyl	H	3	3–6		X	

a O= except in thiamylal and thiopental, where it is replaced by S=.

barbiturates are exceedingly lipid soluble, cross the blood-brain barrier rapidly, and induce sleep within seconds. Because the longer-acting barbiturates are more water soluble, they are slower to penetrate the CNS. Sleep induction with these compounds, therefore, is delayed for 20 to 30 minutes and residual "hangover" is prominent (since the plasma half-lives of most barbiturates vary from 10 to 48 hours).

Urinalysis is used to screen for the presence of barbiturates as well as other psychoactive drugs of abuse. Depending on the specific barbiturate, tests will be positive as short as 30 hours or as long as several weeks after the drug is ingested. When urinalysis is positive for barbiturates, more specific confirmation is needed to determine the exact drug that was taken.

Pharmacological Effects

The barbiturates possess a low degree of selectivity and therapeutic index. Thus, it is not possible to achieve anxiolysis without evidence of sedation. Barbiturates are not analgesic; they may even increase one's reaction to painful stimuli. Hence, they cannot be relied on to produce sedation or sleep in the presence of even moderate pain. In some individuals who are experiencing pain, barbiturates cause overt excitement and even delirium instead of sedation.[1]

This state of overt excitement is caused by the drug-induced brain syndrome. The degree of excitement depends on the person and the circumstances under which the drugs were taken. Physical aggression can be seen during the period of intoxication, especially in individuals experiencing pain or in patients with paranoia or paranoid ideation.

Sleep patterns are especially affected by the barbiturates, with rapid eye movement (REM) sleep being markedly suppressed. Because dreaming occurs during REM sleep, its suppression is nonphysiologic at best. During drug withdrawal, dreaming becomes vivid and excessive. Such rebound increase in dreaming during withdrawal, termed *REM rebound*, is one example of a withdrawal effect following prolonged periods of barbiturate ingestion. Indeed, the vivid nature of the dreams can lead to insomnia, often clinically relieved by restarting the drug and thus negating the attempt at withdrawal. Drowsiness ("hangover") and more subtle alterations of judgment, cognitive functioning, motor skills, and behavior may persist for hours or days until the barbiturate is completely metabolized and eliminated.

Sedative doses of barbiturates have minimal effect on respiration, but overdoses (or combinations of barbiturates and alcohol) can result in death. Barbiturates appear to have no significant effects on the cardiovascular system, the gastrointestinal tract, the kidneys, or other organs until toxic doses are reached. In the liver, barbiturates stimulate the synthesis of enzymes that metabolize these as well as other drugs, an effect that produces significant tolerance to such drugs (see Table 1.3).

Psychological Effects

The behavioral depression and the motor and cognitive dysfunctions caused by barbiturates are similar to those caused by alcohol-induced inebriation and may even be indistinguishable from it. A person may respond to low doses either with relief from anxiety (the expected effect) or with withdrawal, emotional depression, or aggressive and violent behavior. Higher doses (or low doses combined with another depressant) lead to more general behavioral depression and sleep. The person's mental set and his or her physical or social setting can determine whether relief from anxiety, mental depression, aggression, or other unexpected or unpredictable responses are experienced. Driving skills, judgment, insight, and memory all become severely impaired during the period of intoxication.

Adverse Reactions

Side Effects and Toxicity. Drowsiness is one of the primary effects induced by barbiturates and is an inescapable accompaniment to the anxiolytic effect. Drowsiness is often the effect one seeks, especially if the drug was intended to produce either daytime sedation or nighttime sleep.

Barbiturates significantly impair motor and intellectual performance and judgment:

> A person need not be rendered staggering drunk before his motor performance and, probably more important, his judgment are significantly impaired. The most common offending agent in this regard is alcohol. . . . At this time it should be emphasized that all sedatives are equivalent to alcohol in their effects; that all are additive in their effects with alcohol; and that their effects persist longer than might be predicted.[10]

There are no specific antidotes to the serious effects of barbiturate overdosage. Treatment of overdosage is aimed at supporting the respiratory and cardiovascular system until the drug is metabolized and eliminated.

Tolerance. The barbiturates can induce tolerance by either of two mechanisms: (1) the induction of drug metabolizing enzymes in the liver and (2) the adaptation of neurons in the brain to the presence of the drug. With the latter mechanism, tolerance develops primarily to the sedative effects and much less so to the brain stem depressant effects on respiration. Thus, the margin of safety for the person who uses the drug decreases.

Physical Dependence. Normal, clinical doses of barbiturates can induce a degree of physical dependence, usually manifested by sleep difficulties during attempts at withdrawal. The mechanism involved in withdrawal possibly involves an unmasking of the excitatory N-methyl-D-aspartate component of the glutamate receptor complex, which had been suppressed during barbiturate ingestion.[11] REM rebound during withdrawal is common and is accompanied by increased dreaming, which can progress to sleep deprivation, vivid dreams, and nightmares. Withdrawal from high doses of barbiturates may result in hallucinations, restlessness, disorientation, and even life-threatening convulsions.

Psychological Dependence. Psychological dependence refers to a compulsion to use a drug for a pleasurable effect. This phenomenon usually results from an effect of the drug on reward centers in the brain. All CNS depressants are subject to such an effect and are known to be abused compulsively. Because they can relieve anxiety, induce sedation, and produce a state of euphoria, these drugs may be used to achieve a variety of pleasurable psychological states in a variety of abuse situations.

Effects in Pregnancy. Barbiturates, like all psychoactive drugs, are freely distributed to the fetus. Because the newborn has limited metabolizing and excreting systems, it may be depressed for a significant period of time after delivery if the mother ingested barbiturates. Should the drug ingestion have been continuous before delivery, withdrawal signs may be seen in the newborn. Thus, unless special medical situations are present, barbiturates should probably be avoided during pregnancy. Data are limited on whether deleterious fetal abnormalities occur as a result of a pregnant woman taking barbiturates, although there is a suggestion that developmental abnormalities occur. This can be a concern for pregnant females who are epileptic and must take a barbiturate to prevent seizures. The implications are discussed at the end of this chapter.

Miscellaneous Nonbarbiturate Sedative-Hypnotic Drugs

In the early 1950s, three nonbarbiturate sedatives, *glutethimide* (Doriden), *ethchlorvynol* (Placidyl), and *methyprylon* (Noludar) were introduced as anxiolytics, daytime sedatives, and hypnotics. Structurally resembling the barbiturates, they offered few advantages; their toxicity and abuse potential were as great as those of barbiturates. Now considered obsolete, they are rarely encountered in therapeutic use but are seen occasionally as drugs of abuse.

Methaqualone (Quaalude) was another nonbarbiturate depressant that had little to justify its widespread use. During the late 1970s and early 1980s, the popularity and illicit use of methaqualone rose dramatically, and it trailed only marijuana and alcohol in its level of abuse. Such attention was due to an undeserved reputation as an aphrodisiac. Extensive illicit use and numerous deaths led to its removal from sale in 1984. Methaqualone was pharmacologically similar to the barbiturates and, as a sedative drug, was actually an anaphrodisiac. Methaqualone, far from being a "love drug," was merely one of several nonselective depressants that were thought to affect the user favorably when they were taken in the right setting and with a particular set of expectations.[12]

Meprobamate (Equanil, Miltown), now largely of historical interest, was introduced as an antianxiety agent in 1955 as another alternative to the barbiturates for daytime sedation and anxiolysis. Around it developed the term *tranquilizer*, in a marketing attempt to distinguish it from the barbiturates, a distinction that was not borne out in reality. Like the barbiturates, meprobamate produces long-lasting daytime sedation, mild euphoria, and relief from anxiety. Meprobamate is not as potent a respiratory depressant as the barbiturates; attempted suicides from overdosage are seldom successful. Despite a continuing reduction in clinical use, abuse and dependency continue and are difficult to treat.[13]

Chloral hydrate (Noctec) is yet another drug of largely historical interest, having been available clinically since the late 1800s. It is rapidly metabolized to *trichlorethanol* (a derivative of ethyl alcohol), which is a nonselective CNS depressant and the active form of chloral hydrate. It has been noted that REM sleep is not greatly depressed by chloral hydrate, and REM rebound is minimal upon discontinuation. Chloral hydrate appears to be a relatively safe and effective sedative-hypnotic, with a plasma half-life of about 4 to 8 hours. Hangover is less likely to occur than with compounds having longer half-lives. Its liability in producing tolerance and dependence is similar to that of the barbiturates. Withdrawal of the drug may be associated with disrupted sleep and intense nightmares. Occasionally, chloral hydrate is utilized as a bedtime sedative in elderly patients. One interesting aside is that the combination of chloral hydrate with alcohol can produce increased intoxication, stupor, and loss of memory (amnesia or blackout). This mixture is called a "Mickey Finn."

Paraldehyde, introduced into medicine before the barbiturates, is a polymer of acetaldehyde, an intermediate by-product in the body's metabolism of ethyl alcohol. Administered either rectally or orally, paraldehyde is occasionally used to treat delirium tremens (DTs) in hospitalized patients undergoing withdrawal from alcohol (detoxification). The drug is rapidly absorbed (from both rectal and oral routes), sleep ensues within 10 to 15 minutes after hypnotic doses, and the drug is metabolized in the liver to acetaldehyde and eventually to carbon dioxide and water. Some paraldehyde is eliminated through the lungs, producing a characteristic odor to the breath. Individuals dependent on paraldehyde (usually individuals who received paraldehyde as a treatment for alcoholism) suffer a variety of toxicities, primarily to the stomach, liver, and kidneys.

General Anesthetics

General anesthetic agents are potent CNS depressants that produce a loss of sensation accompanied by unconsciousness. General anesthesia is therefore the most severe state of intentional drug-induced CNS depression. The agents that are used as general anesthetics are of two types: (1) those that are administered by inhalation through the lungs and (2) those that are injected directly into a vein to produce unconsciousness.

The *inhalation anesthetics* in current use include one gas (nitrous oxide) and five volatile liquids (isoflurane, halothane, desflurane, enflurane, and sevoflurane), whose vapors are delivered into the patient's lungs by means of an anesthesia machine. These drugs produce a generalized, graded, dose-related depression of all functions of the CNS— an initial period of sedation followed by the onset of sleep. As anesthesia deepens, the patient's reflexes become progressively depressed and both analgesia and amnesia are induced. At that point, a patient is said to be "anesthetized."

Prominent scientists have studied the possible mechanisms of action of the inhaled general anesthetics for more than 100 years.[14] The mechanisms proposed have been so diverse that one recent textbook of pharmacology devotes seven pages to this puzzle.[15] To me, the most plausible explanation for the action of anesthetics involves alteration in the physiochemical processes of nerve membranes. This follows from the linear correlation (see Figure 2.3) between the potency of various drugs as general anesthetic agents and their solubility in lipid. As anesthetics dissolve in the nerve membranes, the structure of the lipid matrix of the membranes becomes distorted, thereby "perturbing" the function of the ion channels and the membrane proteins.[16]

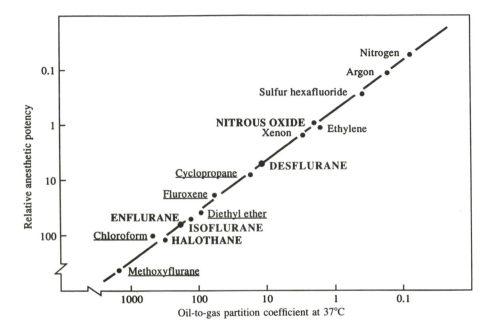

Figure 2.3 Correlation of anesthetic potency with the oil-to-gas coefficient. The correlation is shown for a number of general anesthetic agents and for other inert gases that are not usually used for anesthesia. Note the excellent correlation over a very wide range of fat solubilities and potencies. Agents that are used today in anesthesia are shown in boldface capital letters. Agents that were historically used as anesthetics are underscored.

Occasionally, the inhaled anesthetic agents are subject to misuse. Nitrous oxide, a gas of low anesthetic potency, is an example. Currently used not only in anesthesia but as a carrier gas in cans of whipped cream (e.g., Whippets), nitrous oxide induces a state of behavioral disinhibition, analgesia, and mild euphoria. Since the inhalation of nitrous oxide dilutes the air that a person is breathing, extreme caution must be exercised in order to prevent hypoxia. If the nitrous oxide were mixed only with room air, hypoxia would result, which could produce irreversible brain damage. Other inhaled anesthetics are similarly abused, presuming that the drug abuser can find a supply of the agents. Inhaled as vapors, these drugs produce intoxication, delirium, and eventually unconsciousness. These and other forms of inhalant abuse are discussed in Chapter 3.

Several *injectable anesthetics* are available. Thiopental (Pentothal) and methohexital (Brevital) are ultrashort-acting barbiturates. Propofol

(Diprovan) and etomidate (Amidate) are structurally unique; propofol structurally resembles the neurotransmitter GABA. The mechanism of action of all these anesthetics probably involves intense CNS depression produced secondary both to facilitation of GABA$_A$-receptor activity as well as to depression of excitatory glutamate synaptic transmission. These and other forms of inhalant abuse are discussed in Chapter 3.

Antiepileptic Drugs, Including Those Also Used to Treat Psychological Disorders

Seizures are manifestations of electrical disturbances in the brain. The term *epilepsy* refers to CNS disorders characterized by relatively brief, chronically recurring seizures that have a rapid onset. Epileptic seizures are often associated with focal (or localized) lesions within the brain.

Drugs suppress epileptic seizures by one of two mechanisms.[17] The first is to limit the repetitive firing of neurons (repetitive discharge is thought to initiate or sustain a seizure) by blocking transmembrane channels (see Figure 2.4) through which sodium ions flow (thereby blocking the depolarizing action of sodium ions on the cell). The second mechanism is to enhance GABA-mediated synaptic inhibition[18] by reducing the metabolism of GABA, enhancing the influx of chloride ions (as discussed earlier), or facilitating GABA release from presynaptic nerve terminals.

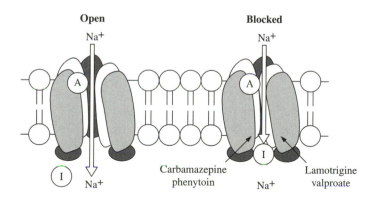

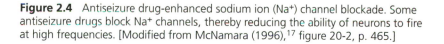

Figure 2.4 Antiseizure drug-enhanced sodium ion (Na$^+$) channel blockade. Some antiseizure drugs block Na$^+$ channels, thereby reducing the ability of neurons to fire at high frequencies. [Modified from McNamara (1996),[17] figure 20-2, p. 465.]

In laboratory animals, epileptic seizures can be induced by a variety of techniques, including "kindling" (repeated low-voltage electrical stimulation of the amygdala or hippocampus to increase the sensitivity of neurons therein). Post and Weiss[19] associate kindling not only with antiepileptic drug action but also with the treatment of bipolar disorders. Others have reported efficacy of antiepileptic drugs (especially valproic aid) in treating conduct disorder, borderline personality disorder, and similar disorders in disturbed nonepileptic psychiatric patients, a use first promulgated two decades ago,[20] when phenytoin (Dilantin) was advocated to treat uncontrolled bouts of mania, panic, and aggression. Another antiepileptic drug, carbamazepine (Tegretol), has been used to treat bipolar disorder, unipolar depression, schizoaffective disorder, dyscontrol syndromes, intermittent explosive disorder, post-traumatic stress syndrome, and atypical psychosis. These nonepileptic uses of valproic acid and carbamazepine are further discussed in Chapter 8.

The observation that both the barbiturates and the benzodiazepines are not only anxiolytic but also antiepileptic encourages the notion that epilepsy, mania, and explosive psychological disorders can be treated with CNS depressants that "stabilize" neuronal membranes either by facilitating inhibition or by limiting excitation.

Relationships between Structure and Activity

The older, traditional antiepileptic drugs belong to one of a relatively small number of chemically similar classes—the barbiturates and the hydantoins (see Figure 2.5). Other structurally similar antiepileptic drugs include *ethosuximide* and *primidone*. In the 1990s, *felbamate, gabapentin,* and *lamotrigine* were introduced as effective new antiepileptic drugs (see Table 2.2).

Felbamate[21] structurally resembles meprobamate, an anxiolytic discussed earlier. To date, nonepileptic, psychological uses of felbamate have not been reported, although the structural resemblance to meprobamate implies an anxiolytic effect. At first thought to be free of serious side effects, felbamate's use was drastically curtailed in late 1994 because of serious hematological reactions. Felbamate is currently used only when the drug is obviously necessary and irreplaceable as an antiepileptic.

Gabapentin, a structural analogue of GABA, was synthesized as a GABA-mimetic drug that crosses the blood-brain barrier. It is an effective antiepileptic drug when used with other drugs for certain types of seizures.[22] In a case report (1995),[23] gabapentin was effective in treating an anxiety disorder (phobia) and pain (reflex sympathetic dystrophy) in

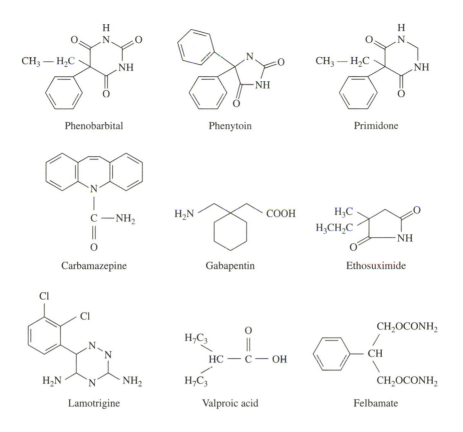

Figure 2.5 Representative drugs used to treat epilepsy.

a female patient. Gabapentin appears to act by promoting the release of GABA from presynaptic nerve terminals.[24]

Lamotrigine (introduced in 1995) acts by inhibiting ion fluxes through sodium channels, thereby stabilizing neuronal membranes and inhibiting the presynaptic release of neurotransmitters, principally glutamate.[25] The drug is rapidly absorbed orally and has a half-life of 30 hours, which decreases to about 14 hours if the patient is taking other antiepileptic drugs that increase the amount of hepatic drug metabolizing enzymes (e.g., carbamazepine, phenobarbital, and phenytoin).[26,27]

Barbiturates

Phenobarbital, the first widely effective antiepileptic drug, replaced the more toxic agent, bromide, which had been used through the nineteenth century. Two other barbiturates are also used occasionally for treating epilepsy—*mephobarbital* (Mebaral) and *metharbital* (Gemonil). Because of their efficacy in reducing seizures, barbiturates are still used occasionally, even though more effective, more specific, and less sedating antiepileptic agents are now the drugs of first choice. Because of their long duration of action, the barbiturates can be administered once each day, sometimes a therapeutic advantage. Epileptic children given barbiturates can display adverse neuropsychological reactions (behavioral hyperactivity and interference with learning ability). *Primidone* (Mysoline), an antiepileptic agent structurally similar to phenobarbital, is metabolized to phenobarbital, which might well be the major active form of the drug.

Hydantoins

Phenytoin (Dilantin) remains a commonly used anticonvulsant. At an effective plasma level (see Table 2.3), phenytoin produces less sedation than barbiturates. The drug is slowly but completely absorbed when taken orally and has a half-life of about 24 hours. Thus, daytime sedation can be minimized if the patient takes the full daily dose at bedtime.

Benzodiazepines

All benzodiazepines possess antiepileptic and anxiolytic properties. Two of them, *clonazepam* (Klonopin) and *clorazepate* (Tranxene), are used to treat seizures, especially types of seizures that are difficult to treat (such as petit mal variant, myoclonic, and akinetic seizures). When used in children, drug-induced personality changes and learning disabilities must be carefully monitored. Both drugs have psychiatric applications that include the treatment of acute mania and other agitated psychotic conditions, usually in combination with other "mood stabilizers" (see Chapter 8). Clonazepam has been referred to as a "behavioral suppressor" rather than a "mood stabilizer."[28]

Carbamazepine

Carbamazepine (Tegretol), as an antiepileptic drug, is used to treat several types of epilepsy. Possibly because of its structural resemblance to imipramine (see Chapter 7), its sedative effect is less intense than that of the other antiepileptic agents. The primary limitations of carbamazepine include rare but potentially serious alterations in the cellular composition of blood (reduced numbers of white blood cells),

TABLE 2.3 Antiepileptic drugs available in the United States

Year introduced	Generic name	Trade name	Half-life (hours)	Therapeutic blood level (mcg/mL)
1912	Phenobarbital	Luminal	50+	15–40
1935	Mephobarbital	Mebaral	—	—
1938	Phenytoin	Dilantin	18+	5–20
1946	Trimethadione	Tridione	6–13	>700
1947	Mephenytoin	Mesantoin	95	—
1949	Paramethadione	Paradione	—	—
1951	Phenacemide	Phenurone	—	—
9152	Metharbital	Gemonil	—	—
9153	Phensuximide	Milontin	8	—
1954	Primidone	Mysoline	5–20	5–40
1957	Methsuximide	Celontin	2–40	
1957	Ethotoin	Peganone	4–9	15–50
1960	Ethosuximide	Zarontin	30+	40–400
1968	Diazepam	Valium	20–50	—
1974	Carbamazepine	Tegretol	18–50	4–12
1975	Clonazepam	Klonopin	18–60	20–80
1978	Valproic acid	Depakene	5–20	50–150
1981	Clorazepate	Tranxene	30–100	—
1981	Lorazepam	Ativan		
1993	Felbamate	Felbatol	22	—
1994	gabapentin	Neuronin	5–7	—
1995	Lamotrigine	Lamictal	33	

— implies data not available
mcg/mL = micrograms of drug per millimeter of blood

presumably secondary to its effects on bone marrow. For nonepileptic, psychiatric use, carbamazepine is being increasingly used in bipolar disorder.[29-31] This use is discussed further in Chapter 8.

Valproic Acid

Valproic acid (Depakene, Depakote, Depacon, divalproex, valproate) is effective and widely used in treating seizure disorders in children, probably by augmenting the postsynaptic action of GABA. Valproic acid is rapidly absorbed, but because it has a short half-life (about 6 to 12 hours), it must be administered several times a day. About 75 percent of epileptic patients receiving valproic acid respond favorably. Serious side effects from valproic acid are rare, but liver failure has been reported.

Valproic acid possesses both antiepileptic action and GABAergic actions, so it is not surprising that the drug is effective in nonepileptic situations as a mood stabilizer, especially in individuals suffering from bipolar disorder (see Chapter 8).[32-34] "Currently, valproic acid is . . . emerging as a highly effective alternate treatment to lithium for acute mania."[35]

Several new and novel classes of drugs are being evaluated for clinical usefulness as antiepileptic agents. Of particular interest are several steroid derivatives, referred to as *epalons*. Epalons are neuroactive endogenous or synthetic steroids, devoid of hormonal action, but which appear to exert anxiolytic, sedative, and anticonvulsant effects by facilitating ion transfer through $GABA_A$ receptors.[36] One such agent, *ganaxolone*, is currently undergoing trials in humans[37] and offers promise as an antiepileptic agent, resembling valproic acid in its clinical profile. Nonepileptic uses are yet to be reported.

Antiepileptic Drugs in Pregnancy

Rates of stillbirth and infant mortality are higher for epileptic mothers. Children of epileptic mothers who received antiseizure medication during the early months of pregnancy have an increased incidence of a variety of birth defects. The risk is approximately 7 percent, compared with 2 percent to 3 percent for the general population.[38]

Pitting this fact against the obvious necessity to control seizures is a therapeutic dilemma in treating pregnant women who have epilepsy. In general, epileptic women of childbearing age should be advised of teratogenic potential. Prior to becoming pregnant, it should be determined whether drugs can be tapered off and discontinued. If this cannot be done safely, one approach is to use a single medication at the lowest possible dose that will control seizures. Divided daily doses may decrease the peak levels in plasma while maintaining an adequate steady state level of the drug in the blood.

NOTES

1. W. R. Hobbs and T. A. Verdoorn, "Hypnotics and Sedatives: Ethanol," in J. G. Hardman, L. E. Limbird, P. B. Molinoff, R. W. Ruddon, and A. G. Gilman, eds., *Goodman and Gilman's The Pharmacological Basis of Therapeutics*, 9th ed. (New York: McGraw-Hill, 1996), 361–396.
2. P. G. Janicak, J. M. Davis, S. H. Preskorn, and F. J. Ayd, Jr., *Principles and Practice of Psychopharmacotherapy* (Baltimore: Williams & Wilkins, 1993), 405.

3. W. Marszalec and T. Narahashi, "Use-Dependent Pentobarbital Block of Kainate and Quisqualate Currents," *Brain Research* 608 (1993), 1–15.

4. B. Tabakoff and P. L. Hoffman, "Ethanol, Sedative Hypnotics, and Glutamate Receptor Function in Brain and Cultured Cells," *Behavior Genetics* 23 (1993): 231–236.

5. Z. Cai and P. P. McCaslin, "Acute, Chronic, and Differential Effects of Several Anesthetic Barbiturates on Glutamate Receptor Activation in Neuronal Culture," *Brain Research* 611 (1993): 181–186.

6. C. F. Zorumski and K. E. Isenberg, "Insights into the Structure and Function of GABA-Benzodiazepine Receptors: Ion Channels and Psychiatry," *American Journal of Psychiatry* 148 (1991): 162–173.

7. P. A. Saunders and I. K. Ho, "Barbiturates and the GABA$_A$ Receptor Complex," *Progress in Drug Research* 34 (1990): 261–286.

8. J. Amin and D. S. Weiss, "GABA$_A$ Receptor Needs Two Homologous Domains of the Beta-Subunit for Activation by GABA but Not by Pentobarbital," *Nature* 366 (1993): 565–569.

9. B. D. Harris, G. Wong, E. J. Moody, and P. Skolnick, "Different Subunit Requirements for Volatile and Nonvolatile Anesthetics at Gamma-Aminobutyric Acid Type A Receptors," *Molecular Pharmacology* 47 (1995): 363–367.

10. H. Meyers, E. Jawetz, and A. Goldfien, *Review of Medical Pharmacology,* 3rd ed. (Los Altos, Calif.: Lange Medical Publications, 1972), 219.

11. M. Rabbani, J. Wright, A. R. Butterworth, Q. Zhou, and H. J. Little, "Possible Involvement of NMDA Receptor-Mediated Transmission in Barbiturate Physical Dependence," *British Journal of Pharmacology* 111 (1994): 89–96.

12. C. V. Wetli, "Changing Patterns of Methaqualone Abuse," *Journal of the American Medical Association* 249 (1983): 621.

13. J. D. Roache and R. R. Griffiths, "Lorazepam and Meprobamate Dose Effects in Humans: Behavioral Effects and Abuse Liability," *Journal of Pharmacology and Experimental Therapeutics* 243 (1987): 978.

14. J. H. Tinker, "Voices from the Past: From Ice Crystals to Fruit Flies in the Quest for a Molecular Mechanism of Anesthetic Action," *Anesthesia and Analgesia* 77 (1993): 1–3.

15. C. M. Smith and A. M. Reynard, *Textbook of Pharmacology* (Philadelphia: Saunders, 1992), 188–194.

16. J. P. Diliger, A. M. Vidal, H. I. Mody, and Y. Liu, "Evidence for Direct Actions of General Anesthetics on an Ion Channel Protein," *Anesthesiology* 81 (1994): 431–442.

17. J. O. McNamara, "Drugs Effective in the Therapy of the Epilepsies," in J. G. Hardman, L. E. Limbird, P. B. Molinoff, R. W. Ruddon, and A. G. Gilman, eds., *Goodman and Gilman's The Pharmacological Basis of Therapeutics,* 9th ed. (New York: McGraw-Hill, 1996), 461–486.

18. P. Granger, B. Biton, C. Faure, X. Vige, H. Depoortere, D. Graham, S. Z. Langer, B. Scatton, and P. Avonet, "Modulation of the Gamma-Aminobutyric Acid Type A Receptor by the Antiepileptic Drugs Carbamazepine and Phenytoin," *Molecular Pharmacology* 47 (1995): 1189–1196.

19. R. M. Post and S. R. B. Weiss, "Sensitization, Kindling, and Anticonvulsants in Mania," *Journal of Clinical Psychiatry* 50, Suppl. 12 (1989): 23–30.

20. J. Dryfus, *The Lion of Wall Street* (Washington DC: Regnery Publishing, 1996).

21. K. J. Palmer and D. McTavish, "Felbamate: A Review of Its Pharmacodynamic and Pharmacokinetic Properties, and Therapeutic Efficacy in Epilepsy," *Drugs* 46 (1993): 1041–1065.

22. R. H. Mattson, ed., "Managing Epilepsy: The Role of Gabapentin," *Neurology* 44, No. 6, Suppl. 5 (1994).

23. G. A. Mellick and M. L. Seng, "The Use of Gabapentin in the Treatment of Reflex Sympathetic Dystrophy and a Phobic Disorder," *American Journal of Pain Management* 5 (1995): 7–9.

24. O. Honmou, J. D. Kocsis, and G. B. Richerson, "Gabapentin Potentiates the Conductance Increase Induced by Nipecotic Acid in CA1 Pyramidal Neurons *In Vitro*," *Epilepsy Research* 20 (1995): 193–202.

25. A. W. Yuen, "Lamotrigine: A Review of Antiepileptic Efficacy," *Epilepsia* 35, Suppl. 5 (1994): S33–S36.

26. J. T. Gilman, "Lamotrigine: An Antiepileptic Agent for the Treatment of Partial Seizures," *Annals of Pharmacotherapy* 29 (1995): 144–151.

27. A. D. Fraser, "New Drugs for the Treatment of Epilepsy," *Clinical Biochemistry* 29 (1996): 97–110.

28. P. G. Janicak, J. M. Davis, S. H. Preskorn, and F. J. Ayd, Jr., *Principles and Practice of Psychopharmacotherapy* (Baltimore: Williams & Wilkins, 1993), 358.

29. Ibid, 369.

30. J. G. Small et al., "Carbamazepine Compared with Lithium in the Treatment of Mania," *Archives of General Psychiatry* 48 (1991): 915–921.

31. N. Coxhead, T. Silverstone, and J. Cookson, "Carbamazepine versus Lithium in the Prophylaxis of Bipolar Affective Disorder," *Acta Psychiatrica Scandinavia* 85 (1992): 114–118.

32. P. G. Janicak, R. Newman, and J. M. Davis, "Advances in the Treatment of Mania and Related Disorders: A Reappraisal," *Psychiatric Annals* 22 (1992): 92–103.

33. H. G. Pope, S. L. McElroy, P. E. Keck, and J. L. Hudson, "A Placebo-Controlled Study of Valproate in Mania," *Archives of General Psychiatry* 48 (1991): 62–68.

34. T. W. Freeman, J. L. Clothier, P. Pazzaglia, M. C. Lesem, and A. C. Swann, "A Double-Blind Comparison of Valproate and Lithium in the Treatment of Acute Mania," *American Journal of Psychiatry* 149 (1992): 108–111.

35. P. G. Janicak, J. M. Davis, S. H. Preskorn, and F. J. Ayd, Jr., *Principles and Practice of Psychopharmacotherapy* (Baltimore: Williams & Wilkins, 1993), 382.

36. K. W. Gee, L. D. McCauley, and N. C. Lan, "A Putative Receptor for Neurosteroids on the $GABA_A$ Receptor Complex: The Pharmacological Properties and Therapeutic Potential of Epalone," *Critical Reviews in Neurobiology* 9 (1995): 207–227.

37. K. W. Gee, "Epalons as Anticonvulsants," *Proceedings of the Western Pharmacology Society* 39 (1996): 55.

38. D. Lindhout and J. G. Omtzigt, "Teratogenic Effects of Antiepileptic Drugs: Implications for the Management of Epilepsy in Women of Childbearing Age," *Epilepsia* 35, Suppl. 4 (1994): S19–S28.

Chapter 3

CENTRAL NERVOUS SYSTEM DEPRESSANTS: ALCOHOL AND THE INHALANTS OF ABUSE

ALCOHOL

When we use the term *alcohol*, we mean ethyl alcohol (ethanol)—a psychoactive drug that is similar in most respects to the sedative-hypnotic compounds; the main difference from the other depressants is that it is used primarily for recreational rather than medical purposes. Because it is the second most widely used psychoactive substance in the world (after caffeine), alcohol has created special problems for both individual users and society in general.

Pharmacology of Alcohol

Pharmacokinetics

Absorption. Alcohol is a simple molecule containing two carbon atoms; a hydroxyl (OH) group is attached to one of those carbons (see Figure 3.1). Alcohol is soluble in both water and fat, and it diffuses easily through biological membranes. Thus, it is rapidly and completely

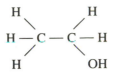

Figure 3.1 Structure of ethanol (CH$_3$CH$_2$OH).

absorbed from the entire gastrointestinal tract, most being absorbed from the upper intestine (because of its large surface area).

The time from the last drink to maximal concentration in blood ranges from 30 to 90 minutes.[1] In a person with an empty stomach, approximately 20 percent of a single dose of alcohol is absorbed directly from the stomach, usually quite rapidly. The remaining 80 percent is absorbed rapidly and completely from the upper intestine; the only limiting factor is the time it takes to empty the stomach. If a person drinks alcohol on a full stomach, gastric emptying is delayed, and the rapid absorption that usually occurs in the upper intestine is slowed. Thus, maximal blood levels may be reached only at the 90 minutes after ingestion is stopped.

Distribution. After absorption, alcohol is evenly distributed throughout all body fluids and tissues. The blood-brain barrier is freely permeable to alcohol. When alcohol appears in the blood and reaches a person's brain, it crosses the blood-brain barrier almost immediately. Alcohol is also freely distributed from a pregnant woman's blood to the fetus. It crosses both the placenta and the infant's blood-brain barrier rapidly and easily. Fetal alcohol levels become the same as those of the drinking mother. Alcohol can be detected on a baby's breath at birth, in amniotic fluid during pregnancy, and in the baby's blood. Research on the impact of maternal alcohol consumption on human infants has demonstrated the occurrence of *fetal alcohol syndrome,* which consists of serious birth defects, in 30 to 50 percent of all babies born to alcoholic mothers. The fetal alcohol syndrome was described more than 20 years ago[2] and is discussed more completely later in this chapter.

Metabolism and Excretion. Approximately 95 percent of the alcohol that a person ingests is enzymatically metabolized by alcohol dehydrogenase. The other 5 percent is excreted unchanged, mainly through the lungs.* This metabolism of alcohol (about 85 percent) occurs primarily in the liver. However, a small but significant amount of alcohol metabolism (up to 15 percent) is carried out by gastric alcohol dehydrogenase enzyme, which is located in the lining of the stomach.[3] This gastric enzyme metabolizes significant amounts of alcohol as the alcohol is absorbed across the stomach wall into the bloodstream. Indeed, gastric metabolism of alcohol can be expected to decrease the blood level of alcohol by about 15 percent, which obviously attenuates its systemic toxicity. Frezza and coworkers[4] reported that when women and men consume comparable amounts of alcohol (after correction for differences in body weight), women have higher blood ethanol concentrations than men. Indeed, women have about 50 percent less gastric metabolism of alcohol than men, because women, whether alcoholic or nonalcoholic, have a lower level of gastric alcohol dehydrogenase enzyme. This factor may increase the vulnerability of some women to both acute intoxication and to the chronic complications of alcoholism.

Once alcohol is absorbed, its metabolism in the liver occurs in two steps (see Figure 3.2). The first step is initiated by the enzyme called *alcohol dehydrogenase*, which converts alcohol to acetaldehyde. In the second step, the enzyme *aldehyde dehydrogenase* helps convert acetaldehyde to acetic acid, which is ultimately broken down into carbon dioxide and water, thus releasing energy (calories). Other than providing calories, alcohol has no nutritional value.

The rate of metabolism of alcohol in the liver is unusual because it is independent of the concentration of alcohol in the blood, is linear with time, and is little increased by raising the concentration of alcohol in the blood.[†] In an adult, approximately 10 milliliters (one-third ounce) of 100 percent ethanol is metabolized per hour regardless of the blood alcohol concentration. In other words, it would take an adult 1 hour to metabolize the amount of alcohol that is contained in a 1-ounce glass of 80-proof whiskey (about 40 percent ethanol), a 4-ounce glass of wine, or a 12-ounce bottle of beer. Thus, consumption of 4 ounces of wine, 12 ounces of beer, or 1 ounce of whiskey per hour would keep the blood lev-

---

*Small amounts of alcohol are excreted from the body through the lungs. Most of us are familiar with the "alcohol breath" that results from exhalation of alcohol. This feature forms the basis for the breath analysis test, because alcohol equilibrates rapidly across the membranes of the lungs. Indeed, in the breathalyzer test, a ratio of 1:2300 exists between alcohol in exhaled air and in venous blood. The blood alcohol concentration is easily extrapolated from the alcohol concentration in the expired air.

†In biochemical terms, this is called "zero-order" metabolism. Virtually all other drugs are metabolized by "first-order" metabolism, which means that the amount of drug metabolized per unit of time depends on the amount (or concentration) of drug in blood (see Chapter 1). Perhaps first-order metabolism occurs because the amount of enzyme (alcohol dehydrogenase and aldehyde dehydrogenase) is limited and becomes "saturated" with only minimal amounts of alcohol in the body.

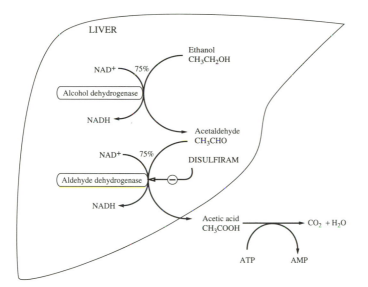

Figure 3.2   Metabolism of ethanol.

els of alcohol in a person fairly constant. If a person ingests more alcohol in any given hour than is metabolized, his or her blood concentrations increase. Consequently, there is a limit to the amount of alcohol that a person can consume in an hour without becoming drunk. These kinetics also allow one not only to estimate one's blood alcohol concentration after drinking a known amount of alcoholic beverage but to estimate the fall in blood concentration over time after drinking ceases.

The following may serve to explain the relationship between the amount of alcohol consumed, the resulting blood levels of alcohol, and the impairment of motor and intellectual functioning (here, driving ability). Most states define a blood alcohol concentration (BAC) of 0.08 grams percent (g%)* as "intoxication," and a person who drives with a BAC above this amount can be charged with driving while under the influence of alcohol. Thus, one might assume that a level of 0.07 g% is acceptable but a level of 0.09 g% is not. However, the behavioral effects of alcohol are not all or none; alcohol (like all sedatives) progressively impairs a person's ability to function. Thus, the 0.08 g% blood level is only a legally established, arbitrary value. Driving ability is minimally impaired at a BAC of 0.01 g%, but at 0.05 to 0.08 g%, a driver has in-

*Grams percent (g%) is the number of grams of ethanol that would be contained in 100 milliliters of blood.

creasingly impaired judgment and reactions and becomes less inhibited. As a result, the risk of an accident quadruples. The deterioration of a person's driving ability continues at a BAC of 0.10 to 0.14 g%, leading to a sixfold to sevenfold increase in the risk of having an accident. At 0.15 g% and higher, a person is 25 times more likely to become involved in a serious accident.

Figure 3.3 illustrates the correlation between alcohol and driving impairment. To use this chart, first glance at the left margin and find the number that is closest to your body weight in pounds. Then, look across the columns to the right and find the column that shows the number of drinks that you have consumed. By matching your body weight with the number of drinks that you have ingested, you can find your BAC. From this number, subtract the amount of alcohol that has been metabolized (remember that approximately 1 drink equivalent is

Blood Alcohol Concentration — A Guide

Drinks   One drink equals 1 ounce of 80 proof alcohol; 12-ounce bottle of beer; 2 ounces of 20% wine; 3 ounces of 12% wine.

Weight (lb)	1	2	3	4	5	6	7	8	9	10
100	.029	.058	.088	.117	.146	.175	.204	.233	.262	.290
120	.024	.048	.073	.097	.121	.145	.170	.194	.219	.243
140	.021	.042	.063	.083	.104	.125	.146	.166	.187	.208
160	.019	.037	.055	.073	.091	.109	.128	.146	.164	.182
180	.017	.033	.049	.065	.081	.097	.113	.130	.146	.162
200	.015	.029	.044	.058	.073	.087	.102	.117	.131	.146
220	.014	.027	.040	.053	.067	.080	.093	.106	.119	.133
240	.012	.024	.037	.048	.061	.073	.085	.097	.109	.122

CAUTION   DRIVING IMPAIRED   LEGALLY DRUNK

Alcohol is "burned up" by your body at .015g% per hour, as follows:

Number of hours since starting first drink	1	2	3	4	5	6
Percent alcohol burned up	.015	.030	.045	.060	.075	.090

Calculate your BAC

Example:

180 lb. man — 8 drinks in 4 hours is .130g% on chart.

Subtract .060g% burned up in 4 hours. BAC equals .070g% — DRIVING IMPAIRED.

Figure 3.3 Relation between blood alcohol concentration, body weight, and the number of drinks ingested. See text for details. [Data supplied by Richard Zylman, Center for Alcohol Studies, Rutgers University, New Brunswick, N.J.]

metabolized in 1 hour). The final figure is your approximate BAC. By calculating this number, you can predict the degree to which your driving ability is impaired.

The following examples illustrate how to use the chart. Consider a 160-pound man who takes 6 drinks in 2 hours. The chart value for the blood alcohol concentration is 0.109 g%. Subtract 0.030 g% for metabolism (0.015 g% in 2 hours). His resulting BAC is 0.079 g%, which is not legally intoxicating but is enough to impair his driving ability. Next, consider a 120-pound woman who takes the same 6 drinks in the same 2 hours. The chart value is 0.145 g%. Subtract the same 0.030 g% for metabolism. Her resulting BAC is 0.115 g%, which is a legally intoxicating value.

Some agencies and organizations have even more stringent BAC standards. For example, the federal Department of Transportation regulations test and limit truck drivers from driving at 0.04 g% and airline pilots from flying at 0.02 g% after 24 hours of abstinence.

Factors that may alter the predictable rate of metabolism of alcohol are usually not clinically significant. With long-term use, however, alcohol can induce drug-metabolizing enzymes in the liver, thereby increasing the liver's rate of metabolizing alcohol (and so inducing tolerance) as well as its rate of metabolizing other compounds that are similar to alcohol (cross tolerance).

Mention should be made here of *disulfiram* (Antabuse), a drug frequently used to treat chronic alcoholism. Disulfiram inhibits aldehyde dehydrogenase, the enzyme responsible for metabolizing acetaldehyde into acetic acid (see Figure 3.2). As a result, acetaldehyde and toxic breakdown products accumulate in the body, causing unpleasant symptoms, such as flushing, coughing, headache, nausea, vomiting, drowsiness, and hangover. Disulfiram makes alcoholics feel so dreadful when they drink that they are discouraged from drinking. To avoid the devastating experience of the acetaldehyde syndrome, an alcoholic cannot drink for at least 3 to 4 days after taking disulfiram. Although disulfiram is occasionally helpful in preventing recurrent bouts of drinking, most alcoholic individuals simply do not take disulfiram regularly.[5]

Pharmacodynamics

Identifying the mechanism of the action of alcohol has been and continues to be difficult because of alcohol's variety of behavioral and neurochemical actions. Indeed, a "unitary hypothesis," where one single neurochemical effect can explain all of alcohol's actions, may not be possible at all. For many years, it was presumed that alcohol acted through a general depressant action on nerve membranes and synapses. Being both water soluble and lipid soluble, ethanol interacts with and dissolves into all body tissues. This property led to a unitary hypothesis of action—that the drug dissolves in membranes, distorting, disorganizing, or "perturbing" the membranes, similar to the action of general anesthetics (see Chapter 2). This dissolving has the result of nonspecifically and indirectly altering membrane processes, such as electrical transmission, transmembrane ion currents, and release of synaptic transmitter chemicals. The neuronal membrane in essence becomes more "fluid," and its functions are disrupted.[5]

Although this membrane hypothesis may correlate with and explain the high-dose or anesthetic properties of alcohol, in the 1990s it was replaced by newer concepts about specific actions on excitatory (glutamate) and inhibitory (GABA) neurotransmitter systems.[1] Regarding the glutamate receptors, Hoffman and Tabakoff (1993)[6] note that ethanol is a potent and selective inhibitor of the function of the N-methyl-D-aspartate (NMDA) subtype of glutamate receptors. The drug appears to exert inhibition by decreasing the frequency of ion channel opening (for sodium ions). The role of such action and the resulting receptor adaptation in the development of physical dependence is discussed later.

Regarding the actions of ethanol on GABA receptors, it appears that ethanol shares with barbiturates and benzodiazepines the capacity to augment GABA-mediated synaptic transmission, by acting at $GABA_A$ receptors.[7] Kushner and coworkers (1996)[8] demonstrated that low doses of ethanol act acutely to reduce both panic and the anxiety surrounding panic. This lends support to the view that drinking by those with panic disorder and anxiety states is reinforced by this GABAergic agonist effect. Thus, the use of alcohol to self-medicate one's panic or anxiety disorder may contribute to the high rate at which alcohol-use disorders cooccur with anxiety and panic disorders.

> Drinking may be both promoted by the short-term anxiolytic effects of alcohol and inhibited by the long-term anxiogenic effects of alcohol. Further, it seems likely that subgroups of those with panic disorder may be more or less prone to escalate drinking aimed at the control of anxiety and panic. Variations in sensitivity to the anxiolytic properties of alcohol, personality dimensions, beliefs about alcohol, and availability of effective coping responses may all influence the likelihood that alcohol is used to control anxiety and panic.[8]

The action of alcohol on the $GABA_A$ receptor differs from that of the barbiturates in that alcohol binds to a different subunit of the GABA receptor that is required for alcohol's enhancing action. This subunit is not necessary for the action of other GABA agonists.[9] A chronic adaptive effect seems to involve changes in intracellular mRNA, suggesting that chronic alcohol can affect gene expression.[10,11] As a result of this GABAergic agonist action, other transmitter systems are affected. Two are of importance here—the cholinergic (acetylcholine) and the dopaminergic (dopamine) systems.

Alcohol inhibits the release of acetylcholine in the central nervous system (CNS), which is an anticholinergic effect. Because the anticholinergic drug *scopolamine* (see Appendix IV) is an exceedingly effective amnesic, and because intact cholinergic mechanisms are necessary for learning and memory, this anticholinergic action may contribute to alcohol's impairment of cognition. Such anticholinergic action is probably indirect, occurring secondary to increased GABA$_A$ inhibition of acetylcholine function.

The GABA agonist action of ethanol has been linked to the positive reinforcing effects of the drug.[12,13] Indeed, the abuse potential of alcohol follows from an ultimate action to augment dopamine neurotransmitter systems, particularly the dopaminergic projection from the ventral tegmental area (VTA) to the nucleus accumbens and to the frontal cortex (see Chapter 14). As Figure 3.4 demonstrates, alcohol

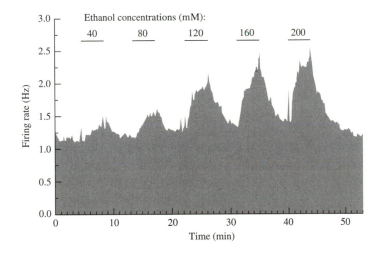

Figure 3.4 This ratemeter record of the firing rate of a single putative dopamine-containing ventral tegmental area (VTA) neuron in a brain slice preparation illustrates the effect of ethanol on spontaneous neuronal activity. Horizontal bars indicate duration of ethanol superfusion. The firing rate was averaged over 12-second intervals, and the height of each vertical bar indicates the mean firing rate in that interval. Concentrations of from 40 to 200 mM ethanol produced a concentration-dependent increase in firing rate. [From Harris, Brodie, and Dunwiddie (1992).[13]]

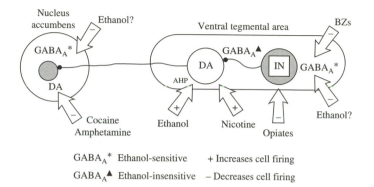

Figure 3.5 Putative substrates of pharmacological reinforcement. This illustrates schematically some of the ways in which drugs of abuse might interact with the ventral tegmental area/nucleus accumbens system. Cocaine and amphetamine are likely to act by potentiating dopamine (abbreviated DA) effects in nucleus accumbens, which would have a primarily depressant effect on cell firing, whereas nicotine appears to have a direct excitatory effect upon DA neurons in the ventral tegmental area. Opiates, benzodiazepines (BZs), and ethanol may all act to inhibit the firing of inhibitory interneurons (IN) via effects on opiate receptors or an ethanol-sensitive GABA$_A$ receptors. Alternatively, ethanol might have a direct excitatory effect upon the DA cells via a mechanism that does not involve a GABAergic receptor. [From Harris, Brodie, and Dunwiddie (1992).[13]]

increases the discharge rate of neurons in the ventral tegmental area. Harris, Brodie, and Dunwiddie (1992) postulate that "the excitatory effects of ethanol on dopamine neurons in the VTA might come about as a result of an inhibition of inhibitory interneurons mediated via GABA$_A$ receptors."[13] The same authors also state that ethanol may act directly on dopamine neurons to increase their firing, not indirectly via the interneurons. These possible effects of ethanol are summarized in Figure 3.5.

Pharmacological Effects

The graded, reversible depression of CNS function is the primary pharmacological effect of alcohol. Respiration, although transiently stimulated at low doses, becomes progressively depressed and, at very high blood concentrations of alcohol, is the cause of death. Alcohol is also anticonvulsant, although it is not clinically used for this purpose. On the other hand, when one stops drinking alcohol, withdrawal is accompanied by a prolonged period of hyperexcitability, and seizures can occur, with the seizure activity peaking approximately 8 to 12 hours after the last drink.*

The effects of alcohol are additive with those of other sedative-hypnotic compounds, resulting in more sedation and greater impairment of driving ability. Other sedatives (especially the benzodiazepines) and marijuana are the drugs that are most frequently combined with alcohol, and they increase its deleterious effects on a person's motor and intellectual skills as well as one's state of alertness.

Alcohol also affects the circulation and the heart. Alcohol dilates the blood vessels in the skin, producing a warm flush and a decrease in body temperature. Thus, it is pointless and possibly dangerous to drink alcohol to keep warm when one is exposed to cold weather. Long-term use of alcohol is also associated with diseases of the heart muscle, which can result in heart failure. Several reports have noted that low doses of alcohol consumed daily (up to 2.5 ounces) may reduce the risk of coronary artery disease. This protective effect occurs because of an alcohol-induced increase in high-density lipoprotein in blood with a corresponding decrease in low-density lipoprotein. (The higher the concentration of high-density lipoprotein and the lower the concentration of low-density lipoprotein, the lower the incidence of coronary heart disease.) Unfortunately, the cardioprotective effect of low doses of alcohol is lost on persons who also smoke cigarettes.

Alcohol exerts a diuretic effect on the body by increasing the excretion of fluids as a result of its effects on renal function, by decreasing the secretion of an antidiuretic hormone, and by the diuretic action produced simply by ingesting large quantities of fluid. Alcohol, however, does not appear to harm either the structure or the function of the kidneys.

Alcohol (like all depressant drugs) is not an aphrodisiac. The behavioral disinhibition induced by low doses of alcohol may appear to cause some loss of restraint, but alcohol depresses body function and actually interferes with sexual performance. As Shakespeare says in *Macbeth*: "It provokes the desire, but it takes away the performance."

Psychological Effects

The short-term psychological and behavioral effects of alcohol are primarily restricted to the CNS. Figure 3.6 correlates the effects of alcohol with levels of the drug measured in the blood. The behavioral reaction

*Hoffman and Tabakoff (1993)[6] postulate that ethanol withdrawal seizures may follow from chronic suppression of the NMDA subtype of glutamate receptors with "upregulation" of these receptors and unmasking of these increasingly sensitive receptors after ethanol ingestion is stopped and withdrawal begins.

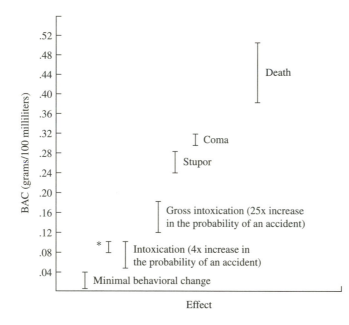

Figure 3.6 Correlation of the blood level of ethanol with degrees of intoxication. The legal level of intoxication (*) varies by state; the range of values is shown. BAC = blood alcohol concentration.

to disinhibition, which occurs at low doses, is unpredictable. It is largely determined by the person, his or her mental expectations, and the environment. In one setting a person may become relaxed and euphoric; in another he or she may become withdrawn or violent. Mental expectations and the physical setting become progressively less important at increasing doses, because the sedative effects increase and behavioral activity decreases.

At low doses, a person may still function (although with less coordination) and attempt to drive or otherwise endanger himself and others. Memory, concentration, and insight are progressively dulled and then lost. As the dose increases, the drinker becomes progressively incapacitated.

Alcohol intoxication, with its resulting disinhibition, plays a major role in a large percentage of violent crimes, including rape, sexual assault, and certain kinds of deviant behaviors.[14] More than 50 percent of crimes and highway accidents are alcohol related, a number that has changed little in 20 years.[15] More than 10 million individuals in the United States currently suffer the consequences of alcohol abuse, which include arrests, traffic accidents, occupational injuries, violence, and health and occupational losses. This number does not include the 10 million individuals considered to be alcohol dependent (with their own suffering of negative consequences). Thus, about 10 percent of our society is personally afflicted with (or suffers the consequences of) another's alcohol use.

Long-term effects of alcohol may involve many different organs of a person's body, depending on whether the drinking is moderate or heavy. Long-term ingestion of moderate amounts of alcohol seems to produce few physiological, psychological, or behavioral changes in a person. But long-term ingestion of larger amounts of alcohol leads to a variety of serious neurological, mental, and physical disorders. These disorders are described in the section on alcoholism.

As stated previously, alcohol is quite caloric but has little nutritional value. Thus, a person may survive for years on a diet of alcohol and not much else, but he or she will slowly develop vitamin deficiencies and nutritional diseases, which may result in physical deterioration. Indeed, alcohol abuse has been suggested as the most common cause of vitamin and trace element deficiencies in adults.[16]

Tolerance and Dependence

The patterns and mechanisms for the development of tolerance, physical dependence, and psychological dependence on alcohol are similar to those for all the depressant compounds. The extent of tolerance depends on the amount, pattern, and extent of alcohol ingestion. Persons who ingest alcohol only intermittently on sprees or more regularly but in moderation develop little or no tolerance; persons who regularly ingest large amounts of alcohol develop marked tolerance. The tolerance that does develop is of three types:

1. Metabolic tolerance, where the liver increases its amount of drug-metabolizing enzyme. This type of tolerance accounts for at most 25 percent of the tolerance that develops to alcohol.

2. Tissue, or functional, tolerance, where neurons in the brain adapt to the amount of drug present. Individuals who develop this type of tolerance characteristically display blood alcohol levels about twice those of a nontolerant individual at a similar level of behavioral intoxication.

3. Associative, contingent, or homeostatic tolerance.[17] A variety of environmental manipulations can counter the effects of ethanol, and these counterresponses are a possible mechanism of tolerance.

The relationship of tolerance to the development of excessive drinking has yet to be determined.[12] No evidence has been demonstrated that any degree of tolerance to the positive reinforcing effects of ethanol develops. Tolerance develops only to the motor-disrupting, hypothermic, sedative, anxiolytic, and anticonvulsant effects.

When physical dependence develops from chronic ingestion of alcohol, withdrawal of the drug results, within several hours, in a period of rebound hyperexcitability that may eventually lead to convulsions. Concomitant with this hyperexcitability is a period of tremulousness, with hallucinations, psychomotor agitation, confusion and disorientation, sleep disorders, and a variety of associated discomforts—a syndrome that is sometimes referred to as *delirium tremens* (DTs).

Side Effects and Toxicity

Many of the side effects and toxicities associated with alcohol have already been mentioned, but let us summarize and expand on them. In acute use, a *reversible drug-induced brain syndrome* is induced. This syndrome is manifested as a clouded sensorium with disorientation, impaired insight and judgment, amnesia ("blackouts"), and diminished intellectual capabilities. The person's affect may be labile, with emotional outbursts precipitated by otherwise innocuous events. With high doses of alcohol, delusions, hallucinations, and confabulations may occur. In social functioning, these alterations result in unpredictable states of disinhibition (drunkenness), alterations in driving performance, and uncoordinated motor behavior.

Liver damage is the most serious physiological long-term consequence of excessive alcohol consumption. Irreversible changes in both the structure and the function of the liver are common. The significance of alcohol-induced liver dysfunction is illustrated by the fact that 75 percent of all deaths attributed to alcoholism are caused by cirrhosis of the liver, and cirrhosis is the seventh most common cause of death in the United States. Cirrhosis appears to result from alcohol-induced interference with normal body immune functions.[18]

Long-term alcohol ingestion may irreversibly cause the *destruction of nerve cells*, producing a permanent brain syndrome with dementia (Korsakoff's syndrome). The digestive system may also be affected. Pancreatitis (inflammation of the pancreas) and chronic gastritis (inflammation of the stomach), with the development of peptic ulcers, may occur.

A great deal of epidemiological evidence now shows that chronic excessive alcohol consumption is a major risk factor for *cancer* in humans. Although ethanol alone may not be carcinogenic, heavy drinking increases a person's risk of developing cancer of the tongue, mouth, throat, voice box, and liver.[19] This cancer-potentiating effect can be explained by the role of alcohol in modifying the action of other cancer-causing agents. Indeed, alcohol clearly exerts a synergistic action with tobacco. For example, the risk of head and neck cancers for heavy drinkers who smoke is 6 to 15 times greater than for those who abstain from both. The risk of throat cancer is 44 times greater for heavy users of both alcohol and tobacco than for nonusers. Thus, alcohol may promote tumor growth—an effect that may follow from its immunosuppressive action and the resultant reduction in body defense mechanisms against tumor cells.[18]

Teratogenic Effects

Alcohol is a clearly delineated teratogen. A *fetal alcohol syndrome* occurs in the offspring of mothers who have high blood levels of alcohol during critical stages of fetal development.[20] Features of the fetal alcohol syndrome include the following:

- CNS dysfunction, including low intelligence and microcephaly (reduced cranial circumference), mental retardation, and behavioral abnormalities (often presenting as hyperactivity and difficulty with social integration).
- Retarded body growth rate.
- Facial abnormalities (short palpebral fissures, short nose, wide-set eyes, and small cheekbones).
- Other anatomical abnormalities (for example, congenital heart defects and malformed eyes and ears).[21]

In the United States, an estimated 2.6 million infants are born annually following significant intrauterine alcohol exposure.[22] At present, the projected incidence of fetal alcohol syndrome may be as high as 1 in every 300 births, while a "lesser degree of damage, termed fetal alcohol effects, may occur in 1 in 100 live births."[22] This would make alcohol ingestion the third leading cause of birth defects with associated mental retardation, following only Down's syndrome and spina bifida. However, fetal alcohol syndrome is the only one of these conditions that is preventable. Indeed, alcohol seems to be the most frequent cause of teratogenically induced mental deficiency known in the Western world.

Even moderate drinking of alcohol is clearly contraindicated during pregnancy.[1] A study of more than 31,000 pregnancies shows that the consumption of only one or two drinks daily can cause a substantially increased risk of a growth-retarded infant.[23] One drink per day has minimal effect but cannot be considered safe. Fetal alcohol syndrome is thought to occur in 1 out of 3 infants of alcoholic mothers.

Despite these statistics, 20 percent of pregnant women continue to consume alcohol.[24] This obviously places the unborn infant at risk of incurring significant damage even before birth. The highest rates of alcohol use during pregnancy occur in women who smoke (37 percent) and in women who are not married (28 percent). These facts suggest that special efforts are needed to convince pregnant women who are smokers, unmarried, less educated, or younger to avoid alcohol.

The effects of paternal drinking or alcoholism on the fetus are unknown. More than 25 percent of pregnant women who are moderate-to-heavy drinkers report that their infants' fathers are also heavy drinkers. This factor may or may not be significant.

Alcoholism

Definition of the term *alcoholism* is relatively recent, as is the recognition of alcoholism as a multifaceted disease process.[25] The founding of Alcoholics Anonymous in 1935 offered a spiritual and behavioral framework for understanding, accepting, and recovering from the compulsion to use alcohol. It was not until the late 1950s that the American Medical Association recognized the syndrome of alcoholism as an illness. In *The Disease Concept of Alcoholism*, E. M. Jellinek presented the hypothesis that alcoholism is a disease.[26] In the mid-1970s, alcoholism was defined as

> a chronic, progressive, and potentially fatal disease. It is characterized by tolerance and physical dependency, or pathologic organ changes, or both—all the direct or indirect consequences of the alcohol ingested.[27]

This definition fails to recognize the biopsychosocial factors that influence the development of alcoholism. Thus, the definition has been revised and expanded as follows:

> Alcoholism is a primary, chronic disease with genetic, psychosocial, and environmental factors influencing its development and manifestations. The disease is often progressive and fatal. It is characterized by impaired control over drinking, preoccupation with the drug alcohol,

use of alcohol despite adverse consequences, and distortions in thinking, most notably denial. Each of these symptoms may be continuous
or periodic.[28]

In this definition, "adverse consequences" involve impairments in such
areas as physical health, psychological functioning, interpersonal functioning, and occupational functioning, as well as legal, financial, and
spiritual problems.[28] "Denial" refers broadly to a range of psychological maneuvers that decrease awareness of the fact that alcohol use is
the cause of a person's problems rather than a solution to those problems. Denial becomes an integral part of the disease and is nearly always a major obstacle to recovery.[28]

Of the 160 million Americans who are old enough to drink legally,
112 million do so.[25,29] As many as 14 million Americans may have serious alcohol problems, and about half that number (7 million) are considered to be alcoholic. The daily consumption of about a half-pint of
80-proof liquor is thought to place a person's health at risk.
Approximately 10 percent of the drinking population ingests the equivalent of this quantity of alcohol as beer, wine, or hard liquor. Older
people who drink are at risk for their own set of problems. In 1996 the
American Medical Association published "Alcohol in the Elderly,"[30] an
update on alcohol use in this population.

Long-term alcoholism may lead to malnutrition and chronic physiological degeneration. This condition causes a bloated look, flabby
muscles, fine tremors, decreased physical capacity and stamina, and
increased susceptibility to infections. Although this state of chronic degeneration is not present in the majority of alcoholics who receive adequate nutrition, nutrition alone does not fully protect the brain, the
liver, or the digestive tract from damage.[31]

There is a reasonably good correlation between drinking habits,
maximum blood concentrations, and the intensity of a withdrawal syndrome. With a low level of dependence, alcohol withdrawal consists of
altered sleep patterns, nausea, anxiety, wakefulness, and mild tremors
that may last for only a day or so. At higher levels of dependence, an alcohol withdrawal syndrome is seen in which these signs are intensified
and accompanied by vomiting, cramps, nightmares, and transient hallucinations. As the dependence progresses, withdrawal may include
confusion, disorientation, agitation, persecutory hallucinations, and
severe tremors or seizures. After recovery, depression, sleep deficits,
cognitive deficits, and other alterations of brain function may persist
for months or even be relatively permanent.

The more recent definition of alcoholism calls it a primary disorder, implying that it is not associated with other pathopsychophysio-
logical states. Goodwin (1995)[27] states:

> A good deal of evidence now indicates that many, if not most, alcoholics do not have primary alcoholism. Their alcoholism is associated with other psychopathology, including addiction to other drugs.

Goodwin further states that 30 to 50 percent of alcoholics meet criteria for major depression; 33 percent have a coexisting anxiety disorder (social phobias in men, agoraphobia in women); many have antisocial personalities (14 percent); some are schizophrenic (3 percent); and many (36 percent) are addicted to other drugs. Indeed, some, if not many, individuals may have first used alcohol and become psychologically dependent on the drug by using it as a self-prescribed medication to treat their primary disorder. Therefore, dual diagnosis must always be presumed (until proven otherwise).

Drugs Used to Treat Alcoholism

> Because alcoholism involves the ingestion of alcohol, eliminating the taking of alcohol is an obvious therapeutic strategy.[36]

A recent study by Vaillant (1996)[32] points to the poor long-term outlook of this prognosis. Vaillant performed a remarkable 50-year follow-up of two cohorts of men who abused alcohol at an early age. One group consisted of Harvard University undergraduates and the second consisted of nondelinquent inner-city adolescents. By 60 years of age, 18 percent of the college alcohol abusers had died, 11 percent were abstinent, 11 percent were controlled drinkers, and 60 percent were still abusing alcohol. By 60 years of age, 28 percent of the inner-city alcohol abusers had died, 30 percent were abstinent, 12 percent were controlled drinkers, and 30 percent were still abusing alcohol. Continued abuse, greater in college-educated males, certainly needs to be addressed, as alcohol use after age 60 can be devastating.[29] This data also questions "controlled drinking" as a therapeutic endpoint.

Today, the *benzodiazepines* (see Chapter 4) are mainstays in the treatment of acute alcohol withdrawal syndrome ("detoxification"). One might question why one potentially addictive drug is substituted for another. One explanation for this is as follows. The short duration of the action of alcohol and its narrow range of safety make it an extremely dangerous drug from which to withdraw. When alcohol ingestion is stopped, it rapidly is metabolized, precipitating withdrawal symptoms. Substituting a long-acting drug prevents or suppresses the withdrawal symptoms.[33–35] The longer-acting benzodiazepine is then either maintained at a level low enough to allow the person to function or is withdrawn gradually. Preferred drugs are the benzodiazepines with long-acting active metabolites (e.g., chlordiazepoxide [Librium] or diazepam [Valium]). Unpublished to date are outcome studies delineating the efficacy of benzodiazepine substitution and/or withdrawal. In other words, if alcoholics withdraw utilizing benzodiazepine substitution and later withdraw from the benzodiazepine, what percentage of individuals, over time, returns to the original drinking patterns and what percentage remains drug free?

Disulfiram (Antabuse) has long been used to treat alcoholism. As discussed above, disulfiram alters the metabolism of alcohol, allowing acetaldehyde to accumulate. Such accumulation results in an acetaldehyde syndrome if the patient ingests alcohol within several days of taking disulfiram. If taken daily, disulfiram can result in total abstinence in the vast majority of patients. Like any effective drug, it does not work if it is not taken![36]

Haloperidol (Haldol) and other antipsychotic agents (see Chapter 9) may be used to treat the hallucinations associated with severe delirium tremens. However, if seizures occur, haloperidol cannot be used because it lowers the seizure threshold. In addition, there is concern that antipsychotics may increase the liver damage caused by alcohol. Therefore, haloperidol is rarely used either in acute alcohol detoxification or in chronic use to reduce the rate of relapse.

Conditioned-avoidance techniques that include the use of emesis-inducing agents (e.g., *apomorphine* or *Ipecac*) have in past years been used to treat alcoholism. The patient takes the emetic agent and then drinks a dose of alcohol shortly thereafter. When nausea and vomiting occur, the patient associates the drinking of alcohol with the unpleasant reaction. Alcohol thus becomes a conditioned stimulus for the production of nausea and vomiting. Although currently out of favor, treatment with low doses of apomorphine has been tried in efforts to reduce the craving for alcohol.[33]

As noted earlier, many alcoholics suffer from a coexisting major depression. Following alcohol withdrawal, the depression may persist and require therapy. *Tricyclic antidepressants* and the newer *serotonin-specific antidepressants* (both classes of antidepressants are discussed in Chapter 7) have been used to treat alcoholics during the months following withdrawal. However, the evidence in favor of therapeutic efficacy is marginal. McGrath and coworkers (1996)[37] reported on the effects of the tricyclic antidepressant *imipramine*:

> Imipramine treatment was safe and associated with improvement in depression. . . . While there was no overall effect on drinking outcome, patients whose mood improved showed decreased alcohol consumption that was more marked in those treated with imipramine [in contrast to nonmedicated controls].

They concluded that:

> Imipramine treatment is effective for primary depression among actively drinking alcoholic outpatients, and may improve alcoholic outcome for those whose depression responds to treatment.

Similarly, Mason and coworkers (1996)[38] reported on the effects of *desipramine*, a related tricyclic antidepressant:

> Major depression secondary to alcohol dependence that is diagnosed after at least one week of abstinence can remain stable in some placebo-treated alcoholics and can respond to desipramine. Treating depression secondary to alcoholism may reduce risk for drinking relapse in some patients. Use of desipramine to reduce relapse in nondepressed alcoholics is not supported.

Antidepressants that selectively inhibit serotonin reuptake can reduce alcohol intake in persons in the early stages of alcoholism;[39,40] *fluoxetine* (Prozac) is the best studied. Studies in male alcoholics[41] confirm a reduction in alcohol intake, but reductions were small (14 percent). Nunes, McGrath, and Quitkin (1995)[42] conclude that while tratment of comorbid anxiety can only rarely cure alcoholism, the anxiety must be addressed and drugs such as bupropion (Chapter 7) used to treat it simultaneously with treatment of alcoholism.

Some investigators have tested a hypothesis that the endogenous opioid system (see Chapter 10) may have a role in in modulating the intake of alcohol.[43] In particular, *naltrexone* (a long-acting, orally administered narcotic antagonist) administered to alcoholics over a 12-week period can reduce alcohol craving and relapse[43,44] and can potentiate the therapeutic effects of learning coping skills and training to prevent relapse.[45] Some but not all of the benefits resulting from short-term treatment with naltrexone persist after discontinuation of treatment.[46] O'Brien (1995)[47] summarized his thoughts on naltrexone:

> Some therapists are opposed in principle to treating alcohol abuse with a drug, and even clinicians who find naltrexone useful know that it is insufficient by itself. Alcoholism is a complex disorder with symptoms that involve the body, brain, emotions, and social relations. Naltrexone should always be used as part of a comprehensive rehabilitation program including psychosocial treatment. Otherwise, our research indicates, patients do not take it consistently and it is of no use.

In 1995 naltrexone was approved by the FDA for use in the treatment of alcoholism in the United States. Spanagel and Zieglgansberger[43] review the potential mechanisms through which naltrexone may exert its anticraving action. They also review another anticraving drug, *acamprosate*, which is available in Europe but not yet in the United States. Acamprosate appears to exerts its anticraving effect by modulating excitatory synapses operated by glutamic acid.[43] Initial clinical reports are encouraging, with the drug appearing to be an effective adjunct to psychosocial rehabilitation programs.[48,49]

Techniques for Treating Alcoholism

As stated by Collins (1993)[25]:

> Contemporary alcoholism treatment is . . . an amalgamation of medical, psychological, psychosocial, and spiritual modalities interacting in a quasi-organized framework to assist the individual in achieving and sustaining lasting, contented sobriety.

It should be emphasized that such treatment can only follow management of alcohol withdrawal symptoms and maintenance of a period of sobriety. Gessner (1992)[50] emphasizes that

> heavy chronic consumption of ethanol induces an impairment of memory and cognitive function. At the same time, a great deal of learning is required to maintain abstinence and even more to achieve stable moderate drinking. Accordingly, it is not surprising that one of the best predictors of treatment outcome is the degree of cognitive impairment patients present upon entry into therapy: the greater the impairment, the less likely the success of therapy. With abstinence there is a partial reversal of such impairment. Accordingly, an initial period of abstinence is therapeutically desirable, whatever the long-term treatment goals.

Following withdrawal and a period of abstinence (probably of at least several weeks duration), treatment has three goals: (1) continued sobriety, (2) amelioration of cooccurring psychiatric conditions, and (3) long-term prevention of relapse.[27] As mentioned in the discussion about drug therapies for alcoholism, no drug or class of drugs has been shown to be universally effective in the long-term prevention of relapse, although benzodiazepine, antidepressant, or naltrexone therapy may be beneficial for some patients in particular circumstances. Certainly, detoxification is relatively easy; the most complicated and frustrating part of treatment is preventing relapse. Indeed:

> Almost any alcoholic can stop drinking temporarily if given the safety of a medically supervised detoxification. The real challenge for patients with alcohol use disorders is not to stop drinking (however

briefly) but to remain abstinent. Ninety percent of alcoholics may experience at least one relapse during the four-year period following treatment. . . . Relapse prevention is the central concern of alcoholism treatment.[38]

One must therefore find clinical strategies to help patients remain abstinent after their initial period of sobriety. Most drug therapies focus on the early periods. Controversy arises regarding longer-term use of psychoactive drugs because of the inherent risk of relapse into chemical dependence (on a benzodiazepine, for example). What is needed is a variety of effective medications that support patients' efforts at remaining abstinent without undesirable mood-altering properties that could place patients at risk for development of a new dependence. For some, antidepressants may be of assistance in relieving comorbid depression. For others, naltrexone may help reduce the craving.

Perhaps most important, it is vital to integrate pharmacotherapy with behavioral and psychological therapy. Indeed, McCrady and Langenbucher (1996)[51] have called for reform of alcohol treatments as part of health care reform, based on their assessment that

1. Alcohol use disorders and problems associated with alcohol use are prevalent and complicated by various comorbid conditions, and they result in large costs to the health care system and to society.

2. Alcohol treatment generally results in reduced drinking and more efficient use of health care resources.

3. Specific treatments have demonstrated effectiveness.

4. Screening and assessment instruments with excellent sensitivity to the heterogeneity of alcohol problems have been developed.

5. Evidence that specific treatments have differential effectiveness with different patient groups is accumulating.

6. Good evidence exists for the effectiveness of brief interventions, particularly with less severe and chronic alcohol problems.[51]

The authors call for the following altered alcohol treatment goals:

• Universal coverage for alcohol treatment, including outpatient care.

• A rational system of assessment and triage for treatment, including an increased emphasis on screening and brief interventions in primary medical care settings.

• A full range of treatment services that vary in intensity.

- Incentives for addiction-treatment providers and contingencies to provide treatments of proven effectiveness.

A call for drastic reform is certainly timely and necessary, although it is certainly bound to meet with controversy.

INHALANTS OF ABUSE

The inhalants of abuse consist of a variety of organic solvents and other chemicals that are volatile at room temperature (they readily vaporize from the liquid state when exposed to air) and when inhaled, produce euphoria, delirium, intoxication, and alterations in mental status, somewhat resembling alcohol intoxication. Inhaled substances include the following:

- Anesthetics, especially nitrous oxide and halothane
- Industrial or household solvents, including paint thinners or solvents, degreasers, and solvents in glues
- Art and office supply solvents, including typewriter correction fluid and marker pen solvents
- Gases used in household or commercial products, including butane lighters, aerosol cream dispensers, and propane tanks
- Household aerosol propellants, including paint, hair spray, and fabric protector sprays
- Aliphatic nitrites and organic solvents, including amyl nitrite capsules

Some of the substances found in these different products are listed in Table 3.1. Abused inhalants are rarely, if ever, administered by routes other than inhalation.[51]

Why Inhalants Are Abused and Who Abuses Them

Why are such substances used for recreational or abuse purposes, what is their attraction, and why do they have the potential for abuse? Yavich and coworkers (1994)[53] investigated in rats the behavior-reinforcing properties of glue vapors (which are a mixture of four organic

TABLE 3.1 Chemicals commonly found in inhalants

	Inhalant	Chemical
ADHESIVES	Airplane glue	Toluene, ethyl acetate
	Other glues	Hexane, toluene, methyl chloride, acetone, methyl ethyl ketone, methyl butyl ketone
	Special cements	Trichloroethylene, tetrachloroethylene
AEROSOLS	Spray paint	Butane, ropane (U.S.), fluorocarbons, toluene, hydrocarbons, "Texas shoe shine" (a spray containing toluene)
	Hair spray	Butane, propane (U.S.), CFCs
	Deodorant, air freshner	Butane, propane (U.S.), CFCs
	Analgesic spray	Chlorofluorocarbons (CFCs)
	Asthma spray	Chlorofluorocarbons (CFCs)
	Fabric spray	Butane, trichloroethane
	PC cleaner	Dimethyl ether, hydrofluorocarbons
ANESTHETICS	Gas	Nitrous oxide
	Liquid	Halothane, enflurane
	Local	Ethyl chloride
CLEANING AGENTS	Dry cleaning	Tetrachloroethylene, trichloroethane
	Spot remover	Xylene, petroleum distillates, chlorohydrocarbons
	Degreaser	Tetrachloroethylene, trichloroethane, trichloroethylene
SOLVENTS AND GASSES	Nail polish remover	Acetone, ethyl acetate
	Pint remover	Toluene, methyl chloride, methanol acetone, ethyl acetate
	Paint thinner	Petroleum distillates, esters, acetone
	Correction fluid and thinner	Trichloroethylene, trichloroethane
	Fuel gas	Butane, isopropane
	Lighter	Butane, isopropane
	Fire extinguisher	Bromochlorodifluoromethane
WHIPPED CREAM	Whipped cream	Nitrous oxide
	Whippets	Nitrous oxide
"ROOM ODORIZERS"	Locker Room, Rush, poppers	Isoamyl, isobutyl, isopropyl or butyl nitrate (now illegal), cyclohexyl

From Sharp (1992),[52] pp. 4–5.

solvents—toluene, benzene, ethyl acetate, and methyl chloride). At low to moderate concentrations of vapor, the motor activity of the rats increased, as did their rates of self-stimulation in the lateral hypothalamus. Increasing the vapor concentration suppressed this activation of brain reward systems and concomitantly brought on behavioral depression. These effects were similar to those produced by ether and chloroform, volatile anesthetics that have been similarly abused since their introduction into medicine in the mid-1800s.

Sharp and Rosenberg (1992)[54] describe the methods of inhalant abuse as follows:

> The practice of "sniffing," "snorting," "huffing," "bagging," or inhaling to get high describes various forms of inhalation. If the substance is glue or some other dissolved solid, the user empties the can's contents into a plastic bag and then holds the bag to the nose and inhales ("bagging"). Another method is to soak a rag with the mixture and then stick the rag in the mouth and inhale the fumes ("huffing"). A simple but more toxic approach is to spray the substance directly into the oral cavities. This allows abusers to be identified by various telltale clues, such as organic odors on the breath or clothes, stains on the clothes or around the mouth, empty spray paint or solvent containers, and other unusual paraphernalia. These telltale clues may enable one to identify a serious problem of solvent abuse before it causes serious health problems or death.

The extent of the problem of solvent abuse is greater than most people acknowledge, both in well developed[55] and in less developed[56] countries. Inhalant abusers are usually from one of three groups: young males between the ages of 14 and 20; inhalant-dependent adults; and multidrug users. The majority of deaths involving use of inhalants occurs in male teenagers; most of the remainder occur in adults in their twenties. About 90 percent of all inhalant-caused deaths occur in males. A relatively high percentage (about 20 percent) of youths have experience with inhalant abuse by the end of the eighth grade. Indeed, while the use of inhalants by young males is exceeded by use of marijuana, alcohol, and cigarettes, the death rate associated with inhalant abuse is abnormally high, with most deaths the result of direct toxic effects of gas fuels (e.g., butane, gasoline) and solvents.[54]

Acute Intoxication and Chronic Effects

As noted in Table 3.1, a variety of volatile substances are abused by inhalation, each with its own pharmacology and toxicology. In general, however, most inhaled vapors produce a rapid onset state of intoxication (or "drunkenness") that resembles alcohol intoxication. Thus, one sees the continuum of sedation (see Chapter 2) with anxiolysis, disinhibition, drowsiness, light-headedness, and euphoria. With increasing intoxication, the user experiences ataxia (staggering), dizziness, delirium, and disorientation. With severe intoxication, there is muscle weakness, lethargy, and signs of light to moderate general anesthesia. With lack of oxygen (hypoxia), hallucinations and behavior changes may occur. When death occurs during acute intoxication, it usually follows from brain anoxia, cardiac arrhythmia, aspiration of vomitus, or trauma.

With chronic abuse of solvents, serious complications include partially reversible symptoms of peripheral and central nervous system dysfunction (e.g., peripheral neuropathies and encephalopathy), liver and/or kidney failure, and severe toxicities to a fetus should a female abuser be pregnant.[57]

Two Nonsolvent Inhalants of Note

Nitrites

The nitrites are a class of volatile liquids that include *butyl nitrite* and *propyl nitrite*, which are found in cans of room deodorizer, and *amyl nitrite*, which has been used historically for the medical treatment of chest pain due to cardiac ischemia (lack of oxygen to the heart, or *angina pectoris*). With amyl nitrite, the nitrite-dilated blood vessels reduce blood pressure and blood return to the heart and the work load of the heart muscle. This ultimately reduces the pain associated with cardiac ischemia.

When inhaled, the nitrites reduce blood pressure and produce cerebral ischemia, dizziness, and a flushed feeling. Nitrites are usually abused in conjunction with sexual activity for a claimed ability to enhance orgasms.[52] One report[58] indicates that nitrites temporarily reduce anger, fatigue, and depression, offering additional insight into the abuse of these compounds.

Nitrous Oxide

Nitrous oxide is a commonly used, low-potency general anesthetic gas, abused by both youths and some medical personnel. In nonanesthetic formulations, nitrous oxide is used as a propellant in cans of whipped cream. With inhalation, disinhibition, anxiolysis, sedation, and euphoria (hence the nickname "laughing gas") dominate. The major risks with nitrous oxide are acute hypoxia and brain anoxia, which result from the dilution of room air by the gas. Although there is evidence of peripheral neuropathies following long-term use, toxicity is controversial.

Extensive reviews of the topic of volatile substance abuse are available.[52,54,59]

NOTES

1. W. R. Hobbs, T. W. Rall, and T. A. Verdoorn, "Hypnotics and Sedatives: Ethanol," in J. G. Hardman, L. E. Limbird, P. B. Molinoff, R. W. Ruddon, and A. G. Gilman, eds., *Goodman and Gilman's The Pharmacological Basis of Therapeutics*, 9th ed. (New York: McGraw-Hill, 1996), 361–396.

2. J. W. Hanson, K. L. Jones, and D. W. Smith, "Fetal Alcohol Syndrome," *Journal of the American Medical Association* 235 (1976): 1458–1460.

3. J. Caballeria, M. Frezza, R. Hernandez-Munoz, C. DiPadova, M. A. Korsted, E. Baraona, and C. S. Lieber, "Gastric Origin of the First-Pass Metabolism of Ethanol in Humans: Effect of Gastrectomy," *Gastroenterology* 97 (1989): 1205–1209.

4. M. Frezza, C. DiPadova, G. Pozzato, M. Terpin, E. Baraona, and C. S. Lieber, "High Blood Alcohol Levels in Women: The Role of Decreased Gastric Alcohol Dehydrogenase Activity and First-Pass Metabolism," *New England Journal of Medicine* 322 (1990): 95–99.

5. A. Goldstein, *Addiction: From Biology to Drug Policy* (New York: W. H. Freeman and Company, 1994), 125–127.

6. P. L. Hoffman and B. Tabakoff, "Ethanol, Sedative-Hypnotics, and Glutamate Receptor Function in Brain and Cultured Cells," *Alcohol and Alcoholism*, Suppl. 2 (1993): 345–351.

7. J. Kotlinska and R. Langwinski, "Influence of CGS 8216 on Some Acute Effects of Ethanol," *Alcohol and Alcoholism* 30 (1995): 601–605.

8. M. G. Kushner, T. B. Mackenzie, J. Fiszdon, D. P. Valentiner, E. Foa, N. Anderson, and D. Wangensteen, "The Effects of Alcohol Consumption on Laboratory-Induced Panic and State Anxiety," *Archives of General Psychiatry* 53 (1996): 264–270.

9. F.-J. Wan, F. Berton, S. G. Madamba, W. Francesconi, and G. R. Siggins, "Low Ethanol Concentrations Enhance GABAergic Inhibitory Postsynaptic Potentials in Hippocampal Pyramidal Neurons Only After Block of $GABA_B$ Receptors," *Proceedings of the National Academy of Sciences* 93 (1996): 5049–5054.

10. P. Montpied, A. L. Morrow, J. W. Karanian, E. I. Ginns, B. M. Martin, and S. M. Paul, "Prolonged Ethanol Inhalation Decreases $GABA_A$ Receptor Alpha Subunit mRNAs in the Rat Cerebral Cortex," *Molecular Pharmacology* 39 (1991): 157–163.

11. K. J. Buck and R. A. Harris, "Neuroadaptive Responses to Chronic Ethanol," *Alcoholism, Clinical and Experimental Research* 15 (1991): 460–470.

12. H. H. Samson and R. A. Harris, "Neurobiology of Alcohol Abuse," *Trends in Pharmacological Sciences* 13 (1992): 206–211.

13. R. A. Harris, M. S. Brodie, and T. V. Dunwiddie, "Possible Substrates of Ethanol Reinforcement: GABA and Dopamine," *Annals of the New York Academy of Sciences* 654 (1992): 61–69.

14. S. C. Woods and J. G. Mansfield, "Ethanol and Disinhibition: Physiological and Behavioral Links," in R. Room and S. Collins, eds., *Alcohol and Disinhibition: Nature and Meaning of the Link* (Washington, D.C.: U.S. Government Printing Office, 1983), 4–23.

15. R. G. Niven, "Alcoholism—A Problem in Perspective," *Journal of the American Medical Association* 252 (1984): 1912–1914.

16. M. J. Edkardt et al., "Health Hazards Associated with Alcohol Consumption," *Journal of the American Medical Association* 246 (1981): 648–666.

17. C. X. Poulos and H. Cappell, "Homeostatic Theory of Drug Tolerance: A General Model of Physiologic Adaptation," *Psychological Review* 98 (1991): 390–408.

18. S. I. Mufti, H. R. Darban, and R. R. Watson, "Alcohol, Cancer, and Immunomodulation," *Critical Reviews in Oncology/Hematology* 9 (1989): 243–261.

19. S. Palmer, "Diet, Nutrition, and Cancer," *Progress in Food and Nutrition Science* 9 (1985): 283–341.

20. U.S. Department of Health, Education, and Welfare, *Alcohol and Health: Third Special Report to the U.S. Congress* (Washington, D.C.: U.S. Government Printing Office, 1978).

21. National Institute on Alcohol and Alcoholism, *Alcohol and Birth Defects: The Fetal Alcohol Syndrome and Related Disorders,* U.S. Department of Health and Human Services Publication Number ADM 87–1531 (Washington, D.C.: U.S. Government Printing Office, 1987), 6–10.

22. L. P. Finnegan and S. R. Kandall, "Maternal and Neonatal Effects of Alcohol and Drugs," in J. H. Lowinson, P. Ruiz, R. B. Millman, and J. G. Langrod, eds., *Substance Abuse: A Comprehensive Textbook,* 2nd ed. (Baltimore: Williams & Wilkins, 1992), 650.

23. J. L. Mills et al., "Maternal Alcohol Consumption and Birth Weight," *Journal of the American Medical Association* 252 (1984): 1875–1879.

24. M. Serdula, D. F. Williamson, J. S. Kendrick, R. F. Anda, and T. Byers, "Trends in Alcohol Consumption by Pregnant Women," *Journal of the American Medical Association* 265 (1991): 876–879.

25. G. B. Collins, "Contemporary Issues in the Treatment of Alcohol Dependence," *Psychiatric Clinics of North America* 16, no. 1 (1993): 33–48.

26. E. M. Jellinek, *The Disease Concept of Alcoholism* (New Haven: Hillhouse Press, 1960).

27. D. W. Goodwin, "Alcohol: Clinical Aspects," in J. H. Lowinson, P. Ruiz, R. B. Millman, and J. G. Langrod, eds., *Substance Abuse: A Comprehensive Textbook,* 2nd ed. (Baltimore: Williams & Wilkins, 1992), 650.

28. R. M. Morse and D. K. Flavin, "The Definition of Alcoholism," *Journal of the American Medical Association* 268 (1992): 1012–1014.

29. G. B. Cloninger, S. H. Dunwiddie, and T. Reich, "Epidemiology and Genetics of Alcoholism," *Annual Reviews of Psychiatry* 8 (1989): 331–346.

30. Council on Scientific Affairs, American Medical Association, "Alcoholism in the Elderly," *Journal of the American Medical Association* 275 (1996): 797–801.

31. U.S. Department of Health and Human Services, *Fifth Special Report to the U.S. Congress on Alcohol and Health* (Washington, D.C.: U.S. Government Printing Office, 1984).

32. G. E. Vaillant, "A Long-Term Follow-up of Male Alcohol Abuse," *Archives of General Psychiatry* 53 (1996): 243–249.

33. H. R. Kranzler and B. Orrok, "The Pharmacotherapy of Alcoholism," *Annual Reviews of Psychiatry* 8 (1989): 397–417.

34. O. Nutt, B. Adinoff, and M. Linniola, "Benzodiazepines in the Treatment of Alcoholism," *Recent Developments in Alcoholism* 7 (1989): 283–313.

35. R. Saitz, M. F. Mayo-Smith, M. S. Roberts, H. A. Redmond, D. R. Bernard, and D. R. Calkins, "Individualized Treatment for Alcohol Withdrawal: A Randomized Double-Blind Controlled Trial," *Journal of the American Medical Association* 272 (1994): 519–523.

36. P. K. Gessner, "Alcohols," in C. M. Smith and A. M. Reynard, *Textbook of Pharmacology* (Philadelphia: Saunders, 1992), 264.

37. P. J. McGrath, E. V. Nunes, J. W. Stewart, D. Goldman, V. Agosti, K. Ocepek-Welikson, and F. M. Quitkin, "Imipramine Treatment of Alcoholics with Primary Depression," *Archives of General Psychiatry* 53 (1996): 232–240.

38. B. J. Mason, J. H. Kocsis, E. C. Ritvo, and R. B. Cutler, "A Double-Blind, Placebo-Controlled Trial of Desipramine for Primary Alcohol Dependence Stratified on the Presence or Absence of Major Depression," *Journal of the American Medical Association* 275 (1996): 761–767.

39. D. A. Gorelick, "Serotonin Uptake Blockers and the Treatment of Alcoholism," *Recent Developments in Alcoholism* 7 (1989): 267–281.

40. C. A. Naranjo, K. E. Kadlee, P. Sanjueze, and D. Woodley-Remus, "Fluoxetine Differentially Alters Alcohol Intake and Other Consummatory Behaviors in Problem Drinkers," *Clinical Pharmacology and Therapeutics* 47 (1990): 490–498.

41. H. R. Kranzler, J. A. Burleson, et al., "Placebo-Controlled Trial of Fluoxetine as an Adjunct to Relapse Prevention in Alcoholics," *American Journal of Psychiatry* 152 (1995): 391–397.

42. E. V. Nunes, P. J. McGrath, and F. M. Quitkin, "Treating Anxiety in Patients with Alcoholism, " *Journal of Clinical Psychiatry* 56, suppl. 2 (1995): 3–9

43. R. Spanagel and W. Zieglgansberger, "Anti-Craving Compounds for Ethanol: New Pharmacological Tools to Study Addictive Processes," *Trends in Neurosciences* 18 (1997): 54–59.

44. J. R. Volpicelli, I. Alterman, M. Hayashida, and C. P. O'Brien, "Naltrexone in the Treatment of Alcohol Dependence," *Archives of General Psychiatry* 49 (1992): 876–880.

45. S. S. O'Malley, A. J. Jaffe, G. Chang, R. S. Schottenfeld, R. E. Meyer, and B. Rounsaville, "Naltrexone and Coping Skills Therapy for Alcohol Dependence," *Archives of General Psychiatry* 49 (1992): 881–887.

46. S. S. O'Malley, A. J. Jaffe, G. Chang, S. Rode, R. Schottenfeld, R. E. Meyer, and B. Rounsaville, "Six-Month Follow-up of Naltrexone and Psychotherapy for Alcohol Dependence," *Archives of General Psychiatry* 53 (1996): 217–224.

47. C. P. O'Brien, "What Are the Uses of Naltrexone in the Treatment of Alcoholism?," *The Harvard Mental Health Letter* 12 (December 1995): 8.

48. A. Whitworth, "Comparison of Acamprosate and Placebo in Long-term Treatment of Alcohol Dependence," *Lancet* 347 (1996): 1438–1442.

49. M. Shuckit, "Recent Developments in the Pharmacotherapy of Alcohol Dependence," *Journal of Consulting and Clinical Psychology* 64 (1996): 669–674.

50. P. K. Gessner, "Alcohols," in C. M. Smith and A. M. Reynard, *Textbook of Pharmacology* (Philadelphia: Saunders, 1992), 267–268.

51. B. S. McCrady and J. W. Langenbucher, "Alcohol Treatment and Health Care System Reform," *Archives of General Psychiatry* 53 (1996): 737–746.

52. C. W. Sharp, "Introduction to Inhalant Abuse," in C. W. Sharp, P. Beauvais, and R. Spence, eds., *Inhalant Abuse: A Volatile Research Agenda*, NIDA Research Monograph 129 (Rockville, Md.: U.S. Department of Health and Human Services, 1992), 1–10.

53. L. Yavich, N. Patkina, and E. Zvartau, "Experimental Estimation of Addictive Potential of a Mixture of Organic Solvents," *European Neuropsychopharmacology* 4 (1994): 111–118.

54. C. W. Sharp and N. L. Rosenberg, "Volatile Substances," in J. H. Lowinson, P. Ruiz, R. B. Millman, and J. G. Langrod, eds., *Substance Abuse: A Comprehensive Textbook*, 2nd ed. (Baltimore: Williams & Wilkins, 1992), 303–327.

55. L. A. Warner, R. C. Kessler, H. Hughes, J. C. Anthony, and C. B. Nelson, "Prevalence and Correlates of Drug Use and Dependence in the United States: Results from the National Comorbidity Survey," *Archives of General Psychiatry* 52 (1995): 219–229.

56. H. A. Miguez, M. C. Pecci, and A. Carrizosa, Jr., "Epidemiology of Alcohol and Drug Abuse in Paraguay," *Acta Psiquiatrica y Psicologica de America Latina* 38 (1992): 19–29.

57. L. Wilkins-Haug and P. A. Gabow, "Toluene Abuse During Pregnancy: Obstetric Complications and Perinatal Outcomes," *Obstetrics and Gynecology* 77 (1991): 504–509.

58. R. J. Mathew, W. H. Wilson, and S. R. Tant, "Regional Cerebral Blood Flow Changes Associated with Amyl Nitrite Inhalation," *British Journal of Addictions* 84 (1989): 293–299.

59. J. C. Garriott, "Death Among Inhalant Abusers," in C. W. Sharp, P. Beauvais, and R. Spence, eds., *Inhalant Abuse: A Volatile Research Agenda*, NIDA Research Monograph 129 (Rockville, Md.: U.S. Department of Health and Human Services, 1992), 181–191.

Chapter 4

DRUG TREATMENT OF ANXIETY DISORDERS: BENZODIAZEPINES AND "SECOND-GENERATION" ANXIOLYTICS

Anxiety can be described as apprehension, tension, or uneasiness related to anticipated danger. It may be a response to external stimuli, or it may be devoid of any apparent precipitating stimulus.[1] Anxiety is also a fundamental emotion, and it is a normal response to an experience that mimics a past experience that posed a significant problem.

Anxiety is a complex of subjective feelings of tension, fear, worry, helplessness, apprehension, and difficulties with thought, concentration, or sleep. The behavioral or physiological signs that accompany anxiety may include headaches, nausea, diarrhea, rapid heart rate, rapid breathing, tremors, muscle tension, restlessness, and fatigue. Certainly these feelings, behaviors, and physical signs are normal, appropriate, and necessary responses for survival in a hostile world (serving as the cognitive and emotional concomitant of a behavioral alarm system), but anxiety can be harmful when carried to extremes.

It is important to recognize the variety of anxiety disorders. The *Diagnostic and Statistical Manual of Mental Disorders*, 4th edition

(DSM-IV),[2] the most recent (1994) official guide to psychiatric disorders and their nomenclature, classifies the following forms of anxiety disorders:

1. Panic disorder (with or without agoraphobia)
2. Specific phobia
3. Social phobia
4. Obsessive-compulsive disorder (OCD)
5. Post-traumatic stress disorder (PTSD)
6. Acute stress disorder
7. Generalized anxiety disorder (GAD)
8. Anxiety disorder due to a general medical condition (for example, hyperthyroidism, Cushing's disease, coronary artery disease)
9. Substance-induced anxiety disorder (for example, from cocaine, caffeine, asthma medications, nasal decongestants, and withdrawal from alcohol or sedatives)
10. Anxiety disorder not otherwise specified

With the prevalence of anxiety disorders in our culture, it is not surprising that anxiolytic drugs are among the most frequently prescribed drugs in medicine. However, *anxiolytic* is a deceptive term for this category of agents. Although the medications discussed in this chapter are commonly known as anxiolytics, they are not the only medications used to treat anxiety disorders either in adults or in children. Indeed, in children, most anxiolytics are of limited use because of their detrimental effects on learning and memory.[3] Thus, while the anxiolytics discussed in this chapter are widely used, other classes of drugs are effective in certain of the DSM-IV classified disorders. They are briefly introduced here because their use is related to treatment in adults as well as in children and adolescents.

In adults,[4] obsessive-compulsive disorder (OCD) is most responsive to serotonin-selective reuptake inhibitors (SSRIs) and to clomipramine (both discussed in Chapter 7). Patients suffering from agoraphobia and panic disorders are best treated with the SSRIs, tricyclic antidepressants, or monoamine oxidase inhibitors (MAOI, see Chapter 7). Individuals suffering from post-traumatic stress syndrome (PTSD) may respond favorably to any of the various classes of antidepressants, to carbamazepine (see Chapter 2) or to lithium (see Chapter 8). Antipsychotic agents (see Chapter 9) may be utilized when delusions and/or hallucinations accompany the anxiety disorder. Thus, several of the above listed anxiety disorders rely heavily for their treatment on drugs not classified as anxiolytics.

In children and adolescents, antidepressants or behavioral stimulants are the long-term treatment of choice for most anxiety disorders, including attention deficit disorders.[3] Similarly, antipsychotics, adrenergic antagonists, and sedative antihistamines (such as diphenhydramine, or Benadryl) are often used for their sedative and anxiolytic effects. Bernstein (1994)[4] addresses the use of adrenergic antagonists, which block the functioning of our adrenergic (or adrenaline) nervous system, in treating anxiety disorders:

> An anxious patient will describe feeling nervous and uncomfortable with or without physiologic signs and symptoms. Most often, however, severe anxiety is accompanied by a variety of autonomic nervous system manifestations, including tachycardia, palpitations, irregular heart rhythm, dizziness, tremor, excessive sweating, dry mouth, diarrhea, abdominal pain, and headache. These physiologic manifestations may be present regardless of the specific type of anxiety disorder. Administration of sedating drugs such as the benzodiazepines, either intermittently or during a prolonged course of therapy, may alleviate symptoms of nervousness and dysphoria, but generally provide only minimal blunting of the physiologic manifestations of anxiety. Numerous clinical studies, however, indicate that beta-adrenergic blocking drugs, such as propranolol, metoprolol, and atenolol, may dramatically inhibit the physiologic manifestations of anxiety, when administered alone or in conjunction with modest doses of benzodiazepines. One major advantage of beta-adrenergic blocking drugs in the treatment of anxiety is their minimal risk of producing mental clouding and their absence of addiction potential.

Despite the use of alternative drugs (adrenergic blockers, antidepressants, antihistamines, antipsychotics, and so on) in the treatment of various anxiety disorders, the anxiolytic drugs discussed in this chapter are the most widely prescribed psychoactive agents in the world; more than 55 million prescriptions for their use are written yearly.

Benzodiazepines

Today, the term *anxiolytic* has become nearly synonymous with the *benzodiazepines*,[3] because these compounds are the drugs of choice for the short-term pharmacological treatment of stress-related anxiety and insomnia. This follows from their ease of use, relatively low toxicity, and tremendous effectiveness in relieving anxiety. The benzodiazepines effectively relieve the psychological distress and the dysphoria associated with anxiety. However, their adverse effects and their potential for producing dependency is generally conceded to limit their therapeutic use to relatively short periods of time, perhaps 1 to 6 weeks, and only for conditions where such short-term therapy is beneficial. Such conditions include acute situational grief, acute incapacitating stress reactions, and insomnia caused by anxiety over short-lived external events. In the DSM-IV list at the beginning of the chapter, these conditions would fall into the category of acute stress disorder.

Benzodiazepines are generally not utilized for chronic anxiety disorders or endogenous depression, in situations requiring fine motor or cognitive skills or mental alertness or situations where alcohol or other central nervous system (CNS) depressants will be used, and with the elderly, children or adolescents, or individuals prone to drug misuse. Despite these limitations, some feel that strong attitudes against the use of these drugs may be depriving many anxious patients of appropriate treatment.[5]

Mechanism of Action: The Benzodiazepine-GABA Receptor

Neuroanatomically, the *amygdala* has long been associated with the production of behavioral responses to fearful stimuli, because electrical stimulation of this structure evokes behavioral and physiological responses that are associated with fear and anxiety. Lesions of the amygdala result in an anxiolytic effect. PET scanning of the brain demonstrates increased amygdalar blood flow concomitant with anxiety responses; MRI scanning of the brain demonstrates amygdalar abnormalities in panic disorder patients. In rats, blockade of GABAergic function elicits anxiogenic-like effects, with both behavioral and physiologic alterations similar to symptoms of human anxiety states. Saunders, Morzarati, and Shekhar (1995) "primed" or "kindled" the amygdala of rats by chronically blocking $GABA_A$-receptor function (by injecting a $GABA_A$-receptor antagonist directly into the amygdala).[6] Results indicated that this increased activity of amygdalar function (with lowered GABAergic inhibition of function) produced anxiogenic responses as measured both in animal models of anxiety and by increases in heart rate and blood pressure. Thus, hypofunctional $GABA_A$-receptor activity may sensitize (or "prime") the amygdala to anxiogenic responses to what might otherwise be considered nondistressing stimuli. As stated by Saunders and coworkers (1995)[6]: "This could be one potential mechanism for developing pathological emotional responses, such as chronic, high levels of anxiety." As we will see, drugs that facilitate $GABA_A$-receptor function—such as the benzodiazepines—may reset the threshold of the amygdala to a more normal level of responsiveness.

In Chapter 2 we introduced the $GABA_A$ receptor as a site of barbiturate action. It is now clear that most, if not all, of the actions of the benzodiazepines (as sedatives, hypnotics, anxiolytics, muscle relaxants, amnestics, and anticonvulsants) are mediated through binding to a specific site on $GABA_A$ receptors; this binding facilitates the binding of the neurotransmitter GABA.[7] GABA, in turn, depresses neuronal excitability by selectively increasing the transmembrane conductance of chloride ions; that is, GABA opens chloride channels in the nerve membrane of $GABA_A$ receptors, allowing an influx of chloride ions into the postsynaptic cell and hyperpolarizing the cell membrane, which decreases cellular activity and responsiveness (see Figure 4.1).

To complicate matters, there may be five or more types of GABA receptors; $GABA_A$ and $GABA_B$ receptors are the most studied. Kerr and Ong (1995)[8] and Johnston (1996),[9] respectively, review the physiology and pharmacology of $GABA_B$ and $GABA_C$ receptors. Hobbs, Rall, and Verdoorn (1996)[10] elaborate in detail the molecular biology of the interaction between benzodiazepines and $GABA_A$ receptor function.

A recently introduced benzodiazepine antagonist (flumazenil) exerts antagonistic action by competitively occupying the benzodiazepine binding site on the $GABA_A$ receptor. Through this action, it competes with the benzodiazepine for its binding site, displacing the benzodiazepine from its receptors (see Figure 4.1). Flumazenil is discussed later in this chapter.

Pharmacokinetics

Fifteen benzodiazepine derivatives are currently available in the United States (see Table 4.1) and still more are available in other countries. These agents are marketed as sedatives, anxiolytics, muscle relaxants, intravenous anesthetics, and anticonvulsants. They differ from each other mainly in their pharmacokinetic parameters, which include rates of metabolism to pharmacologically active intermediates and plasma half-lives of both the parent drug and any active metabolites. Of the benzodiazepines commercially available in the United States, 14 are available in a dosage form for oral ingestion, 2 (diazepam and lorazepam) are also available for parenteral use, and 1 (midazolam) is available only in parenteral formulation.

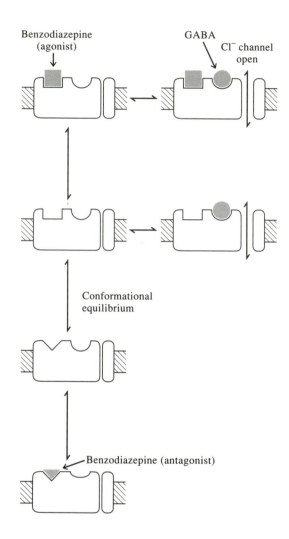

Figure 4.1 Benzodiazepine-GABA receptor interaction. Benzodiazepine agonists (e.g., diazepam) and antagonists (e.g., flumazenil) are believed to bind to a site on the GABA receptor that is distinct from the GABA binding site. A conformational equilibrium exists between states in which the benzodiazepine receptor exists in its *agonist binding* conformation (*top*) and in its *antagonist binding* conformation (*bottom*). In the latter state, the GABA receptor has a much reduced affinity for GABA, so the chloride channel remains closed. [Modified from H. P. Rang and M. M. Dale (1991),[11] figure 25.6.]

The basic structure of the benzodiazepines is shown in Figure 4.2, with a list of currently available derivatives. Note that all these drugs share the same basic structure, differing only in their substituent groups.

TABLE 4.1 Benzodiazepines

Drug name		Dosage form		Active metab-olite	Active compounds in blood	Mean elimination half-life in hours (range)
Trade	Generic	Oral	Parent-eral			
LONG-ACTING AGENTS						
Valium	Diazepam	X	X	Yes	Diazepam	24 (20–50)
					Nordiazepam	60 (50–100)
Librium	Chlordiazepoxide	X		Yes	Chlordiaze-poxide	10 (8–24)
					Nordiazepam	60 (50–100)
Dalmane	Flurazepam	X		Yes	Desalkylflura-zepam	80 (70–160)
Paxipam	Halazepam	X		Yes	Halazepam	14 (10–20)
					Nordiazepam	60 (50–100)
Centrax	Prazepam	X		Yes	Nordiazepam	60 (50–100)
Tranxene	Chlorazepate	X		Yes	Nordiazepam	60 (50–100)
INTERMEDIATE-ACTING AGENTS						
Ativan	Lorazepam	X	X	No	Lorazepam	15 (10–24)
Klonopin	Clonazepam	X		No	Clonazepam	30 (18–50)
Dormalin	Quazepam	X		Yes	Quazepam	35 (25–50)
					Desalkylflura-zepam	80 (70–160)
ProSom	Estazolam	X		Yes	Hydroxyesta-zolam	18 (13–35)
SHORT-ACTING AGENTS						
Versed	Midazolam		X	No	Midazolam	2.5 (1.5–4.5)
Serax	Oxazepam	X		No	Oxazepam	8 (5–15)
Restoril	Temazepam	X		No	Temazepam	12 (8–35)
Halcion	Triazolam	X		No	Triazolam	2.5 (1.5–5)
Xanax	Alprazolam	X		No	Alprazolam	12 (11–18)

Absorption and Distribution

Benzodiazepines are well absorbed when they are taken orally; peak plasma concentrations are achieved in about one hour. Some (e.g., ox-azepam and lorazepam) are absorbed more slowly, while others (e.g., triazolam) are absorbed more rapidly. Clorazepate is metabolized in gastric juice to an active metabolite (nordiazepam) which is com-pletely absorbed.[10]

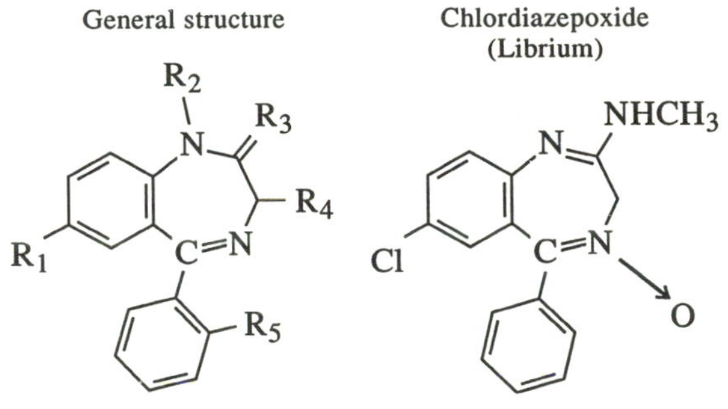

Drug	R_1	R_2	R_3	R_4	R_5
Diazepam	Cl	CH_3	$=O$	H_2	H
Nitrazepam	NO_2	H	$=O$	H_2	H
Flurazepam	Cl	$(CH_2)_2N(C_2H_5)_2$	$=O$	H_2	H
Flunitrazepam	NO_2	H	$=O$	H_2	F
Oxazepam	Cl	H	$=O$	OH	H
Temazepam	Cl	CH_3	$=O$	H_2	H
Clonazepam	NO_2	H	$=O$	H_2	Cl
Lorazepam	Cl	H	$=O$	OH	Cl
Clorazepate	Cl	H	$=O$	COOH	H
Nordiazepam	Cl	H	$=O$	H_2	H

Figure 4.2 Structures of some benzodiazepines.

Metabolism and Excretion

Usually, psychoactive drugs are metabolized to pharmacologically in-active, water-soluble products, which are then excreted in urine (see Chapter 1). While this holds true for some benzodiazepines, several of them are first biotransformed to intermediate products that are phar-macologically active; these, in turn, must be detoxified by further me-tabolism before they can be excreted (see Figure 4.3). As can be seen from Table 4.1 and Figure 4.3, several long-acting compounds are bio-transformed into long-lasting pharmacologically active metabolites, primarily nordiazepam, the half-life of which is about 60 hours. Figure 4.4 demonstrates the buildup and slow metabolism of active metabolite in a human volunteer who was given diazepam (Valium) daily for 14 days. Thus, the long-acting benzodiazepines are so because much of their anxiolytic activity is provided not by the parent (original) drug but by its pharmacologically active, long-half-life metabolite. In con-trast, the short-acting benzodiazepines are short-acting because they

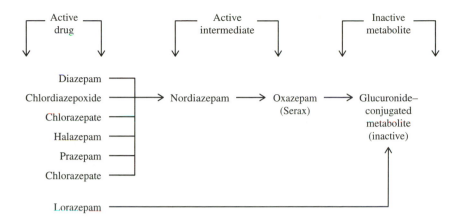

Figure 4.3 Metabolism of benzodiazepines. The intermediate metabolite nordiazepam is formed from many agents. Oxazepam (Serax) is commercially available and is also an active intermediate in the metabolism of nordiazepam to its inactive products.

are metabolized directly into inactive products. As Hobbs, Rall, and Verdoorn (1996)[10] state:

> Because active metabolites are generated that are biotransformed more slowly than the parent compound, the duration of action of many benzodiazepines bears little relationship to the half-time of elimination of the drug that has been [originally] administered. . . . Conversely, the rate of biotransformation of those agents that are inactivated by the initial reaction is an important determinant of their duration of action; these agents include oxazepam, lorazepam, temazepam, triazolam, and midazolam.

The elderly have a reduced ability to metabolize long-acting benzodiazepines and their active metabolites. In this population, the elimination half-life (for both the parent drug and the active metabolite) is often 7 to 10 days. Since it takes about six half-lives to rid the body completely of a drug (see Chapter 1), it may take an elderly patient one month or longer to become completely drug-free after even a single dose of diazepam. Because these drugs can induce a "brain syndrome," elderly patients can become profoundly and persistently drug-demented as a result. In general, no long-acting benzodiazepine should be administered to an elderly patient. As Rang and Dale (1991)[11] state:

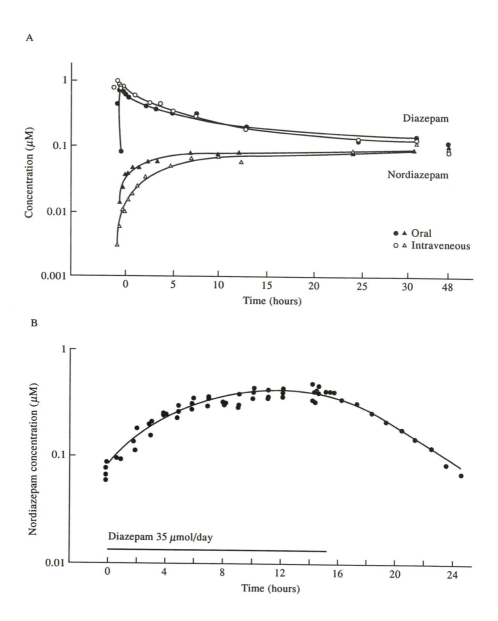

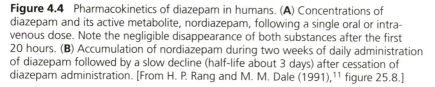

Figure 4.4 Pharmacokinetics of diazepam in humans. (**A**) Concentrations of diazepam and its active metabolite, nordiazepam, following a single oral or intravenous dose. Note the negligible disappearance of both substances after the first 20 hours. (**B**) Accumulation of nordiazepam during two weeks of daily administration of diazepam followed by a slow decline (half-life about 3 days) after cessation of diazepam administration. [From H. P. Rang and M. M. Dale (1991),[11] figure 25.8.]

> At the age of 91, the grandmother of one of the authors was growing increasingly forgetful and mildly dotty, having been taking nitrazepam for insomnia regularly for years. To the author's lasting shame, it took a canny general practitioner to diagnose the problem. Cancellation of the nitrazepam prescription produced a dramatic improvement.

My own 85-year-old grandmother experienced the identical problem with diazepam. Two months after discontinuation of the drug, her dementia disappeared and she remained lucid until her death 10 years later.

Because of the long elimination times, a person who has been using one of these drugs for prolonged periods may maintain detectable urinary concentrations of the drug for many days to several weeks after discontinuing its use.

Pharmacological Effects

The clinical and behavioral effects of the benzodiazepines all occur as a result of facilitation of GABA-induced neuronal inhibition at the various locations of GABA$_A$ receptors throughout the CNS. Indeed, all benzodiazepines that exert actions similar to those exerted by diazepam are termed *complete agonists* because they faithfully facilitate GABA binding as a result of their attachment to the benzodiazepine binding site on the GABA$_A$ receptor. Low doses of complete-agonist benzodiazepines alleviate anxiety, agitation, and fear by their actions on receptors located in the amygdala. The mental confusion and amnesia follow action on GABA neurons located in the cerebral cortex and the hippocampus. The mild muscle-relaxant effects of the benzodiazepines are probably caused both by their anxiolytic actions and by effects on GABA receptors located in the spinal cord, cerebellum, and brain stem. The antiepileptic actions seem to follow from actions on GABA receptors located in the cerebellum and the hippocampus. The behavioral rewarding effects and thus the abuse potential and psychological dependency probably result from actions on GABA receptors that modulate the discharge of neurons located in the ventral tegmentum and the nucleus accumbens (see Figure 3.5).

Given a number of subgroups of GABA$_A$ receptors, we may eventually find benzodiazepine derivatives that bind to various substituents of different types of GABA$_A$ receptors, perhaps with less than complete agonist action. Such drugs would be called *partial agonists*, and, hopefully, some might have specificity of action (e.g., anxiolysis without sedation). For example, the drug *zolpidem* (Ambien) was marketed in the mid-1990s. This drug, discussed later in this chapter, is structurally not a benzodiazepine, but it binds to a subclassification of $GABA_A$ receptors (the $GABA_{A-1}$ receptor) and exhibits primarily a hypnotic effect rather than an anxiolytic one.

Uses

The major indication for benzodiazepine therapy is to treat anxiety that is so debilitating that the patient's lifestyle, work, and interpersonal relationships are severely hampered. As already stated, administration of benzodiazepines, either intermittently or during a prolonged regular course of therapy, may alleviate the symptoms of nervousness, dysphoria, and psychological distress without necessarily blocking the physiological correlates accompanying the state of anxiety. Usually, resolution of the psychological distress is accompanied by amelioration of the physiological symptoms. Since benzodiazepines are not specific anxiolytics, they possess many of the characteristics of the barbiturates. Thus, they are effectively used as hypnotics for the treatment of insomnia. Here, agents with rapid onset, a 2- to 3-hour half-life, and no active metabolites (which persist in the body into the next day) may be preferred in order to minimize daytime sedation. However, when daytime sedation or next-day anxiolysis is desired, the long-acting drugs with active metabolites might be preferred.

Because increased GABA activity inhibits neuronal function, the benzodiazepines have been used as "muscle relaxants," both to directly reduce states associated with increased muscle tension and to reduce the psychological distress that can predispose to muscle tension.

Benzodiazepines are among the best agents available to produce antegrade amnesia (amnesia that starts at the time of drug administration and ends at the time when the blood level of drug decreases to a point where memory function is regained). For this use, either of two injectable benzodiazepines is perhaps most reliable—lorazepam, when long-lasting amnesia is desirable, and midazolam, when shorter periods of amnesia are desirable. Examples of situations where amnesia might be a therapeutic goal include during surgical procedures or preanesthetic medication before surgery. Occasionally, the amnestic effect may be undesirable. For example, recently much concern has been expressed about an illegally imported "date-rape" drug, which is actually a benzodiazepine that is commercially marketed outside the United States. This drug, *flunitrazepam* (Rohypnol, or "roofies," "rochas"), is pharmacologically similar to triazolam (Halcion; Table 4.1), producing anxiolysis, sedation, and amnesia, especially when taken with alcohol. When so ingested by an unknowing victim, the effect closely resembles the "Mickey Finn" discussed in Chapter 2.

Panic attacks and phobias can be treated with benzodiazepines, such as alprazolam.[12] Here, however, the efficacy of benzodiazepines may be less than that of the antidepressants, such as imipramine. Davidson (1997)[13] reviewed the use of benzodiazepines, noting their advantages of rapid onset, anxiolysis, low-level side effects, and good patient acceptance. Disadvantages noted include impaired psychomotor performance and alertness and the potential for dependence and abuse. Treatment efficacy is therefore not without some controversy.

Because benzodiazepines can substitute for alcohol, they are used both in treating acute alcohol withdrawal and in long-term therapy to reduce the rate of relapse to previous drinking habits.[14]

All benzodiazepines exert antiepileptic actions because they raise the threshold for generating seizures. In general, however, benzodiazepines are used as secondary drugs or as adjuvants to other, more specific anticonvulsants (see Chapter 2).

Side Effects and Toxicity

Common acute side effects associated with benzodiazepine therapy are usually dose-related extensions of the intended actions. These include sedation, drowsiness, ataxia, lethargy, mental confusion, motor and cognitive impairments, disorientation, slurred speech, amnesia, and induction or extension of the symptoms of dementia. At higher doses, impairments continue and become dominated by continuing mental and psychomotor dysfunction progressing to hypnosis.

Respiration is not seriously depressed, even at high doses. Indeed, attempted suicides by overdose are rarely successful unless the benzodiazepine is taken along with another CNS depressant, such as alcohol. This combination can cause a most serious (and potentially fatal) drug interaction. Sleep patterns can be altered markedly. When short-acting agents are taken at bedtime, both early-morning wakening and rebound insomnia for the next night are common. When long-acting agents (or agents with active metabolites) are taken at bedtime, daytime sedation can be a problem. Impairment of motor abilities—especially a person's ability to drive an automobile—is common. This impairment is compounded by the drug-induced suppression of one's ability to assess his or her own level of physical and mental impairment.

The cognitive deficits associated with benzodiazepine use are significant. We stated that, as $GABA_A$ agonists, these drugs are exceedingly effective amnestic agents—a desirable effect when used in anesthesia but a potentially serious side effect when the retention of mental capacity is important. In both children and adults, benzodiazepines can significantly interfere with learning behaviors.

Side effects associated with long-term, chronic use of benzodiazepines include the dementing effects of the drugs, especially in the elderly. In this population, memory and cognition can be severely affected to the point where an elderly individual taking a benzodiazepine can appear demented. Because of the long half-lives of the drugs and their metabolites, a prolonged period of drug abstinence is required in order to determine accurately an individual's normal mental capacity.

Tolerance and Dependence

Although benzodiazepines have a reputation for causing only a low incidence of abuse and dependence, the possibility of this adverse complication of chronic use must not be overlooked.[10] When benzodiazepines are taken for prolonged periods of time, a pattern of dependence can develop, even following only therapeutic dosages.[15,16] Early withdrawal signs include a return (and possible intensification) of the anxiety state for which the drug was originally given.[17] Rebound increases in insomnia, restlessness, agitation, irritability, and unpleasant dreams gradually appear. In rare instances, hallucinations, psychoses, and seizures have been reported. Most of these withdrawal symptoms subside within one to four weeks.

Regarding compulsive abuse of the benzodiazepines, Hobbs, Rall, and Verdoon (1996) state:[10]

> Patients who have histories of drug or alcohol abuse are most apt to use these agents inappropriately, and abuse of benzodiazepines usually occurs as part of a pattern of abuse of multiple drugs. In such individuals, benzodiazepines seldom are preferred to barbiturates or even alcohol, but they often are combined with those drugs to either accentuate their effect (e.g., alcohol and opiates) or reduce their toxicity (e.g., cocaine).

Thus, benzodiazepines rarely are primary drugs of abuse—people rarely use them alone to produce intoxication.[18] As part of a multidrug pattern, benzodiazepines (especially diazepam and alprazolam) may be taken for a euphoriant effect or to enhance the euphoriant effect of narcotics.[18] In patients who take methadone as part of treatment protocols for opioid dependency (see Chapter 10), benzodiazepines can reduce the anxiety that is often present. Many alcohol and cocaine abusers take benzodiazepines, presumably for their reinforcing and anxiolytic properties and to self-medicate symptoms of cocaine toxicity.

Tolerance to benzodiazepines can develop, which can necessitate small increases in dose. This tolerance, however, is not as marked as that which occurs following long-term use of the barbiturates.

Benzodiazepines administered during the first trimester of pregnancy have been reported to cause fetal abnormalities. Other data dispute this relationship.[19] It does appear, however, that a fetus can develop benzodiazepine dependence, and withdrawal may occur in the newborn. As with all psychoactive drugs, unless it is absolutely necessary, benzodiazepines should be avoided during pregnancy.

Flumazenil: A GABA$_A$ Antagonist

Flumazenil (Romazicon) is a benzodiazepine derivative that binds with high affinity to benzodiazepine receptors on the GABA$_A$ complex (see Figure 4.1), but, after binding, it exhibits no intrinsic activity. As a consequence, flumazenil competitively blocks the access of pharmacologically active benzodiazepines to the receptor, effectively reversing the antianxiety and sedative effects of any benzodiazepines administered before flumazenil.

Flumazenil is metabolized quite rapidly in the liver and has a short half-life (about 50 to 70 minutes). Because this half-life is much shorter than that of most benzodiazepines, the benzodiazepine effects can reappear as flumazenil is lost, thus necessitating reinjection. Flumazenil is utilized as an antidote whenever benzodiazepine ingestion is suspected. There is also indication that flumazenil may be useful in the differential diagnosis of some cognitive disorders and in the diagnosis of panic disorder.[20]

"SECOND-GENERATION" ANXIOLYTICS

Zolpidem

Zolpidem (Ambien) is a nonbenzodiazepine that was first marketed in 1993 for the short-term treatment of insomnia.[21] Although chemically unrelated to the benzodiazepines, it binds to a specific subtype (type 1) of the GABA$_A$ receptor,[22] and it displays some, but not all, of the actions of all other benzodiazepine agonists. Thus, it might be classified pharmacologically as an incomplete or "partial" agonist of benzodiazepine receptors. Zolpidem possesses relatively strong sedative actions, which tend to overwhelm any anxiolytic effects. Thus, the drug is marketed for use as a sedative-hypnotic agent rather than as an anxiolytic.

Before initiating discussion of zolpidem as a hypnotic agent, it might be pertinent to review the role of drugs in sleep disorders.[23,24] Insomnia, the experience of poor quality or quantity of sleep, is quite common. Approximately 65 million adults (36 percent of the population) in the United States complain of poor sleep. Of this group, 25 percent have insomnia on a chronic basis. Chronic insomniacs have difficulty with concentration, memory, and the ability to cope with minor problems. They have a 2.5 times greater risk of fatigue-related automobile accidents. Despite its ubiquity, insomnia is often inadequately treated. Short-acting benzodiazepines are advocated for transient insomnia of three weeks or shorter duration and for patients with chronic insomnia where nondrug therapies are insufficient. The putative adverse effects of benzodiazepines must be weighed against the severe health problems caused by continued sleep impairment. Short-term or intermittent use is advocated. Benzodiazepines, antidepressants, and zolpidem are effective pharmacologic agents.[24] Studies demonstrate that the adverse effects of short-acting benzodiazepines (amnesia and daytime sedation or "hangover") differ little among agents or between those drugs and zolpidem. These drugs should not be thought of as the sole treatment for insomnia and should be used in conjunction with nondrug techniques, such as biofeedback therapy, stimulus control, sleep restriction, and good sleep hygiene.[24]

Pharmacokinetics

Zolpidem is rapidly and completely absorbed from the gastrointestinal tract after oral administration. Peak plasma levels are reached in about one hour. Following metabolism in the liver, the end products are excreted by the kidneys. The metabolic half-life is about two hours[25] (longer in the elderly) with no active metabolites. Because of this short half-life, the drug is usually compared to triazolam (Halcion).[26]

Pharmacodynamics

At doses of 5 to 10 milligrams, zolpidem produces sedation and promotes a physiological pattern of sleep in the absence of anxiolytic, anticonvulsant, or muscle-relaxant effects. It is claimed that at these doses memory is less affected than after comparable doses of triazolam, even in the elderly.[27] Wesensten and coworkers (1995)[28] reported that flumazenil would effectively reverse any memory impairments induced by zolpidem (as well as those produced by triazolam). Of additional interest in this report was that flumazenil tended to improve learning and memory function above levels seen with a placebo, denoting a possible role of some sort of "endogenous benzodiazepines" in limiting memory function. It is interesting conjecture that flumazenil might have acted as a "cognitive enhancer," a term sometimes applied to inhibitors of GABA function.[29,30]

Adverse Effects

Dose-related adverse effects include drowsiness, dizziness, and nausea. In the elderly taking 20 milligrams or more, confusion, falls, memory loss, and psychotic reactions have been reported. A high-dose incidence of nausea and vomiting may tend to limit overdosage, such as in suicide attempts. Overdoses to 400 milligrams (20 times the high-dose therapeutic amount) have not been fatal.

In conclusion, zolpidem is an effective nonbenzodiazepine hypnotic that binds to benzodiazepine receptors in the brain. Its minimal effect on the stages of sleep is a claimed advantage over benzodiazepine hypnotics. Zolpidem probably results in similar levels of daytime sedation and cognitive impairment as would triazolam, one of the shortest half-life benzodiazepines.[31] The potential for the drug to induce tolerance or be abused remains to be determined.

Buspirone

Buspirone (BuSpar) is an anxiolytic drug that differs from the benzodiazepines both structurally and pharmacologically. It is not only an effective therapy for certain anxious patients but also a useful tool for investigating the neurochemistry of anxiety. Buspirone relieves anxiety in a unique fashion:

- Its anxiolysis occurs without significant sedation, drowsiness, or hypnotic action, even in overdosage.

- Amnesia, mental confusion, and psychomotor impairment are minimal or absent.

- It does not potentiate the CNS depressant effects of alcohol, benzodiazepines, or other CNS sedatives (i.e., synergism does not occur).

- It does not substitute for benzodiazepines in treating anxiety or benzodiazepine withdrawal.

- It does not exhibit cross tolerance or cross dependence with benzodiazepines.

- It exhibits little potential for addiction or abuse.

- It exhibits an antidepressant effect in addition to its anxiolytic effect, making it potentially useful in depressive disorders with accompanying anxiety.

- Its effect has a gradual onset rather than the immediate onset of the action of the benzodiazepines.

- It is ineffective as a hypnotic to promote the onset of sleep.

Mechanism of Action

To this point, we have correlated anxiolytic action with drug binding to $GABA_A$ receptors. Buspirone is unique as an anxiolytic in that it selectively binds to a subgroup of serotonin (5-hydroxytryptamine, or 5-HT) receptors. Because this subclass is called the 1-A group, the receptors are called 5-HT_{1A}. After binding, buspirone exerts a weak stimulant action; the drug is therefore termed a *weak agonist* of 5-HT_{1A} receptors. As a result, it exerts an anxiolytic action (and possibly an antidepressant action as well; this role of 5-HT_{1A} receptors in depression is discussed in Chapter 7). Electrical lesions of these seritonergic neurons are accompanied by a loss of anxiolytic action.[32] Furthermore, this selective receptor binding is confined to areas of the brain thought to be involved in mechanisms of anxiety, especially the hippocampus.[33,34]

Clinical Uses

Buspirone is considered an effective drug for the treatment of generalized anxiety disorder (addressed later as a special topic). It has also been recommended for many patients of all ages who suffer from mixed symptoms of anxiety and depression, as well as in elderly individuals with agitated dementia.[35] Buspirone is most helpful in anxious patients who do not demand immediate gratification or the immediate response they associate with the benzodiazepine response. Slower and more gradual onset of anxiety relief is balanced by the increased safety and lack of dependency-producing aspects of buspirone.

To see clinical effects takes several weeks of continuous, three-times-per-day treatment. Patients who have previously been taking benzodiazepines do poorly on buspirone. This has led to an impression in some clinicians that buspirone, despite lower toxicity, may possess lower clinical efficacy. Harvey and Balon (1995)[36] summarize the efficacy of buspirone in several psychological disorders, including depression, panic disorder, obsessive-compulsive disorder, schizophrenia, and anxiety. They conclude that the major usefulness of buspirone in treating these disorders may be for the augmentation of the beneficial effects of other psychotropic medications. Preliminary results of a study in children[37] indicate that buspirone may reduce irritability, aggression, and temper outbursts in children with developmental disorders and may significantly potentiate the effects of behavioral stimulants in children and adolescents with comorbid attention deficit and oppositional defiant disorders. Similarly,[38] buspirone has enhanced the effects of cognitive behavioral therapy on individuals with panic disorder with agoraphobia; the panic attacks were largely unaffected by the drug alone.

ANXIOLYTICS: SPECIAL TOPICS

Use of Anxiolytics in Individuals at the Extremes of Age

As discussed earlier, anxiolytics are rarely indicated for use in *children and adolescents* because of their adverse effects on learning and memory (inhibiting cognitive functioning), on behavior (producing paradoxical excitement, perhaps intensifying anxiety), and on considerations relevant to dependence and compulsive abuse. Albano and Chorpita (1995)[39] reviewed the pharmacologic and nonpharmacologic treatment of anxiety disorders of childhood. The prevalence of such disorders in children and adolescents ranges from 1.1 percent for social phobias to about 13 percent for separation anxiety disorder. The primary agents of drug therapy utilized are any of the various classes of antidepressants (see Chapter 7). However, for treatment of social phobias and avoidance disorders, the benzodiazepine *alprazolam* (Xanax) has been reported to be useful.[40]

In the treatment of *obsessive-compulsive disorder (OCD)* in children, again the antidepressants produce moderate to marked improvement in up to 75 percent of children diagnosed with the disorder.[41,42] Drug effectiveness in *post-traumatic stress syndrome (PTSS)* in children has not been adequately studied to summarize effectiveness. *Panic disorder* has also been poorly studied; however, antidepressants and possibly high-potency benzodiazepines may be useful.[39] In all these instances, a benzodiazepine is not used without knowledge of the potential adverse effects and remains at the discretion of the prescriber.

Sheikh and Saltzman (1995),[43] Jeneke (1996),[44] and Folks and Fuller (1997)[35] review the pharmacologic treatment of anxiety disorders in the *elderly*. In this population, anxiety disorders are common, and their origins can often be traced back to early adulthood. Virtually all of the various anxiolytics have been used. As a general rule:

> Numerous compounds belonging to several different classes have been used as anxiolytic agents during the past few decades. These classes include the benzodiazepines, antihistamines, antidepressants, neuroleptic agents, beta blockers, and azapirones (buspirone). When prescribing any medication for the elderly, one needs to consider age-related physiologic changes in absorption, distribution, protein binding, metabolism, and excretion of drugs. These changes can alter significantly plasma levels of drugs, lead to excessive accumulation of medications in various body tissues, and make elderly patients particularly prone to experiencing toxic effects, even at doses that are average for the general population. Hence the adage, "Start low and go slow."[43]

Catterson, Preskorn, and Martin[45] add a third admonition: "Keep it [the drug regime] as simple as possible."

In general, for most of the anxiety disorders, psychological interventions (e.g., cognitive behavioral therapy) are probably to be preferred over pharmacologic intervention. However, anxiolytics can be useful. For example, in the treatment of panic disorder in the elderly, high-potency benzodiazepines (e.g., alprazolam and clonazepam) are effective for symptom control, although adrenergic blockers may likewise alleviate symptoms with the disadvantages of CNS depression.

Generalized anxiety disorder (GAD) in the elderly presents special problems; some reliable estimates project the one-year prevalence to be as high as 7.1 percent.[43] GAD often exists as a comorbid disorder with depression.[46] Benzodiazepines have traditionally been prescribed for people with this combination, but utilization should be restricted to drugs without active intermediates, because their half-lives are not unduly prolonged in the elderly. Constant vigilance for signs and symptoms of drug-induced impairment is necessary. As Sheikh and Salzman (1995)[43] state:

> The four primary areas of impairment associated with benzodiazepine toxicity in the elderly are decreased arousal, cerebellar toxicity (increasing the risks of falls), reduced psychomotor speed and accuracy, and impaired attention and short-term recall. Additional areas of concern in the elderly are medical comorbidity, polypharmacy, and noncompliance as a result of forgetfulness and confusion, regarding various medication schedules.

Buspirone has less detrimental effects in the elderly, but therapeutic response is somewhat inconsistent.[43] When pharmacologic intervention is necessary in the elderly for the treatment of PTSD, OCD, and phobias, antidepressants are generally the drugs of first choice.

Regarding the extent of use of benzodiazepines in the elderly, Zisselman, Rovner, and Shmuely (1996)[47] studied 131 consecutively admitted elderly patients to an inpatient psychiatry unit. Fifty-nine of these patients were taking prescribed benzodiazepines; in 38 of the 59, use was outside generally approved guidelines, and 30 of 76 patients diagnosed with depression disorders had received benzodiazepines as sole treatment of depression prior to their admission. Obviously, their depressive disorder had been pharmacologically mismanaged.

Long-Term Use of Anxiolytics

The wide use of benzodiazepines attests to their clinical efficacy and overall safety. We have already alluded to the attentional, psychomotor, cognitive, and memory impairments that can accompany the acute (short-term) use of these drugs. We have not addressed, however, the risks of their long-term use.[48,49]

First, it appears that therapy with stable (nonincreasing) doses for more than eight weeks results in the development of tolerance to most of the adverse effects of the benzodiazepines, although it is unclear whether persistent intellectual and psychomotor deficits might impair one's ability to execute complex "real-world" tasks.[48] And, of course, untreated anxiety may impair a person to as great or greater an extent than might long-term benzodiazepine therapy.[49] Thus, even with slight drug-induced impairments, there might be a net gain in ability to function.

Certainly, benzodiazepines have a potential for recreational abuse, although the degree or extent of drug craving is much lower than that for most other drugs of abuse.[50] Indeed, actual abuse seems to occur primarily in abusers of other drugs, to ameliorate anxiety associated with either stimulants or narcotics. Physical dependence, with a resulting withdrawal syndrome, can occur following abrupt withdrawal from a benzodiazepine.[13] However, the signs and symptoms of withdrawal (nervousness, insomnia, restlessness, and so on) are confused by the probable return of the anxiety symptoms for which the drug was originally prescribed. Withdrawal signs can, therefore, be lessened by combining withdrawal with psychological therapies (for treatment of the underlying disorder) and by gradual tapering of dose. Severe withdrawal anxiety may indicate a need for continuation of drug therapy until such time as interventional therapies can be instituted, the necessity for continued long-term drug therapy excluded, and alternative methods of withdrawal assessed.

Future Directions in the Pharmacology of Anxiety

As Kunovac and Stahl (1995)[51] state:

> The benzodiazepines possess a number of properties that limit their use as ideal anxiolytic agents. Not only can they be sedating, induce memory impairment, and increase the intoxicating potency of alcohol, but they may be subject to abuse and possess dependence potential after long-term use.

Thus, the search continues for new anxiolytics without these undesirable properties. To achieve this goal, several research approaches continue and some are likely to be successful within the not-too-distant future.

The first involves identifying partial agonists at the benzodi-azepine binding site on the $GABA_A$ receptor. Remembering that benzo-diazepines are full (complete) agonists and that flumazenil is a full (complete) antagonist at this site, a partial (incomplete) agonist would have some of the desirable properties of the classic benzodiazepines, perhaps with fewer of the undesired effects. Partial agonists are cur-rently under intense investigation.

The second approach is to identify possibly superior drugs that act by affecting different subtypes of the $GABA_A$ receptor. Zolpidem (dis-cussed earlier) is one example: its sedative property appears to follow from action upon the $GABA_{A-1}$ receptor subtype. A similar drug, avail-able in Europe and marketed under the name *alpidem*, is a partial ago-nist at both $GABA_{A-1}$ and $GABA_{A-3}$ receptors, is more anxiolytic, with little sedation, tolerance, or physical dependence, and did not interact with ethanol.[52–54] Unfortunately, some recent reports of drug-induced hepatitis may temper the enthusiasm for this drug. Costa and Guidotti[55] discuss other experimental GABAergic anxiolytics, including imidazenil, a new-generation anxiolytic that "has minimal disruptive effects on learning and memory and is virtually devoid of the tolerance liability and other unwanted side effects of classic benzodiazepines."

Third, as discussed in Chapter 2, certain neuroactive (nonhor-monal) neurosteroids act at $GABA_A$ receptors as agonists.[56] As a result, when administered to rats, these drugs (termed *epalons*) display anxi-olytic and hypnotic activities. They also regulate gene expression at the receptor. As Rupprecht et al. (1996)[57] state:

> These findings extend the concept of a "cross-talk" between mem-brane and nuclear hormone effects and provide a new role for the therapeutic application of these steroids in neurology and psychiatry.

Fourth, *abecarnil* is a new drug (of a class of drugs called *beta-carbo-lines*) effective in the treatment of GAD. Mechanistically, abecarnil binds to benzodiazepine receptors but is a partial agonist at other binding sites. Preliminary studies indicate that the drug possesses anx-iolytic activity comparable to that exerted by alprazolam and that it may have less potential for developing tolerance or dependence and less potential for compulsive abuse.[58]

Fifth, *bretazenil* is a derivative of the benzodiazepine antagonist flumazenil.[51] Bretazenil is classified as a *weak (partial) agonist* at ben-zodiazepine receptors; it exhibits anxiolytic and antiepileptic activity with lower abuse potential than full agonist benzodiazepines.[59] Future studies with this agent may be interesting.

Last, several lines of investigation are leading toward serotonin receptors as a target for anxiolytic drug development. This follows from the successful development of buspirone (discussed earlier). The subclass of serotonin receptors that is of most interest is the 5-HT$_{1A}$ receptor. Kunovac and Stahl (1995)[51] review these studies in detail, as well as other, more novel, approaches to anxiolytic drug development. Chapter 7 discusses the role of the 5-HT$_{1A}$ receptor in antidepressant and anxiolytic action of *nefazodone* (Serzone), a new antidepressant compound.

NOTES

1. American Medical Association, "Drugs Used for Anxiety and Sleep Disorders," in *Drug Evaluations Annual 1994* (Milwaukee, Wis.: American Medical Association, 1993), 219.

2. American Psychological Association, *Diagnostic and Statistical Manual of Mental Disorders*, 4th ed. (DSM-IV) (Washington, D.C.: American Psychological Association, 1994), 393–394.

3. D. R. Rosenberg, J. Holttum, and S. Gershon, *Textbook of Pharmacotherapy for Child and Adolescent Psychiatric Disorders* (New York: Brunner/Mazel Publishers, 1994), 309.

4. J. G. Bernstein, *Drug Therapy in Psychiatry*, 3rd ed. (St. Louis: Mosby, 1995), 49–50.

5. H. Unlenhuth, H. DeWit, M. B. Balter, C. E. Johanson, and G. D. Mellinger, "Risks and Benefits of Long-term Benzodiazepine Use," *Journal of Clinical Psychopharmacology* 8 (1988): 161–167.

6. S. K. Saunders, S. L. Morzorati, and A. Shekhar, "Priming of Experimental Anxiety by Repeated Subthreshold GABA Blockade in the Rat Amygdala," *Brain Research* 699 (1995): 250–259.

7. A. Breier and S. M. Paul, "The GABA-A/Benzodiazepine Receptor: Implications for the Molecular Basis of Anxiety," *Journal of Psychiatric Research* 24, Suppl. 2 (1990): 91–104.

8. D. I. B. Kerr and J. Ong, "GABA$_B$ Receptors," *Pharmaceutical Therapeutics* 67 (1995): 187–246.

9. G. A. R. Johnston, "GABA$_C$ Receptors: Relatively Simple Transmitter-Gated Ion Channels," *Trends in Pharmaceutical Sciences* 17 (1996): 319–323.

10. W. R. Hobbs, T. W. Rall, and T. A. Verdoorn, "Hypnotics and Sedatives; Ethanol," in J. G. Hardman, L. E. Limbird, P. B. Molinoff, R. W. Ruddon, and A. G. Gilman, eds., *Goodman and Gilman's The Pharmacological Basis of Therapeutics*, 9th ed. (New York: McGraw-Hill, 1996), 365–367.

11. H. P. Rang and M. M. Dale, *Pharmacology*, 2nd ed. (Edinburgh: Churchill Livingstone, 1991), 637.

12. D. J. Greenblatt, J. S. Harmatz, and R. I. Shader, "Plasma Alprazolam Concentrations: Relation to Efficacy and Side Effects in the Treatment of Panic Disorder," *Archives of General Psychiatry* 50 (1993): 715–722.

13. J. R. T. Davidson, "Use of Benzodiazepines in Panic Disorder," *Journal of Clinical Psychiatry* 58, Suppl. 2 (1997): 26–28.

14. R. Saitz, M. F. Mayo-Smith, M. S. Roberts, H. A. Redmond, D. R. Bernard, and D. R. Calkins, "Individualized Treatment for Alcohol Withdrawal: A Randomized Double-Blind Controlled Trial," *Journal of the American Medical Association* 272 (1994): 519–523.

15. R. L. DuPont, "A Practical Approach to Benzodiazepine Discontinuation," *Journal of Psychiatric Research* 24, Suppl. 2 (1990): 81–90.

16. D. J. Greenblatt, L. G. Miller, and R. L. Shader, "Benzodiazepine Discontinuation Syndromes," *Journal of Psychiatric Research* 24, Suppl. 2 (1990): 73–80.

17. American Psychiatric Association, *Benzodiazepine Dependence, Toxicity, and Abuse: A Task Force Report of the American Psychiatric Association* (Washington, D.C.: American Psychiatric Association, 1990).

18. American Psychiatric Association, "Abuse Liability of Benzodiazepines," in *Benzodiazepine Dependence, Toxicity, and Abuse: A Task Force Report of the American Psychiatric Association* (Washington, D.C.: American Psychiatric Association, 1990), 49–53.

19. L. S. Cohen, V. C. Heller, and J. F. Rosenbaum, "Treatment Guidelines for Psychiatric Drug Use in Pregnancy," *Psychosomatics* 30 (1989): 25–33.

20. D. J. Nutt, P. Glue, C. Lawson, and S. Wilson, "Flumazenil Provocation of Panic Attacks: Evidence for Altered Benzodiazepine Receptor Sensitivity in Panic Disorder," *Archives of General Psychiatry* 47 (1990): 917–925.

21. "Zolpidem for Insomnia," *The Medical Letter on Drugs and Therapeutics* 35, no. 895 (Apr. 30, 1993): 35–36.

22. D. Ruana, J. Benavides, A. Machado, and J. Vitorica, "Regional Differences in the Enhancement by GABA of [3H]Zolpidem Binding to Omega-1 Sites in Rat Brain Membranes and Sections," *Brain Research* 600 (1993): 134–140.

23. W. B. Mendelson and B. Jain, "An Assessment of Short-Acting Hypnotics," *Drug Safety* 13 (1995): 257–270.

24. D. J. Kupfer and C. F. Reynolds, "Management of Insomnia," *New England Journal of Medicine* 336 (1997): 341–346.

25. P. Salva and J. Costa, "Clinical Pharmacokinetics and Pharmacodynamics of Zolpidem," *Clinical Pharmacokinetics* 29 (1995): 142–153.

26. J. M. Jonas, B. S. Coleman, A. Q. Sheridan, and R. W. Kalinske, "Comparative Clinical Profiles of Triazolam Versus Other Shorter-Acting Hypnotics," *Journal of Clinical Psychiatry* 53, suppl. (1992): 19–31.

27. M. Roger, P. Attali, and J. P. Coquelin, "Multicenter, Double-Blind, Controlled Comparison of Zolpidem and Triazolam in Elderly Patients with Insomnia," *Clinical Therapeutics* 15 (1993): 127–136.

28. N. J. Wesensten, T. J. Balkin, H. Q. Davis, and G. L. Belenky, "Reversal of Triazolam- and Zolpidem-Induced Memory Impairment by Flumazenil," *Psychopharmacology* 121 (1995): 242–249.

29. H. Bittiger, W. Froestl, S. J. Mickel, and H.-R. Olpe, "GABA$_B$ Receptor Antagonists: From Synthesis to Therapeutic Applications," *Trends in Pharmacological Sciences* 14 (1993): 391–394.

30. C. Mondadori, J. Jaekel, and G. Preiswerk, "CGP 36742: The First Orally Active GABA$_B$ Blocker Improves the Cognitive Performance of Mice, Rats, and Rhesus Monkeys," *Behavioral and Neural Biology* 60 (1993): 62–68.

31. I. Hindmarch and D. B. Fairweather, "Assessing the Residual Effects of Hypnotics," *Acta Psychiatrica Belgica* 94 (1994): 88–95.

32. D. P. Taylor and S. L. Mood, "Buspirone and Related Compounds as Alternative Anxiolytics," *Neuropeptides* 19, suppl. (1991): 15–19.

33. F. D. Yocca, "Neurochemistry and Neurophysiology of Buspirone and Gepirone: Interactions at Presynaptic and Postsynaptic 5-HT$_{1A}$ Receptors," *Journal of Clinical Psychopharmacology* 10, Suppl. 3 (1990): 6S–12S.

34. H. Chen, L. Zhang, D. R. Rubinow, and D. M. Chuang, "Chronic Buspirone Treatment Differentially Regulates 5-HT$_{1A}$ and 5-HT$_{2A}$ Receptor mRNA and Binding Sites in Various Regions of the Rat Hippocampus," *Brain Research, Molecular Brain Research* 32 (1995): 348–353.

35. D. G. Folks and W. C. Fuller, "Anxiety Disorders and Insomnia in Geriatric Patients," *The Psychiatric Clinics of North America* 20 (1997): 137–164.

36. K. V. Harvey and R. Balon, "Augmentation with Buspirone: A Review," *Annals of Clinical Psychiatry* 7 (1995): 143–147.

37. M. D. Gross, "Buspirone in ADHD with ODD," *Journal of the American Academy of Child and Adolescent Psychiatry* 34 (1995): 1260.

38. J. Cottraux, I.-D. Note, C. Cungi, P. Legeron, F. Heim, L. Chneiweiss, G. Bernard, and M. Bouvard, "A Controlled Study of Cognitive Behavior with Buspirone or Placebo in Panic Disorder with Agoraphobia," *British Journal of Psychiatry* 167 (1995): 635–641.

39. A. M. Albano and B. F. Chorpita, "Treatment of Anxiety Disorder of Childhood," *The Psychiatric Clinics of North America* 18 (1995): 767–784.

40. J. C. Simeon, H. B. Ferguson, V. Knott, et al., "Clinical, Cognitive, and Neurophysiological Effects of Alprazolam in Children and Adolescents with Overanxious and Avoidant Disorders," *Journal of the American Academy of Child and Adolescent Psychiatry* 31 (1992): 29–33.

41. G. J. DeVaugh, G. Moroz, J. Bierderman, et al., "Clomipramine Hydrochloride in Childhood and Adolescent Obsessive-Compulsive Disorder—A Multicenter Trial," *Journal of the American Academy of Child and Adolescent Psychiatry* 31 (1992): 45–49.

42. H. L. Leonard, S. Swedo, M. C. Lenane, "A 2- to 7-Year Follow-up Study of 54 Obsessive-Compulsive Children and Adolescents," *Archives of General Psychiatry* 50 (1993): 429–439.

43. J. I. Sheikh and C. Salzman, "Anxiety in the Elderly: Course and Treatment," *The Psychiatric Clinics of North America* 18 (1995): 871–883.

44. M. A. Jeneke, "Geriatric Psychopharmacology," *The Psychiatric Clinics of North America* 3 (1996): 151–203.

45. M. L. Catterson, S. H. Preskorn, and R. L. Martin, "Pharmacodynamic and Pharmacokinetic Considerations in Geriatric Psychopharmacology," *The Psychiatric Clinics of North America* 20 (1997): 205–218.

46. C. Salzman, "Pharmacologic Treatment of the Anxious Elderly," in C. Salzman and B. D. Lebowitz, eds. *Anxiety in the Elderly* (New York: Springer-Verlag, 1991), 251–265.

47. M. H. Zisselman, B. W. Rovner, and Y. Shmuely, "Benzodiazepine Use in the Elderly Prior to Psychiatric Hospitalization," *Psychosomatics* 37 (1996): 38–42.

48. J. H. Woods, J. L. Katz, and G. Winger, "Benzodiazepines: Use, Abuse, and Consequences," *Pharmacological Reviews* 44 (1992): 151–347.

49. E. Schweizer, "Generalized Anxiety Disorder: Longitudinal Course and Pharmacologic Treatment," *The Psychiatric Clinics of North America* 18 (1995): 843–857.

50. S. G. McCracken, H. deWit, E. H. Uhlenhuth, et al., "Preference for Diazepam in Anxious Adults," *Journal of Clinical Psychopharmacology* 10 (1990): 190–196.

51. J. L. Kunovac and S. M. Stahl, "Future Directions in Anxiolytic Pharmacotherapy," *The Psychiatric Clinics of North America* 18 (1995): 895–909.

52. G. Perrault, E. Morel, D. J. Sanger, and B. Zivkovic, "Repeated Treatment with Alpidem, a New Anxiolytic, Does Not Induce Tolerance or Physical Dependence," *Neuropharmacology* 32 (1993): 855–863.

53. L. Frattola, M. Garreau, R. Piolti, S. Bassi, M. G. Albizzati, C. Borghi, and P. L. Morselli, "Comparison of the Efficacy, Safety, and Withdrawal of Alpidem and Alprazolam in Anxious Patients," *British Journal of Psychiatry* 165 (1994): 94–100.

54. D. J. Sanger and B. Zivkovic, "Discriminative Stimulus Effects of Alpidem, a New Imidazopyridine Anxiolytic," *Psychopharmacology* 113 (1994): 395–403.

55. E. Costa and A. Guidotti, "Benzodiazepines on Trial: A Research Strategy for Their Rehabilitation," *Trends in Pharmacological Sciences* 17 (1996): 192–200.

56. K. W. Gee, L. D. McCauley, and N. C. Lan, "A Putative Receptor or Neurosteroids on the $GABA_A$ Receptor Complex: The Pharmacological Properties and Therapeutic Potential of Epalons," *Critical Reviews in Neurobiology* 9 (995): 207–227.

57. R. Rupprecht, C. A. Hauser, T. Trapp and F. Holsboer, "Neurosteroids: Molecular Mechanisms of Action and Psychopharmacological Significance," *Journal of Steroid Biochemistry and Molecular Biology* 56 (1996): 163–168.

58. G. K. Mumford, C. R. Rush and R. R. Griffiths, "Abecarnil and Alprazolam in Humans: Behavioral, Subjective, and Reinforcing Effects," *Journal of Pharmacology and Experimental Therapeutics* 272 (1995): 570–580.

59. U. Busto, H. L. Kaplan, L. Zawertailo, "Pharmacological Effects and Abuse Liability of Bretazenil, Diazepam, and Alprazolam in Humans," *Clinical Pharmacology and Therapeutics* 55 (1994): 451–463.

Chapter 5

PSYCHOSTIMULANTS: COCAINE AND THE AMPHETAMINES

Cocaine and the amphetamines are powerful psychostimulants that markedly affect one's mental functioning and behavior. All of the psychostimulants act through various mechanisms to ultimately augment the synaptic action of the *catecholamine, dopamine,* and, to a lesser extent, *norepinephrine neurotransmitters,* producing, in addition to other actions, a direct action upon the *nucleus accumbens,* a structure we earlier associated with behavioral reinforcement, compulsive abuse, and drug dependency. In addition, the psychostimulants also have limited (but continuing) therapeutic use, and all have significant side effects, toxicities, and patterns of abuse.

Cocaine and the amphetamine-like drugs (see Figure 5.1) elevate mood, induce euphoria, increase alertness, reduce fatigue, provide a sense of increased energy, decrease appetite, improve task performance, and relieve boredom. Anxiety, insomnia, and irritability are common side effects. At higher doses, irritability and anxiety become more intense, and a pattern of psychotic behavior may appear. Indeed, cocaine and the amphetamines produce remarkably similar behavioral effects. At low doses, psychostimulants evoke an alerting, arousing, or behavior-activating response that is not unlike a normal reaction to an emergency or to stress. Blood pressure and heart rate increase, pupils dilate, blood flow shifts from skin and internal organs to muscle, and

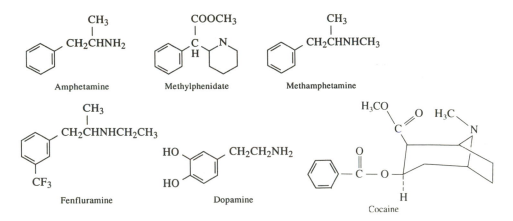

Figure 5.1 Structures of amphetamines, dopamine, and cocaine.

oxygen levels rise, as does the level of glucose in the blood. These effects occur because these drugs augment or potentiate the action of dopamine and norepinephrine both in the body and in the brain. This action mimics and overwhelms the natural release of biological amines (e.g., adrenaline) as part of our normal alerting or activating response.

COCAINE

The leaves of *Erythroxylon coca* (a tree indigenous to Peru and Bolivia) have been used for centuries for religious, mystical, social, euphoriant, and medicinal purposes—most notably to increase endurance, promote a sense of well-being, induce euphoria, and alleviate hunger. The active alkaloid in *E. coca* was isolated in 1859 and named *cocaine*. Used as an endurant by natives, who chewed the leaves, the usual total daily dose of cocaine in the plant material was up to about 200 milligrams, a point that will become more important later in this discussion. Today, the relevant clinical issues related to cocaine's history have to do largely with the changes over time in dosage, route of administration, patterns of use, and technology of production.[1]

In 1884 Sigmund Freud advocated the use of cocaine to treat depression and to alleviate chronic fatigue. Freud described cocaine as a "magical drug"; he even wrote a "Song of Praise" to it. In the same year, Carl Koller demonstrated cocaine's local anesthetic properties and introduced the drug for use in ophthalmologic surgery. Freud, while using cocaine to relieve his own depression, described cocaine as inducing exhilaration and lasting euphoria, which in no way differs from the normal euphoria of the healthy person. However, he did not immediately perceive its side effects—tolerance, dependence, a state of psychosis, and withdrawal depression. In his later writings, Freud called cocaine the "third scourge" of humanity, after alcohol and heroin. This is perhaps an appropriate description.

In the United States, around 1885, cocaine was incorporated (along with caffeine) in numerous patent medicines, including the beverage Coca-Cola. Until 1903 Coca-Cola contained approximately 60 milligrams of cocaine per 8-ounce serving.[1] In the late 1800s, however, concern about cocaine's toxicities increased. By 1891 at least 200 reports of cocaine intoxication and 13 deaths were reported. About 1910 President William H. Taft proclaimed cocaine as Public Enemy Number 1, and in 1914 the Harrison Narcotic Act banned the incorporation of cocaine in patent medicines and beverages.[2] In 1924 the American Medical Association reviewed 43 deaths of patients who had been under local anesthesia induced by cocaine and attributed 26 of those deaths to cocaine toxicity. Guidelines for the safe use of cocaine in medicine were then established.

The use of cocaine rose during the 1920s and then decreased during the 1930s, when amphetamines became available and cost less and produced longer-lasting yet similar effects. Thus, cocaine was not used much again until the late 1960s, when tight federal restrictions on amphetamine distribution raised the cost of amphetamines, once again making cocaine attractive.*

More recently, the smoking of concentrated preparations of cocaine ("free base" or "crack" cocaine) has introduced a new era in the abuse of cocaine, characterized by high-dose, rapid-onset effects with the rapid development of both toxicity and dependency. One of the most addictive and reinforcing of the abused drugs, cocaine is used by an estimated 20 to 30 million people in the United States. About 4.5 million people have used cocaine within the past year, and about 1.3 million persons report frequent use, defined as use at least monthly.[3] Of those who used cocaine at least once in the past year, 77 percent "snorted" (used the drug nasally) cocaine hydrochloride, 36 percent smoked crack cocaine, and 7 percent injected (intravenously) cocaine hydrochloride.[4]

---

*Because their net effects can be nearly indistinguishable, cocaine and the amphetamines can be used almost interchangeably as euphoriants. Availability, price, and sociocultural considerations now largely determine the comparative popularity of the two.

Cocaine addicts are typically young (12 to 39 years of age), dependent on at least three drugs, and male (75 percent). Addicts tend to have coexisting psychopathology (30 percent have anxiety disorders, 67 percent suffer from clinical depression, and 25 percent exhibit paranoia). About 85 to 90 percent are alcohol dependent. Cocaine use is associated with a range of violent premature deaths, including homicides, suicides, and accidents.[1] In addition, more people are using illicit amphetamines (e.g., methamphetamine and its smokable form "ICE"), the increased use of which may be negating any reductions in cocaine use.

Chemistry

The leaf of *E. coca* contains about 0.5 to 1.0 percent cocaine. When the leaves are soaked and mashed, cocaine is extracted in the form of coca paste (60 to 80 percent cocaine). Because persons who smoke coca paste may experience a high incidence of psychopathological states, extreme toxicity, and severe dependence, coca paste is usually treated to form the less potent hydrochloride salt before it is exported. Then it is diluted (to increase its bulk and decrease its potency) and sold illicitly in powdered form as cocaine hydrochloride ("crystal" or "snow"). Inhaled ("snorted") in this form, a "line" of cocaine hydrochloride provides a dose of about 25 milligrams; thus, a user might sniff about 50 to 100 milligrams of drug at a time.

Until recently the diluted hydrochloride salt preparation was the most common form of cocaine. For a more rapid onset and greater intensity of effect, a smokable form of cocaine was developed. For this use, the hydrochloride salt of the drug was not suitable, because cocaine in this form decomposes at the temperature of the smoke.[4] To resolve this problem, the hydrochloride form is chemically altered to its "base" form by boiling the drug in a solution of baking soda or ammonia until the water evaporates. The residue is a form of cocaine base that is commonly called *crack*, from the cracking sound it makes when heated.

"Freebasing" is a less common method of creating the base from the hydrochloride salt. Here, the alkaline water-cocaine mixture is extracted into ether; evaporating the ether phase by heating yields a similar smokable product. The base form of cocaine does not decompose at the temperature of smoke, and the vaporized particles can be inhaled by using a heated pipe.[5] The smoking of crack cocaine yields average doses in the range of 250 milligrams to 1 gram (see Table 5.1). The consequences of these higher doses are severe, as will become apparent later in this chapter.

TABLE 5.1 Effects of cocaine administration

Route	Administration Mode	Initial onset of action (s)	Duration of "high" (min)	Average acute dose (mg)	Peak plasma levels (ng/ml)	Purity (percent)	Bioavailability (percent absorbed)
Oral	Coca leaf chewing	300–600	45–90	20–50	150	0.5–1	25
Oral	Cocaine HCI	600–1800		100–200	150–200	20–80	20–30
Intranasal	"Snorting" cocaine HCI	120–180	30–45	5×30	150	20–80	20–30
Intravenous	Cocaine HCI	30–45	10–20	25–50	300–400	$7–100 \times 58$	100
				>200	1000–1500		
Smoking	Coca paste	8–10	5–10	60–250	300–800	40–85	6–32
	Free base	8–10	5–10	250–1000	800–900	90–100	6–32
	Crack	8–10	5–10	250–1000	?	50–95	6–32

From Gold (1992),[1] table 16.5, p. 209.

Pharmacokinetics

Cocaine is absorbed from all sites of application, including mucous membranes, the gastrointestinal tract, and the lungs. It is detoxified both in plasma and in the liver. Only small amounts are excreted unchanged. Further pharmacokinetic details follow.

Absorption

The three principal routes through which cocaine is commonly taken are intranasal (snorting), intravenous, and inhalation (smoking), the latter effective only with the base form of cocaine. Table 5.1 presents some pharmacokinetic data for each method of administration.

Snorted intranasally, cocaine, as the hydrochloride salt, poorly crosses the mucosal membranes. Also, because cocaine constricts blood vessels, such vasoconstriction limits its own absorption. Thus, only about 20 to 30 percent of the snorted drug is absorbed through the nasal mucosa into blood, with plasma peaking within 30 to 60 minutes. The time course of the pharmacological effects (the subjective "high") parallels the blood levels, as well as the amount of drug actually in brain tissue (see Figure 5.2).

When cocaine (base) is vaporized and smoked, some particles become trapped in the nose while others pass through the nasal pharynx into the trachea and onto lung surfaces, from which absorption is rapid and quite complete. Onset of effects is within seconds, peaks at 5 minutes, and persists for about 30 minutes. Only about 6 to 32 percent of the initial amount reaches plasma.

Obviously, intravenous injection of cocaine hydrochloride bypasses all the barriers to absorption, placing the total dose of drug immediately into the bloodstream. The 30- to 60-second delay in onset of action simply reflects the time it takes the drug to travel from the site of injection to the brain.

Distribution

Cocaine penetrates the brain rapidly; initial brain concentrations far exceed the concentrations in plasma. After it penetrates the brain, cocaine is rapidly redistributed to other tissues. Cocaine freely crosses the placental barrier, achieving levels in the unborn equal to those in the mother.

Metabolism and Excretion

Cocaine has a biological half-life of 30 to 90 minutes; it is rapidly and almost completely metabolized by enzymes located both in plasma and

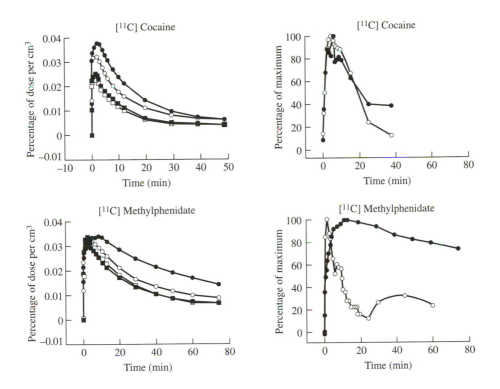

Figure 5.2 (*Top left*) Time course of cocaine in cerebral cortex (circles) and cerebellum (squares) before (solid circles) and after (open circles) methylphenidate. (*Bottom left*) Time course of methylphenidate in cerebral cortex (circles) and cerebellum (squares) before (solid circles) and after (solid squares) cocaine. (*Top right*) Time course of cocaine in cerebral cortex (solid circles) and the subjective experience of being "high" after cocaine administration (open circles). Note the parallelism between the "high" after cocaine administration and the kinetics of the drug in cerebral cortex. (*Bottom left*) Time course of methylphenidate in cerebral cortex (solid circles) and the subjective experience of being "high" after methylphenidate administration (open circles). Note the dissociation between the persistence of methylphenidate in brain tissue and the short-lived "high." Persistence of methylphenidate (*lower right*) may prevent a "high" from subsequent doses. [Adapted from Volkow et al. (1995),[68] p. 457.]

in the liver. Urine can test positive for cocaine for only about 12 hours. The major metabolite is the inactive compound *benzoylecgonine*, which can be detected in the urine for about 48 hours and much longer (up to 2 weeks) in chronic users.[5] Urine detection of benzoylecgonine forms the basis of drug testing for cocaine use. The persistence of the metabolite in urine implies that high-dose, long-term users might accumulate drug in their body tissues.

Several reports in the early 1990s have documented an interesting metabolic interaction between cocaine and ethanol. In individuals who use cocaine and drink alcohol concurrently, a unique ethyl ester of benzoylecgonine is produced by the liver enzymes that metabolize these two drugs.[6] This metabolite (*cocaethylene*) is pharmacologically as active as cocaine in blocking the presynaptic dopamine reuptake transporter, potentiating the euphoric effect of cocaine, increasing the risk of dual dependency, and increasing the severity of withdrawal with chronic patterns of use.[7] The cocaethylene metabolite is actually more toxic than cocaine and exacerbates cocaine's toxicity.[8]

Pharmacodynamics

Pharmacologically, cocaine has three prominent actions that account for virtually all of its physiological and psychological effects:

1. It is a potent *local anesthetic.*

2. It is a *vasoconstrictor,* strongly constricting blood vessels.

3. It is a powerful *psychostimulant* with strong reinforcing qualities.

It is the psychostimulant property that contributes to the compulsive abuse of the drug. Therefore, we focus on the actions that lead to its psychostimulation and its behavior-reinforcing properties. The vaso-constrictive and local anesthetic actions contribute to its severe cardio-vascular toxicities (discussed later).

Cocaine has long been known to potentiate the synaptic actions of dopamine, norepinephrine, and serotonin, secondary to cocaine's ability to block the active reuptake of these three transmitters back into the presynaptic nerve terminals from which they were released (see Figure 5.3). By 1990 cocaine's action on the *dopaminergic neurons* (rather than on the norepinephrine or serotonin neurons) was known to be crucial to its behavior-reinforcing and psychostimulant properties.[9]

Dopaminergic pathways originating from neurons located in the midbrain (see Figure IV.17) are emerging as central to many of the behavioral manifestations of cocaine, especially those concerning reinforcement and hyperactivity. The ventral tegmental area of the midbrain contains dopamine-containing neurons whose axons project to mesolimbic brain areas, including the medial prefrontal cortex and nucleus accumbens, as well as the amygdala and hippocampus. The

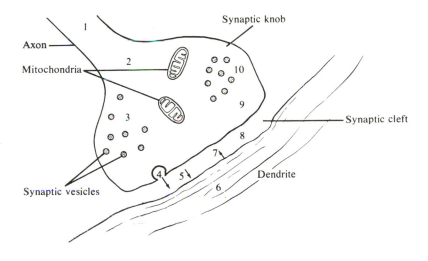

Figure 5.3 Schematic diagram of a dopamine (DA) synapse within the central nervous system. The steps in neurotransmission are numbered. (1) Conduction of an action potential down the presynaptic axon. (2) Arrival of the action potential at the nerve terminal with electrically induced increases in calcium ion influx. (3) Synthesis of DA and its storage in the synaptic vesicles (this may occur before steps 1 and 2). (4) Release of DA (because of the calcium ion influx) from synaptic vesicles into the synaptic cleft. (5) Diffusion of DA across the synaptic cleft. (6) Activation of the postsynaptic activity by DA. (7) Release of DA from the postsynaptic receptor back into the synaptic cleft. (8) Metabolism of some of the DA in the synaptic cleft by extracellular enzymes. (9) Binding of DA to the presynaptic reuptake transporter protein and active reuptake of DA into the presynaptic nerve terminal. (10) Uptake of DA in the presynaptic nerve terminal into the presynaptic vesicle. Cocaine blocks step 9. The amphetamines initiate step 4. The exact mechanisms by which they do this is unknown.

activity of cocaine on the presynaptic nerve terminals of dopamine-releasing axons in these latter projection sites (see Figure 3.5) is proposed as the key to the reinforcing properties of the drug.[10]

Several studies have advanced our understanding of this action on the dopaminergic system.[10–13] These studies demonstrate that both dopamine and cocaine decrease the discharge rate of neurons located in both the ventral tegmental area and the nucleus accumbens, indicating that dopamine exerts inhibitory effects on the postsynaptic receptors (i.e., dopamine is primarily an inhibitory neurotransmitter). Cocaine markedly potentiates this dopamine-induced decrease in discharge rate, such potentiation occurring secondary to cocaine-induced blockade of dopamine reuptake (into the presynaptic nerve terminal), thus increasing the extracellular (synaptic) concentration of dopamine, potentiating its inhibitory action on postsynaptic receptors.[14] How this inhibitory

synaptic transmitter action of dopamine translates into behavioral reinforcement is still unclear, but it likely involves disinhibition of frontal
cortical activity from chronic dopaminergic inhibition.

In 1991 the presynaptic "transporter" protein for dopamine, which
is blocked by cocaine, was cloned and characterized.[15–16] This transporter protein is a 619-amino-acid protein with 12 putative membrane-
spanning regions; both termini of the protein are located in the intracellular cytoplasm of the presynaptic neuron (see Figure 5.4). Cocaine
probably competes with dopamine for this receptor, the cocaine blocking the binding of dopamine and prolonging its presence in the synaptic cleft. Cocaine also inhibits the reuptake of norepinephrine into
presynaptic nerve terminals. Similarly, cocaine may bind to certain
serotonin receptors in the brain. The significance of these two actions
is unclear, because cocaine has poor antidepressant properties.

Finally, the question arises about neuronal and neurochemical alterations during cocaine withdrawal, changes that might shed light
on the mechanisms of cocaine-induced tolerance and dependency.
Kuhar and Pilotte (1996)[17] note that *presynaptic* dopamine trans-

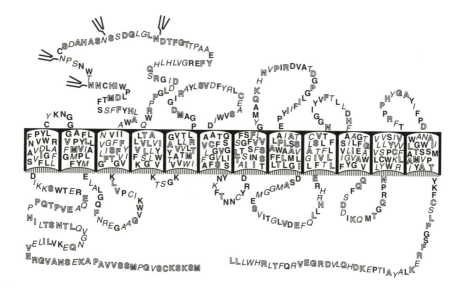

Figure 5.4 Schematic representation of the dopamine transporter showing proposed orientation in the plasma membrane, amino acids conserved in GABA,
dopamine (DA), and norepinephrine (NE) transporters amino acids conserved in DA
and NE transporters (italic letters), or amino acids found only in DA transporters
(open letters). [From Shimada et al. (1991),[15] figure 1, p. 577.]

porter levels in the nucleus accumbens and ventral tegmentum increase in the days following cessation of cocaine administration and decrease for several months thereafter. Such biphasic action during cocaine withdrawal is also reflected in a biphasic increase and then persistent decrease in both frontal cortical blood flow and glucose metabolism. As they state:

> Both a primary and a protracted abstinence syndrome are associated with cocaine withdrawal, at least at the biochemical level. What could the significance of these changes be? As the mesolimbic neurons are involved in reward and reinforcement, significant dysfunction of these neurons could mediate anhedonia, craving, or other events reported in humans who stop abusing drugs.[17]

It is also clear that chronic exposure of *postsynaptic* receptors to the increased amounts of dopamine that are available (after its active reuptake has been blocked) leads to a decrease in the number of postsynaptic dopamine receptors,[11] with the development of a twofold increase in the amount of dopamine necessary to produce a postsynaptic action (i.e., tolerance develops[18]).

Side Effects of Short-Term, Low-Dose Use

Low dose (e.g., 25 to 100 milligrams) nontoxic, *physiological responses* to cocaine include increased alertness, motor hyperactivity, tachycardia, vasoconstriction, hypertension, bronchodilation, increased body temperature, pupillary dilation, increased glucose availability, and shifts in blood flow from the internal organs to the muscles. *Psychological effects* of low doses include an immediate euphoria, giddiness, enhanced self-consciousness, and a forceful boastfulness that last only about 30 minutes. This period is followed by one of milder euphoria mixed with anxiety, which can last for 60 to 90 minutes, followed by a more protracted anxious state that spans hours. During acute and subacute intoxication, thoughts typically race and speech becomes talkative and rapid, often pressured, even garrulous, with tangential and incoherent speech.

Appetite is markedly suppressed but later rebounds. Sleep is delayed; fatigue is postponed but later rebounds. Conscious awareness and mental acuity are increased but are followed with depression. Motor activity is increased, with agitation, restlessness, and a feeling of constant motion. Perhaps most important, as a potent behavioral reinforcer, cocaine promotes one's desire to take more cocaine, even instead of such important reinforcers as food.

Cocaine functions as a discriminative stimulus in several species,[14] a fundamental mechanism by which a drug can control behavior. Also, cocaine administration has been reported to be followed by an increase in cocaine craving, "an effect that may, like its positive reinforcing effect, increase the likelihood of additional cocaine consumption."[14] In fact, even when self-administering cocaine is punished, a person on cocaine will still tend to want more of the drug.[18] After the "high" ends, anxiety, depression, and paranoia follow. This rapid shift causes the user to crave more drug in an attempt to regain the euphoria felt just minutes ago. Such drug craving becomes intense and "forms a distinct part of the withdrawal syndrome associated with cocaine."[1] At higher doses all these effects are intensified, as is the depressive rebound that follows. There is a progressive loss of coordination, followed by tremors and eventually seizures. Central nervous system (CNS) stimulation is followed by depression, dysphoria, anxiety, somnolence, and drug craving.

Although one's sexual interest may be heightened by using cocaine and high doses (injected or smoked) are sometimes described as orgasmic, cocaine is not an aphrodisiac. Sexual dysfunction is common in heavy users. Further, when dysfunction is combined with the isolation that cocaine-dependent individuals experience, normal interpersonal, sensual, and sexual interactions are compromised.

Specific medical complications are also associated with the method of administering cocaine. When cocaine is snorted, chronic rhinitis, perforations of the nasal septum, and a loss of the sense of smell can occur. When cocaine is taken intravenously, diseases transmitted by needle (e.g., hepatitis and AIDS) and infectious endocarditis (infections of the heart and its valves) are not uncommon. Smoking crack cocaine can cause pulmonary difficulties, black sputum, and burns on the lips and tongue.

Toxic and Psychotic Effects of Long-Term, High-Dose Use

Although low doses of cocaine cause CNS stimulation that is mostly pleasurable or euphoric, higher doses produce toxic symptoms, including anxiety, sleep deprivation, hypervigilance, suspiciousness, paranoia, and persecutory fears. Persons taking cocaine may become hyperreactive, paranoid, and impulsive, and may display a repetitive, compulsive pattern of behavior. Such persons can have a markedly altered perception of reality, and they can become aggressive or homicidal in response to imagined persecution.[3] These behaviors make up what is called a *toxic paranoid psychosis.*

Other high-dose, long-term effects of cocaine use include interpersonal conflicts (resulting from the sense of isolation and paranoia), depression, dysphoria, and bizarre and violent psychotic disorders that can last days or weeks after a person stops using the drug. As summarized by Johanson and Fischman (1989)[18].

> One of the most significant consequences of cocaine abuse is the development of behavioral pathology in chronic users. In its most extreme form, a cocaine psychosis can be produced, characterized by paranoia, impaired reality testing, anxiety, a stereotyped compulsive repetitive pattern of behavior, and vivid visual, auditory, and tactile hallucinations, including delusions of insects crawling under the skin. More subtle changes in behavior ... may include irritability, hypervigilance, extreme psychomotor activation, paranoid thinking, impaired interpersonal relations, and disturbances of eating and sleeping.

An acutely toxic dose of cocaine has been estimated to be about 1 to 2 milligrams per kilogram of body weight. Thus, 70 to 150 milligrams of cocaine is a toxic, one-time dose for a 150-pound (70-kilogram) person. Serious physiological toxicity follows higher doses.

A 1993 symposium on acute cocaine intoxication addressed the cardiovascular[19] and neurovascular[20] sequelae of cocaine use, including strokes in healthy, young individuals, persistent alterations in blood perfusion of the brain, oxygen deprivation to the heart, cardiac arrhythmias, and seizures. Billman (1995)[21] reviewed the causes of cocaine-induced cardiac toxicity, ascribing it to a combination of local anesthetic (cardiac depressant) and adrenaline-induced cardiac irritability, both of which predispose to fatal cardiac arrhythmias. Intense coronary artery vasoconstriction reduces blood flow to the hard-working, irritable heart muscle; the combination of vasoconstriction and peripheral hypertension predisposes to inadequate oxygenation of heart muscle, leading to ischemia and "heart attacks" in predisposed individuals.

Chronic cocaine use produces virtually every psychiatric syndrome: affective disorders (mania and depression), schizophrenia-like syndromes, personality disorders, and so on. Rounsaville and coworkers (1991)[22] studied 300 cocaine abusers seeking treatment for substance abuse. They found that 56 percent met current criteria and 73 percent met lifetime criteria for the presence of a neuropsychological disorder (major depression, anxiety disorder, bipolar affective disorder, antisocial personality, or history of childhood attention deficit hyperactivity disorder). Thus, toxic symptoms may indicate either high-dose drug toxicities or the onset of symptoms of a coexisting neuropsychological disorder (or both). According to one report:

Cocaine addicts, like alcoholics and heroin addicts, often show a certain profile on personality tests—they are reckless, rebellious, and have a low tolerance for frustration and a craving for excitement. In fact, most of them have been or will be alcoholics or heroin addicts as well. They use opiates and alcohol either to enhance the effects of cocaine or to medicate themselves for unwanted side effects—calming jitters, dulling perceptions, and reducing paranoia to indifference. Intravenous drug users often take cocaine and heroin together in a mixture known as a speedball. Probably more than half of people treated for cocaine abuse are also alcoholic, and the rate of alcoholism in the families of cocaine addicts is high.[23]

Weddington (1993)[5] goes on to say that:

With repeated or chronic intoxication, tolerance develops. Accompanying a diminishing intensity of euphoria, chronic cocaine users regularly report increasing dysphoria, anxiety, a sense of loss of control with decreased self-esteem, suspiciousness increasing to paranoia, aggressiveness, and confusion. In addition, environmental consequences to cocaine addiction, such as social and family dissolution, financial loss, or legal contingencies, may contribute to an addict's growing dysphoria and despair associated with chronic cocaine abuse.

Fetal Effects

One of tragedies of the late twentieth century is the birth of hundreds of thousands of infants who have been injured *intra utero* by drugs and who are born into poor nutritional and social environments. Prominent among these drugs is cocaine, a drug that produces infants with "jittery baby syndrome" and infants known as "crack babies." Because of the wide spectrum of fetal effects, a "fetal cocaine syndrome" cannot be well defined, because most fetal effects may be related to vasoconstriction, hypertension, and cerebral infarcts at any time during gestation and in any structure.[24]

To determine effects of cocaine on the fetus, one must be aware of both the direct as well as the indirect effects of the drug on fetal development (see Figure 5.5). Indirect effects of cocaine on the fetus result from its vasoconstrictive action on the mother's blood vessels, which decreases blood flow to the uterus and reduces fetal oxygenation. Adverse effects include placental detachment, placental insufficiency, preterm or precipitous labor, fetal death (stillbirths), low birth weight, intrauterine growth retardation, small head size (microcephaly), and possible aberrations in brain and heart development. As reviewed by

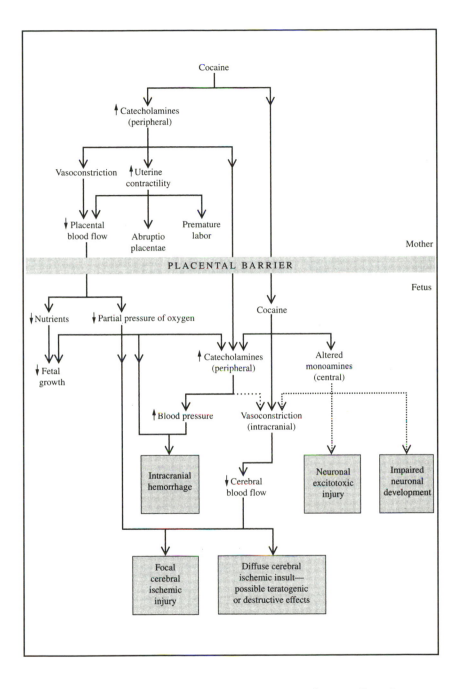

Figure 5.5 Deleterious effects of maternal cocaine use on fetuses. Effects that appear plausible on the basis of current information but whose confirmation requires more supporting evidence are indicated by dotted lines. ↑ denotes increased and ↓ decreased. [From J. J. Volpe (1992),[26] figure 1, p. 401.]

Kain, Rimer, and Barash (1993):[25] "Virtually any body organ in the neonate can be affected if blood flow to that organ is reduced during fetal development." Volpe (1992),[26] reviewing the direct fetotoxic effects of cocaine, notes that, as the brain develops, exposure of the fetus to cocaine may promote serious destructive lesions, leading to a neonatal neurological syndrome typified by abnormal sleep patterns, tremors, poor feeding, irritability, occasional seizures, and an increased risk or incidence of sudden infant death syndrome (SIDS).

Undoubtedly, any fetal cocaine syndrome is not as clearly defined as the fetal alcohol syndrome (see Chapter 3), and cocaine use by the mother "is only one of many undesirable influences in the children's lives. . . . Neglect and abuse by addicted parents are a greater danger."[27] Therefore, babies born into a drug-using environment, and possibly into poverty, experience little physical or emotional nurturing, and so bonding is incomplete or absent.

The statistics on cocaine use and newborns include the facts that 50,000 to 100,000 babies are born each year to mothers who have used at least some cocaine during pregnancy,[27] and 5 to 7 percent of pregnant women have used cocaine during pregnancy, with much higher rates in low income, inner-city women.[28] Birnbach and coworkers (1997)[29] noted in a New York City study that 68 percent of pregnant women who were admitted to labor and delivery without previous prenatal care tested positive for cocaine, placing both the pregnant woman and her fetus at risk for life-threatening cardiovascular and CNS complications. Improved prenatal care and drug treatment both contribute to improved fetal outcomes.[28]

As cocaine-impaired children enter the school system, they have difficulty developing attachments or dealing effectively with multiple stimuli. They may become either aggressive or withdrawn when they are overstimulated. They have difficulty with unstructured play and a low tolerance for frustration. They also structure input and information poorly, displaying a high incidence of attention deficit hyperactivity disorder (ADHD). These children may form a cohort whose combined physiological damage and extrinsic socioeconomic disadvantage is determined from birth.

Treatment of Cocaine Abuse

A variety of psychological, behavioral, and pharmacological approaches have been suggested for treating cocaine abuse,[1,5,9,17] but as yet there is no consensus regarding any generally accepted treatment for such abuse. Several major problems complicate attempts at therapy. First, there is the intensity of both the drug effect and the behavior-reinforcing action of cocaine. Second is the pronounced tendency toward relapse, with cocaine acting as a cue to an increased craving for the drug. The third problem is the fact that virtually all cocaine addicts have a coexisting disease, involving additional drug dependencies and/or psychiatric disorders, including major depression, an anxiety disorder, bipolar disorder, borderline personality disorder, and/or antisocial personality disorder. Given these complications, the needs of the cocaine addict are at least fivefold:

1. Immediate abstinence
2. Diagnosis of any coexisting disorders
3. Determination whether the cocaine addiction is a primary disorder or is secondary to other disorders
4. Maintenance of abstinence for long enough to diagnose and begin treatment of coexisting disorders
5. Prevention of relapse

Approaches to treatment are many, from classic "12-step" recovery programs resembling that of Alcoholics Anonymous to experimental interventions utilizing psychopharmacotherapy, psychotherapy, cognitive-behavioral, or behavioral reinforcement approaches.[5,30] In all cases, abstinence is usually considered essential and must be monitored by frequent, random, unannounced urine tests to screen for cocaine and other drugs of abuse.

In the mid-1980s, Gawin and Kleber (1986)[31] developed a three-phase model of abstinence symptomatology related to cocaine abuse. The phases, called the "crash," "withdrawal," and "extinction," may have important implications for treatment. The crash phase is quite short (9 hours to 4 days); during this period the user is generally uninterested in abstaining from or using cocaine, appearing quite depressed and somnolent. This period likely represents the time period of drug elimination with concomitant depletion of dopamine at its receptors, combined with a period of postsynaptic receptor hyposensitivity persisting after drug cession. The withdrawal phase, which lasts 1 to 10 weeks, is the period of maximal relapse potential and drug craving, which, as discussed earlier, may be associated with reduced dopamine transporter levels and reduced frontal cortical activity. The extinction phase is of unlimited duration; here patients require continued monitoring because conditioned cues, which must be extinguished, can still trigger craving and result in relapse.

Psychopharmacotherapy could, at least theoretically, be used in treating cocaine abuse for any of four reasons:

1. To antagonize or block the effects of cocaine at its receptors
2. To produce an aversive (Antabuse-like) reaction if cocaine is taken in the presence of the aversive agent
3. To treat any coexisting psychological disorder
4. To reduce cocaine craving and prevent relapse

Regarding goals 1 and 2, to date no specific cocaine antagonists are available, nor are there any aversive drugs. Therefore, drug therapy is aimed at utilizing drugs to treat coexisting disorders or to attenuate the craving for cocaine.

Regarding goal 3, many patients who abuse cocaine have a past or present history of major depression episodes and a positive family history for affective illness.[32] Because cocaine inhibits the presynaptic reuptake of dopamine, it somewhat resembles the pharmacologic actions of the antidepressants (see Chapter 7). Thus, cocaine may have been (at least initially) used by some individuals as self-treatment for their depressive disorder. Indeed, several studies have reported favorable effects of tricyclic antidepressants, such as *desipramine* and *imipramine*, in improving mood and prolonging abstinence in patients (with coexisting depression) who have withdrawn from cocaine. Similarly, the serotonin-specific antidepressant *fluoxetine* (Prozac; see Chapter 7) has been reported to alleviate comorbid depression and reduce cocaine use. Other psychotherapeutic drugs have been reported to be useful in treating comorbid affective disorders, including *lithium* and *carbamazepine* (see Chapters 2 and 8).[32] In their review of this topic, however, Mendelson and Mello (1996)[3] conclude that fluoxetine, lithium, and carbamazepine are all ineffective, while the adverse effects of imipramine are more severe than those of desipramine. Because withdrawal from cocaine is accompanied by depletion of dopamine stores, administration of an antidepressant that enhances dopamine neurotransmission might help alleviate both depression and drug craving. *Buproprion* (Wellbutrin, see Chapter 7) is such an agent and is thought to be useful in some patients. This claim, however, has been disputed by Margolin and coworkers (1995).[33]

Regarding goal 4, the memory of cocaine euphoria is so powerful that drug craving, even after months or years of abstinence, can be overwhelming. To date, no specific agents have been shown to be effective in decreasing cocaine craving, although numerous agents have been suggested,[34] including the dopamine receptor agonists *amantadine, bromocriptine,* and *pergolide* and the amino acids *tryptophan* (which may increase serotonin levels in the brain) and *tyrosine* (a precursor in the synthesis of dopamine). While the dopamine agonists may have some usefulness, the amino acids have not been demonstrated to be effective (see Mendelson and Mello[3] for review). Chapter 14 reviews the potential usefulness of *ibogaine* to reduce cocaine craving.

Carroll and coworkers (1994)[35] evaluated the effectiveness of cognitive-behavioral treatment (based on relapse prevention principles), clinical management, and desipramine, alone and in randomized combination, in treating ambulatory cocaine abusers. All treatments significantly reduced cocaine use. Desipramine was not as effective as nonpharmacological treatment, although desipramine as a short-term adjunct appeared to facilitate the effectiveness of psychotherapy. Severe cocaine abusers appeared to respond best to relapse-prevention therapy. Lower-intensity approaches (such as desipramine without concomitant psychotherapy) were effective only with less severe abusers. The American Psychiatric Association (1996)[36] has published practice guidelines for the treatment of cocaine-related disorders.

Mendelson and Mello (1996)[3] conclude:

> At present, no drug therapy is uniquely effective in treating cocaine abuse and dependence. A number of medications that were initially developed to treat other disorders have been used to treat the behavioral disorders often associated with cocaine abuse and dependence. Unfortunately, none are considered to be highly effective for either cocaine detoxification or the maintenance of abstinence. However, the limitations of the medications currently available should not lead investigators to give up their search, because medication is only one element of humane and comprehensive therapy for persons with drug dependence. There is compelling evidence that many cocaine abusers have had major psychological and psychosocial impairments that contributed to and may have been compounded by subsequent problems of drug dependence. These impairments include cognitive and learning disorders, interpersonal and social problems, and legal and financial difficulties. [We] stressed the heterogeneity among cocaine abusers and the need to develop specialized treatment for clinically distinct subgroups. It is axiomatic that treatment should be selected on the basis of all biomedical and psychosocial factors associated with the patient's illness.

AMPHETAMINES AND RELATED DRUGS

Amphetamine (see Figure 5.1) and a variety of compounds either structurally or pharmacologically similar to amphetamine produce a variety of effects on both the CNS and the autonomic nervous system.* These drugs are also called *sympathomimetic agents* because they mimic the actions of adrenaline (epinephrine, one of the transmitters of our "sympathetic" nervous system). They produce vasoconstriction, hypertension, tachycardia, and other signs and symptoms of our normal alerting response. The drugs also stimulate the CNS, producing tremor, restlessness, increased motor activity, agitation, insomnia, and loss of appetite (anorexia). These actions result from an indirect action involving the presynaptic release of dopamine and norepinephrine and, to a lesser extent, direct stimulation of postsynaptic catecholamine receptors.

At one time or another (continuing until today), these drugs have been used therapeutically to treat a multitude of disorders. Between 1935 and 1946, a list of 39 conditions for which amphetamine could be used in treatment was developed. The list included schizophrenia, morphine addiction, tobacco smoking, heart block, head injury, radiation sickness, hypotension, seasickness, severe hiccups, and caffeine dependence. During World War II amphetamine was used as an aid to fight fatigue and enhance the performance of servicemen.

In some individuals, therapeutic use can lead to compulsive abuse. Large-scale abuse (usually oral ingestion of amphetamine tablets) began in the late 1940s, primarily by students and truck drivers in efforts to maintain wakefulness, temporarily increase alertness, and delay sleep. Amphetamines continued to be used (and abused) as appetite suppressants, despite the fact that the anoretic effect persists only over the first two weeks of treatment, after which time it diminishes. In the late 1960s, the abuse pattern of amphetamines changed with the advent of injectable forms of amphetamine. These injectable products (by legitimate manufacturers) have been discontinued.

---

*The *autonomic nervous system* (ANS) is frequently called the "visceral" nervous system because it regulates and maintains the homeostasis of the body's internal organs. It controls the function of the heart, the flow of blood, and the functioning of the digestive tract, and it regulates other internal functions that are essential for maintaining the balance necessary for life. The ANS is divided into two subdivisions—the *sympathetic* and the *parasympathetic*. The latter can be viewed as maintaining our "vegetative" functions, while the former functions to handle the body's response to stress, fright, fear, or other responses that demand an immediate alerting response. Neurotransmitters in the sympathetic division of the ANS include epinephrine (adrenaline), norepinephrine, and dopamine.

Today, interest in amphetamine-like compounds involves two separate areas: (1) therapeutic use in the treatment of narcolepsy, attention deficit disorder, and obesity and (2) compulsive misuse and dependency, especially with the amphetamine derivative *methamphetamine* in its various illicit forms and routes of administration (including the smoking of free-based methamphetamine, termed *ICE*).

Mechanism of Action

The amphetamines exert virtually all of their CNS effects by causing the release of newly synthesized catecholamines (especially dopamine) from presynaptic storage sites in nerve terminals.[37,38] The behavioral stimulation and increased psychomotor activity appear to follow from the resulting stimulation of the dopamine receptors in the mesolimbic system (including the nucleus accumbens). The high-dose stereotypical behavior (including constant repetition of meaningless acts) appears to involve dopamine neurons in the caudate nucleus and putamen of the basal ganglia.

The actions leading to an increase in aggressive behavior are complex. Clinically, such behavioral stimulant action is seen primarily in adults, often observed as increases in stereotypical, repetitive behaviors; in children, amphetamines are used therapeutically to reduce aggressive behavior and activities characteristic of ADHD, although in adults with a history of ADHD, behavioral calming can occur.[38]

Pharmacological Effects

The various amphetamines exert their peripheral and central actions largely by causing the release of newly synthesized norepinephrine and dopamine from presynaptic nerve terminals[37] (see Figure 5.3). All the physical and behavioral effects of the amphetamines follow from this action. Note that the release of dopamine increases the amount of dopamine available to the postsynaptic receptor, much as does cocaine. Thus, because both drugs have the net effect of increasing the amount of dopamine available (albeit through two different mechanisms), the net effects of the two drugs are quite similar. Indeed, individuals who have used cocaine have difficulty distinguishing between the subjective effects of 8 to 10 milligrams of cocaine and 10 milligrams of dextroamphetamine when both are administered intravenously.

The pharmacological responses to amphetamines vary with the specific drug, the dose, and the route of administration. In general, with amphetamine itself, effects may be categorized as those observed at low to moderate doses (5 to 50 milligrams), usually administered orally, and those observed at high doses (more than approximately 100 milligrams), often administered intravenously. These dose ranges are not the same for all amphetamines. For example, dextroamphetamine is three to four times more potent than amphetamine. Low to moderate doses of dextroamphetamine range from 2.5 to 20 milligrams, while high doses are 50 milligrams or more. Because methamphetamine is even more potent, dose ranges must be lowered even more.

At low doses, all amphetamines increase blood pressure, slow heart rate, relax bronchial muscle, and produce a variety of other responses that follow from the body's alerting response. In the CNS, amphetamine is a potent psychomotor stimulant, producing increased alertness, euphoria, excitement, wakefulness, a reduced sense of fatigue, loss of appetite, mood elevation, increased motor and speech activity, and a feeling of power. Although task performance is improved, dexterity may deteriorate. When short-duration, high-intensity energy output is desired, such as during an athletic competition, a user's performance may be enhanced, despite the fact that his or her dexterity and fine motor skills may be impaired. Amphetamines are excreted in the urine and are easily detectable for up to 48 hours after use.

At moderate doses (20 to 50 milligrams), additional effects of amphetamine include stimulation of respiration, slight tremors, restlessness, a greater increase in motor activity, insomnia, and agitation. In addition, amphetamines prevent fatigue, suppress appetite, promote wakefulness, and cause sleep deprivation.

Persons who chronically use high doses of amphetamine suffer from a different set of drug effects. Stereotypical behaviors include continual, purposeless, repetitive acts; sudden outbursts of aggression and violence; paranoid delusions; and severe anorexia. The harmful effects that are seen in the high-dose user include psychosis and abnormal mental conditions, weight loss, skin sores, infections resulting from neglected health care, and a variety of other consequences that occur both because of the actions of the drug itself and because of poor eating habits, lack of sleep, or the use of unsterile equipment for intravenous injections. Most high-dose users show a progressive deterioration in their social, personal, and occupational affairs. Also seen is amphetamine psychosis with paranoid ideation; many addicts must be hospitalized intermittently for treatment of episodes of psychosis. Today, psychosis is especially seen in people who abuse methamphetamine.

The toxic dose of amphetamine varies widely. Severe reactions can occur from low doses (20 to 30 milligrams). On the other hand, persons who have not developed tolerance have survived doses of 400 to

500 milligrams. Even larger doses are tolerated by chronic users. The slogan "speed kills" not only refers to a direct fatal effect of single doses of amphetamine but also to the deteriorating mental and physical condition that occurs in the addicted user.

Dependence and Tolerance

As a potent psychomotor stimulant and behavior-reinforcing agent, the amphetamines are prone to compulsive abuse. Physical dependence is readily induced in both man and laboratory animals and follows a classical positive conditioning model (the positive reward leads to further drug use). Once drug use is stopped, the individual experiences a withdrawal syndrome, although it is less dramatic than the withdrawal associated with either narcotics (see Chapter 10) or barbiturates (see Chapter 2). As Bernstein (1995)[32] states:

> Withdrawal symptoms associated with the amphetamines include increased appetite, weight gain, decreased energy, and increased need for sleep. Patients may develop a voracious appetite and sleep for several days after amphetamines are discontinued. Paranoid symptoms may persist during drug withdrawal, but generally do not develop as a result of withdrawal. The patient suddenly discontinuing amphetamine use may develop severe depression and become suicidal. Management of amphetamine withdrawal does not require detoxification, but does require appropriate and cautious clinical observation of the patient, recognition of depression, and treatment with an appropriate antidepressant drug if clinically necessary. ... High potency antipsychotic drugs, such as haloperidol [see Chapter 9], generally in relatively low doses, may be necessary [to treat paranoid reactions].

Tolerance rapidly develops and can necessitate higher and higher doses, which starts a vicious circle of drug use and withdrawal. At this point, tolerance to the euphoriant effects develops, and periods of prolonged "binging" begin. This tolerance combined with the memory of drug-induced highs leads to further drug intake, social withdrawal, and a focus on procuring drugs.

"ICE": A "Free Base" Form of Methamphetamine

Methamphetamine is a more potent drug than dextroamphetamine, and it is easily synthesized in clandestine laboratories from readily obtainable chemicals. In animals, methamphetamine has been implicated as a neurotoxic agent, although such toxicity has not been demonstrated in humans. As a drug of abuse, methamphetamine is also known as "speed," "crystal," "crank," "go," and "ICE," with considerable overlap in nomenclature with other amphetamines except for ICE, which refers to the smokable form of methamphetamine.[39]

Like cocaine, methamphetamine (as the hydrochloride salt) is broken down at the temperatures that must be achieved for it to be vaporized for smoking. However, when converted to its base, methamphetamine can be effectively vaporized and inhaled in smoke. Methamphetamine hydrochloride is used orally, by intravenous injection, and by snorting; the base form (ICE) is administered by smoking. Absorbed rapidly through the lungs and mucous membranes, the rapidity of ICE's absorption approaches the rapidity of action that follows intravenous injection of methamphetamine hydrochloride. Thus, ICE is to methamphetamine as crack is to cocaine, the free-base, concentrated, high-potency smokable form of the parent compound. Unlike crack, methamphetamine has an extremely long half-life, resulting in an intense drug action that can persist for many hours.

Abuse of ICE began in Hawaii, spread to Japan (where it is called "shabu"), then came to California and spread throughout the United States.[39] As a form of methamphetamine, ICE is between 90 and 100 percent pure. It is more potent and longer lasting than cocaine, and chronic use can result in serious and persistent psychiatric, cardiovascular, metabolic, and neuromuscular changes.

Pharmacokinetics

Smoking ICE results in its near-immediate absorption into plasma, with additional absorption continuing over the next 4 hours. The blood level then progressively declines.[40] The biological half-life of methamphetamine is more than 11 hours.[41] After distribution to the brain, about 60 percent of the methamphetamine is slowly metabolized in the liver, and the end products are excreted through the kidneys, along with unmetabolized methamphetamine (about 40 percent is excreted unchanged) and small amounts of the pharmacologically active metabolite amphetamine.

Effects and Toxicity

The effects of methamphetamine closely resemble and are frequently indistinguishable from those of cocaine. Both are potent psychomotor stimulants and positive reinforcers; self-administration is extremely difficult to control and modify, especially in abusers who use the drug either by injection or by smoking. Repeated high doses of methamphetamine are associated with violent behavior and paranoid psychosis. Such doses cause long-lasting decreases in dopamine and serotonin in the brain. These changes appear to be irreversible, because the chemical effects can persist for more than a year after drug administration. This toxic effect is directed at the neurons that manufacture dopamine and serotonin, and the biochemical changes do not appear to be expressed in gross behavioral changes. Permanent neurochemical alterations, however, may be expressed as alterations in sleep or sexual function, depression, movement disorders, or schizophrenia.

As discussed earlier, prolonged cocaine use can result in psychoses resembling paranoid schizophrenia. A similar pattern of acute delusional and psychotic behavior occurs after smoking ICE. However, unlike cocaine, ICE-induced psychosis can persist for days or weeks and can occur much earlier. Fatalities reported to date have resulted from cardiac toxicity manifested as either pulmonary edema or heart failure.[42] A recent case report has associated the smoking of ICE with recurrent corneal ulcerations.[43] Undoubtedly, more information on methamphetamine toxicity will come to light as the use of ICE increases in the United States.

Therapeutic Uses of Amphetamines and Related Stimulants

The medical uses of amphetamines today are limited and include (1) treatment of narcolepsy, (2) treatment of attention deficit disorder, and (3) treatment of obesity.

Narcolepsy

Narcolepsy is a relatively uncommon condition characterized by attacks of irresistible sleepiness that disrupts the patient's daily life. The pathologic sleepiness is sometimes accompanied by *cataplexy*, which is a bilateral, sudden loss of muscle tone (motor paresis) without loss of consciousness. Preceding or accompanying sleep attacks can be *hypnagogic hallucinations*, which are vivid, often terrifying, usually visual, hallucinatory experiences; the hallucinations can lead to delusional behavior that has been misdiagnosed as schizophrenia.[44] In 1994 standard recommendations for the diagnosis and treatment of narcolepsy were published.[45]

Treatment of narcolepsy consists of both nonpharmacologic and pharmacologic interventions. Nonpharmacologic interventions are reviewed by Garma and Marchand (1994)[46] and consist of behavioral management (sleep habit training and daytime naps), medical and psychiatric care, and treatment addressing the psychosocial impact of narcolepsy. Pharmacologic interventions rely primarily on the utilization of behavioral stimulants. Drugs with well-documented clinical efficacy include methylphenidate (Ritalin), dextroamphetamine (Dexedrine), pemoline (Cylert), and methamphetamine (Methedrine).[47-50] Other, less frequently used drugs reported to have successfully treated narcolepsy include the clinical antidepressants (see Chapter 7) imipramine[51] and fluoxetine,[52] as well as selegeline (Eldepryl; see Appendix III),[53] a drug also used in the treatment of Parkinson's disease.

Attention Deficit Hyperactivity Disorder (ADHD)

Amphetamines have been used since about 1936 for treating attention deficit hyperactivity disorder (ADHD) in children and adolescents. Treatment started with the use of amphetamine and dextroamphetamine and has progressed over the years to the extensive use of methylphenidate (Ritalin), pemoline (Cylert), several of the clinical antidepressants, a variety of other compounds, including clonidine, lithium, carbamazepine, guanfacine, and bupropion, and (in 1997) to a return to amphetamine use (Adderall).

Background. ADHD is the most common psychological disorder of childhood, estimated to affect 3 percent to 9 percent of school-age children.[54,55] Today, 1.29 million children are being treated with stimulant medication.[56] ADHD is characterized by age-inappropriate problems with attention, learning, impulse control, and (usually) hyperactivity. ADHD persists beyond childhood and into adulthood in about 40 to 60 percent of affected individuals.[57] It is associated with a tenfold increase of antisocial personality disorder, up to a fivefold increased risk of drug abuse, a twenty-fivefold increase in risk for institutionalization for delinquency, and up to a ninefold increased risk for incarceration.[54]

> ADHD . . . in adults is associated with considerable disability and distress; it remains an underdiagnosed and undertreated adult psychiatric disorder. . . . Adult ADHD is an orphan diagnosis in both adult and child clinics. Child clinicians do not usually follow up patients into adulthood, and adult ADHD often is not considered in adult psychiatric settings.[54]

There is a remarkable incidence of comorbid or concomitant disease in individuals affected with ADHD. As many as two-thirds of elementary school-age children with ADHD who are referred for clinical evaluation have at least one other diagnosable psychiatric disorder.[55] Concomitant diseases include conduct disorder, oppositional defiant disorder,[58] learning disorders, anxiety disorders, and mood disorders (especially depression[59]). Cantwell (1996)[55] states that "The internalizing problems such as anxiety and mood disorders may be underreported by parents and teachers, who are better able to see the externalizing behaviors."

Several recent reports address some of the issues predisposing a person to ADHD and comorbid disorders.[60–62] Youths whose parents have experienced affective disorders or other psychopathology and/or who come from families that are disorganized or suffer familial dysfunction are at high risk for ADHD and/or affective disorder. The high incidence of familial linkage with childhood ADHD implies not only environmental influences but also a possible genetic component with an underlying demonstrable neurological deficit. Indeed, in a laboratory model of ADHD, altered dopaminergic function has been demonstrated in the prefrontal cortex and nucleus accumbens.[63] Levy (1991)[64] reviews a dopamine hypothesis of ADHD, invoking a "disorder of polysynaptic dopaminergic circuits, between prefrontal and striate centers." This theory is consistent with our discussion of the mechanism of action of amphetamine and cocaine in the nucleus accumbens. Pliska, McCracken, and Maas (1996)[65] further review this concept and present a multistage hypothesis that emphasizes the interaction of central catecholamine transmitters in the modulation of attention and impulse control (see Figure 5.6). In ADHD there may be a dysregulation of this system so that a "posterior attention system" is not effectively "primed" to sensory input, and an "anterior executive attention system," involving dopamine, becomes disinhibited through reduced dopaminergic activity.[65] Such a system is in agreement with the data of Coull (1994)[66] and explains, as we will see next, the utility of behavioral stimulants in treating ADHD.

Pharmacological Treatment. Stimulant drugs improve behavior and learning ability in 60 to 80 percent of children who are correctly diagnosed.[58,67] The agents differ primarily in terms of their pharmacokinetics (see Table 5.2). As Cantwell (1996)[55] states:

> The primary psychopharmacological agents used to treat ADHD are the CNS stimulants. The prototype drugs are dextroamphetamine, methylphenidate, and pemoline. There are a number of amphetamines, including methamphetamine and dextroamphetamine, but dextroamphetamine probably enjoys the greatest use. Methylphenidate is probably used more than any of the other stimulants.

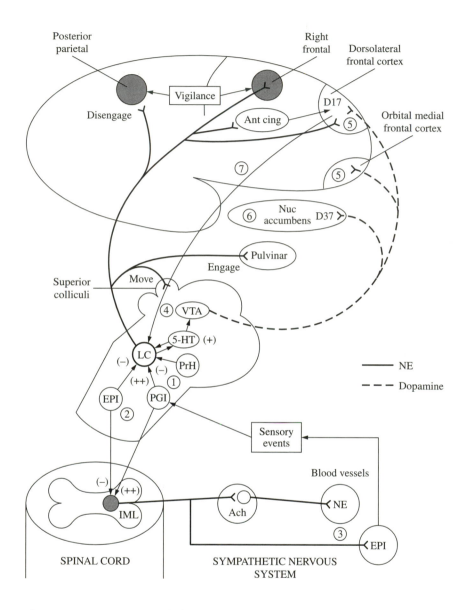

Figure 5.6 Interacting catecholamine systems in ADHD. Ant cing = anterior cingulate gyrus; Nuc accumbens = nucleus accumbens; VTA = ventral tegmental area; 5-HT = serotonin; LC = locus ceruleus; PrH = propositus hypoglossi; EPI = epinephrine; PGI = paragigantocellularis; IML = intermediolateral cell column; Ach = acetylcholine; NE = norepinephrine. [Adapted from Pliska, McCracken, and Maas (1996),[65] figure 1, p. 266.]

TABLE 5.2 Psychostimulants used to treat attention deficit hyperactivity disorder

Feature	Methylphenidate	Pemoline	Dextro-amphetamine
Elimination half-life	2–3	2–12	6–7
Time to peak plasma concentration (T_{max})	1–3	1–5	3–4
Onset of behavioral effect	1	3–4 weeks	1
Duration of behavioral effect	3–4	Not available	4
Daily dose range			
mg/kg/day	0.6–0.7	0.5–3.0	0.3–1.25
mg/day	10–60	37.5–112.5	5–40

From P. G. Janicak, J. M. Davis, S. H. Preskorn, and F. J. Ayd, Jr., *Principles and Practice of Psychopharmacotherapy* (Baltimore: Williams & Wilkins, 1993), tab. 14.1, p. 493.
Note: All time values are given in hours unless otherwise noted.

Of these drugs, *methylphenidate* accounts for 90 percent of the medication given to children for the treatment of ADHD. Methylphenidate is of rapid onset and short duration; thus, it must be administered at both breakfast time and lunchtime. It is not administered in the evening to permit the blood level to drop, allowing for normal sleep. The short half-life is a problem in some children who experience an end-of-dose rebound in dysfunctional behavior. Sustained-release preparations of methylphenidate have been disappointing.

Because methylphenidate as a behavioral stimulant resembles both the amphetamines and cocaine, concern has arisen about the potential reinforcing effects and its abuse liability. Because both cocaine and methylphenidate potentiate dopamine neurotransmission, Volkow et al. (1995)[68] studied the effects of the two drugs, comparing their concentrations in the brain with the subjective "high." The data for cocaine in Figure 5.2 illustrate that the decline in the high parallels its fast removal from the brain. In contrast, the rate of clearance of methylphenidate from the brain is extremely slow (also shown in Figure 5.2), with an obvious dissociation between its clearance and the decline of the high. The authors speculate that this slow rate of clearance is a limiting factor in promoting its frequent self-administration. In other words, the persistence of drug in the brain reduces the potential of subsequent doses to induce the high that leads to compulsive abuse. Spencer et al. (1995)[59] report on the efficacy of methylphenidate in adults with a history of childhood-onset ADHD.

Pemoline (Cylert) has a much longer but more variable half-life and can be effective in once-daily dosage. There is a clinical impression that pemoline is somewhat less effective than methylphenidate and that its extremely slow onset of effect limits clinical usefulness. Pelham et al. (1995)[69] dispute this impression, offering clinical evidence of rapid-onset (2-hour), long-lasting (7-hour) improvements on measures of classroom behavior and academic performance, if the doses used are high enough to achieve efficacy. One limitation of pemoline is potentially fatal liver damage in children receiving the drug. Although the incidence is low (1 to 3 percent) and any damage is reversible if recognized early, this toxicity limits use of pemoline to instances where other drug and nondrug therapies have failed.

Amphetamines still provide a treatment option to methylphenidate; both *dextroamphetamine* (Dexedrine) and *amphetamine* (Adderall) are promoted for use.

Even though the stimulant drugs are considered drugs of first choice in the treatment of ADHD, about 10 to 30 percent of ADHD individuals do not respond adequately and are considered to be "treatment resistant." Therefore, recent research has focused on the clinical evaluation of nonstimulant agents. Antidepressants (especially *nortriptyline*, a tricyclic antidepressant) have been extensively studied. In one study of "nonresponders" to other medications, 84 percent of which had at least one comorbid diagnosis with ADHD, 76 percent were claimed to respond positively to nortriptyline.[70] However, rare cases of potentially fatal cardiac toxicities associated with tricyclic antidepressant use in adolescents pose a considerable limitation.[58,67] Initial reports on other antidepressants indicate some usefulness of *fluoxetine* (Prozac) and *buproprion* (Wellbutrin), although effectiveness is generally less than that obtained with the stimulants.[71] All these antidepressants are discussed in Chapter 7.

Other drugs reported to have positive effects in the treatment of ADHD include *carbamazepine* (Tegretol)[72] and two CNS-acting antihypertensive (blood pressure–lowering), catecholamine agonists (stimulants)—*clonidine* (Catapres)[73] and *guanfacine* (Tenex).[74,75] Use of these agents in combination with methylphenidate may result in improved therapy at a lower dose of the stimulant. Indeed, the increasingly recognized comorbidity of ADHD with other psychiatric disorders is leading to increasing utilization of combined pharmacotherapy in individuals less than adequately responsive to a single agent.[76]

In summary, the treatment of childhood and adolescent ADHD remains controversial, especially the management of "treatment-resistant" youths. No well-designed, long-term study comparing the efficacy of various treatments has yet been published. However, Greenhill et al.[77] discuss one soon-to-be-published study. Designed to be completed in 1997 and published in 1998, the National Institute of Mental Health (NIMH) Collaborative Multisite Multimodel Treatment Study of Children with Attention-Deficit/Hyperactivity Disorder will be the largest psychiatric treatment study of children to date. Hopefully, it will provide answers regarding indications for and efficacy of the various approaches to the pharmacotherapy of childhood and adolescent ADHD.

Obesity

Obesity is a major public health problem affecting more than 40 percent of Americans, in whom it is associated with increased risk of diabetes and cardiovascular diseases, among others. At least 47 million Americans are 30 percent or more above ideal body weight and are considered to be seriously obese, and obesity contributes to over 300,000 deaths per year.* Obesity is an ongoing, chronic disease, and it is appropriately treated as a chronic disease. Obesity is rarely cured; palliation is a realistic goal. Weight gain (relapse) following cessation of drug therapy is not necessarily a sign of drug failure but simply a sign that when a drug is not taken, it does not work.[78] Any planned drug therapy must be combined with behavior modification, diet correction, and exercise.

For decades, the amphetamines were used in treating obesity, but their use has always been extremely controversial. Side effects, dependency, addiction, and the rapid development of tolerance have always been considered impediments to their use. As stated in the package insert of each of these compounds:

> The natural history of obesity is measured in years, whereas [all studies reviewed] are restricted to a few weeks duration: Thus, the total impact of drug-induced weight loss over that of diet alone must be considered clinically limited.

Compounds acting through dopamine-augmented anorexia have been commercially available for many years and include

---

*Obese individuals who lose even small amounts of weight are likely to lower their blood pressure, reduce abnormally high levels of blood glucose, bring down levels of cholesterol and triglycerides, reduce sleep apnea or irregular breathing during sleep, decrease the risk of osteoarthritis of the weight-bearing joints, decrease depression, and increase self-esteem.[74]

- benzphetamine (Didrex)
- phendimetrazine (Anorex, Oblan, Phendiet, Wehless)
- diethylpropion (Tenuate, Tepanol)
- mazindol (Mazenor, Sanorex)
- phentermine (Fastin, Ionamin, Phentrol, Adipex-P, Oby-Trim)
- phenylpropanolamine (Dexatrim)
- dextroamphetamine/amphetamine combination (Obetrol)

One researcher stated, "No clinical need exists for any of these drugs in the treatment of obesity."[78] Nonetheless, one of these dopaminergic agents (*phentermine*) has found recent popularity used in combination with a serotonin-potentiating agent (*fenfluramine*); the combination is known as *fen-phen*. Another drug, *sibutramine* (Meridia), acts as both a norepinephrine- and a serotonin-reuptake inhibitor and reduces weight in obese patients.[79] In animals, *sibutramine* enhances satiety and increases energy expenditure. However, the U.S. Food and Drug Administration (FDA) in late 1996 delayed the manufacturer's request to market the drug because of a worrisome side-effect—small but significant increases in blood pressure, increases that could, at least theoretically, increase cardiovascular toxicity in obese patients. The drug will probably appear on the commercial market shortly.

Among the serotonin-potentiating anti-obesity agents (discussed in Chapter 7), drugs such as *fenfluramine* (Pondimin) act to "partially inhibit the reuptake of serotonin and to release serotonin from nerve endings. This increased serotonin in the neuronal [synaptic] cleft is believed to reduce food intake."[78] Furthermore, "fenfluramine combined with phentermine [as fen-phen] enhanced the magnitude of weight loss over and above what could be achieved with the best behavior modification, exercise, and nutrition program, and the effect continued for nearly four years."[78,80] Weintraub and coworkers (1992)[80] concluded that fen-phen can help a person lose weight and maintain the weight loss for prolonged periods of time with little fear of developing abuse patterns of drug ingestion.

In 1996 the active isomer of fenfluramine, *dexfenfluramine* (Redux), was approved by the FDA as an aid to diet for treatment of obesity and maintenance (for up to one year) of weight loss.[81] Dexfenfluramine appears to promote serotonin release and inhibit serotonin reuptake by acting on presynaptic serotonin-releasing neurons. The active metabolite, dex-norphenfluramine, appears to directly stimulate postsynaptic serotonin receptors, further augmenting serotonin neurotransmission.[82] These actions are thought to suppress appetite and (through an antidepressant action) promote a feeling of self-worth. Both the drug and the metabolite have long half-lives, in the range of 17 and 32 hours, respectively. Curson, Gibson, and Oluyomi (1997)[83] critically review the serotonin theory of dexfenfluramine, challenging the assumption that it reduces food intake by blocking serotonin reuptake. The drug activates postsynaptic $5\text{-}HT_{2\text{-}C}$ receptors, potentiates dopamine neurotransmission, and may inhibit the appetite-stimulating action of *neuropeptide Y,* a brain protein.

Despite this rather optimistic and beneficial action to reduce food cravings and improve psychological well-being, dexfenfluramine's safety may be in question, because it possesses a rare but serious and potentially fatal side effect—the drug produces pulmonary hypertension (increased blood pressure in the blood vessels perfusing the lungs) in small numbers of patients (about 18 occurrences per million patients treated).[84] Because obese patients may develop life-threatening pulmonary hypertension without the drug (probably secondary to obesity-related sleep apnea and airway obstruction), the addition of dexfenfluramine may place patients at increased risk for this lethal complication. Since the appetite-suppressing effects of other serotonin-acting antidepressants appear to dissipate after a few weeks, it remains to be seen both whether or not the small amounts of weight loss achieved through use of dexfenfluramine persist during (or after) therapy and also whether any weight loss is worth the risk of developing pulmonary hypertension. Davis and Faulds (1996)[85] reviewed the pharmacology of dexfenfluramine and its role in the management of obesity.

To summarize the current status of antiobesity drug research, it was recently stated:

> With more than a third of the U.S. population alone now deemed clinically obese, the market for new drugs indicated for the modulation of food intake, energy balance, and the regulation of body weight is, to say the least, enormous. Add to the equation their potential applications in the treatment of obesity-related comorbidities, and few would argue that the market for these agents may well represent *the largest target population in the history of modern medicine* [italics added]. But despite decades of intensive research, the "magic bullet" continues to elude us.[86]

NOTES

1. M. S. Gold, "Cocaine (and Crack): Clinical Aspects," in J. H. Lowinson, P. Ruiz, R. B. Millman, and J. G. Langrod, eds., *Substance Abuse: A Comprehensive Textbook,* 2nd ed. (Baltimore: Williams & Wilkins, 1992), 205.

2. G. Das, "Cocaine Abuse in North America: A Milestone in History," *Journal of Clinical Pharmacology* 33 (1993): 296–310.

3. J. H. Mendelson and N. K. Mello, "Management of Cocaine Abuse and Dependence," *New England Journal of Medicine* 334 (1996): 965–972.

4. D. K. Hatsukami and M. W. Fishman, "Crack Cocaine and Cocaine Hydrochloride: Are the Differences Myth or Reality?," *Journal of the American Medical Association* 276 (1996): 1580–1588.

5. W. W. Weddington, "Cocaine: Diagnosis and Treatment," *Psychiatric Clinics of North America* 16 (1993): 88.

6. P. Jatlow, J. D. Elsworth, C. W. Bradberry, et al., "Cocaethylene: A Neuropharmacologically Active Metabolite Associated with Concurrent Cocaine-Ethanol Ingestion," *Life Sciences* 8 (1991): 1787–1794.

7. W. L. Hearn, D. D. Flynn, G. W. Hime, et al., "Cocaethylene: A Unique Cocaine Metabolite Displays High Affinity for the Dopamine Transporter," *Journal of Neurochemistry* 56 (1991): 698–701.

8. W. L. Hearn, S. Rose, J. Wagner, et al., "Cocaethylene Is More Potent than Cocaine in Mediating Lethality," *Pharmacology, Biochemistry, and Behavior* 39 (1991): 531–533.

9. F. H. Gawin, "Cocaine Addiction, Psychology, and Neurophysiology," *Science* 251 (1991): 1580–1586.

10. J.-T. Qiao, P. M. Dougherty, R. C. Wiggins, and N. Dafny, "Effects of Microiontophoretic Application of Cocaine, Alone and with Receptor Antagonists, upon the Neurons of the Medial Prefrontal Cortex, Nucleus Accumbens and Caudate Nucleus of Rats," *Neuropharmacology* 29 (1990): 379–385.

11. S. L. Peterson, S. A. Olsta, and R. T. Matthews, "Cocaine Enhances Medial Prefrontal Cortex Neuron Response to Ventral Tegmental Area Activation," *Brain Research Bulletin* 24 (1990): 267–273.

12. L. C. Einhorn, P. A. Johansen, and F. J. White, "Electrophysiological Effects of Cocaine in the Mesoaccumbens Dopamine System: Studies in the Ventral Tegmental Area," *Journal of Neuroscience* 8 (1988): 100–112.

13. N. Uchimura and R. A. North, "Actions of Cocaine on Rat Nucleus Accumbens Neurons in Vitro," *British Journal of Pharmacology* 99 (1990): 736–740.

14. W. L. Woolverton and K. M. Johnson, "Neurobiology of Cocaine Abuse," *Trends in Pharmacological Sciences* 13 (1992): 193–200.

15. S. Shimada, S. Kitayama, C.-L. Lin, et al., "Cloning and Expression of a Cocaine-Sensitive Dopamine Transporter Complementary DNA," *Science* 254 (1991): 576–578.

16. J. E. Kilty, D. Lorang, and S. G. Amara, "Cloning and Expression of a Cocaine-Sensitive Rat Dopamine Transporter," *Science* 254 (1991): 578–580.

17. M. J. Kuhar and N. S. Pilotte, "Neurochemical Changes in Cocaine Withdrawal," *Trends in Pharmacological Sciences* 17 (1996): 260–264.

18. C.-E. Johanson and M. W. Fischman, "The Pharmacology of Cocaine Related to Its Abuse," *Pharmacological Reviews* 41 (1989): 35.

19. L. R. Goldfrank and R. S. Hoffman, "The Cardiovascular Effects of Cocaine—Update 1992," in H. Sorer, ed., *Acute Cocaine Intoxication:*

Current Methods of Treatment, NIDA Research Monograph 123, Pub. No. 93-3498 (Rockville, Md.: National Institutes of Health, 1993), 70–109.

20. B. L. Miller, F. Chiang, L. McGill, T. Sadow, M. A. Goldberg, and I. Mena, "Cerebrovascular Complications from Cocaine: Possible Long-Term Sequelae," in H. Sorer, ed., *Acute Cocaine Intoxication: Current Methods of Treatment,* NIDA Research Monograph 123, Pub. No. 93-3498 (Rockville, Md.: National Institutes of Health, 1993), 129–146.

21. G. E. Billman, "Cocaine: A Review of Its Toxic Actions on Cardiac Function," *Critical Reviews in Toxicology* 25 (1995): 113–132.

22. B. J. Rounsaville, S. F. Anton, K. Carroll, et al., "Psychiatric Diagnoses of Treatment-Seeking Cocaine Abusers," *Archives of General Psychiatry* 48 (1991): 43–51.

23. "Update on Cocaine, Part II," *The Harvard Mental Health Letter* 10, no. 3 (September 1993): 2.

24. R. J. Konkol and G. D. Olsen, *Prenatal Cocaine Exposure* (Boca Raton, Fla.: CRC Press, 1996).

25. Z. N. Kain, S. Rimar, and P. G. Barash, "Cocaine Abuse in the Parturient and Effects on the Fetus and Neonate," *Anesthesia and Analgesia* 77 (1993): 835–845.

26. J. J. Volpe, "Effects of Cocaine Use on the Fetus," *New England Journal of Medicine* 327 (1992): 399–407.

27. "Update on Cocaine, Part I," *The Harvard Mental Health Letter* 10, no. 2 (August 1993): 3.

28. C. Chazotte, J. Youchah and M. C. Freda, "Cocaine Use During Pregnancy and Low Birth Weight: The Impact of Prenatal Care and Drug Treatment," *Seminars in Perinatology* 19 (1995): 293–300.

29. D. J. Birnbach, D. J. Stein, A. Grunebaum, B. I. Danzer, and D. M. Thys, "Cocaine Screening of Parturients Without Prenatal Care: An Evaluation of a Rapid Screening Assay," *Anesthesia and Analgesia* 84 (1997): 76–79.

30. K. Silverman, S. T. Higgins, R. K. Brooner, et al., "Sustained Cocaine Abstinence in Methadone Patients Through Voucher-Based Reinforcement Therapy," *Archives of General Psychiatry* 53 (1996): 409–415.

31. F. H. Gawin and H. D. Kleber, "Abstinence Symptomatology and Psychiatric Diagnoses in Cocaine Abusers," *Archives of General Psychiatry* 43 (1986): 107–113.

32. J. G. Bernstein, *Drug Therapy in Psychiatry,* 3rd ed. (St. Louis: Mosby, 1995), 494–498.

33. A. Margolin, T. R. Kosten, S. K. Avants, et al., "A Multicenter Trial of Buproprion for Cocaine Dependence in Methadone-Maintained Patients," *Drug and Alcohol Dependence* 40 (1995): 125–131.

34. D. J. Calcagnetti, B. J. Keck, L. A. Quatrella, and M. D. Schechter, "Blockade of Cocaine-Induced Conditioned Place Preference: Relevance to Cocaine Abuse Therapeutics," *Life Sciences* 56 (1995): 475–483.

35. K. M. Carroll, B. J. Bruce, J. Rounsaville, et al. "Psychotherapy and Pharmacotherapy for Ambulatory Cocaine Abusers," *Archives of General Psychiatry* 51 (1994): 177–187.

36. Work Group on Substance Use Disorders, "Practice Guidelines for the

Treatment of Patients with Substance Use Disorders: Alcohol, Cocaine, Opioids," *Practice Guidelines* (Washington, D.C.: American Psychiatric Association, 1996), 209–319.

37. P. M. Groves, L. J. Ryan, M. Diana, S. Y. Young, and L. J. Fisher, "Neuronal Actions of Amphetamine in the Rat Brain," in K. Saqhar and E. DeSouza, eds., *Pharmacology and Toxicology of Amphetamine and Related Designer Drugs*, NIDA Research Monograph 94 (Rockville, Md.: National Institute on Drug Abuse, 1989), 127–145.

38. G. R. King and E. H. Ellinwood, Jr., "Amphetamines and Other Stimulants," in J. H. Lowinson, P. Ruiz, R. B. Millman, and J. G. Langrod, eds., *Substance Abuse: A Comprehensive Textbook*, 2nd ed. (Baltimore: Williams & Wilkins, 1992), 247–266.

39. D. K. Beebe and E. Walley, "Smokable Methamphetamine ('ICE'): An Old Drug in a Different Form," *American Family Physician* 51 (1995): 449–453.

40. R. M. Perez, W. R. White, S. A. McDonald, J. M. Hill, and A. R. Jeffcoat, "Clinical Effects of Methamphetamine Vapor Inhalation," *Life Sciences* 49 (1991): 953–959.

41. C. E. Cook, A. R. Jeffcoat, J. M. Hill, et al., "Pharmacokinetics of Methamphetamine Self-Administration to Human Subjects by Smoking S-(+)-Methamphetamine Hydrochloride," *Drug Metabolism and Disposition: The Biological Fate of Chemicals* 21 (1993): 717–723.

42. R. Hong, E. Matsuyama, and K. Nur, "Cardiomyopathy Associated with the Smoking of Crystal," *Journal of the American Medical Association* 265 (1991): 1152–1154.

43. R. S. Chuck, J. M. Williams, M. A. Goldberg, and A. J. Lubniewski, "Recurrent Corneal Ulcerations Associated with Smokable Methamphetamine Abuse," *American Journal of Ophthalmology* 121 (1996): 571–572.

44. A. B. Douglass, J. E. Shipley, R. F. Haines, et al., "Schizophrenia, Narcolepsy, and HLA-DR15, DQ6," *Biological Psychiatry* 34 (1993) 773–780.

45. American Sleep Disorders Association, Standards of Practice Committee, "Practice Parameters for the Use of Stimulants in the Treatment of Narcolepsy," *Sleep* 17 (1994): 348–351.

46. L. Garma and F. Marchand, "Non-Pharmacological Approaches to the Treatment of Narcolepsy," *Sleep* 17, Suppl. 8 (1994): S97–S102.

47. G. E. Francisco and C. B. Ivanhoe, "Successful Treatment of Post-Traumatic Narcolepsy with Methylphenidate: A Case Report," *American Journal of Physical Medicine & Rehabilitation* 75 (1996): 63–65.

48. M. M. Mitler, "Evaluation of Treatment with Stimulants in Narcolepsy," *Sleep* 17, Suppl. 8 (1994): S103–106.

49. M. M. Mitler, M. S. Aldrich, G. F. Koob, and V. P. Zarcone, "Narcolepsy and Its Treatment with Stimulants: ASDA Standards of Practice," *Sleep* 17 (1994): 352–371.

50. M. M. Mitler, R. Hajdukovic, and M. K. Erman, "Treatment of Narcolepsy with Methamphetamine," *Sleep* 16 (1993): 306–317.

51. D. Parks, "Introduction to the Mechanism of Action of Different Treatments of Narcolepsy," *Sleep* 17, Suppl. 8 (1994): S93–S96.

52. Y. K. Wing, S. Lee, H. F. Chiu, C. K. Ho, and C. N. Chen, "A Patient with Coexisting Narcolepsy and Morbid Jealousy Showing Favourable Response to Fluoxetine," *Postgraduate Medical Journal* 70 (1994): 34–36.

53. G. Mayer, K. Ewert-Meier, and K. Hephata, "Selegeline Hydrochloride Treatment in Narcolepsy: A Double-Blind, Placebo-Controlled Study," *Clinical Neuropharmacology* 18 (1995): 306–319.

54. M. H. Teicher, Y. Ito, C. A. Glod, and N. I. Barber, "Objective Measurement of Hyperactivity and Attentional Problems in ADHD," *Journal of the American Academy of Child and Adolescent Psychiatry* 35 (1996): 334–342.

55. D. P. Cantwell, "Attention Deficit Disorder: A Review of the Past 10 Years," *Journal of the American Academy of Child and Adolescent Psychiatry* 35 (1996): 978–987.

56. K. O'Toole, A. Abramowitz, R. Morris, and M. Dulcan, "Effects of Methylphenidate on Attention and Nonverbal Learning in Children with Attention-Deficit Hyperactivity Disorder," *Journal of the American Academy of Child and Adolescent Psychiatry* 36 (1997): 531–538.

57. T. Spencer, T. Wilens, J. Biederman, et al., "A Double-Blind, Crossover Comparison of Methylphenidate and Placebo in Adults with Childhood-Onset Attention-Deficit Hyperactivity Disorder," *Archives of General Psychiatry* 52 (1995): 434–443.

58. R. B. Eiraldi, T. J. Power, and C. M. Nezu, "Patterns of Comorbidity Associated with Subtypes of Attention-Deficit/Hyperactivity Disorder Among 6- to 12-Year-Old Children," *Journal of the American Academy of Child and Adolescent Psychiatry* 36 (1997): 503–514.

59. C. Z. Garrison, J. L. Waller, S. P. Cuffe, et al.,"Incidence of Major Depressive Disorder and Dysthymia in Young Adolescents," *Journal of the American Academy of Child and Adolescent Psychiatry* 36 (1997): 458–465.

60. J. Biederman, S. Milberger, S. V. Faraone, et al., "Family-Environment Risk Factors for Attention-Deficit Hyperactivity Disorder," *Archives of General Psychiatry* 52 (1995): 464–470.

61. J. Biederman, S. Faraone, S. Milberger, et al., "Predictors of Persistence and Remission of ADHD into Adolescence: Results from a Four-Year Prospective Follow-up Study," *Journal of the American Academy of Child and Adolescent Psychiatry* 35 (1996): 343–351.

62. W. R. Beardslee, M. B. Keller, R. Seifer, et al., "Prediction of Adolescent Affective Disorder: Effects of Prior Parental Affective Disorders and Child Psychopathology," *Journal of the American Academy of Child and Adolescent Psychiatry* 35 (1996): 279–288.

63. V. Russell, A. deVilliers, and T. Sagvolden, "Altered Dopaminergic Function in the Prefrontal Cortex, Nucleus Accumbens, and Caudate-Putamen of an Animal Model of Attention-Deficit Hyperactivity Disorder: The Spontaneously Hypertensive Rat," *Brain Research* 676 (1995): 343–351.

64. F. Levy, "The Dopamine Theory of Attention Deficit Hyperactivity Disorder," *Australian and New Zealand Journal of Psychiatry* 25 (1991): 277–283.

65. S. R. Pliska, J. T. McCracken, and J. W. Maas, "Catecholamines in Attention-Deficit Hyperactivity Disorder: Current Perspectives," *Journal of*

the American Academy of Child and Adolescent Psychiatry 35 (1996): 264–272.

66. J. T. Coull, "Pharmacological Manipulations of the Alpha 2-Noradrenergic System: Effects on Cognition," *Drugs and Aging* 5 (1994): 116–126.

67. M. Campbell and J. E. Cueva, "Psychopharmacology in Child and Adolescent Psychiatry: A Review of the Past Seven Years, Part I," *Journal of the American Academy of Child and Adolescent Psychiatry* 34 (1995): 1124–1132.

68. N. D. Volkow, Y.-S. Ding, J. S. Fowler, et al., "Is Methylphenidate Like Cocaine?" *Archives of General Psychiatry* 52 (1995): 456–463.

69. W. E. Pelham, J. M. Swanson, M. B. Furman, and H. Schwindt, "Pemoline Effects on Children with ADHD: A Time-Response by Dose-Response Analysis of Classroom Measures," *Journal of the American Academy of Child and Adolescent Psychiatry* 34 (1995): 1504–1513.

70. T. E. Wilens, J. Biederman, D. E. Geist, R. Steingard, and T. Spencer, "Nortriptyline in the Treatment of ADHD: A Chart Review of 58 Cases," *Journal of the American Academy of Child and Adolescent Psychiatry* 32 (1993): 343–349.

71. C. K. Conners, C. D. Casat, T. Gualtieri, et al., "Bupropion Hydrochloride in Attention Deficit Disorder with Hyperactivity," *Journal of the American Academy of Child and Adolescent Psychiatry* 35 (1996): 1314–1321.

72. R. R. Silva, D. M. Munoz, and M. Alpert, "Carbamazepine Use in Children and Adolescents with Features of Attention-Deficit Hyperactivity Disorder: A Meta-Analysis," *Journal of the American Academy of Child and Adolescent Psychiatry* 35 (1996): 352–358.

73. H. S. Singer, J. Brown, S. Quaskey, et al., "The Treatment of Attention-Deficit Hyperactivity Disorder in Tourette's Syndrome: A Double-Blind Placebo-Controlled Study with Clonidine and Desipramine," *Pediatrics* 95 (1995): 74–81.

74. R. D. Hunt, A. F. T. Arnsten, and M. D. Asbell, "An Open Trial of Guanfacine in the Treatment of Attention-Deficit Hyperactivity Disorder," *Journal of the American Academy of Child and Adolescent Psychiatry* 34 (1995): 50–54.

75. P. B. Chappell, M. A. Riddle, L. Scahill, et al., "Guanfacine Treatment of Comorbid Attention-Deficit Hyperactivity Disorder and Tourette's Syndrome: Preliminary Clinical Experience," *Journal of the American Academy of Child and Adolescent Psychiatry* 34 (1995): 1140–1146.

76. T. E. Wilens, T. Spencer, J. Biederman, J. Wozniak, and D. Connor, "Combined Pharmacotherapy: An Emerging Trend in Pediatric Psychopharmacology," *Journal of the American Academy of Child and Adolescent Psychiatry* 34 (1995): 110–112.

77. L. L. Greenhill, H. B. Abikoff, E. Arnold, et al., "Medication Treatment Strategies in the MTA Study: Relevance to Clinicians and Researchers," *Journal of the American Academy of Child and Adolescent Psychiatry* 35 (1996): 1304–1313.

78. G. A. Bray, "Use and Abuse of Appetite-Suppressant Drugs in the Treatment of Obesity," *Annals of Internal Medicine* 119 (1993): 708–709.

79. D. H. Ryan, P. Kaiser, and G. A. Bray, "Sibutramine: A Novel New Agent For Obesity Treatment," *Obesity Research* 3, Suppl. 4 (November 1995): 553S–559S.

80. M. Weintraub, P. R. Sundaresan, M. Madan, et al., "Long-term Weight Control Study: I–VII," *Clinical Pharmacology and Therapeutics* 51 (1992): 581–646.

81. "Dexfenfluramine For Obesity," *The Medical Letter* 38 (July 19, 1996): 64–65.

82. M. Spedding, C. Ouvry, M. Millan, J. Duhault, and C. Dacquet, "Neural Control of Dieting," *Nature* 380 (1996): 488.

83. G. Curson, E. L. Gibson, and A. O. Oluyomi, "Appetite Suppression by Commonly Used Drugs Depends on 5-HT Receptors but Not on 5-HT Availability," *Trends in Pharmacological Sciences* 18 (1997): 21–25.

84. P. Cacoub, R. Dorent, P. Nataf, et al., "Pulmonary Hypertension and Dexfenfluramine," *European Journal of Clinical Pharmacology* 48 (1995): 81–83.

85. R. Davis and D. Faulds, "Dexfenfluramine: An Updated Review of Its Therapeutic Use in the Management of Obesity," *Drugs* 52 (1996): 696–724.

86. T. Bliss, organizer, *The 1996 International Conference on Anti-Obesity Drug Targets* (Cambridge, Mass.: The BioScience Advisory Council, 1996).

Chapter 6

PSYCHOSTIMULANTS: CAFFEINE AND NICOTINE

CAFFEINE

Caffeine, the most popular and widely consumed drug in the world, is found in significant concentrations in coffee, tea, cola drinks, chocolate candy, and cocoa. As shown in Table 6.1, the average cup of coffee contains about 50 to 150 milligrams of caffeine. A 12-ounce bottle of cola contains between 35 and 55 milligrams of caffeine, much of which is added as a supplement by the manufacturer. The caffeine content of chocolate may be as high as 25 milligrams per ounce. The annual consumption of coffee in the United States is estimated at about 15 million pounds, with the daily per capita intake of caffeine averaging between 170 and 200 milligrams. Eighty percent of adults consume between three and five cups of coffee every day.

Why is there such massive consumption of a legal, widely used, and socially acceptable psychoactive drug? Certainly, caffeine must be reinforcing; otherwise there would be no compulsion to ingest the drug. If caffeine is reinforcing, does the reinforcement mechanism involve the mesolimbic system described for cocaine and the amphetamines, or is its behavioral reinforcement exerted through another mechanism? Also, given the almost universal dependence on caffeinated beverages, what is caffeine's potential for producing toxicities or physical dependency?

TABLE 6.1 Caffeine content in beverages, foods, and medicines

Item	Caffeine content	
	Average (mg)	Range
Coffee (5-ounce cup)	100	50–150
Tea (5-ounce cup)	50	25–90
Cocoa (5-ounce cup)	5	2–20
Chocolate (semisweet, baking) (1 ounce)	25	15–30
Chocolate milk (1 ounce)	5	1–10
Cola drink (12 ounces)	40	35–55
OTC stimulants (No Doz, Vivarin)	100+	
OTC analgesics (Excedrin)	65	
(Anacin, Midol, Vanquish)	33	
OTC cold remedies (Coryban-D, Triaminicin)	30	
OTC diuretics (Aqua-ban)	100	

Note: OTC, over the counter.

Pharmacokinetics

Taken orally, caffeine is rapidly absorbed; significant blood levels of caffeine are reached in 30 to 45 minutes. Complete absorption occurs over the next 90 minutes, with levels in plasma peaking in about 2 hours.

Caffeine is freely and equally distributed throughout all the water in the body. Thus, caffeine is found in almost equal concentrations in all parts of the body and the brain. Most caffeine is metabolized by the liver before it is excreted by the kidneys. Only about 10 percent of the drug is excreted unchanged. The half-life of caffeine is about 3.5 to 5 hours in most adults; it is longer in infants, pregnant women, and the elderly and shorter in smokers. Like all psychoactive drugs, caffeine freely crosses the placenta to the fetus. Eskenazi (1991)[1] states:

> Caffeine has a longer half-life in the human fetus than in the adult because the fetus does not have the liver enzymes for detoxifying caffeine. The half-life of caffeine in the pregnant woman increases from 3 to 10 hours by the latter part of pregnancy.

Concentrations of caffeine in breast milk equal or may even exceed the level that exists in the mother's plasma.

Pharmacological Effects

Behavioral Effects

Caffeine is an effective psychostimulant, ingested to "obtain a rewarding effect, usually described as feeling more alert and competent."[2] The cortex, being more sensitive to caffeine than brain stem structures, is affected first. Only at toxic doses of caffeine is the spinal cord stimulated. As a result of cerebral cortical stimulation, the earliest behavioral effects of caffeine include increased mental alertness, a faster and clearer flow of thought, wakefulness, and restlessness. Fatigue is reduced and the need for sleep is delayed.

This increased mental awareness may result in sustained intellectual effort for prolonged periods of time without significant disruption of coordinated intellectual or motor activity. However, tasks that involve delicate muscular coordination and accurate timing or arithmetic skills may be adversely affected. The effects on the cerebral cortex occur after oral doses that are as small as 100 or 200 milligrams, that is, one to two cups of coffee. Heavy consumption (12 or more cups a day, or 1.5 grams of caffeine) can cause more intense effects, such as agitation, anxiety, tremors, rapid breathing, and insomnia.

Only after massive doses (2 to 5 grams) does the spinal cord become stimulated. The lethal dose of caffeine is about 10 grams, which is equivalent to 100 cups of coffee. Thus, death from caffeine is highly unlikely, and the drug is usually considered to be relatively nontoxic. The syndrome of "caffeinism" is discussed later.

Physical Effects

Caffeine has a slight stimulant action on the heart, increasing cardiac contractility and output and dilating the coronary arteries. It should be noted, however, that caffeine exerts an opposite effect on the cerebral blood vessels; it constricts these vessels, thus decreasing blood flow to the brain. Such action can afford striking relief from headaches, especially migraines. Cardiac arrhythmias after ingesting caffeine are not uncommon, although they are rarely serious.* Other physical actions of caffeine include bronchial relaxation (an antiasthmatic effect), increased secretion of gastric acid, and increased urine output.

---

*Chopra and Morrison (1995)[3] discuss a case involving nonfatal cardiac arrhythmias after ingestion of *20 grams* of caffeine (in a suicide attempt). Although the cardiac rhythm was described as "chaotic," blood pressure was maintained and the arrhythmia was effectively resolved with standard antiarrhythmic therapy.

Mechanism of Action

The mechanism of action of caffeine involves a dose-related attachment to and blockade of adenosine receptors in the central nervous system (CNS).[4–6] Caffeine is therefore called a *competitive antagonist of adenosine* at its receptors, which are located on cell membranes both in the CNS and in the peripheral nervous system. Fredholm[7] says, "Of the known biochemical actions of caffeine, only inhibition of adenosine receptors occurs at concentrations achieved during normal human consumption of the drug." To understand the pharmacology of caffeine, we should therefore briefly examine the role of adenosine in the CNS.

Adenosine is an *autacoid** that acts on specific receptors on the surface of cells to produce behavioral sedation, to regulate the delivery of oxygen to cells, to dilate cerebral and coronary blood vessels, to produce bronchospasm (asthma), and to regulate other metabolic processes. There do not appear to be discrete adenosine pathways in the CNS; instead, adenosine, through attachment to caffeine-sensitive receptors, indirectly inhibits the release of many classes of neurotransmitters, including norepinephrine, dopamine, acetylcholine, glutamate, and GABA. The blockade of adenosine receptors by caffeine appears to increase the activity of such neurotransmitters, especially dopamine and acetylcholine. The dopaminergic augmentation is indicated by potentiation of the CNS effects of cocaine and the amphetamines and by the mild behavioral reinforcing effects of the drug, including augmentation of ventral tegmental activity but not of nucleus accumbens activity.[5,8]

Regarding the acetylcholine ("cholinergic") system:

> Acetylcholine release in the hippocampus is under tonic (continuous) inhibitory control by the neuromodulator adenosine. Orally administered caffeine enhances acetylcholine release by antagonism of local adenosine receptors. Thus, there is a possible link between adenosine receptors in the hippocampus, increased cholinergic activity, and the psychostimulant effects of caffeine.[9]

Blockade of adenosine receptors by caffeine (note the structural similarity between caffeine and adenosine in Figure 6.1) would thus account

---

*The term *autacoid*, derived from the Greek *autos* (self) and *akos* (medicine or remedy), refers to a variety of locally acting, hormone-like or neurotransmitter-like substances that regulate cellular functions. Studies involving adenosine and caffeine suggest a neuromodulatory role for adenosine, indicating that adenosine-releasing neurons constitute an important CNS depressant system that is blocked by caffeine.

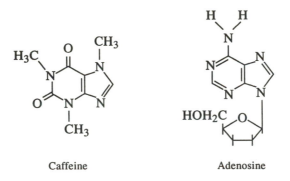

Figure 6.1 Structures of caffeine and adenosine.

for the variety of caffeine's behavioral effects. At the levels obtained after drinking a few cups of coffee, caffeine occupies 50 to 70 percent of adenosine receptors, antagonizing adenosine-induced neuronal inhibition. Shi and coworkers (1993)[10] reported that chronic administration of very high doses of caffeine (100 mg/kg/day) to mice increased the density of cerebral cortical adenosine receptors (adenosine-1 receptors), implying that chronic ingestion may increase the numbers of receptors in order to overcome their chronic drug-induced blockade (a possible mechanism of caffeine tolerance).

Side Effects

There is little evidence that caffeine plays a role in the cause of cancer in humans.[11-13] Some years ago, it was thought that caffeine use by women might be associated with the formation or enlargement of benign (noncancerous) lumps (fibrocystic lesions) in the breasts; current opinion is that no causative relationship exists.[13]

Caffeinism

Caffeinism is a clinical syndrome, characterized by both CNS and peripheral symptoms, produced by the overuse of caffeine. CNS symptoms include anxiety, insomnia, and mood changes. Peripheral symptoms include tachycardia, hypertension, cardiac arrhythmias, and gastrointestinal disturbances. Caffeinism is usually dose related, with doses higher than about 500 to 1,000 milligrams (1 gram) per day (5 to 10 cups of coffee per day) causing the most unpleasant effects.[4] Cessation of caffeine ingestion resolves these symptoms.

Panic Attacks

Patients who have a history of panic disorders may be particularly sensitive to the effects of caffeine. Indeed, in an older study,[14] moderate doses of caffeine (about 4 to 5 cups of coffee) precipitated panic attacks in about half the subjects. Here the implications are twofold: (1) In a person who experiences panic attacks, caffeine should be investigated as a possible, treatable cause, and (2) any person who has a history of panic attacks should be counseled to avoid caffeine-containing products or, at least, to use them in moderation and to be alert for signs of drug-induced precipitation of an attack. Greden and Walters (1992)[4] feel that caffeine does not induce panic attacks in normal individuals. However, in persons predisposed to panic disorders, the peripheral and the CNS effects of caffeine can be exaggerated.[15–16]

Cardiovascular Risks

The cardiovascular effects of caffeine are rarely harmful, although they might be detrimental to some individuals with heart disease. In both males and females without heart disease, the use of caffeinated coffee and the total daily intake of caffeine does not appreciably increase the risk of coronary artery disease or stroke.[17,18] Coffee consumption is strongly associated with cigarette smoking,[19] and increased rates of coronary heart disease in heavy coffee drinkers who smoke occur as a result of the cigarette smoking, not the caffeine consumption. Thus, while a conservative view is that caffeine should be used in moderation by people who are at risk for heart disease, the coffee is not necessarily "bad." As stated by Chou and Benowitz (1994)[20]: "Contrary to common belief, the published literature provides little evidence that coffee and/or caffeine in typical dosages increases the risk of infarction, sudden death, or arrhythmias."

Reproductive Effects

> Is caffeine safe during pregnancy? Caffeine, the most widely used psychotropic drug, is consumed by at least 75 percent of pregnant women via caffeinated beverages. Despite its widespread use, the safety of this habit during pregnancy is unresolved.[1]

For more than 30 years, it has been known that massive quantities of caffeine may induce chromosomal aberrations in a variety of nonhuman species.[21] As early as 1980, the U.S. Food and Drug Administration cautioned pregnant women to minimize their intake of caffeine. On the other hand, D'Ambrosio (1994)[22] reviewed the published literature on the genetic toxicity of caffeine, concluding that "it is difficult to implicate caffeine, even at the highest levels of daily consumption, as a genotoxin to humans."

Data in this area have always been both conflicting and controversial. Indeed, in 1993 the *Journal of the American Medical Association* published two studies on this issue that arrived at contradictory conclusions. The first article reported that caffeine was relatively safe in moderate doses (less than 300 milligrams per day, or less than 3 medium-sized cups of coffee per day).[23] At higher levels, an increased incidence of intrauterine growth retardation was seen. The second study[24] reported that low doses of caffeine (about 160 milligrams per day) in the first trimester of pregnancy increased the risk of intrauterine growth retardation; high consumption (greater than 300 milligrams per day), even in the month before pregnancy, "nearly doubled the risk of spontaneous abortion." Miller and coworkers (1994)[25] assessed the cardiovascular effects of caffeine ingestion in pregnant females and their fetuses. The authors noted that in both mothers and fetuses, caffeine increased heart rate, blood pressure, and the velocity of blood flow. Thus, caffeine does affect the fetal cardiovascular system just as it does the mother's; however, there was no implication that these effects were in any way detrimental to either the mothers or their fetuses.

Tolerance and Dependence

Chronic use of caffeine "is often associated with habituation and tolerance, and . . . discontinuation may produce a withdrawal syndrome."[4] In one study, "those who drank the most coffee complained of headache, drowsiness, fatigue, and a generally negative mood state on awakening the morning after placebo had been drunk, but not the morning after caffeine."[2] These are certainly signs of mild withdrawal and, therefore, indications of the development of a state of mild dependency. Other reported withdrawal signs include impaired intellectual and motor performance, difficulty with concentration, drug (caffeine) craving, and other psychological complaints.[26] Caffeine may cause an increase in the number of adenosine receptors in the CNS, a situation associated with an increased sensitivity to adenosine.[10] Because about 80 percent of American adults consume more than 200 milligrams of caffeine daily, there is almost universal dependence on caffeine. This seems to be of minimal consequence, however, because "no toxic effects of any kind have been associated with modest use of caffeine. . . . And, when caffeine is used on a long-term basis—unlike alcohol or tobacco—it causes no evident organ damage."[2]

NICOTINE

Together with caffeine and ethyl alcohol, nicotine is one of the three most widely used psychoactive drugs in our society. Despite the fact that nicotine has little or no therapeutic application in medicine, its potency, its widespread use, and its toxicity give it immense importance. Indeed, nicotine and the other ingredients in tobacco are responsible for a wide variety of health problems, including the deaths of more than 1,100 Americans every day![27]

From the end of World War II to the mid-1960s, cigarette smoking was considered chic. Today, after almost 30 years of U.S. government reports on the adverse health consequences of cigarettes, cigarette smoking is being increasingly shunned both in the United States[28,29] and throughout the Americas.[30] Nevertheless, each day 3,000 children become regular smokers, and almost 1,000 of them will eventually die from diseases related to smoking. Also, 9 in 10 smokers become addicted before age 21. Today, in the United States, 3 million adolescents are smokers.

On the positive side, half of all persons who have ever smoked cigarettes have quit, and the proportion of American adults who smoke has fallen from 50 percent in 1965 to 26 percent in 1995. About one million potential deaths have been averted or postponed by persons who have quit smoking. Millions more deaths will be avoided or postponed during the 1990s and into the twenty-first century.[28] As stated by the surgeon general, "Smoking will continue as the leading cause of preventable, premature death for many years to come."[11]

In this discussion, it is important to note that nicotine, the primary active ingredient in tobacco, is only 1 of about 4,000 compounds released by the burning of cigarette tobacco. Nicotine accounts only for the acute pharmacological effects of smoking and for the dependence on cigarettes. The adverse, long-term cardiovascular, pulmonary, and carcinogenic effects of cigarettes are related to other compounds contained in the product.

Pharmacokinetics

According to Jarvik and Schneider (1992),[31] "Nicotine is readily absorbed from every site on or in the body, including the lungs, buccal and nasal mucosa, skin, and gastrointestinal tract." This easy and complete absorption forms the basis for the recreational abuse of smoked or chewed tobacco, as well as the medical use of nicotine (in treating nicotine dependency) in gums, nasal sprays, transdermal skin patches, and smokeless inhalers (discussed later).

Nicotine is suspended in cigarette smoke in the form of minute particles ("tars"), and it is quickly absorbed into the bloodstream from the lungs when the smoke is inhaled. Most cigarettes contain between 0.5 and 2.0 milligrams of nicotine, depending on the brand. Approximately 20 percent (between 0.1 and 0.4 milligrams) of the nicotine in a cigarette is actually inhaled and absorbed into the smoker's bloodstream. Indeed, the physiological effects of smoking a single cigarette can be closely duplicated by the intravenous injection of these amounts of nicotine. Furthermore, the smoker can readily avoid acute toxicity, because inhalation as a route of administration offers exceptional controllability of the dose. The user-controlled frequency of breaths, the depth of inhalation, the time the smoke is held in the lungs, and the total number of cigarettes smoked all allow the smoker to regulate the rate of drug intake and thus control the blood level of nicotine. When nicotine is administered orally in the form of snuff, chewing tobacco, or gum, blood levels of nicotine are comparable to those achieved by smoking (see Figure 6.2).

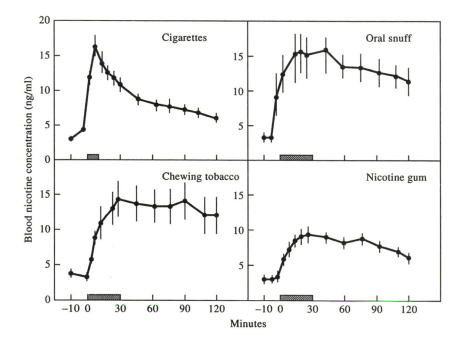

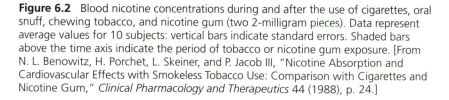

Figure 6.2 Blood nicotine concentrations during and after the use of cigarettes, oral snuff, chewing tobacco, and nicotine gum (two 2-milligram pieces). Data represent average values for 10 subjects: vertical bars indicate standard errors. Shaded bars above the time axis indicate the period of tobacco or nicotine gum exposure. [From N. L. Benowitz, H. Porchet, L. Skeiner, and P. Jacob III, "Nicotine Absorption and Cardiovascular Effects with Smokeless Tobacco Use: Comparison with Cigarettes and Nicotine Gum," *Clinical Pharmacology and Therapeutics* 44 (1988), p. 24.]

Nicotine is quickly and thoroughly distributed throughout the body, rapidly penetrating the brain, crossing the placental barrier, and appearing in all bodily fluids, including breast milk. The liver metabolizes approximately 80 to 90 percent of the nicotine administered to a person either orally or by smoking before it is excreted by the kidneys. The elimination half-life of nicotine in a chronic smoker is about two hours, necessitating frequent administration of the drug to avoid withdrawal symptoms or drug craving.

Pharmacological Effects

Nicotine is the only pharmacologically active drug in tobacco smoke apart from carcinogenic tars. It exerts powerful effects on the brain, the spinal cord, the peripheral nervous system, the heart, and various other body structures.

In the early stages of smoking, nicotine causes nausea and vomiting by stimulating both the vomiting center in the brain stem and the sensory receptors in the stomach. Tolerance to this effect develops rapidly. Nicotine stimulates the hypothalamus to release a hormone, antidiuretic hormone (ADH), which causes fluid retention. Nicotine reduces the activity of afferent nerve fibers coming from the muscles, leading to a reduction in muscle tone. This action may be involved (at least partially) in the relaxation that a person may experience as a result of smoking. Nicotine also reduces weight gain, probably by reducing appetite.

Nicotine stimulates specific acetylcholine receptors ("nicotinic" receptors) in the CNS, including the cerebral cortex, producing increases in psychomotor activity,[33] cognitive function,[34] sensorimotor performance, attention, and memory consolidation.[35] The drug can also induce tremors and, in toxic overdosage, seizures. As with all stimulant drugs, a period of depression follows.

Recent papers have reported antidepressant effects of nicotine as well as the comorbidity of childhood attention deficit hyperactivity disorder (ADHD)[34] and depression[35] with cigarette use and of adult depressive disorders and nicotine dependence. Salin-Pascual and coworkers (1996),[36] noting a high frequency of cigarette smoking among individuals with major depression, found that, in nonsmokers, transdermal nicotine patches produced short-term improvement in depression (see Figure 6.3). They postulated that the high rate of smoking among depressed individuals may, in part, represent an attempt at self-medication to assist in dealing with some of their depressive symptoms. In agreement with this concept, Fergusson and coworkers (1996),[37] in a study of 16-year-olds reported:

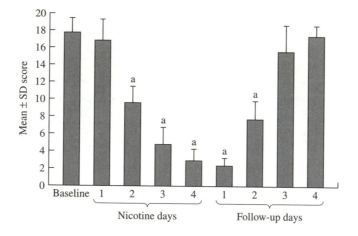

Figure 6.3 Hamilton rating scale for depression ratings of 10 depressed patients before, during, and after administration of nicotine patches. A significant reduction was observed on the second day of nicotine patches and continued until the second follow-up day. [From R. J. Salin-Pascual et al. (1996),[36] figure 2, p. 388.]

There was evidence of clear comorbidity between depressive disorders and nicotine dependence in this cohort of 16-year-olds; subjects with depression had odds of nicotine dependence that were more than 4.5 times the odds for those without depression. This relationship was similar for male and female subjects. These results suggest that comorbidities between nicotine dependence and depression are well established by the age of 16 years.

Nicotine exerts a potent reinforcing action, especially in the early phases of drug use. The reinforcing action of nicotine probably involves indirect activation of midbrain dopamine neurons.[34] This is discussed further in the next section.

In the veteran smoker, the reinforcing action appears to diminish, and the user smokes primarily to relieve or avoid withdrawal symptoms. In the later stages, smokers adjust their nicotine intake to maintain nicotine levels between about 30 to 40 nanograms of nicotine per milliliter of plasma.[31] Because of nicotine's short half-life, there is a very low residual level of nicotine in the blood and brain after a night's sleep. In essence, the smoker wakes each morning in a state of drug withdrawal. "The first cigarette of the morning has a powerful [reinforcing] effect because it brings relief of withdrawal discomfort. Thereafter, each cigarette produces a sharp increase in the nicotine concentration bathing the brain."[32]

In addition to its effects on the CNS, normal doses of nicotine can increase heart rate, blood pressure, and cardiac contractility. In nonatherosclerotic coronary arteries, nicotine initiates vasodilation, increasing blood flow to meet the increased oxygen demand of the heart muscle. In atherosclerotic coronary arteries (which cannot dilate), however, cardiac ischemia can result when the oxygen supply fails to meet the oxygen demand created by the drug's cardiac stimulation. This occurrence can precipitate angina or myocardial infarction (a heart attack).

Mechanism of Action

Nicotine exerts most of its CNS and peripheral effects by activating certain specific acetylcholine receptors ("nicotinic" receptors). In the peripheral nervous system, activation of these receptors causes an increase in blood pressure and heart rate, causes release of epinephrine (adrenaline) from the adrenal glands, and increases the tone and activity of the gastrointestinal tract.

In the CNS, the nicotine-sensitive acetylcholine receptors are widely distributed and may be located on the presynaptic nerve terminals of dopamine- and serotonin-secreting neurons. Activation of these acetylcholine neurons by nicotine appears to facilitate the release of dopamine and serotonin, accounting for the behavioral reinforcement, stimulant, and antidepressant actions of nicotine.

Tolerance and Dependence

Nicotine does not appear to induce any pronounced degree of biological tolerance. Indeed, as discussed earlier, smokers seem to learn how to dose themselves so as to maintain a blood level of nicotine within a reasonably narrow range (30 to 40 nanograms per milliliter). To achieve this can take anywhere from 10 to 50 cigarettes per day, as a result of the many variables associated with self-dosing through inhalation.

Nicotine clearly induces both physiological and psychological dependence. Indeed, as early as 1988, the surgeon general of the United States made the following conclusions:

- Cigarettes and other forms of tobacco are addicting.
- Nicotine is the drug in tobacco that causes addiction.
- The pharmacologic and behavioral processes that determine tobacco addiction are similar to those that determine addiction to drugs such as heroin and cocaine.

- More than 300,000 cigarette-addicted Americans die yearly* as a consequence of their addiction.[31]

In 1995, the *Journal of the American Medical Association* accused the tobacco industry of concealing its own research demonstrating that tobacco is addicting and fatally toxic.[40] This led U.S. FDA Commissioner David Kessler to propose classifying cigarettes as drug-delivery devices, giving the FDA regulatory control over their promotion, sale, and distribution. As might be expected in such an emotionally, financially, and politically charged arena, there was much opposition (even from a 1996 candidate for president of the United States!), and positive moves to control tobacco were defeated. The 1997 regulatory situation is more encouraging and is discussed in Chapter 14. Today, the scientific case that nicotine is addictive is overwhelming:

> Patterns of use by smokers and the remarkable intractability of the smoking habit point to compulsive use as the norm. Studies in both animal and human subjects have shown that nicotine can function as a reinforcer, albeit under a more limited range of conditions than with some other drugs of abuse. In drug discrimination paradigms, there is some cross-generalization between nicotine on the one hand, and amphetamine and cocaine on the other. A well-defined withdrawal syndrome has been delineated which is alleviated by nicotine replacement. Nicotine replacement also enhances outcomes in smoking cessation, roughly doubling success rates. In total, the evidence clearly identifies nicotine as a powerful drug of addiction, comparable to heroin, cocaine, and alcohol.[39]

Withdrawal from cigarettes is characterized by an abstinence syndrome. This includes a craving for nicotine, irritability, anxiety, anger, difficulty in concentrating, restlessness, impatience, increased appetite, and insomnia.[41] The period of withdrawal may be intense and persistent, often lasting for many months.[41] The difficulty in handling cigarette dependence is illustrated by the fact that cigarette smokers who seek treatment for other drug and alcohol problems often find it harder to quit cigarette smoking than to give up the other drugs. Even in the late 1800s, "Freud ... continued his cigar habit [20/day] until death, in spite of an endless series of operations for mouth and jaw cancer [the jaw was eventually totally removed], persistent heart problems that were exacerbated by smoking, and numerous attempts at quitting."[42]

---

*As of 1997, this number had increased to 435,000 deaths per year.

In 1994 Swanson and coworkers[43] raised an interesting point that abstinent smokers displaying signs of withdrawal often tend to increase their caffeine (coffee) consumption. Indeed, blood caffeine levels increase and remain elevated for as long as 6 months. In addition: "A review of 86 studies of nicotine withdrawal, caffeine withdrawal, and caffeine toxicity suggests that the symptoms are similar enough to be confused, and that reported nicotine withdrawal symptoms may be a mixture of nicotine withdrawal and caffeine toxicity."[43]

Toxicity

The toxic substances in cigarette smoke are nicotine, carbon monoxide, and tars. Of the more than 435,000 persons in the United States who die annually from tobacco use, 82,000 deaths are caused by noncancerous lung diseases, 112,000 are caused by lung cancer, 30,000 are caused by cancers of other body organs, and more than 200,000 result from heart and vascular diseases. A person's life is shortened 14 minutes for every cigarette smoked. In other words, a person who smokes two packs of cigarettes a day for 20 years loses an estimated 8 years of his or her life. More than 50 million people (one out of every five Americans) alive today will die prematurely from the effects of smoking cigarettes. Cigarette smoking, the nation's greatest public health hazard, is, ironically, the nation's most preventable cause of premature death, illness, and disability.[44–45] Internationally, similar statistics are appearing; according to estimates, global tobacco use is responsible for nearly 2.5 million deaths per year.[46]

Cardiovascular Disease

Carbon monoxide decreases the amount of oxygen delivered to the heart muscle, while nicotine increases the amount of work that the heart must do (by increasing the heart rate and blood pressure). Both carbon monoxide and nicotine increase the incidence of atherosclerosis* (narrowing) and thrombosis (clotting) in the coronary arteries.

---

*Atherosclerosis first appears as fatty deposits inside large arteries and progresses to occlusion of the arteries throughout the body; the result is clinically manifested as strokes or peripheral vascular ischemic disease. In a large study of arteries collected from young men who had died of violent causes, a history of cigarette smoking was associated with a threefold to fourfold increase in atherosclerosis of the coronary arteries and abdominal aorta.[47] This was the first report of cigarette-induced, severe atherosclerosis in persons under 25 years of age. It emphasizes that in males, cigarette-induced atherosclerosis begins at a young age, and it reinforces the fact that smoking must be controlled for the long-range prevention of adult vascular disease.

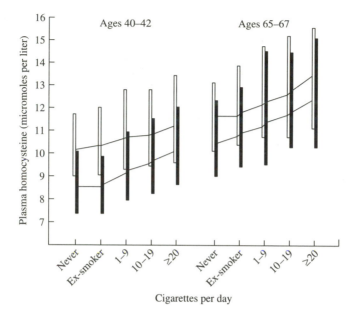

Figure 6.4 Total plasma homocysteine levels according to the extent of smoking in young and old men and women. The group aged 40 to 42 years comprised 5,918 men and 6,348 women, and the group aged 65 to 67 years included 1,386 men and 1,932 women. The solid lines are median values, and the shaded area indicates the 95 percent coincidence intervals, while the boxes show the 25th to 75th percentile intervals and are open for men and darkly shaded for women. [Adapted from O. Nygard et al. (1995),[48] figure 3, p. 1531.]

These three actions (and others as well) seem to underlie the fivefold to nineteenfold increase in the risk of death from coronary heart disease in smokers as compared to nonsmokers. If a smoker has preexisting hypertension or diabetes, the risk is magnified.

In recent studies, a relationship has been shown between elevations of the amount of the amino acid *homocysteine* in blood plasma and the early onset of arterial wall thickening and premature vascular disease in the coronary, cerebral, and peripheral arteries. In 1995 Nygard and coworkers[48] demonstrated that current smokers have a distinctly higher plasma homocysteine level that increased almost linearly with the daily number of cigarettes smoked (see Figure 6.4). Because the plasma homocysteine level is inversely related to the level of folic acid in plasma,[49,50] cigarette smoking may produce low folate levels, and folic acid dietary supplementation may delay the onset of cigarette-induced vascular disease.

Pulmonary Disease

In the lungs, chronic smoking results in a smoker's syndrome, characterized by difficulty in breathing, wheezing, chest pain, lung congestion, and increased susceptibility to infections of the respiratory tract. Cigarette smoking impairs ventilation and greatly increases the risk of emphysema (a form of irreversible lung damage). About 9 million Americans suffer from cigarette-induced chronic bronchitis and emphysema. Indeed, 70 percent of pulmonary diseases and deaths are tobacco-related; 57,000 deaths per year result from emphysema. The effects of cigarettes on cancers of the lungs are discussed next.

Cancer

The relation between smoking and cancer is now beyond question. Cigarette smoking is the major cause of lung cancer in both men and women, causing approximately 112,000 deaths in the United States every year. Denissenko and coworkers (1996)[51] identified a biological link between a chemical in cigarette smoke as a causative agent in cigarette-induced lung cancers:

> Benzo[a]pyrene, which occurs in amounts of 20–40 nanograms per cigarette, is . . . one of the most potent mutagens and carcinogens known. The compound requires metabolic activation to become the ultimate carcinogenic metabolite, BPDE (benzo[a]pyrene diol epoxide).

This metabolite, BPDE, damages a cancer suppressor gene (the *P53* gene),* resulting in the cancer-causing transformation of human lung tissue. This fact "provides a direct link between a defined cigarette smoke carcinogen and human cancer mutations."[51]

Levi and coworkers (1997)[52] made an interesting observation that a new lung cancer epidemic has started, resulting from the switch from high-tar to low-tar, filtered cigarettes. Whereas in the time period 1974–1994 *squamous cell carcinomas* accounted for the majority of cigarette-induced lung cancer deaths, in the time period 1995–1997 *adenocarcinomas* caused the majority of cigarette-induced lung cancer deaths. Squamous cell carcinomas attack the upper trunks of the lungs, while adenocarcinomas attack the smaller, outer branches of the lungs. Both cancers are fatal.

Smoking is also a major cause of cancers of the mouth, voice box, and throat. Concomitant alcohol ingestion greatly increases the incidence of these problems. In addition, cigarette smoking is a primary cause of more than 50 percent of the nearly 10,000 deaths every year

*For a discussion of the *P53* gene, see *Newsweek* (Dec. 23, 1996), 42–50.

that result from bladder cancer, it is a primary cause of pancreatic cancer, and it increases the risk of cancer of the uterine cervix twofold. Of all cancer deaths in the United States, 30 percent (154,000 annually) would be prevented if people stopped smoking.[53]

Effects of Passive Smoke

In addition to the direct effects of cigarettes on smokers, the environmental pollution caused by smokers can have adverse consequences for nonsmokers.[53] Indeed, 4,000 Americans die annually from lung cancer caused by other persons' smoking (so-called passive smoke), and an additional 37,000 deaths every year follow from heart disease contracted as a result of inhaling passive smoke. Subsequently, Wells (1994)[54] recalculated earlier data and estimated that in 1985 there were 62,000 deaths due to coronary artery disease caused by passive smoking. Wells further concluded that nonsmokers exposed to passive smoking have a coronary death rate 20 to 70 percent higher than nonsmokers not exposed to passive smoking.

Effects During Pregnancy

Cigarette smoking adversely affects the developing fetus and leads to increases in the rates of spontaneous abortion, stillbirth, and early postpartum death. The risk of intrauterine growth retardation is increased 40 percent, prematurity rates are 50 percent higher, and ectopic pregnancy risk is increased twofold. More than 2,000 infant deaths per year are attributed to maternal smoking. There is evidence that infants born of smoking mothers may be growth retarded compared to those born of nonsmoking mothers.

Cigarette smoking reduces oxygen delivery to the developing fetus, causing fetal hypoxia, which can result in long-term, irreversible intellectual and physical deficiencies. Indeed, Milberger and coworkers (1996)[55] presented evidence that school-age children born of mothers who smoked during pregnancy have lower intelligence quotients (IQs) and an increased prevalence of ADHD when compared with children born of nonsmoking mothers.

Government Response

Despite three decades of advice from experts (surgeon generals, FDA commissioners, and so on) and from multitudes of health professionals, the federal government had, until 1997, failed to implement meaningful policy that would serve both to decrease the attractiveness of cigarettes and to reduce the promotion of smoking to impressionable youth. The community is slowly recognizing the dangers of smoking, as shown by smoke-free zones and the offering of programs to help people quit smoking. The strength of the tobacco industry, combined with its continued denial of cigarette-induced toxicity and addictive potential (see note 40), had led to inaction on the part of most elected representatives. In 1985 C. Everett Koop, M.D., then surgeon general, challenged the United States to become a smoke-free society by the year 2000. Because of the addictive potential of cigarettes and nicotine, Dr. Koop's dream will probably not be realized; even the goal of a smoking rate of 15 percent of the U.S. population by the year 2000 may be unattainable.

In 1994 Henningfield, Kozlowski, and Benowitz[56] proposed labeling cigarettes much as food products are labeled with nutritional information. The proposed label would include an improved warning statement and information on the yields of nicotine, tar, carbon monoxide, and harmful chemicals, as well as information about nicotine delivery. In 1996 President Clinton proposed granting the Food and Drug Administration authority to regulate tobacco products, including formally classifying tobacco as a "drug." In 1997 authority was granted, and hopefully positive moves will be forthcoming. Annas (1997)[57] reviews the current status of antismoking litigation.

Therapy for Nicotine Dependence

The 1990s have seen dramatic advances both in the recognition of nicotine dependence and in its treatment. Perhaps the most important advance has been the development and clinical application of nicotine replacement therapies, specifically nicotine-containing gum, transdermal nicotine-containing patches, and nicotine-containing nasal spray and inhalers.[58] Other adjunctive agents that have been tried in attempts either to reduce cigarette cravings or to relieve withdrawal symptoms (such as anxiety, depression, and sleep disorders) include clonidine, antidepressants (see Chapter 7), and buspirone (see Chapter 4).

In addition to the availability of nicotine-replacement delivery systems, there has been a need for critical analysis and specific guidelines for the treatment of nicotine-dependent individuals. In 1996 this need was answered with the publication of two major professional treatises. The first was compiled by the U.S. Agency for Health Care Policy and Research (AHCPR)* and titled *Smoking Cessation Clinical Practice*

---

*The AHCPR publication can be ordered from any branch of a U.S. government bookstore or through the AHCPR website on the Internet (http://www.ahcpr.gov). The APA publication can be ordered from the APA, 1400 K Street, NW, Washington, D.C. 20005. See also "Practice Guidelines" in Chapter 15.

Guideline,[59] with a consensus statement summarizing the key recommendations of the *Guideline* published in the *Journal of the American Medical Association.*[60] The second major treatise was published in late 1996 by the American Psychiatric Association (APA) and is titled *Practice Guidelines for the Treatment of Patients with Nicotine Dependence.*[61]

Regarding the use of pharmacologic agents, the AHCPR panel of experts

> identified nicotine replacement therapy [nicotine patches and nicotine gum] as the only pharmacotherapy currently shown to be effective as an aid to smoking cessation. The panel recommends that, unless there is a clear medical contraindication, all patients planning a quit attempt should be offered nicotine replacement therapy. While both the nicotine patch and nicotine gum were found to be efficacious, the panel felt the patch is preferable for routine clinical use because of greater compliance and ease of use.[59]

For professionals working with clients/patients who smoke, the AHCPR and APA guidelines and the AMA consensus statement are necessary reading.

NOTES

1. B. Eskenazi, "Caffeine During Pregnancy: Grounds for Concern," Journal of the American Medical Association 270 (1993): 2973–2974.
2. A. Goldstein, *Addiction: From Biology to Drug Policy* (New York: W. H. Freeman and Company, 1994), 179–189.
3. A. Chopra and L. Morrison, "Resolution of Caffeine-Induced Complex Dysrhythmia with Procainamide Therapy," *Journal of Emergency Medicine* 13 (1995): 113–117.
4. J. F. Greden and A. Walters, "Caffeine," in J. H. Lowinson, P. Ruiz, R. B. Millman, and J. G. Langrod, eds., *Substance Abuse: A Comprehensive Textbook,* 2nd ed. (Baltimore: Williams & Wilkins, 1992), 357–370.
5. J. W. Daly, "Mechanism of Action of Caffeine," in S. Garattini, ed., *Caffeine, Coffee, and Health* (New York: Raven Press, 1993).
6. G. B. Kaplan, D. J. Greenblatt, M. A. Kent, et al., "Caffeine-Induced Behavioral Stimulation Is Dose-Dependent and Associated with A1 Adenosine Receptor Occupancy," *Neuropsychopharmacology* 6 (1992): 145–153.
7. B. B. Fredholm, "Adenosine, Adenosine Receptors, and the Actions of Caffeine," *Pharmacology and Toxicology* 76 (1995): 93–101.
8. L. Pulvirenti, N. R. Swerdlow, and G. F. Koob, "Nucleus Accumbens NMDA Antagonist Decreases Locomotor Activity Produced by Cocaine, Heroin, or Accumbens Dopamine, but Not Caffeine," *Pharmacology, Biochemistry, and Behavior* 40 (1991): 841–845.

9. A. J. Carter, W. T. O'Connor, M. J. Carter, and U. Ungerstedt, "Caffeine Enhances Acetylcholine Release in the Hippocampus *in vivo* by a Selective Interaction with Adenosine A1 Receptors," *Journal of Pharmacology and Experimental Therapeutics* 273 (1995): 637–642.

10. D. Shi, O. Nokodijevic, K. A. Jacobson, and J. W. Daly, "Chronic Caffeine Alters the Density of Adenosine, Adrenergic, Cholinergic, GABA, and Serotonin Receptors and Calcium Channels in Mouse Brain," *Cellular & Molecular Neurobiology* 13 (1993): 247–261.

11. S. J. Smith, J. M. Deacon, and C. E. Chilvers, "Alcohol, Smoking, Passive Smoking, and Caffeine in Relation to Breast Cancer Risk in Young Women. UK National Case-Control Study Group," *British Journal of Cancer* 70 (1994): 112–119.

12. M. L. Slattery and D. W. West, "Smoking, Alcohol, Coffee, Tea, Caffeine, and Theobromine: Risk of Prostate Cancer in Utah," *Cancer Causes and Control* 4 (1993): 559–563.

13. A. R. Folsom, D. R. McKenzie, K. M. Bisgard, L. H. Kushi, and T. A. Sellers, "No Association Between Caffeine Intake and Postmenopausal Breast Cancer Incidence in the Iowa Women's Health Study," *American Journal of Epidemiology* 138 (1993): 380–383.

14. D. S. Charney, G. R. Heniger, and P. L. Jatlow, "Increased Anxiogenic Effects of Caffeine in Panic Disorders," *Archives of General Psychiatry* 42 (1985): 233–243.

15. L. Christensen, A. Bourgeois, and R. Cockcroft, "Electroencephalographic Concomitants of a Caffeine-Induced Panic Reaction," *Journal of Nervous and Mental Disease* 181 (1993): 327–330.

16. F. Newman, M. B. Stein, J. R. Trettau, R. Coppola, and T. W. Uhde, "Quantitative Electroencephalographic Effects of Caffeine in Panic Disorder," *Psychiatry Research* 45 (1992): 105–113.

17. D. E. Grobbee, E. B. Rimm, E. Giovannucci, et al., "Coffee, Caffeine, and Cardiovascular Disease in Men," *New England Journal of Medicine* 323 (1990): 1026–1032.

18. W. C. Willett, M. J. Stampfer, J. E. Manson, et al., "Coffee Consumption and Coronary Heart Disease in Women: A Ten-Year Follow-up," *Journal of the American Medical Association* 275 (1996) 458–462.

19. J. A. Swanson, J. W. Lee, and J. W. Hopp, "Caffeine and Nicotine: A Review of Their Joint Use and Possible Interactive Effects in Tobacco Withdrawal," *Addictive Behaviors* 19 (1994): 229–256.

20. T. M. Chou and N. L. Benowitz, "Caffeine and Coffee: Effects on Health and Cardiovascular Disease," *Comparative Biochemistry and Psychology. Part C: Pharmacology, Toxicology, Endocrinology* 109 (1994): 173–189.

21. L. Dlugosz and M. S. Bracken, "Reproductive Effects of Caffeine: A Review and Theoretical Analysis," *Epidemiology Review* 14 (1992): 83–100.

22. S. M. D'Ambrosio, "Evaluation of the Genotoxicity Data on Caffeine," *Regulatory Toxicology & Pharmacology* 19 (1994): 243–281.

23. J. L. Mills et al., "Moderate Caffeine Use and the Risk of Spontaneous Abortion and Intrauterine Growth Retardation," *Journal of the American Medical Association* 269 (1993): 593–597.

24. C. Infante-Rivard, A. Fernandez, R. Gauthier, M. David, and G.-E. Rivard, "Fetal Loss Associated with Caffeine Intake Before and During Pregnancy," *Journal of the American Medical Association* 270 (1993): 2940–2943.

25. R. C. Miller, W. J. Watson, A. C. Hackney, and J. W. Seeds, "Acute Maternal and Fetal Cardiovascular Effects of Caffeine Ingestion," *American Journal of Perinatology* 11 (1994): 132–136.

26. R. R. Griffiths, S. M. Evans, S. J. Heishman, et al., "Low-Dose Caffeine Physical Dependence in Humans," *Journal of Pharmacology and Experimental Therapeutics* 255 (1990): 1123–1132.

27. J. Cocores, "Nicotine Dependence: Diagnosis and Treatment," *Psychiatric Clinics of North America* 16 (1993): 49.

28. U.S. Department of Health and Human Services, "Reducing the Health Consequences of Smoking: 25 Years of Progress. A Report of the Surgeon General" (Rockville, Md.: U.S. Department of Health and Human Services, 1989), iv.

29. U.S. Department of Health and Human Services, "The Health Benefits of Smoking Cessation. A Report of the Surgeon General" (Rockville, Md.: U.S. Department of Health and Human Services, 1990).

30. U.S. Department of Health and Human Services, "Smoking and Health in the Americas," DHHS Publication No. (CDC) 92–8419 (Atlanta, Ga: U.S. Department of Health and Human Services, Centers for Disease Control, Office on Smoking and Health, 1992).

31. M. E. Jarvik and N. G. Schneider, "Nicotine," in J. H. Lowinson, P. Ruiz, R. B. Millman, and J. G. Langrod, eds., *Substance Abuse: A Comprehensive Textbook,* 2nd ed. (Baltimore: Williams & Wilkins, 1992), 339–340.

32. E. D. Levin, "Nicotine Systems and Cognitive Function," *Psychopharmacology* 108 (1992): 417–431.

33. D. M. Warburton, J. M. Rusted, and J. Fowler, "A Comparison of the Attentional and Consolidation Hypothesis for the Facilitation of Memory by Nicotine," *Psychopharmacology* 108 (1992): 443–447.

34. S. Milberger, J. Biederman, S. V. Faraone, L. Chen, and J. Jones, "ADHD Is Associated with Early Initiation of Cigarette Smoking in Children and Adolescents," *Journal of the American Academy of Child and Adolescent Psychiatry* 36 (1997): 37–44.

35. R. A. Brown, P. Lewinsohn, J. R. Seeley, and E. F. Wagner, "Cigarette Smoking, Major Depression, and Other Psychiatric Disorders among Adolescents," *Journal of the American Academy of Child and Adolescent Psychiatry* 35 (1996): 1602–1610.

36. R. J. Salin-Pascual, M. Rosas, A. Jimenez-Genchi, et al., "Antidepressant Effect of Transdermal Nicotine Patches in Nonsmoking Patients with Major Depression," *Journal of Clinical Psychiatry* 57 (1996): 387–389.

37. D. M. Fergusson, M. T. Lynskey, and L. J. Horwood, "Comorbidity Between Depressive Disorders and Nicotine Dependence in a Cohort of 16-Year-Olds," *Archives of General Psychiatry* 53 (1996): 1043–1047.

38. M. C. Fiore, "Trends in Cigarette Smoking in the United States: The Epidemiology of Tobacco Use," *The Medical Clinics of North America* 76 (March 1992): 289–304.

39. I. P. Stolerman and M. J. Jarvis, "The Scientific Case that Nicotine Is Addictive," *Psychopharmacology* 117 (1995): 2–10.
40. S. A. Glantz, D. E. Barnes, L. Bero, P. Hanauer, and J. Slade (in varying orders), "Looking Through a Keyhole at the Tobacco Industry," "Nicotine and Addiction: The Brown and Williamson Documents," "Lawyer Control of Internal Scientific Research to Protect Against Product Liability Lawsuits," "Lawyer Control of the Tobacco Industry's External Research Program," "Environmental Tobacco Smoke: The Brown and Williamson Documents," "The Brown and Williamson Documents: The Company's Response," all in the *Journal of the American Medical Association* 274 (1995): 219–258.
41. J. R. Hughes, S. W. Gust, K. Skoog, R. M. Keenan, and J. W. Fenwick, "Symptoms of Tobacco Withdrawal: A Replication and Extension," *Archives of General Psychiatry* 48 (1991): 52–59.
42. P. K. Gessner, "Substance Abuse Treatment," in C. M. Smith and A. M. Reynard, eds., *Textbook of Pharmacology* (Philadelphia: Saunders, 1992), 1160.
43. J. A. Swanson, J. W. Lee, and J. W. Hopp, "Caffeine and Nicotine: A Review of Their Joint Use and Possible Interactive Effects in Tobacco Withdrawal," *Addictive Behaviors* 19 (1994): 229–256.
44. U.S. Department of Health and Human Services, "Reducing the Health Consequences of Smoking: 25 Years of Progress. A Report of the Surgeon General" (Rockville, Md.: U.S. Department of Health and Human Services, 1989), 16–17.
45. Ibid., 98–99.
46. M. Barry, "The Influence of the U.S. Tobacco Industry on the Health, Economy, and Environment of Developing Countries," *New England Journal of Medicine* 324 (1991): 917–920.
47. Pathobiological Determinants of Atherosclerosis in Youth (PDAY) Research Group, "Relationship of Atherosclerosis in Young Men to Serum Lipoprotein Cholesterol Concentrations and Smoking," *Journal of the American Medical Association* 264 (1990): 3018–3024.
48. O. Nygard, S. E. Vollset, H. Refsum, et al., "Total Plasma Homocysteine and Cardiovascular Risk Profile," *Journal of the American Medical Association* 274 (1995): 1526–1533.
49. C. J. Boushey, S. Beresford, G. S. Omenn, and A. G. Motulsky, "A Quantitative Assessment of Plasma Homocysteine as a Risk Factor for Vascular Disease," *Journal of the American Medical Association* 274 (1995): 1049–1057.
50. H. I. Morrison, D. Schaubel, M. Desmeules, and D. T. Wigle, "Serum Folate and Risk of Fatal Coronary Heart Disease," *Journal of the American Medical Association* 275 (1996): 1893–1896.
51. M. F. Denissenko, A. Pao, M. Tang, and G. P. Pfeifer, "Preferential Formation of Benzo[a]pyrene Adducts at Lung Cancer Mutational Hotspots in *P53*," *Science* 274 (Oct. 18, 1996): 430–432.
52. F. Levi, S. Franceschi, C. LaVecchia, L. Randimbison, and V.-C. Te, "Lung Carcinoma Trends by Histologic Type in Baud and Neuchatel, Switzerland, 1974–1994," *Cancer* 79 (1997): 906–914.

53. H. Witschi, J. P. Joad, and K. E. Pinkerton, "The Toxicology of Environmental Tobacco Smoke," *Annual Review of Pharmacology and Toxicology* 37 (1997): 29–52.

54. A. J. Wells, "Passive Smoking as a Cause of Heart Disease," *Journal of the American College of Cardiology* 24 (1994): 546–554.

55. S. Milberger, J. Biederman, S. V. Faraone, L. Chen, and J. Jones, "Is Maternal Smoking During Pregnancy a Risk Factor for Attention Deficit Hyperactivity Disorder in Children?," *American Journal of Psychiatry* 153 (1996): 1138–1142.

56. J. E. Henningfield, L. T. Kozlowski, and N. L. Benowitz, "A Proposal to Develop Meaningful Labeling for Cigarettes," *Journal of the American Medical Association* 272 (July 27, 1994): 312–314.

57. G. J. Annas, "Tobacco Litigation as Cancer Prevention: Dealing with the Devil," *New England Journal of Medicine* 336 (1997): 304–308.

58. K. A. Perkins, J. E. Grobe, D. D'Amico, et al., "Low-Dose Nicotine Nasal Spray Use and Effects During Initial Smoking Cessation," *Experimental and Clinical Psychopharmacology* 4 (1996): 157–165.

59. M. C. Fiore, D. W. Wetter, W. C. Bailey, et al., *Smoking Cessation Clinical Practice Guideline* (Rockville, Md: Agency for Health Care Policy and Research, Public Health Service, U.S. Department of Health and Human Services, 1996).

60. Consensus Statement, Agency for Health Care Policy and Research, "Smoking Cessation Clinical Practice Guideline," *Journal of the American Medical Association* 275 (Apr. 24, 1996): 1270–1280.

61. American Psychiatric Association, "Practice Guidelines for the Treatment of Patients with Nicotine Dependence," *American Journal of Psychiatry* 153, suppl. (October 1996), 1–31.

Chapter 7

ANTIDEPRESSANT DRUGS: FOUR DECADES OF CONTINUING PROGRESS

Anxiety, depression, and bipolar disorders are affective (mood) disorders, in contrast to schizophrenia, which is primarily a thought disorder. Mood disorders are characterized by extreme or prolonged disturbances of mood, such as anxiety, sadness, apathy, or extreme elation. The occurrence of manic symptoms distinguishes bipolar disorders from depressive, or unipolar, disorders. Because of this difference, pharmacological therapies for bipolar disorder and depressive disorder are quite different, but overlap does exist because of the anxiety component often seen in depressive disorder and the depressive component of bipolar disorder. In this and the next chapter, however, we will treat the two disorders as largely separate entities.

Confusion is confounded by the fact that many of the anxiety disorders listed in Chapter 4 (e.g., panic disorder, obsessive-compulsive disorder [OCD], post-traumatic stress disorder [PTSD], and so on) are pharmacologically treated with certain of the antidepressant drugs rather than with the anxiolytics. Anxiety disorders in children and adolescents are treated rarely if at all with anxiolytics (which impair learning and memory), but instead are treated with the antidepressants discussed in this chapter. To a degree, this same limitation applies to the use of anxiolytics in the elderly (because of their clouding effect on consciousness).[1] Thus, antidepressants, are therapeutically useful in the treatment of a variety of affective disorders in both adults and children.

Episodes of depression are characterized by dysphoria, or loss of interest or pleasure in all (or almost all) of a person's usual activities or pastimes. Accompanying this condition are feelings of intense sadness and despair; diminished energy; decreased sexual drive; mental slowing and loss of concentration; pessimism; feelings of helplessness, worthlessness, or self-reproach; inappropriate guilt; recurrent thoughts of death, suicide, and hopelessness; blunted affect; anorexia; fatigue; and insomnia. About 15 percent of persons suffering from depression die by suicide. Certainly, sadness is a normal human emotion in response to various life events. However, depression that has no known cause or unremitting depression that interferes with normal activity is pathological. Nearly 8 percent of the U.S. population will develop a mood disorder at some time during their lives; nearly 5 percent of the population will develop major depression, occurring twice as often in women as in men.

One report[2] states:

> Depression afflicts about 5% of the adult population in the United States at any given time. . . . Over a lifetime, about 30% of the adult population will have suffered from depression. Also, if left untreated, 25% to 30% of adult depressives will commit suicide. . . . More than 50% of suicides saw a physician in the month before their death. These patients, however, were not diagnosed as being depressed. Data . . . show that there were 30,000 reported suicides. Depression is the eighth leading cause of death in the U.S.

Major depression typically has an onset in individuals in their middle to late twenties, although it can occur at any age, even in the elderly. More than 50 percent of persons experiencing an episode of major depression have recurrences, with the average number of episodes being five or six in a lifetime.

> Depression is a disease resulting from biochemical changes in the brain. It is undertreated. Surveys . . . show that about 70% of depressed patients do NOT get treatment for their disease. . . . The vast majority of people respond to the excellent treatments that we have available. About 85% can be treated successfully.[2]

In addition to the use of antidepressants to treat acute attacks of major depression and prevent their recurrence, individuals formerly regarded as having anxiety neurosis have now been reconceptualized as having an affective disorder (i.e., dysthymia) responsive to antidepressant) medication.[3] The need for pharmacotherapy for dysthymia was recently articulated by Shelton and coworkers (1997),[4] Friedman and Kocis (1996)[5] and Thase and coworkers (1996)[6]:

> Dysthymia . . . affects 3% to 6% of the adult population of the United States and as many as 36% of patients who seek treatment at psychiatric outpatient clinics. The symptoms of dysthymia are less severe than those observed in patients with major depression, and hence dysthymia is often considered to be a disorder of subsyndromal intensity. Nevertheless, patients with this disorder experience considerable social dysfunction and disability. Dysthymics . . . are more likely to take nonspecific psychotropic drugs, such as minor tranquilizers and sedatives. . . . More than 75% of dysthymics have coexisting psychiatric disorders, including anxiety disorders and substance abuse. Approximately 40% of dysthymics have coexisting major depression—a combination termed *double depression*. Untreated dysthymia rarely improves spontaneously over time. Dysthymia has historically been underrecognized and undertreated.

Evolution of Antidepressant Drug Therapy

Forty years ago, while investigating the potential antipsychotic efficacy of structural modifications of antipsychotic drugs (the *phenothiazines*; see Figure 7.1), the antidepressant properties of imipramine were first described. Imipramine belongs to a group of drugs later called the *tricyclic antidepressants* (TCAs), now expanded to include seven products (plus clomipramine, discussed later) currently available in the United States (see Table 7.1). Soon thereafter, a class of drugs called the *monoamine amine oxidase inhibitors* (MAOIs) were discovered, three of which became commercially available. For many years, these two classes of drugs were the primary agents used to treat major depression.

> Both classes of compounds are very effective in the treatment of major depression (TCAs) and atypical depression (MAOIs), but possess considerable disadvantages because of their adverse effect profile. TCAs carry a high incidence of anticholinergic effects and cardiotoxicity, extremely important in (suicidal) overdoses; MAOIs may cause hypertensive crises if sympathomimetic agents, e.g., certain other drugs or tyramine in foodstuffs, are additionally taken. These problems precipitated the search for new, effective antidepressants that were better tolerated and less toxic.[7]

In the years that followed, attempts were made to identify drugs with antidepressant properties that might have a lesser degree of

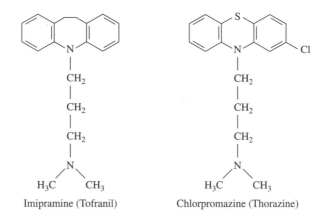

Imipramine (Tofranil)   Chlorpromazine (Thorazine)

Figure 7.1 Chemical structures of imipramine (a tricyclic antidepressant) and chlorpromazine (an antipsychotic). Slight structural differences produce remarkably different receptor affinities: imipramine blocks the presynaptic catecholamine transporter, and chlorpromazine blocks postsynaptic dopamine$_2$ receptors.

bothersome and potentially fatal side effects. This led first to a class of antidepressants that were structurally unrelated to the TCAs (the so-called "second-generation" or "atypical" antidepressants; see Figure 7.2) and, from the late 1980s to the mid-1990s, to a class of antidepressants called *serotonin-specific reuptake inhibitors* (SSRIs), the first of which was fluoxetine (Prozac); additional agents are now available (see Table 7.1).

In the last half of the 1990s, recognizing the limitations and side effects of the SSRIs (discussed later), antidepressant drug research has progressed in two directions. The first provided selective, reversible inhibitors of the MAO-type A enzyme (e.g., moclobimide, marketed outside the United States as Aurorix), and the second identified compounds that combine SSRI activity with either norepinephrine reuptake blockade (e.g. venlafaxine, marketed as Effexor) or postsynaptic serotonin-type 2 receptor (5-HT$_2$) antagonism (e.g., nefazodone, marketed as Serzone, and mirtazapine, marketed as Remeron).

To date, all of these modifications have not yet reduced the number of "treatment-resistant" individuals with major depression.[8] In other words, the newer antidepressants are not necessarily more effective than the older TCAs; rather, they merely alter the profile of side effects, including a reduction in overdose cardiotoxicity. It is likely that many more antidepressants will appear in the next few years:

TABLE 7.1 Drugs used in affective disorders: Antidepressants

Drug name Generic (trade)	Sedative activity	Anticholinergic activity[a]	Elimination half-life (hr)	Reuptake inhibition		
				Norepinephrine	Serotonin	Dopamine
TRICYCLIC COMPOUNDS						
Imipramine (Tofranil)	Moderate	Moderate	10–20	++	++	0
Desipramine (Norpramin)	Low	Low	12–75	+++	+	0
Trimipramine (Surmontil)	High	Moderate	8–20	+	+	0
Protriptyline (Vivactil)	Low	Moderate	55–125	+++	+	0
Nortriptyline (Pamelor, Aventil)	Moderate	Low	15–35	++	++	0
Amitriptyline (Elavil)	High	High	20–35	++	+++	0
Doxepin (Adapin, Sinequan)	High	High	8–24	++	++	0
Clomipramine (Anaframil)	Low	Low	19–37	++	++++	0
SECOND-GENERATION (ATYPICAL) COMPOUNDS						
Amoxapine (Asendin)[b]	Low	Moderate	8–10	++	+	0
Maprotiline (Ludiomil)	Moderate	Moderate	27–58	+++	0	0
Trazodone (Desyrel)	Moderate	Low	6–13	0	++	0
Bupropion (Wellbutrin)	Low	Low	8–14	0/+	0/+	++

[a]Anticholinergic side effects include dry mouth, blurred vision, tachycardia, urinary retention, and constipation.
[b]Also has antipsychotic effects due to blockage of dopamine receptors (Chapter 7).
0 = no effect; + = mild effect; ++ = moderate effect; +++ = strong effect; ++++ = maximal effect.

TABLE 7.1 (continued) Drugs used in affective disorders: Antidepressants

Drug name Generic (trade)	Sedative activity	Anticholinergic activity[a]	Elimination half-life (hr)	Reuptake inhibition		
				Norepinephrine	Serotonin	Dopamine
SEROTONIN-SPECIFIC REUPTAKE INHIBITORS						
Fluoxetine (Prozac)	None	None	24–96	0	++++	0
Sertraline (Zoloft)	None	None	26	0	++++	0
Paroxetine (Paxil)	None	None	24	+	++++	0
Venlafaxine (Effexor)	None	None	3–11	++	++++	0
Fluvoramine (Luvox)	None	None	15	0	++++	0
DUAL-ACTION ANTIDEPRESSANTS						
Nefazodone (Serzone)	Low	None	3–4	0	++++	0
Mirtazapine (Remeron)	High	Low	20–40	++	++++	0
MAO INHIBITORS: IRREVERSIBLE						
Phenelzine (Nardil)	Low	None	2–4[c]	0	0	0
Isocarboxazid (Marplan)	None	None	1–3[c]	0	0	0
Tranylcypromine (Parnate)	None	None	1–3[c]	0	0	0
MAO INHIBITORS: REVERSIBLE						
Moclobemide (NA) (Aurorix)	None	Low	1–3[c]	0	0	0
Brofaramine (NA)[d]	None	Low	12–15[c]	0	0	0
Cimoxatone (NA)[d]	None	Low	9–16[c]	0	0	0

[a]Half-life does not correlate with clinical effect (see text). [d]Trade name not available; not available for use in the United States.
0 = no effect; + = mild effect; ++ = moderate effect; +++ = strong effect; ++++ = maximal effect.

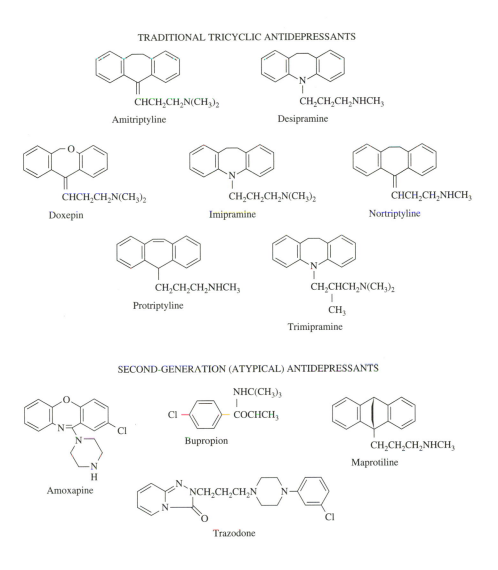

Figure 7.2 Chemical structures of tricyclic and second-generation antidepressants.

Three main therapeutic needs have still to be met: (i) superior efficacy to tricyclic antidepressants; (ii) a faster onset of action; and (iii) reliable effectiveness in the treatment of therapy-resistant depression.[7]

Antidepressant drug research in the latter half of the 1990s appears to be focusing on the development of "dual-action" antidepressants that combine the antidepressant efficacy of serotonin *potentiation* (via blockade of its presynaptic reuptake) with a *blockade* of certain subtypes of postsynaptic serotonin receptors, which, when activated by SSRIs, lead to some of the unpleasant side effects associated with the SSRIs.[9–11] These side effects are discussed later.

Mechanism of Action

The role of brain norepinephrine and dopamine function in the mechanism of action of antidepressant drugs has been the subject of intensive research during the past three decades.[12,13] Most investigators agree that a neurochemical imbalance is involved in depression and that, in some cases, it is genetically determined. Pharmacological evidence points to an involvement of at least two, and perhaps three, biological amines (norepinephrine, serotonin, and possibly dopamine).

The *biological amine theory* of mania and depression was first postulated in the mid-1960s. According to this theory, depression is caused by a functional deficit of specific transmitters (originally thought to be norepinephrine) at certain sites in the brain, while mania results from a functional excess of the same transmitters. Several bits of evidence support this claim. First, reserpine, an older drug that induces severe emotional depression, concomitantly depletes norepinephrine and serotonin from the neurons that release them. Second, the antidepressant drugs exert important actions on both of these transmitters to potentiate their neurotransmitter action. Third, strong evidence for the genetic predisposition toward depression has led to the belief that major depressive episodes may include an abnormally low functioning of the neurotransmission of norepinephrine and serotonin or of the receptors for these transmitters. Appendix IV discusses these neurotransmitters in detail.

Although reasonable correlations have been found between drug-induced increases in the levels of norepinephrine and serotonin and positive, mood-elevating effects in persons who are depressed, several limitations and inconsistencies in this pattern have also been seen. One major difficulty is that the time course of action is vastly different for the biochemical effect and the clinical response. Although neurotransmission of norepinephrine and serotonin is augmented soon after the drug is taken, the clinical antidepressant effect may not appear for 2 to 4 weeks. Thus, increasing the amounts of neurotransmitter may only be an initial step in relieving depression. A more complex series of cellular events may then occur that eventually results in secondary, adaptive changes.

A second problem in correlating antidepressive activity with levels of neurotransmitters is that cocaine and the amphetamines augment biological amine neurotransmission, but they are seldom effective in the treatment of clinical states of depression, even though certain individuals may have tried these behavioral stimulants in self-medication attempts to alleviate symptoms of depression. Perhaps the preference of amphetamines and cocaine for dopamine neurons (rather than for norepinephrine and serotonin neurons) accounts for this discrepancy. According to Baldessarini (1995)[12]:

> A few tentative generalizations may be made from studies with animal models and from the clinical and behavioral effects of antidepressant drugs. First, blockade of dopamine transport seems to be associated with stimulant rather than antidepressant activity. Second, inhibition of serotonin uptake may well contribute to antidepressant activity. Finally, inhibition of the uptake of norepinephrine seems to yield antidepressant activity consistently. However, inhibition of the uptake of norepinephrine or serotonin *per se* may not be a sufficient explanation for the antidepressant action of these drugs.

Postsynaptic receptor desensitization is a late 1980s refinement of the biological amine theory. This hypothesis posits that depression, rather than being the result of a hypoadrenergic state, may be due to a hyperresponsiveness of postsynaptic receptors caused by the decreased availability of norepinephrine.[14] Thus, by blocking norepinephrine reuptake, presynaptic activity normalizes (normal amounts of transmitter become available at the receptor), and slowly the postsynaptic receptors down-regulate to a normal level of responsiveness. Such an adaptive change accounts for the slow onset of clinical effect but allows for an action subsequent to blockade of reuptake.

The *serotonin hypothesis* is a 1990s variation of the receptor desensitization theory. This hypothesis holds that blocking the reuptake of serotonin is more clinically efficacious than blocking the reuptake of norepinephrine. Furthermore, the adaptive changes in serotonin receptors would explain the slow onset of clinical antidepressant effect. While the older TCAs are generally more potent at blocking reuptake of norepinephrine, the newer SSRIs are generally more effective at blocking the reuptake of serotonin. Paul (1990)[15] states:

> Alterations in serotonin neurotransmission have been postulated to be involved in a variety of neuropsychiatric disorders including depression, generalized anxiety disorder, and obsessive-compulsive disorder, although the precise role of serotonin in either the etiology or the pathogenesis of these disorders is still unclear. . . . Augmentation

> of serotonergic neurotransmission may mediate, at least in part, the therapeutic actions of a variety of psychotherapeutic drugs, including antidepressants. . . . Virtually all effective antidepressant treatments augment serotonergic neurotransmission, and, therefore, the serotonergic system may represent a "final common pathway" underlying the therapeutic effects of these drugs.

Thus, alteration in serotonin neurotransmission may be vital in the action of the antidepressants. Indeed, all the different types of antidepressant treatments may ultimately enhance the neurotransmission of serotonin, albeit via different mechanisms.

That alterations in serotonin activity may not represent the final common pathway of antidepressant drug therapy was discussed by Miller and coworkers (1996)[13]:

> The primary abnormality of depression, like the mechanism of action of antidepressant treatments, may result from an abnormality in a neuronal system, which remains to be discovered, that is highly regulated by the brain's monoamine system. . . . The complexity and interdependency in neurotransmitter, neuropeptide, receptor, and intracellular messenger systems in [the] brain suggest that antidepressant action may not lie in the modification of a single neurotransmitter or neuropeptide, but involves the up-regulation or down-regulation of the expression of multiple proteins in multiple neuronal cell types. The key brain structures involved in antidepressant action need to be identified.

To further this concept, Garcia-Sevilla and coworkers[16] in late 1996 expanded on the role of a newly identified class of receptors (the *imidazoline receptors*) in the amine hypothesis of affective disorders. Here, amine-secreting neurons have located on their presynaptic terminals imidazoline receptors, the activity of which inhibits the release of norepinephrine. These authors present evidence that the levels of these receptors are elevated in depressed patients and are down-regulated by both TCAs (desipramine) and SSRIs (fluoxetine). These data "support a role for the newly discovered imidazoline receptors in the pathogenesis of depression and in the mechanism of action of antidepressant drugs."[16]

Until 1991 there was little information on the structure and regulation of the presynaptic reuptake transporter for serotonin, although it was thought that the transporter might resemble the dopamine transporter, which is blocked by cocaine (see Figure 5.5). Then, in 1991, Blakely and coworkers[17] verified the resemblance: the transporter is a 653-amino-acid protein with 12 putative transmembrane domains. It strongly resembles the GABA, dopamine, and norepinephrine presynaptic transporters, but it is significantly different from the postsynaptic serotonin receptor, which is not affected by antidepressant drugs. The latter receptor is a 420-amino-acid chain with 7 membrane-spanning regions (see Figure IV.12).

Shortly after the presynaptic serotonin reuptake transporter was identified, the activity of this transporter was shown to be under the influence of abnormal and as yet uncharacterized regulatory effects during episodes of depressive illness.[18] (Perhaps this represents the influence of the newly described imidazoline receptors.) In other words, this receptor protein can be either up- or down-regulated during periods of depression or remission or in response to the presence or absence of antidepressant medication.

TABLE 7.2 Potency and selectivity of various antidepressants

Drug	Potency[a]			Selectivity[b]
	Norepinephrine	Serotonin	Dopamine	
Amitriptyline	4.2	1.5	0.043	0.36[c]
Amoxapine	23	0.21	0.053	0.0091
Bupropion	0.043	0.0064	0.16	0.15
Clomipramine	3.6	18	0.057	5.3[d]
Desipramine	110	0.29	0.019	0.0026
Doxepin	5.3	0.36	0.018	0.067
Fluoxetine	0.36	8.3	0.063	23
Imipramine	7.7	2.4	0.020	0.31
Maprotiline	14	0.030	0.034	0.0021
Nortriptyline	25	0.38	0.059	0.015
Paroxetine	3.0	136	0.059	45
Protriptyline	100	0.36	0.054	0.0036
Sertraline	0.46	29	0.38	64
Trazodone	0.020	0.53	0.0070	26
Trimipramine	0.20	0.040	0.029	0.20
REFERENCE COMPOUND				
d-Amphetamine[e]	2.00	—	1.2	

From Richelson (1993),[2] table 2, p. 468, with permission.
[a]10^{27} 3 $1/K_i$, where K_i = inhibitor constant in molarity.
[b]Ratio of potency of serotonin uptake blockade to potency of norephinephrine uptake blockade.
[c]Indicates that amitriptyline as about 2.8 (1/0.36) times more potent at blocking uptake of norepinephrine than uptake of serotonin.
[d]Indicates that clomipramine is about 5 times more potent at blocking uptake of serotonin than uptake of norepinephrine.
[e]This is not an antidepressant but is shown here for comparison.

Table 7.2 compares how effectively various antidepressant drugs block the reuptake of norepinephrine, serotonin, and dopamine (in an experimental model) and calculates the selectivity for serotonin over norepinephrine. Most of the newer drugs (fluoxetine, sertraline, paroxetine, clomipramine, and venlafaxine) have serotonin selectivity; one new drug (bupropion) does not, as it selectively blocks dopamine reuptake.

With this background, we can now undertake discussion of each of the classes of antidepressant drugs. Chapter 15 discusses the use of these drugs in the clinical management of specific affective disorders.

Tricyclic Antidepressants

The term *tricyclic antidepressant* describes a class of drugs that all have a characteristic three-ring molecular core (see Figure 7.2) and relieve depression in persons who experience major depressive illness.[12] TCAs are, historically, the drugs of first choice for the treatment of major depression even though the SSRIs, which are extremely popular in the 1990s, are equally effective and exhibit less cardiac toxicity when taken in overdosage. Because of this, the current use of the TCAs is often overshadowed by the use of SSRIs and other, newer antidepressants. TCAs, however, remain the standard against which other antidepressants are compared;[20] no other group of antidepressants has yet been demonstrated to be either more clinically effective or capable of exerting a more rapid onset of antidepressant effect.

Imipramine (Tofranil) is the prototype TCA, but, in fact, another clinically available TCA, *desipramine* (Norpramin), is the pharmacologically active intermediate metabolite of imipramine. Likewise, *amitriptyline* (Elavil) has an active intermediate metabolite, *nortriptyline* (Pamelor, Aventil). In fact, these active intermediates may actually be responsible for much of the antidepressant effect of both imipramine and amitriptyline.

All the TCAs attach to and inhibit (to varying degrees) the presynaptic transporter proteins for both norepinephrine and serotonin (see Table 7.2). The traditional TCAs, however, have three clinical limitations. First, they are claimed to have a slow onset of action, although Soares and Gershon (1996)[19] state that "overall, they [TCAs] seem to start acting as fast as other available compounds, provided that comparable dosage strategies can be tolerated." Second, the TCAs exert a wide variety of effects on the central nervous system (CNS), causing a variety of bothersome side effects (discussed later) not shared with use of the SSRIs. Third, in overdosage (as in suicide attempts), TCAs are cardiotoxic and potentially fatal.

Because TCAs do not produce euphoria or other pleasurable effects and have few discernible psychological effects in normal patients, they have no recreational or behavior-reinforcing value. Thus, abuse and psychological dependence are not a concern. The clinical choice of TCA is determined by effectiveness, tolerance of side effects, and duration of action. In depressed patients, TCAs elevate mood, increase physical activity, improve appetite and sleep patterns, and reduce morbid preoccupation. They are useful in treating acute episodes of major depression as well as in preventing their relapses. In addition, they are clinically effective in the long-term therapy of dysthymia,[5] although SSRIs may be equally effective and better tolerated.[6] In children and adolescents, TCAs have been used in the treatment of behavioral disorders accompanied by depression, as well as in a variety of anxiety states. Wilens and coworkers (1996)[20] evaluated protriptyline in a small study of ADHD (attention deficit hyperactivity disorder) children and reported the drug effective in only 45 percent of patients; half the children discontinued the drug because of adverse effects.

In a related study, Wilens and coworkers (1995)[21] reviewed the effectiveness of TCAs in the treatment of adult ADHD. In a group of 37 patients receiving either desipramine or nortriptyline, the TCA relieved ADHD symptoms in 25. Positive responders received "robust doses" of the TCA, and most patients also received adjunctive agents, especially behavioral stimulants such as methylphenidate. This survey concluded that additional evaluations of TCAs in adult ADHD are warranted.

Pharmacological Effects

Central Nervous System. The therapeutic effects of the TCAs result from drug-induced blockade of presynaptic serotonin, dopamine, and norepinephrine receptors (see Table 7.3); the down-regulation of these receptors accounts for therapeutic effectiveness. In addition to blocking these presynaptic transporters, the TCAs, to varying degrees, block postsynaptic receptors at acetylcholine and histamine neurons. The blockade of acetylcholine receptors results in dry mouth, confusion, memory impairments, and blurred vision. The blockade of histamine receptors results in drowsiness, an effect similar to the sedation seen after administration of the classic CNS-acting antihistamine diphenhydramine (Benadryl).

In the patient on long-term therapy with TCAs, tolerance develops to most of these side effects, but choosing a particular drug with an awareness of its side effects can turn a disadvantage into a therapeutic advantage. For example, amitriptyline and doxepin are the most sedating of the TCAs, making them useful in treating individuals with agitation as

TABLE 7.3 Affinity of antidepressants for neurotransmitter receptors of human brain

Drug	Histamine (H$_1$)[a]	Acetylcholine (Muscarinic)	Norepinephrine (α_1-Adrenoceptor)	Dopamine (D$_2$)
Amitriptyline	91	5.6	3.7	0.10
Amoxapine	4.0	0.10	2.00	0.62
Bupropion	0.015	0.0021	0.022	0.00048
Clomipramine	3.2	2.7	2.63	0.53
Desipramine	0.91	0.50	0.77	0.030
Doxepin	420	1.2	4.2	0.042
Fluoxetine	0.016	0.050	0.0169	0.015
Imipramine	9.1	1.1	1.1	0.050
Maprotiline	50	0.18	1.1	0.29
Nortriptyline	10	0.7	1.7	0.083
Paroxetine	0.0045	0.93	0.029	0.0031
Protriptyline	4.0	4.0	0.77	0.043
Sertraline	0.0041	0.16	0.27	0.0093
Trazodone	0.29	0.00031	2.8	0.026
Trimipramine	370	1.7	4.2	0.56

REFERENCE COMPOUNDS[b]

Drug	Histamine (H$_1$)[a]	Acetylcholine (Muscarinic)	Norepinephrine (α_1-Adrenoceptor)	Dopamine (D$_2$)
Diphenhydramine	7.1	—	—	—
Atropine	—	42	—	—
Phentolamine	—	—	6.7	—
Haloperidol	—	—	—	26

From Richelson (1993),[2] table 3, p. 469, with permission.
[a]10^{27} 3 1/K$_d$, where K$_d$ = equilibrium dissociation constant in molarity.
[b]These are not antidepressants but are shown here for comparison.

well as depression or where improved sleep is desirable. Table 7.4 lists the clinical consequences that can follow blockade of each type of receptor.

Of additional importance are the possible effects of TCAs on memory and cognitive function. Here, one must distinguish between the direct effects of these drugs on cognition, which are related to their intrinsic properties, and indirect effects, which result from the improvement in mood. TCAs with either sedative (antihistamine) effects or anticholinergic effects can directly impair attention, motor speed, dexterity, and memory.[22] Relatively nonsedating compounds with low degrees of anticholinergic side effects cause very little direct

TABLE 7.4 Pharmacological properties of antidepressants and possible clinical consequences

Property	Possible clinical consequences
Blockade of norepinephrine uptake at nerve endings	Tremors Tachycardia Erectile and ejaculatory dysfunction Blockade of the antihypertensive effects of guanethidine (Ismelin and Esimil and guanadrel (Hylorel) Augmentation of pressor effects of sympathomimetic amines
Blockade of serotonin uptake at nerve endings	Gastrointestinal disturbances Increase or decrease in anxiety (dose dependent) Sexual dysfunction Extrapyramidal side effects Interactions with L-tryptophan monoamine oxidase inhibitors, and fenfluramine
Blockade of dopamine uptake at nerve endings	Psychomotor activation Antiparkinsonian effect Aggravation of psychosis
Blockade of histamine H_1 receptors	Potentiation of central depressant drugs Sedation drowsiness Weight gain Hypotension
Blockade of acetylcholine receptors	Blurred vision Dry mouth Sinus tachycardia Constipation Urinary retention
Blockade of norepinephrine receptors	Memory dysfunction Potentiation of the antihypertensive effect of prazosin (Minipress), terazosin (Hytrin) doxazosin (Cardura), labetalol (Normodyne) Postural hypotension, dizziness Reflex tachycardia
Blockade of dopamine D_2 receptors	Extrapyramidal movement disorders Endocrine changes Sexual dysfunction (males)

From Richelson (1993),[2] table 4, p. 471, with permission.

impairment of psychomotor or memory functions. The very young and the elderly may be more susceptible to the anticholinergic-induced impairment of memory, although in the elderly such impairments are "mild and are not similar to those of Alzheimer's patients."[23] Individuals at the extremes of age, if treated with TCAs, should probably receive a drug with low degrees of antihistaminic and (especially) anticholinergic effects. In contrast to these direct effects, relief from depression indirectly improves attention, cognition, and memory.[24]

Antidepressant drugs are effective *analgesics* (pain relievers) in a variety of clinical pain syndromes. Indeed, TCAs (as well as SSRIs) can consistently be demonstrated to be superior to a placebo in the treatment of chronic pain, in particular in improving pain complaints and symptoms.[25,26] Analgesia follows from a direct spinal cord mechanism, as is explained in Chapter 10. The antidepressant action no doubt adds a feeling of well-being to the analgesic action, improving the affect as well as reducing physical discomfort.

Peripheral Nervous System. The TCAs exert a variety of effects on the peripheral nervous system. Here, the effects of TCAs on the heart deserve special mention, since TCAs cause both cardiac depression and increased electrical irritability (as evidenced by cardiac arrhythmias). Cardiac depression can be life threatening when an overdose is taken, as in suicide attempts. In such a situation, the patient commonly exhibits excitement, delirium, and convulsions, followed by respiratory depression and coma, which can persist for several days. Cardiac arrhythmias can lead to ventricular fibrillation, cardiac arrest, and death. These arrhythmias are extremely difficult to treat. Thus, all TCAs can be lethal in doses that are commonly available to depressed patients. For this reason, "it is unwise to dispense more than a week's supply of an antidepressant to an acutely depressed patient."[12]

Popper and Elliott (1990)[27] reported on three cases of sudden death in children receiving desipramine for the treatment of ADHD or depression. Two additional deaths were later reported, and Varley and McClennan (1997)[28] reported two more (one child was being treated with desipramine, the other with imipramine). These seven deaths in the 1990s are certainly cause for concern in using TCAs to treat depression in children where therapeutic efficacy is questionable anyway (e.g., in treating major depression). In cases where efficacy is more demonstrable (e.g., enuresis [bed-wetting], OCD, and ADHD), use is appropriate, but caution is warranted. Biederman and coworkers (1997)[29] studied plasma levels of desipramine in children and made recommendations for therapeutic plasma levels (200 to 300 nanograms per ml) that may avoid cardiac toxicity.

Pharmacokinetics

The TCAs are well absorbed when they are administered orally. Because most of them have relatively long half-lives (see Table 7.1), they should only be taken once a day at bedtime to minimize unwanted side effects, especially the persistent sedation. The TCAs are metabolized in the liver, and, as discussed earlier, two TCAs are converted into pharmacologically active intermediates that are detoxified later (see Figure 7.3). This combination of a pharmacologically active drug and active metabolite results in a clinical effect lasting up to 4 days, and even longer in elderly patients.

TCAs readily cross the placental barrier. However, *in utero* exposure does not affect global IQ, language development, or behavioral development in preschool children.[30] No fetal abnormalities from these drugs has yet been reported.

Second-Generation (Atypical) Antidepressants

Efforts from the late 1970s to the mid-1980s to find structurally different agents that might overcome some of the disadvantages of the TCAs (slow onset of action, limited efficacy, and significant side effects) produced the so-called *second-generation* (or "atypical") *antidepressants* (see Figure 7.2). Their pharmacokinetic data and a comparison with standard TCAs are listed in Tables 7.1 and 7.5. Further efforts resulted in the development of both the *serotonin-specific reuptake inhibitors* (SSRIs) and the newer *"dual-action" antidepressants*, both of which are described after the description of the atypical agents.

Maprotiline (Ludiomil) was one of the first clinically available antidepressants that modified the basic tricyclic structure (see Figure 7.2). It has a long half-life, blocks norepinephrine uptake, and is as efficacious as imipramine (the "gold standard" of TCAs). However, it offers few, if any, therapeutic advantages. A major limitation of maprotiline is that it tends (albeit rarely) to cause seizures, presumably because of the accumulation of active metabolites. Maprotiline does not appear to cause deterioration in cognitive functions.

Amoxapine (Asendin) was another early antidepressant agent that was structurally different from the tricyclics. It is primarily a norepineph-rine-reuptake inhibitor and is as effective as imipramine; although amoxapine may be slightly more effective in relieving any accompanying anxiety and agitation. The use of amoxapine can be associated with parkinsonian-like, neuroleptic side effects (it blocks dopamine receptors), sometimes even after therapy has stopped. The drug is metabolized to an active intermediate, 8-hydroxy-amoxapine; this intermediate may be

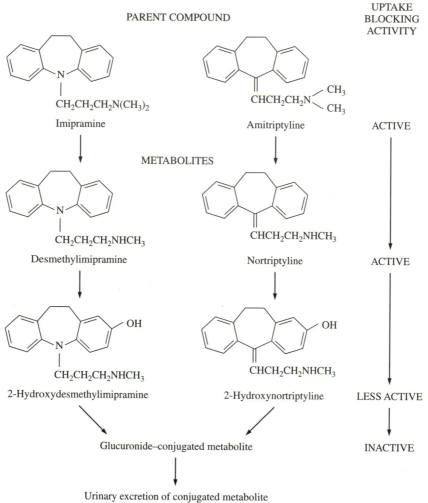

Figure 7.3 Metabolism of imipramine and amitriptyline. Note that the two active intermediates are marketed commercially.

TABLE 7.5 Anvantages and disadvantages of second-generation antidepressants compared to tricyclic antidepressants

Drug	Advantages	Disadvantages
Maprotiline	Sedating and may be useful for agitation Does not antagonize anti-hypertensive effects of clonidine	Increased incidence of seizures Increased lethality in overdose Has long half-life, therefore accumulates Increased incidence of rashes
Amoxapine	Low in sedative effects Low in anticholinergic effects Possibly effective for monotherapy for psychotic depression Has possible rapid onset	Can promote parkinsonian side effects and tardive dyskinesia Cannot separate anti-depressant from "antipsychotic" effect Increased lethality in overdose
Trazodone	Relatively safe in overdose Sedating (may be useful in controlling agitation and hostility in geriatric patients) Useful as a hypnotic in conjunction with MAO inhibitors	Efficacy not clearly established May induce or exacerbate ventricular arrhythmia Can promote priapism
Fluoxetine	Low in sedative, anticholinergic, and hypotensive side effects Does not promote weight gain, maybe helps weight loss No prolonging of cardiac conduction Effective in obsessive-compulsive disorders	Causes anxiety, nausea, and insomnia Has long half-life, therefore accumulates Unknown efficacy in panic Possibly has indirect dopamine blocking effects Has pharmacokinetic interactions with tricyclics and benzodiazepines
Bupropion	Low in sedative, hypotensive, and anticholinergic side effects Does not promote weight gain Lack of ECG changes	Tends to "overstimulate," with insomnia, terror Not effective for panic; unknown effectiveness for obsessive-compulsive disorders Increased incidence of seizures in bulimia May induce perceptual abnormalities and psychosis Causes increase in prolactin

responsible for the dopamine-receptor blockade and neuroleptic effects. Like TCAs, overdosage can result in fatalities.

Trazodone (Desyrel) is yet another chemically unique antidepressant (see Figure 7.2). It is as therapeutically efficacious as the TCAs. Its mechanism of antidepressant action is unclear, because it is not a potent reuptake blocker of either norepinephrine or serotonin. However, it (or its active metabolite) does block a subclass of serotonin receptors (the serotonin$_2$, or 5-HT$_2$, receptor), and it appears to down-regulate either the norepinephrine or serotonin receptors. Trazodone has a short onset of action (about a week), but 2 to 5 weeks are still required to produce an optimal effect. Drowsiness, its most common side effect, occurs in about 20 percent of all patients. In rare instances, priapism (prolonged and painful penile erections) limits its use in males. The effect of trazodone on cognitive functions is controversial; one report indicated sedation and psychomotor impairments,[31] while another report noted no detriment in the cognitive skills of depressed patients.[32]

Bupropion (Wellbutrin) is an antidepressant that is sometimes effective in depressed individuals who do not respond to other agents. Bupropion differs from the other antidepressants in that it selectively inhibits dopamine reuptake (a cocaine-like action), but it does not seem to exert a reinforcing action in animals.[33] Because of its potentiation of dopamine, it has been used to treat children with ADHD[34] (see Chapter 5), although a high incidence of severe skin rashes in children treated with bupropion is disconcerting.[35] Side effects include anxiety, restlessness, tremor, and insomnia. Its potential for compulsive abuse is unclear, because the drug may resemble the behavioral stimulants more than it resembles the antidepressants. More serious side effects include the induction of psychosis *de novo* and generalized seizures. Bupropion is not effective in the treatment of panic disorder. Patients suffering sexual dysfunction as a side effect of SSRIs may recover their capacity for orgasm and feel greater sexual satisfaction without becoming depressed again if they are switched to bupropion.[36] Bupropion is also finding use in the treatment of nicotine craving after smoking cessation. For this use, an extended-release form of bupropion will shortly be available under the trade name Zyban.

Serotonin-Specific Reuptake Inhibitors (SSRIs)

As discussed, it is generally agreed that there is a correlation between diminished serotonin neurotransmission (or receptor responsiveness) and episodes of major depression.[37] This suggested that drugs potentiating serotonin neurotransmission by inhibiting its active presynaptic reuptake might be clinically useful in treating major depression. This idea assumed, of course, that a cause-and-effect relationship exists and that the correlation is not just coincidental. Today, the correlation is of such strength that one author writes:

> The only known common final effect of antidepressant treatments is an enhancement of 5-HT neurotransmission in the CNS upon their long-term administration. . . . Stimulation of 5-HT$_1$ type receptors is probably associated with antidepressant and anxiolytic effects, while stimulation of 5-HT$_2$ and 5-HT$_3$ type receptors is related to adverse effects. Stimulation of 5-HT$_2$ receptors is associated with insomnia, anxiety, agitation, and sexual dysfunction, whereas stimulation of 5-HT$_3$ receptors is associated with nausea.[10]

Six SSRIs are currently available for use in treating major depression (see Figure 7.4): sertraline, fluvoxamine, paroxetine, fluoxetine,

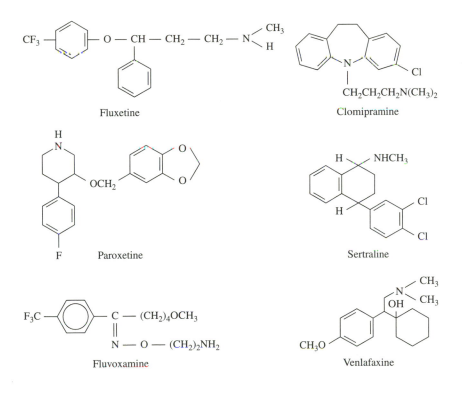

Figure 7.4 Chemical structures of serotonin-specific reuptake inhibitor (SSRI) antidepressants. Note that clomipramine is included here (because of its serotonin specificity), rather than as one of the TCAs, of which it structurally is a member (see Table 7.1).

clomipramine, and venlafaxine. These drugs all block serotonin reuptake; they do not appear to block reuptake of other neurotransmitters to any significant degree, nor do they block postsynaptic serotonin receptors (of any subtype). Such "purity" of effect has led to both their popularity and their constellation of side effects.

Fluoxetine (Prozac) became clinically available in the United States in 1988 as the first antidepressant of the class now known as the *SSRIs*. Fluoxetine is also the first of the non-TCAs that could be considered an antidepressant of first choice (not just for patients who have failed therapy with TCAs), particularly for patients who do not have severe depression (where the SSRIs are generally thought to be somewhat less effective than the TCAs). Fluoxetine's efficacy is generally comparable to that of the TCAs; more important, it is not fatal in overdosage, because it is devoid of the TCA-caused cardiac toxicity.

Fluoxetine has a fairly long half-life (2 to 4 days), but its active metabolite (norfluoxetine) has a half-life of about 14 days. The antidepressant action of the drug and its metabolite thus tend to build with repeated doses over about 2 months, presumably because both compounds continue to accumulate. This may at least partially explain the slow onset of peak therapeutic effect, the late onset of side effects, and the prolonged duration of action following drug discontinuation. With time, doses are stabilized at a low daily level. As a result of the long half-lives of fluoxetine and norfluoxetine, a 5-week drug-free interval is recommended between cessation of fluoxetine administration and the initiation of another drug therapy.

Stanford (1996)[38] discussed the medical and social popularity and the commercial success of fluoxetine, concluding: "Ironically, fluoxetine might be distinctive in that it is the *least* selective SSRI and has marked effects on catecholamine functions in the brain." Regardless, fluoxetine is considered the prototype SSRI, with a side-effect profile characteristic of this class of drugs.

Fluoxetine and other SSRIs demonstrate few anticholinergic or antihistaminic side effects. Thus, they cause little or no sedation and little impairment of learning, memory, or cognition, although there are side effects, including headache, gastrointestinal discomfort, nervousness, insomnia, tremor, and sweating. At the extreme, a "serotonin syndrome" is characterized by agitation, diaphoresis, diarrhea, fever, hyperreflexia, incoordination, mental status changes (confusion and hypomania), myoclonus, shivering, hypothermia, and tremors.[39] In addition, sexual dysfunction has been reported in up to 40 to 60 percent of patients taking fluoxetine or other SSRIs.[40] Sexual dysfunction may contribute significantly to noncompliance with drug therapy and may significantly impair the patient's quality of life.[41] Because of the long half-life of the fluoxetine metabolite, a "drug holiday" is ineffective in alleviating sexual dysfunction, although such a "holiday" may effectively reduce the sexual dysfunction accompanying the use of other, shorter half-life SSRIs.[41] A recently published symposium[42] addresses the issue of sexual dysfunction (anhedonia and anorgasmia) in patients taking SSRI antidepressants.

Sertraline (Zoloft) was the second SSRI approved for clinical use in the United States because it is as effective as TCAs. It is also effective and well tolerated in the elderly. Sertraline is four to five times more potent than fluoxetine in blocking serotonin reuptake and is more selective. Steady-state levels of the drug in plasma are achieved within 4 to 7 days, and its metabolites are less cumulative and less pharmacologically active. Sertraline has fewer anticholinergic, antihistaminic, and cardiovascular adverse effects than the TCAs, as well as a low risk of toxicity in overdose. Sertraline is effective in the treatment of dysthymia and, in general, is better tolerated than imipramine.[6] Mammen and coworkers (1997)[43] documented the presence of sertraline in infants of breast-feeding mothers, and no adverse consequences resulted.

Paroxetine (Paxil) was the third SSRI available for clinical use in treating depression. Therapeutically, it is comparable to the TCAs in efficacy, being clearly superior to a placebo. Paroxetine is effective in the presence or absence of anxiety, agitation, retardation, and reactive and endogenous features. It is highly effective in reducing anxiety, a common symptom in depressive illness.[44] In mid-1996 paroxetine received formal FDA approval for use not only in depression and OCD, but also in the treatment of panic disorder. It was the first SSRI to receive FDA approval for this use.* Like sertraline, paroxetine is more selective than fluoxetine in blocking serotonin reuptake. Also, paroxetine's metabolites are relatively inactive, and steady state is achieved within about 7 days. The metabolic half-life is about 24 hours. The symposium edited by Boyer and Feighner (1992)[45] discusses the antidepressant properties of paroxetine.

Clomipramine (Anafranil), structurally a TCA, has been used in Europe and Canada for many years to treat OCD; the drug was introduced

---

*FDA "approval" does not necessarily mean that paroxetine is more effective than any other SSRI for the treatment of panic disorder. It means that the manufacturer applied for approval and demonstrated sufficient efficacy and safety to justify the formal approval. It is likely that all of the SSRIs are similarly effective in treating panic disorder, although direct comparisons are unavailable. If any drug (antidepressant or otherwise) is used for a therapeutic purpose for which it is not formally FDA "approved," such use is considered an "off-label" use, which is not illegal but must be defensible by the prescribing physician.

in the United States in 1990 for this purpose. About 40 to 75 percent of patients with OCD respond favorably but are seldom completely cured. Behavioral therapy helps maximize the response. The drug has also been used around the world in the treatment of depression, panic disorder, and phobic disorders. Clomipramine is approximately equal to the TCAs in both its efficacy and its profile of side effects. Despite its tricyclic structure, it is one of the most selective inhibitors of serotonin reuptake.

In 1994 *venlafaxine* (Effexor) was introduced as the fifth antidepressant that is thought to exert its effect by blocking active serotonin reuptake. Structurally unique (see Figure 7.4), it also blocks the active reuptake of norepinephrine (see Table 7.1), with little effect on dopamine reuptake.[46] Moller and Volz (1996)[7] refer to venlafaxine as a "combined noradrenalin- and serotonin-reuptake inhibitor," resembling TCAs but lacking their anticholinergic and antihistaminic effects. In this regard, venlafaxine more closely resembles fluoxetine than it resembles either sertraline or paroxetine. Unlike the TCAs, effects on cardiac conduction are minimal.[47] Sanger and Schulte (1996)[48] discuss a patient in whom ventafaxine was superior to sertraline in the management of chronic back pain.

The primary metabolite of venlafaxine is pharmacologically active; the half-lives of the parent compound and the primary metabolite are 5 hours and 11 hours, respectively. Its clinical effectiveness compares favorably with that of other SSRIs. Venlafaxine produces improvements in psychomotor and cognitive function, likely due to the relief of depression in the absence of detrimental sedative and anticholinergic effects.

In 1995 *fluvoxamine* (Luvox), a structural derivative of fluoxetine (see Figure 7.4), became available in the United States for the treatment of OCD.[49,50] Like all SSRIs, fluvoxamine also has well-described antidepressant properties, comparable in efficacy to the TCA imipramine,[51] but is devoid of adverse cardiac effects when compared with maprotiline.[52] A recent symposium (*Journal of Clinical Psychiatry* 57, Suppl. 8, 1996) discusses a variety of clinical uses of fluvoxamine (e.g., treatment of PTSD, dysphoria, and panic disorder).

Other SSRI agents, including *citalopram* (see Figure 7.5) may be introduced for the treatment and preventive maintenance of major depression, social phobias, panic disorder, and OCD.

SSRIs in Children and Adolescents

Popper (1995),[34] DeVane and Sallie (1996),[53] and Leonard and coworkers have reviewed the use of SSRIs in children and adolescents. While these drugs have been reported to be useful for the treatment of at

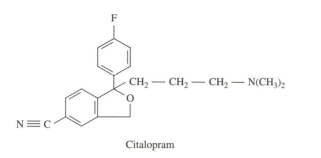

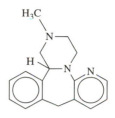

Citalopram   Mirtazapine (Remeron)

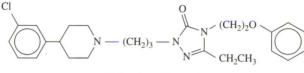

Nefazodone (Serzone)

Figure 7.5 Chemical structures of dual-action antidepressants. Of these three, nefazodone (Serzone) and mirtazapine (Remeron) are approved for clinical use in the United States.

least 13 different conditions (e.g., autism, anorexia, bulimia, ADHD), clinical evidence of efficacy is strongest to support their use in depression and OCD. Birmaher and coworkers (1996)[55] also review the pharmacotherapy of childhood and adolescent depression and arrive at a different conclusion. They state that in this disorder, 40 percent to 70 percent of children and adolescents respond to placebo therapy:

> Taken together, these studies suggest that TCAs are no more effective than placebo for the treatment of major depressive disorder in children and adolescents. . . . [While] open studies have reported 70% to 90% response to fluoxetine [a SSRI] for the treatment of adolescents with major depressive disorder . . . a double-blind, placebo-controlled study . . . did not find significant differences between placebo and fluoxetine. . . . Despite the successful response to fluoxetine, many patients had only partial improvement, suggesting that the ideal treatment may involve variation in dose or length of treatment, or a combination of pharmacological and psychosocial treatments.

Controlled studies are not yet available to support widespread use of SSRIs for other disorders of childhood. Popper (1995)[35] cautions:

SSRIs appear to be changing the treatment philosophy of child and adolescent psychiatrists. Almost as quickly as these new drugs became available, psychiatrists began to prescribe them in adolescents and children for a variety of presumed indications. In contrast to the caution characteristic of the past, children and adolescents in large numbers have been exposed to these new agents—despite the lack of a lengthy track record to demonstrate their safety in adults. . . . Whatever their merits and liabilities may turn out to be, SSRIs have led many psychiatrists to feel comfortable in prescribing newly developed medications in children, although long-term and even many short-term issues were still largely unclear. By breaking this barrier, psychiatrists have perhaps become blasé about playing with newly found fire.

Dual-Action Antidepressants

Nefazodone (Serzone)

In late 1995, *nefazodone* (see Figure 7.5) was introduced as a new, unique antidepressant, unrelated to TCAs or MAOIs and differing from the SSRIs by a *dual action* on the serotonin synapse.

Nefazodone's mode of action is different from that of other currently available antidepressants. Its strongest pharmacological action is 5-HT_{2A} receptor blockade. Nefazodone also has activity as a serotonin reuptake inhibitor at its therapeutic dose. Both actions are thought to be responsible for the effective antidepressant activity of nefazodone, and the 5-HT_{2A} blockade is thought to be responsible for nefazodone's particular benefit on sleep disturbances and anxiety often seen in depressed patients and the lack of induced sexual dysfunction with ongoing treatment.[56]

Regarding both its efficacy as a clinical antidepressant and the tolerability of its side effects, Baldwin and coworkers (1996)[57] demonstrated that both nefazodone and paroxetine (a SSRI) had similar efficacy in relieving major depression and both were well tolerated. Feiger and coworkers (1996)[58] compared nefazodone and seretraline (another SSRI) and reported equal efficacy as antidepressants, but sertraline had detrimental effects on sexual function and performance in both men and women, whereas nefazodone did not.

Since anxiety commonly coexists with depression, the worsening of anxiety symptoms with SSRIs can be a therapeutic limitation to their use. Nefazodone, by blocking 5-HT_{2A} receptors, may reduce anxiety symptoms, in essence combining the actions of a TCA and a benzodiazepine anxiolytic without their side effects.[59] Sedation can be bothersome or limiting with nefazodone therapy. Other reported side effects include nausea, dry mouth, dizziness, and light-headedness. Nefazodone appears to be quite effective in the treatment of depression-related insomnia and nighttime awakenings.[7] Wilens and coworkers (1997)[60] reported successful treatment of juvenile mood disorders, especially depression, in seven "treatment-resistant" youths to whom nefazodone was administered for periods of 6 to 24 weeks.

In treating depressed patients, nefazodone has not been shown to have therapeutic superiority over TCAs or SSRIs or faster onset of action. Davis, Whittington, and Bryson (1997)[61] have reviewed the pharmacology and efficacy of nefazodone.

Mirtazapine (Remeron)

Mirtazapine (see Figure 7.5) is a new antidepressant, introduced into clinical use in the United States in 1997. According to Kasper (1996)[62]:

> In line with the concept that severe depression may respond better to drugs with a dual rather than a single mode of action, mirtazapine is a noradrenergic and specific serotonergic antidepressant. It has a different mode of action from TCAs, SSRIs, and MAOIs, because it increases noradrenergic and serotonergic neurotransmission via a blockade of the central alpha$_2$-autoreceptors and heteroreceptors. The increased release of serotonin, via increased cell firings of 5-HT neurons, stimulates only the 5-HT$_1$ type receptors, because 5-HT$_2$ and 5-HT$_3$ type receptors are specifically blocked by mirtazapine.

The concept of an autoreceptor is described in Appendix IV; here, suffice the Kasper quotation to mean that mirtazapine blocks catecholamine receptors located on the presynaptic nerve terminals, receptors that normally modulate the amount of transmitter released from the nerve terminals. Antagonism of these modulatory receptors results in increased release of NE and 5-HT and, therefore, enhanced NE and 5-HT activity. Fraser (1997)[63] reviews these new concepts in antidepressant drug action. Shader and coworkers (1997)[64] review even more novel concepts regarding the mechanism of action of antidepressants.

Mirtazapine is a potent antagonist of postsynaptic 5-HT$_2$ and 5-HT$_3$ receptors, preventing the described side effects of SSRIs (especially anxiety, insomnia, agitation, nausea, and sexual dysfunction). Mirtazapine is also a potent blocker of histamine receptors, causing drowsiness as a prominent side effect. Such sedation may be advantageous in depressed patients with symptoms of anxiety and insomnia, a common occurrence.

Mirtazapine is rapidly absorbed orally, with peak blood levels occurring 2 hours after administration. The elimination half-life is 20 to 40 hours, allowing once-a-day administration, usually at bedtime in order to maximize sleep and minimize daytime sedation. Kasper (1997),[65] Delbressine and Ria (1997),[66] and Burrows and Kremer (1997)[67] review the pharmacology and clinical efficacy of mirtazapine.

Monoamine Oxidase Inhibitors (MAOIs)

The traditional monoamine oxidase (MAO) inhibitors have long been considered alternative drugs for treating major depressive illnesses; their limitations include their serious side effects and their limited efficacy. Introduced during the late 1950s, they have a checkered and controversial history. Soon after their introduction, they were noted to have serious, frequently fatal, interactions with certain foods and medicines. The latter included adrenaline-like drugs found in nasal sprays, antiasthma medications, cold medicines, cocaine, and so on. The foods included those that contain tyramine, a by-product of fermentation, such as many cheeses, wines, beers, liver, and some beans. As a result of the interaction, blood pressure increases severely, occasionally enough to be fatal. Thus, for about 20 years these drugs were considered dangerous, but with strict dietary restrictions, they can be used safely. Gardner et al (1996)[68] discuss at length the MAOI diet and its appropriate presentation to patients. This diet is presented in Tables 7.6 and 7.7. Today, the MAOIs are experiencing a resurgence in use for several reasons:

- With appropriate dietary restrictions, they can be as safe or safer than TCAs.
- They can work in many patients who respond poorly to both TCAs and SSRIs.
- They are excellent drugs for the treatment of atypical depression, which presents primarily with anxiety and phobic symptoms, masked depression (such as hypochondriasis), anorexia nervosa, bulimia, bipolar depression, dysthymia, depression in the elderly, panic disorder, and phobias.

Monoamine oxidase (MAO) is an enzyme that breaks down normal neurotransmitters in the body, including norepinephrine and serotonin. There are two types of the enzyme: MAO-A (here, the "good" MAO) is found in norepinephrine and serotonin nerve terminals; MAO-B (here,

TABLE 7.6 Relative restrictions of food and beverages with MAOI use

Restriction	Foods
Absolute	Aged cheeses; aged and cured meats; banana peel; broad bean pods; improperly stored or spoiled meats, poultry, and fish; Marmite; sauerkraut; soy sauce and other soybean condiments; tap beer
Moderate	Red or white wine; bottled or canned beer (including nonalcoholic varieties)
Unnecessary	Avocados; bananas; beef/chicken bouillon; chocolate; fresh and mild cheeses, e.g., ricotta, cottage, cream cheese, processed slices; fresh meat, poultry, or fish; gravy (fresh); monosodium glutamate; peanuts; properly stored pickled or smoked fish, e.g., herring; raspberries; soy milk; yeast extracts (except Marmite)

Reproduced with permission from Gardner et al. (1996).[68]

the "bad" MAO) is found in dopamine-secreting neurons. Pharmacologically, drug-induced inhibition of MAO-A is presumably responsible for the antidepressant activity, while inhibition of MAO-B is responsible for the side effects, including serious drug interactions.

Drug-induced blockade of MAO (especially MAO-A) allows large amounts of transmitters to accumulate in the nerve terminals. As a result, more transmitter is released when the neurons are stimulated. Three MAO inhibitors have been available for many years, and all three are both nonselective and irreversible in their inhibition of both MAO-A and MAO-B. Short-acting, reversible MAO-A inhibitors are newer and as yet clinically unavailable in the United States, although one (moclobemide, discussed later) is available in Canada and Europe.

Irreversible MAOIs

The two MAO inhibitors currently available, *phenelzine* (Nardil) and *tranylcypromine* (Parnate), both irreversibly block both MAO-A and MAO-B. Irreversible effects are unusual in pharmacology; most drugs discussed to this point exert reversible actions, usually by competing for receptors with naturally occurring neurotransmitters. The irreversible MAO inhibitors form a chemical bond with part of the MAO enzyme, a bond that cannot be broken; enzyme function returns only as new enzyme is biosynthesized.

TABLE 7.7 Sunnybrook Health Science Center MAOI diet

Several foods and beverages contain tyramine and may interact with medication. The patient must follow the dietary instructions below from the day taking the medication begins until 2 weeks after you start stopping it.
Note: All foods must be fresh or properly frozen. Patients should avoid foods if storage conditions are not known.

	Food to avoid	Food allowed
Cheese	All matured or aged cheese All casseroles made with these cheeses, i.e., pizza, lasagna, etc. Note: All cheeses are considered matured or aged except those listed opposite	Fresh cottage cheese, cream cheese, ricotta cheese, and processed cheese slices. All fresh milk products that have been stored properly (e.g., sour cream, yogurt, ice cream)
Meat, fish, and poultry	Fermented/dry sausage: pepperoni, salami, mortadella, summer sausage, etc. Improperly stored meat, fish, or poultry Improperly stored pickled herring	All fresh packaged or processed meat (e.g., chicken loaf, hot dogs), fish, or poultry Store in refrigerator immediately and eat as soon as possible
Fruits and vegetables	Fava or broad bean pods (not beans) Banana peel	Banana pulp All others except those listed opposite
Alcoholic beverages	All tap beers	Alcohol: No more than *two* domestic bottled or canned beers or 4-fl.-oz. glasses of red or white wine per day; this also applies to nonalcoholic beer; note that red wine may produce headache unrelated to a rise in blood pressure
Miscellaneous foods	Marmite concentrated yeast extract Sauerkraut Soy sauce and other soybean condiments	Other yeast extracts (e.g., brewer's yeast) Soy milk

Reproduced with permission from Gardner et al. (1996).[68]

Pharmacokinetics and Mechanism of Action. As shown in Figure 7.6, the elimination half-life of tranylcypromine is about 2 hours. This rapid rate of elimination results in a rapid decline in plasma levels of the drug (Figure 7.6A), but not in the degree of MAO inhibition (Figure 7.6B). The reason for this lack of correlation is that after tranylcypromine is absorbed, it is metabolized to a reactive intermediate compound. This compound then binds irreversibly with MAO-A and MAO-B in a tight covalent bond. Excess drug that is not converted to the intermediate compound is rapidly metabolized and then excreted.[69] This course of events is illustrated in Figure 7.6B. Here, the upper graph reflects the rapid rise and fall in the blood (plasma) levels of tranylcypromine given orally three times a day for seven days. There is little drug accumulation because the liver rapidly metabolizes the drug. The irreversible inhibition of MAO occurs slowly; a level of 70 percent inhibition is reached by day 7. After the patient stops taking the drug, MAO activity returns very slowly, reflecting the synthesis of new, biologically active enzyme.

Efficacy. The nonselective, irreversible MAO inhibitors were the first clinically effective drugs for treating major depression, preceding the TCAs by about 10 years. Their fall from favor was not from lack of efficacy but from fear of adverse reactions. Indeed, their efficacy is comparable to that of the TCAs.[70] Importantly, MAO inhibitors can be effective in patients in whom therapy with TCAs and SSRIs has failed. Therefore, when administered with dietary counseling,[68] these drugs can be used relatively safely. Needed, however, are MAO inhibitors with shorter durations of clinical action and an increased margin of safety.

Reversible MAOIs

Several short-acting, selective, reversible MAO inhibitors have been developed, but they are not available in the United States. Such agents include *brofaromine, pirlindole, toloxatone,* and (the best studied) *moclobemide.* These drugs are highly selective in their ability to reversibly inhibit MAO-A. Thus, they are much safer than the irreversible MAO inhibitors because they have minimal interaction with the tyramine in food. Fulton and Benfield (1996)[71] review moclobemide (Aurorix) and its therapeutic efficacy (see Figure 7.7). To summarize, moclobemide is as effective as the TCAs, with similar onset of antidepressant action and (reportedly) with fewer side effects.

Figure 7.6 demonstrates that the half-lives and plasma decay curves of moclobemide and tranylcypromine are virtually identical. With moclobemide (administered orally 3 times a day for 7 days), however, the inhibition of MAO is correlated with the plasma concentration

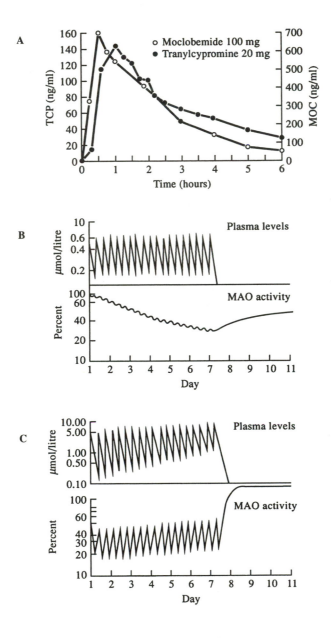

Figure 7.6 (**A**) Concentration profiles of moclobemide (MOC) and tranylcypromine (TCP) after an oral dose. (**B**) Tranylcypromine (10 mg three times a day) plasma levels and MAO activity. (**C**) Moclobemide (150 mg three times a day) plasma levels and MAO activity. [From R. Amrien et al. (1989).[69]]

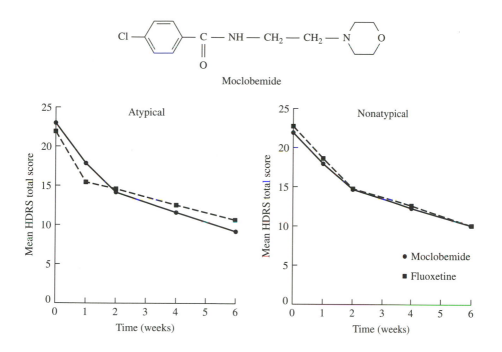

Figure 7.7 Structural formula of moclobemide (*top*) and comparison of the efficacy of moclobemide and fluoxetine. Mean Hamilton Depression Rating scale (HDRS) scores in patients with depressive disorders (DSM-III-R) classified as atypical ($n = 53$) or nonatypical ($n = 156$) and treated with moclobemide 300 to 450 mg/day or fluoxetine 20 to 40 mg/day for six weeks. [Reproduced and adapted with permission from B. Fulton and P. Benfield (1996).[71]]

of the drug (see Figure 7.6C). With each dose, MAO activity fell and then returned as the drug was metabolized and its plasma level fell. When therapy ended, MAO activity rapidly returned to normal. This pattern is like that of most drugs; unlike tranylcypromine, moclobemide does not form an irreversible, covalent bond. Figure 7.6C shows that MAO inhibition is at a maximum after a single dose of moclobemide. Drug effects can be controlled easily, plasma concentration parallels pharmacological effects, and the effect has a short duration with no aftereffects. Because of the specificity of enzyme blockade (MAO-A), side effects are minimal.

Moclobemide does not appear to cause deterioration in cognitive functions but appears to improve vigilance, attention, and some crucial components of memory. These improvements may be related to inhibition of MAO-A as well as to the lack of any anticholinergic action.

Fulton and Benfield (1996)[71] review its superior efficacy in the treatment of social phobias.

In conclusion, the newer, selective, reversible MAO-A inhibitors offer distinct advantages over the older agents. Presumably, clinical usefulness and tolerability will be increased. Indeed, one author has referred to these agents as the "gentle MAO inhibitors."[72]

Drug Administration: Special Topics

Chapter 15 discusses the use of antidepressant drugs in the clinical management of patients with a variety of affective disorders. Here, we comment briefly on special topics not covered in either Chapter 7 or Chapter 15.

To begin, we reiterate the goals of antidepressant therapy for major depression, the long-term treatment of dysthymia, chronic major depression, and "double depression."[3] The first goal is short-term efficacy in controlling acute episodes or exacerbations of major depression:

> Tricyclic antidepressants, selective serotonin reuptake inhibitors, serotonin-2 receptor antagonists, and a reversible inhibitor of monoamine oxidase have now demonstrated efficacy in the short-term treatment of patients.[4]

Short-term efficacy must be measured against "placebo" treatment, which characteristically also shows patient improvement over time. Figure 7.8 summarizes data for TCAs and MAOIs compared with placebo treatment; the response to most antidepressants is about 60 to 70 percent, with placebo response in the range of 25 to 30 percent. Quitkin and coworkers (1996)[73] address the issue of the 30 to 40 percent of patients who do not respond to a trial of drug treatment, factoring in the several-week delay in onset of therapeutic effect:

> Our data suggest that treatments should be changed at the end of four weeks for patients whose conditions never minimally improve, changed at the end of five weeks for patients whose conditions were unimproved but minimally improved in a prior week, and continued for at least six weeks for patients whose conditions were minimally improved at the end of five weeks. At this point, augmentation strategies or a change to a new drug class should be considered.

Figure 7.9 summarizes results of one-year treatment of patients with major depression with either fluoxetine, sertraline, citalopram, or paroxetine, compared with control patients treated with placebo.

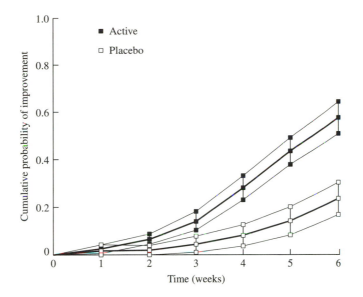

Figure 7.8 Improvement in the state of depression in groups of patients receiving an active drug (TCAs or MAOIs) or placebo for a 6-week period. Approximately 60 to 70 percent of drug-treated patients improved clinically over the 6 weeks, while 30 percent improved while receiving placebo. The figure illustrates the comparative responses to drug and placebo, as well as the lag time to clinical response for both drug and placebo. [Reproduced from F. M. Quitkin et al. (1996).[73]]

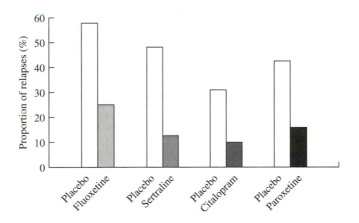

Figure 7.9 Overview of prophylactic trials with selective serotonin uptake inhibitors (SSRIs). All studies were performed for 12 months with the exception of citalopram, which lasted only 6 months. This is also the reason for the relatively small placebo-relapse rate in this trial. The mean relapse rates in the SSRI groups amount to 16 percent and in the placebo groups to 45 percent. [From H.-J. Moller and H.-P. Volz (1996).[7]]

As illustrated, with continuing therapy, the mean relapse rates in the SSRI-treated patients amounted to 16 percent and in the placebo groups to 45 percent. This illustrates that therapy continued beyond the time of resolution of an acute episode of major depression is therapeutically effective in decreasing the probability of recurrence.

Kocis and coworkers (1996)[3] also addressed the issue of whether or not antidepressant therapy reduces the rate of relapse. In their report, outpatients with chronic depression were treated with a TCA (desipramine), and those who positively responded were continued on desipramine for four months, then randomized to placebo or active drug (desipramine) for up to two years. As shown in Figure 7.10, relapse rates during the study phase were 52 percent for the placebo group and 11 percent for the active desipramine group:

> Long-term maintenance treatment with desipramine appeared to be effective in the prevention or postponement of relapse of depression in patients who responded to desipramine during the acute and continuation phases.

Unfortunately, the high rate of relapse in the placebo group demonstrates that cessation of drug therapy is usually followed by relapse of the depression. Kocis and coworkers (1996)[3] state that patients who

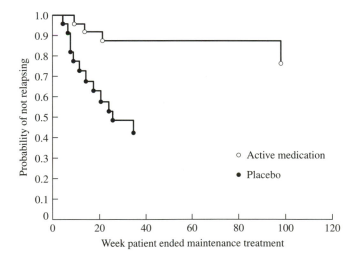

Figure 7.10 Time (in weeks) to relapse of depression in two groups of desipramine-responsive depressed patients; one group continued on desipramine and the other on placebo. [From J. H. Kocis et al. (1996).[3]]

discontinue antidepressant medication have a 50 percent chance of relapse in the first 6 months after therapy is stopped. Future work should focus on those who relapse, on crossover to other medications, and to combinations of psychotherapeutic interventions combined with pharmacotherapy. The volume edited by Hornig-Rohan and Amsterdam (1996)[8] addresses this issue of treatment resistance in these difficult cases.

Sussman (1996)[74] addresses the problem of "treatment-resistant" or "nonresponding" patients by suggesting a number of strategies for enhancing response to treatment. Strategies include dose increase, drug substitution,[75] addition of lithium (see Chapter 8), combinations of antidepressants with different mechanisms of action, use of electroconvulsive therapy, addition of clozapine or risperidone[76] (see Chapter 9), and augmentation of effects with drugs that act on the serotonin 5-HT$_{1A}$ receptor. An example of the latter type of agent is buspirone (BuSpar), discussed in Chapter 4. Sussman (1996)[74] reviews studies demonstrating that the addition of buspirone to standard antidepressants either enhances response or converts nonresponders to responders. Because of its high margin of safety (see Chapter 4), it may be a reasonable choice of supplemental medication to augment the activity of antidepressant medications.

NOTES

1. D. G. Folks and W. C. Fuller, "Anxiety Disorders and Insomnia in Geriatric Patients, *The Psychiatric Clinics of North America* 20 (1997): 137–164.

2. E. Richelson, "Treatment of Acute Depression," *The Psychiatric Clinics of North America* 16 (1993): 462.

3. J. H. Kocis, R. A. Friedman, J. C. Markowitz, et al., "Maintenance Therapy for Chronic Depression," *Archives of General Psychiatry* 53 (1996): 769–774.

4. R. C. Shelton, J. Davidson, K. A. Yonkers, et al., "The Undertreatment of Dysthymia," *Journal of Clinical Psychiatry* 58 (1997): 59–65.

5. R. A. Friedman and J. H. Kocis, "Pharmacotherapy of Chronic Depression," *The Psychiatric Clinics of North America* 19 (1996): 121–132.

6. M. E. Thase, M. Fava, U. Halbreich, et al., "A Placebo-Controlled, Randomized Clinical Trial Comparing Sertraline and Imipramine for the Treatment of Dysthymia," *Archives of General Psychiatry* 53 (1996): 777–784.

7. H.-J. Moller and H.-P. Volz, "Drug Treatment of Depression in the 1990s: An Overview of Achievements and Future Possibilities," *Drugs* 52 (1996): 625–638.

8. M. Hornig-Rohan and J. D. Amsterdam, eds., "Treatment Resistant Depression," *The Psychiatric Clinics of North America* 19:2 (June 1996).

9. S. Kasper, "Treatment Options in Severe Depression" (556–558), in "Controversies in the Treatment and Diagnosis of Severe Depression," *Journal of Clinical Psychiatry* 57 (1996): 554–561.

10. C. DeMontigny, "The Pharmacological Profile of Mirtazapine" (558–559), in "Controversies in the Treatment and Diagnosis of Severe Depression," *Journal of Clinical Psychiatry* 57 (1996): 554–561.

11. T. DeBoer, "The Pharmacological Profile of Mirtazapine," *Journal of Clinical Psychiatry* 57, Suppl. 4 (1996): 19–25.

12. R. J. Baldessarini, "Drugs and the Treatment of Psychiatric Disorders: Depression and Mania," in J. G. Hardman, L. E. Limbird, P. B. Molinoff, R. W. Ruddon, and A. G. Gilman, eds., *Goodman and Gilman's The Pharmacological Basis of Therapeutics*, 9th ed. (New York: McGraw-Hill, 1995), 437.

13. H. L. Miller, P. L. Delgado, R. M. Salomon, et al., "Clinical and Biochemical Effects of Catecholamine Depletion on Antidepressant-Induced Remission of Depression," *Archives of General Psychiatry* 53 (1996): 117–128.

14. P. G. Janicak, J. M. Davis, S. H. Preskorn, and F. J. Ayd, Jr., *Principles and Practice of Psychopharmacotherapy* (Baltimore: Williams & Wilkins, 1993), 211–219.

15. S. M. Paul, "Introduction: Serotonin and Its Effects on Human Behavior," *Journal of Clinical Psychiatry* 51, no. 4, suppl. (April 1990): 3.

16. J. A. Garcia-Sevilla, P. V. Escriba, M. Sastre, et al., "Immunodetection and Quantitation of Imidazoline Receptor Proteins in Platelets of Patients with Major Depression and in Brains of Suicide Victims," *Archives of General Psychiatry* 53 (1996): 803–810.

17. R. D. Blakely, H. E. Berson, R. T. Fremeau, Jr., et al., "Cloning and Expression of a Functional Serotonin Transporter from Rat Brain," *Nature* 354 (1991): 66–70.

18. S. C. Risch and C. B. Nemeroff, "Neurochemical Alterations of Serotonergic Neuronal Systems in Depression," *Journal of Clinical Psychiatry* 53, suppl. (October 1992): 3–7.

19. J. C. Soares and S. Gershon, "Prospects for the Development of New Treatments with a Rapid Onset of Action in Affective Disorders," *Drugs* 52 (1996): 477–482.

20. T. E. Wilens, J. Biederman, A. M. Abantes, and T. J. Spencer, "A Naturalistic Assessment of Protriptyline for Attention-Deficit Hyperactivity Disorder," *Journal of the American Academy of Child and Adolescent Psychiatry* 35 (1996): 1485–1490.

21. T. E. Wilens, J. Biederman, E. Mick, and T. J. Spencer, "A Systematic Assessment of Tricyclic Antidepressants in the Treatment of Adult Attention-Deficit Hyperactivity Disorder," *Journal of Nervous and Mental Diseases* 183 (1995): 48–50.

22. H. V. Curran, M. Sakulsripong, and M. Lader, "Antidepressants and Human Memory: An Investigation of Four Drugs with Different Sedative and Anticholinergic Profiles," *Psychopharmacology* 95 (1988): 520–527.

23. B. A. Marcopulos and R. E. Graves, "Antidepressant Effect on Memory in Depressed Older Persons," *Journal of Clinical and Experimental Neuropsychology* 12 (1990): 655–663.

24. B. Spring, A. J. Gelenberg, R. Garvin, and S. Thompson, "Amitriptyline, Clovoxamine and Cognitive Function: A Placebo-Controlled Comparison in Depressed Outpatients," *Psychopharmacology* 108 (1992): 327–332.

25. R. G. Godfrey, "A Guide to the Understanding and Use of Tricyclic Antidepressants in the Overall Management of Fibromyalgia and Other Chronic Pain Syndromes," *Archives of Internal Medicine* 156 (1996): 1047–1052.

26. D. Stein, T. Peri, E. Edelstein, A. Elizur, and Y. Floman, "The Efficacy of Amitriptyline and Acetaminophen in the Management of Acute Low Back Pain," *Psychosomatics* 37 (1996): 63–70.

27. C. W. Popper and G. R. Elliott, "Sudden Death and Tricyclic Antidepressants: Clinical Considerations for Children," *Journal of Child and Adolescent Psychopharmacology* 1 (1990): 125–132.

28. C. K. Varley and J. McClellan, "Case Study: Two Additional Sudden Deaths With Tricyclic Antidepressants," *Journal of the American Academy of Child and Adolescent Psychiatry* 36 (1997): 390–394.

29. J. Biederman, S. V. Faraone, R. J. Baldessarini, et al., "Predicting Desipramine Levels in Children and Adolescents: A Naturalistic Clinical Study," *Journal of the American Academy of Child and Adolescent Psychiatry* 36 (1997): 384–389.

30. I. Nulman, J. Rovet, D. E. Stewart, et al., "Neurodevelopment of Children Exposed In Utero to Antidepressant Drugs," *New England Journal of Medicine* 336 (1997): 258–262.

31. M. Sakulsripong, H. V. Curran, and M. Lader, "Does Tolerance Develop to the Sedative and Amnesic Effects of Antidepressants? A Comparison of Amitriptyline, Trazodone, and Placebo," *European Journal of Clinical Pharmacology* 40 (1991): 43–48.

32. J. L. Fudge, P. J. Perry, M. J. Garvey, and M. W. Kelly, "A Comparison of the Effect of Fluoxetine and Trazodone on the Cognitive Functioning of Depressed Outpatients," *Journal of Affective Disorders* 18 (1990): 275–280.

33. J. A. Ascher, J. O. Cole, C. Jean-Noel, et al., "Bupropion: A Review of Its Mechanism of Antidepressant Action," *Journal of Clinical Psychiatry* 56 (1995): 395–401.

34. L. L. Barrickman, P. J. Perry, A. J. Allen, et al., "Bupropion versus Methylphenidate in the Treatment of Attention-Deficit Hyperactivity Disorder," *Journal of the American Academy of Child and Adolescent Psychiatry* 34 (1995): 649–657.

35. C. W. Popper, "Balancing Knowledge and Judgment," *Child and Adolescent Psychiatry Clinics of North America* 4 (1995): 483–513.

36. W. Parks, "Improvement in Fluoxetine-Associated Sexual Dysfunction in Patients Switched to Bupropion," *Journal of Clinical Psychiatry* 54 (1993): 459–465.

37. J. J. Mann, K. M. Malone, D. J. Diehy, et al., "Demonstration *in vivo* of Reduced Serotonin Responsivity in the Brain of Untreated Depressed Patients," *American Journal of Psychiatry* 153 (1996): 174–182.

38. S. C. Stanford, "Prozac: Panacea or Puzzle," *Trends in Pharmacological Sciences* 17 (1996): 150–154.

39. T. M. Brown, B. P. Skop, and T. R. Mareth, "Pathophysiology and Management of the Serotonin Syndrome," *Annals of Pharmacotherapy* 30 (1996): 527–533.

40. J. B. Herman, A. W. Brotman, M. H. Pollack, et al., "Fluoxetine-Induced Sexual Dysfunction," *Journal of Clinical Psychiatry* 51 (1990): 25–27.

41. A. J. Rothschild, "Selective Serotonin Reuptake Inhibitor-Induced Sexual Dysfunction: Efficacy of a Drug Holiday," *American Journal of Psychiatry* 152 (1995): 1514–1516.

42. INTERCOM, "The Experts Converse," *Journal of Clinical Psychiatry* 57 (1996): 1–12.

43. O. K. Memmen, J. M. Perel, G. Randolph, et al., "Sertraline and Norsertraline Levels in Three Breastfed Infants," *Journal of Clinical Psychiatry* 58 (1997): 100–103.

44. A. V. Ravindran, R. Judge, B. N. Hunter, et al., "A Double-Blind, Multicenter Study in Primary Care Comparing Paroxetine and Clomipramine in Patients with Depression and Associated Anxiety," *Journal of Clinical Psychiatry* 58 (1997): 112–228.

45. W. F. Boyer and J. P. Feighner, "An Overview of Paroxetine," *Journal of Clinical Psychiatry* 53, Suppl. 2 (1992): 3–6.

46. C. Bolden-Watson and E. Richelson, "Blockade by Newly Developed Antidepressants of Biogenic Amine Uptake into Rat Brain Synaptosomes," *Life Sciences* 52 (1993): 1023–1029.

47. S. A. Montgomery, "Venlafaxine: A New Dimension in Antidepressant Pharmacotherapy," *Journal of Clinical Psychiatry* 54 (1993): 119–126.

48. D. A. Sanger and H. Schulte, "Venlafaxine for the Treatment of Chronic Pain," *American Journal of Psychiatry* 153 (1996): 737.

49. W. K. Goodman, M. J. Kozak, M. Liebowitz, and K. L. White, "Treatment of Obsessive-Compulsive Disorder with Fluvoxamine: A Multicentre, Double-Blind Placebo-Controlled Trial," *International Journal of Psychopharmacology* 11 (1996): 21–29.

50. L. M. Koran, S. L. McElroy, J. R. Davidson, et al., Fluvoxamine Versus Clomipramine for Obsessive-Compulsive Disorder: A Double-Blind Comparison," *Journal of Clinical Psychopharmacology* 16 (1996): 121–129.

51. J. L. Claghorn, C. Q. Earl, D. D. Walczak, et al., "Fluvoxamine Maleate in the Treatment of Depression: A Single-Center, Double-Blind, Placebo-Controlled Comparison with Imipramine in Outpatients," *Journal of Clinical Psychopharmacology* 16 (1996): 113–120.

52. W. Hewer, W. Rost, and W. F. Gattaz, "Cardiovascular Effects of Fluvoxamine and Maprotiline in Depressed Patients," *European Archives of Psychiatry and Clinical Neuroscience* 246 (1995): 1–6.

53. C. L. DeVane and F. R. Sallee, "Serotonin Selective Reuptake Inhibitors in Child and Adolescent Psychopharmacology: A Review of Published Experience," *Journal of Clinical Psychiatry* 57 (1996): 55–66.

54. H. L. Leonard, J. March, K. C. Rickler, and A. J. Allen, "Pharmacology of the Selective Serotonin Reuptake Inhibitors in Children and Adolescents," *Journal of the American Academy of Child and Adolescent Psychiatry* 36 (1997): 725–736.

55. B. Birmaher, N. D. Ryan, D. E. Williamson, D. A. Brent, and J. Kaufman, "Childhood and Adolescent Depression: A Review of the Past 10 Years, Part II," *Journal of the American Academy of Child and Adolescent Psychiatry* 35 (1996): 1575–1583.

56. S. H. Preskorn, "Nefazodone: An Effective Antidepressant" (377–379), in "New Perspectives in the Management of Depression," *Journal of Clinical Psychiatry* 57 (1996): 377–383.

57. D. S. Baldwin, C. J. Hawley, R. T. Abed, et al., "A Multicenter, Double-Blind Comparison of Nefazodone and Paroxetine in the Treatment of Outpatients with Moderate to Severe Depression," *Journal of Clinical Psychiatry* 57, Suppl. 2 (1996): 46–52.

58. A. Feiger, A. Kiev, R. K. Shrivastava, et al., "Nefazodone Versus Sertraline in Outpatients with Major Depression: Focus on Efficacy, Tolerability, and Effects on Sexual Function and Satisfaction," *Journal of Clinical Psychiatry* 57, Suppl. 2 (1996): 53–62.

59. M. B. Keller, "Anxiety in Depression: Focus on Nefazodone" (382–383), in "New Perspectives in the Management of Depression," *Journal of Clinical Psychiatry* 57(1996): 377–383.

60. T. E. Wilens, T. J. Spencer, J. Biederman, and D. Schleifer, "Case Study: Nefazodone for Juvenile Mood Disorders," *Journal of the American Academy of Child and Adolescent Psychiatry* 36 (1997): 481–485.

61. R. Davis, R. Whittington, and H. M. Bryson, "Nefazodone: A Review of its Pharmacology and Clinical Efficacy in the Management of Major Depression," *Drugs* 53 (1997): 608–636.

62. S. Kasper, "Treatment Options in Severe Depression (556–558), in "Controversies in the Diagnosis and Treatment of Severe Depression," *Journal of Clinical Psychiatry* 57 (1996): 554–561.

63. A. Frazer, "Pharmacology of Antidepressants," *Journal of Clinical Psychopharmacology* 17, Suppl. 1 (1997): 2S–18S.

64. R. I. Shader, S. M. Fogelman, and D. J. Greenblatt, "Newer Antidepressants: Further Reflections," *Journal of Clinical Psychopharmacology* 17 (1997): 75–77.

65. S. Kasper, "Efficacy of Antidepressants in the Treatment of Severe Depression: The Place of Mirtazapine," *Journal of Clinical Psychopharmacology* 17, Suppl. 1 (1997): 19S–28S.

66. L. P. C. Delbressine and R. M. E. Vos, "The Clinical Relevance of Preclinical Data: Mirtazapine, a Model Compound," *Journal of Clinical Psychopharmacology* 17, Suppl. 1 (1997): 29S–33S.

67. G. D. Burrows and C. M. E. Kremer, "Mirtazapine: Clinical Advantages in the Treatment of Depression," *Journal of Clinical Psychopharmacology* 17, Suppl. 1 (1997): 34S–39S.

68. D. M. Gardner, K. I. Shulman, S. E. Walker, and S. Tailor, "The Making of a User-Friendly MAOI Diet," *Journal of Clinical Psychiatry* 57 (1996): 99–104.

69. R. Amrien, S. R. Allen, T. W. Guentert, et al., "The Pharmacology of Reversible Monoamine Oxidase Inhibitors," *British Journal of Psychiatry* 155, Suppl. 6 (1989): 66–71.

70. A. C. Swann, C. L. Bowden, J. Rush, et al., "Desipramine Versus Phenelzine in Recurrent Unipolar Depression: Clinical Characteristics and Treatment Response," *Journal of Clinical Psychopharmacology* 17 (1997): 78–83.
71. B. Fulton and P. Benfield, "Moclobemide: An Update of Its Pharmacological Properties," *Drugs* 52 (1996): 450–474.
72. R. G. Priest, "Antidepressants of the Future," *British Journal of Psychiatry* 155, Suppl. 6 (1989): 7–8.
73. F. M. Quitkin, P. J. McGrath, J. W. Stewart, et al., "Chronological Milestones to Guide Drug Change: When Should Clinicians Switch Antidepressants?," *Archives of General Psychiatry* 53 (1996): 785–792.
74. N. Sussman, "Augmentation of Antidepressant Effect with Buspirone" (607–610), in A. J. Rush, chairperson, "Ongoing Needs in Depression," *Journal of Clinical Psychiatry* 57 (1996): 600–610.
75. M. E. Thase, S. L. Blomgren, M. A. Birkett, et al., "Fluoxetine Treatment of Patients with Major Depressive Disorder Who Failed Initial Treatment with Sertraline," *Journal of Clinical Psychiatry* 58 (1997): 16–21.
76. D. J. Stein, C. Bouwer, S. Hawkridge, and R. A. Emsley, "Risperidone Augmentation of Serotonin Reuptake Inhibitors in Obsessive-Compulsive and Related Disorders," *Journal of Clinical Psychiatry* 58 (1997): 119–122.

Chapter 8

PHARMACOTHERAPY OF BIPOLAR DISORDER: ANTIMANIC DRUGS

Bipolar disorder (bipolar depression, manic-depressive disorder) is characterized by recurrent episodes of mania and depression.[1] The disorder requires therapeutic intervention when the mood changes are severe enough to disrupt the patient's life or the lives of people associated with the patient. It is a major medical disorder, occurring in more than 2 percent of the population; a patient is defined as having suffered at least one manic, hypomanic, or mixed episode.[2] If the episode was severe enough to require hospitalization or to seriously interfere with normal functioning, the disorder is classified as *bipolar I*; if the manic episode was less severe, the disorder is classified as *bipolar II*. *Cyclothymia* is defined as recurrent mood swings between depression and elation but of lower severity than bipolar II. Cyclothymia is therefore a part of a continuum from normal to bipolar and can be termed a "bipolar spectrum disorder."[3] Bipolar patients who have had four illness episodes in a 12-month period are termed "rapid cyclers." Such cycling may not be permanent; it may appear and disappear during the course of the illness. As Silverstone and Romans (1996)[3] state:

> Bipolar I disorder can lead to the destruction of a patient's livelihood, marriage, social relationships, or even life. The course of the illness is usually episodic, with periods of mania and/or depression alternating

223

with intervening well periods of varying duration. The great majority of patients experience several episodes during the course of their lives and the risk of recurrence remains ever present.

Thus, bipolar disorder is a chronic, disabling, and even life-threatening disorder. A person who experiences onset of bipolar disorder at age 25 and remains untreated will lose about 9 years of life, 14 years of effective activity, and 12 years of normal health. It is estimated that one of every four or five untreated or inadequately treated patients commits suicide during the course of the illness. An increase in deaths secondary to accidents or intercurrent illnesses (especially substance abuse) also contributes to the greater mortality rate seen in this disorder. Unfortunately, epidemiological studies have indicated that only one-third of bipolar patients are in active treatment despite the availability of effective therapies.[4] It is generally agreed that a patient who exhibits at least two episodes of mania is a candidate for long-term (i.e., lifetime) treatment with an antimanic ("mood stabilizing") drug.

A patient with bipolar disorder can present initially either mania or depression; reduction of depressive symptoms may require an antidepressant, reduction of manic symptoms, an antipsychotic drug. However, successful management of both phases of the disorder is best accomplished by use of a mood stabilizer, classically lithium, the primary drug used to treat this disorder.* In refractory cases, either of two alternative drugs (carbamazepine or valproate) can be substituted or added. In 1994, the American Psychiatric Association published a practice guideline for the treatment of patients with bipolar disorder;[5] this guideline was reprinted in book form in 1996, when it was also expanded as an algorithm to assist the practitioner with specific recommendations in answer to specific questions regarding bipolar therapy.[6] In 1997, the American Academy of Child and Adolescent Psychiatry published practice parameters for the assessment and treatment of children and adolescents with bipolar disorder.[7]

The major objectives of pharmacologic intervention are to treat acute episodes of mania and to reduce the frequency of recurrence of these episodes. Additional goals of therapy are to maintain compliance with therapy, treat accompanying depression, psychosis, and substance abuse, and institute psychosocial treatments appropriate to the

---

*For a historical overview of lithium therapy and commentaries on lithium's status in 1997, see four related letters by M. Schou, by D. J. Kupfer and E. Frank, by S. Gershon and J. C. Soares, and by M. J. Gitlin and L. L. Altshuler in *Archives of General Psychiatry* 54 (1997): 9–23.

patient's needs. Therefore, as stated by Silverstone and Romans (1996)[3]:

> To produce the best clinical results, [one] needs to have a good knowledge of the potentially effective drugs, to offer full and empathetic understanding of the patient's problems, and to provide continuous professional support to the patient and his or her care givers.

Lithium

Lithium is the most commonly recommended drug for treating bipolar disorder and reducing its rate of relapse. Unfortunately, its clinical effectiveness is less than that predicted by clinical trials; relapse often occurs because of patient noncompliance with therapy.[3] Therefore, the pharmacology of lithium and reasons for patient noncompliance with lithium therapy must be clearly understood and alternative drug therapies closely examined.

Lithium (Li^+) is the lightest of the alkali metals (Figure 8.1) and shares some characteristics with sodium (Na^+). In nature, it is abundant in some alkaline mineral-spring waters.[8] Devoid of psychotropic effects in normal individuals, lithium is effective in treating 60 to 80 percent of all acute hypomanic and manic episodes, although in recent years, the limitations, side effects, relapse, and compliance issues associated with its use have become increasingly appreciated. Thus, a brief review of its history of use in treating bipolar illness is helpful.

History

Lithium was used in the 1920s as a sedative-hypnotic compound and as an anticonvulsant drug. During the late 1940s, lithium chloride was

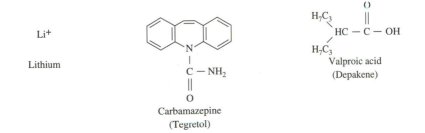

FIGURE 8.1   Drugs used in the treatment of bipolar disorder.

employed as a salt substitute for patients with heart disease. Wide use for this purpose resulted in cases of severe toxicity and death, causing medicine to abandon use of the drug. In 1949, however, Australian scientist J. Cade noted that when lithium was administered to guinea pigs, the animals became lethargic. Taking an intuitive leap, he administered lithium to patients with acute mania, noting somewhat remarkable improvement. However, because of the earlier problems with lithium as a salt substitute, the medical community took more than 20 years to accept this agent as an effective treatment for mania. It was not until the late 1960s that lithium was introduced into the United States by S. Gershon for the treatment of bipolar disorder. Double-blind studies in the 1970s found lithium to be clearly superior to placebo in the prophylaxis of bipolar disorder; fewer than a third of lithium-treated patients relapsed, compared with 80 percent of placebo-treated patients.[3]

Today, lithium's efficacy is again being questioned. Long-term studies are reporting poorer results than expected, with less than 40 percent of treated patients remaining well.[9] Guscott and Taylor (1994)[10] distinguish between the demonstrated *efficacy* of lithium in controlled studies and its poor *effectiveness* in actual clinical practice, a situation that is highly dependent upon compliance in taking the medication. Despite these limitations, lithium is still generally recommended (and so presented in treatment algorithms) as the drug of first choice for both the treatment of acute manic attacks[11] and the long-term management of bipolar disorder,[6] although for acute manic attacks valproic acid (divalproex, discussed later) is being increasingly recommended (see Figure 8.2).

Pharmacokinetics

Lithium is absorbed rapidly and completely when it is administered orally. Peak blood levels are reached within 3 hours, with complete absorption by 8 hours. Its therapeutic efficacy is directly correlated to its level in the blood (discussed later). Lithium crosses the blood-brain barrier slowly and incompletely. There also can be a twofold variation in the concentration of lithium in the brain when compared with its concentration in plasma;[12] the clinical significance of this observation is unclear.

Lithium is excreted by the kidneys in two phases: about half an oral dose is excreted within 18 to 24 hours and the rest (which represents the amount of lithium that is taken up by cells) is excreted over the next 1 to 2 weeks. Thus, when therapy is initiated, lithium accumulates slowly over about 2 weeks until a steady state (or plateau) in both plasma and brain is reached. With this long half-life, once-daily dosage is appropriate for many individuals.

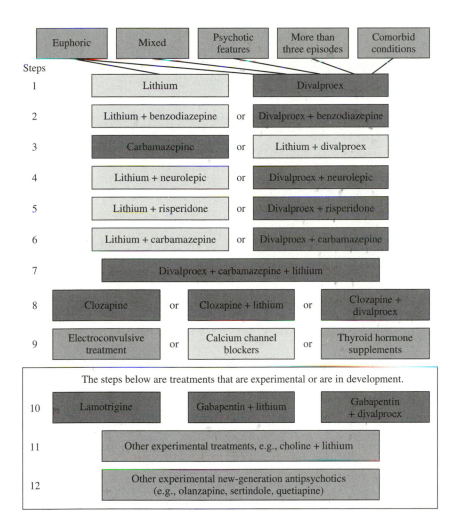

FIGURE 8.2 Pharmacologic treatments of acute mania. When the patient responds, treatment should be continued. If after 3 to 4 weeks of treatment the patient does not respond, has a partial response, or experiences intolerable side effects, the next step should be undertaken. Some of the drugs listed in steps 9 through 12 are not discussed in this chapter. [Data from INTERCOM, "The Experts Converse."[9]]

The therapeutic dose of lithium is determined by closely monitoring blood levels of the drug. Indeed, lithium has a very narrow "therapeutic window," below which the drug fails to have therapeutic effect and above which side effects and toxicity dominate. Older reports and even modern textbooks[8,13] claim that a therapeutic effect is achieved at

0.75 to 1.4 milliequivalents per liter (mEq/L) of blood, with toxicity becoming more severe at levels above 2 mEq/L. After the acute manic episode is controlled, blood levels between 0.5 and 0.9 mEq/L are a recommended "target" level. As Silverstone and Romans (1996)[3] state:

> A level much below this is likely to be associated with a greater likelihood of relapse, while a higher one is frequently accompanied by more adverse effects, leading to an increased risk of noncompliance.

Because lithium is an inorganic ion, it is not metabolized in the body. Rather, it is excreted unchanged in the urine. About 80 percent of the amount of lithium initially filtered into the renal tubules is passively reabsorbed back into plasma (see Chapter 1). This tends to delay excretion and accounts for the long half-life of the drug. Because lithium closely resembles normal salt, when a patient lowers his or her salt intake or loses excessive amounts of salt (such as through sweating), lithium blood levels rise and intoxication may inadvertently follow. Consequently, patients taking lithium should avoid marked changes in sodium intake or excretion.

Pharmacodynamics

In therapeutic concentrations, lithium has almost no discernible psychotropic effect in normal persons.[8] It does not induce sedation, depression, or euphoria, which differentiates it from other psychoactive drugs. Indeed, it exhibits few effects on the brain aside from its specific action on mania. Its detrimental effects on memory and cognition are discussed later.

The mechanism through which lithium exerts its antimanic effect is a matter of speculation and ongoing research. A basic problem is to explain how a simple ion could have such complex effects on multiple transmitter systems and, in particular, have "mood stabilizing" effects in the treatment of both manic and depressive aspects of bipolar illness.[14] Lithium has been shown to affect nerve membranes, pre- and postsynaptic receptors, and the postsynaptic intracellular "second-messenger" impulse transduction systems.[15] Here, we will attempt to summarize some of these actions.

1. Lithium, as a sodium-like ion, may increase the presynaptic reuptake of norepinephrine and serotonin, an action consistent with the biological amine theory of mania and depression, because removing these neurotransmitters from the synaptic space should reduce mania and prevent its recurrence.

2. Lithium may decrease the release of both norepinephrine, and, again, this action is consistent with the biological amine theory. This may occur as a result of lithium-induced attenuation of norepinephrine and dopamine autoreceptors, "possibly via alteration in presynaptic G-protein mediated mechanisms of transmitter release."[15] Manji and coworkers (1991),[16] however, suggest that such presynaptic mechanisms are probably not the primary sites of action of lithium.

3. Lithium may interfere with the movements of intracellular calcium ions, suppressing intracellular calcium ion movement by enhancing the extrusion of intracellular calcium, reducing its intracellular concentration, and, perhaps, thus depressing cellular responsiveness.[17]

4. Lithium may interfere with second-messenger systems in the postsynaptic neuron, reducing the responsiveness of postsynaptic neurons to biological amines.[18] Indeed, of various second-messenger systems in the brain, the cyclic guanosine monophosphate production was most sensitive to lithium attenuation.[19] Risby and associates (1991)[15] summarize as follows:

> Lithium's effects (augmentation) on adenylate cyclase activity are specific with respect to tissue and brain region and . . . lithium may interfere with guanine nucleotide binding (G) protein function. . . . Lithium had significant effects on measures associated with signal transduction that might be contrasted to its more subtle effects on neuronal function (norepinephrine release). . . . Lithium's primary site of action may be on signal transduction mechanisms. These effects subsequently may be manifested in changes in neurotransmitter function that may be important to lithium's mood-stabilizing actions.

In late 1996 a series of research reports described these membrane-stabilizing effects in great detail,[20–22] concluding that:

> Signal transduction pathways are targets for the actions of mood-stabilizing agents; given their key roles in the amplification and integration of signals in the central nervous system, these findings have clear implications not only for research into the etiology/pathophysiology of manic-depressive illness, but also for the development of innovative treatment strategies.[21]

Side Effects and Toxicity

Because lithium has an extremely narrow therapeutic range, blood levels of the drug must be closely monitored. The occurrence and intensity of side effects are, in most cases, directly related to plasma concentrations of lithium. When levels of lithium in plasma fall below 0.5 to 0.6 mEq/L, side effects are usually minimal; they become much more bothersome at levels of 1.0 mEq/L or higher. At levels above 2.0 mEq/L, toxicity becomes severe and potentially fatal.

The main toxic effects involve the gastrointestinal tract, the kidneys, the thyroid, the cardiovascular system, the skin, and the nervous system. At plasma levels of 1.5 to 2.0 mEq/L (and sometimes at lower levels), most reactions involve the gastrointestinal tract, resulting in nausea, vomiting, diarrhea, and abdominal pain. Neurological side effects commonly seen at this level of lithium include a slight tremor, lethargy, impaired concentration, dizziness, slurred speech, ataxia, muscle weakness, and nystagmus. Difficulty with memory is another frequent complaint, as is weight gain with continued treatment.[3] Indeed, in long-term therapy, "up to 30 percent of patients became frankly obese, a prevalence of obesity three times greater than in the general population."[3]

With long-term lithium therapy, the thyroid may become enlarged; rashes or some other kind of skin eruption may occur. In addition, about 60 percent of patients taking lithium experience an increase in urine output (due to an impairment of renal concentrating ability), along with increased thirst and water intake. Although kidney function should be assessed periodically, permanent damage is rare.

As stated, chronic lithium therapy may have adverse effects on memory and cognitive functioning, although these effects are hard to describe because of methodological differences in experiments. Some researchers report improvements in motor performance, cognition, and creative ability after lithium withdrawal, implying detrimental effects of lithium in these areas during drug therapy.[23] Others report few significant cognitive deficits associated with lithium therapy. Richter-Leven and coworkers (1992)[24] and Manji and coworkers (1993)[25] offer some hypotheses involving neurochemical activity to explain possible cognitive, memory, and psychomotor deficits associated with lithium. Richter-Leven and coworkers point out, however, that compensatory mechanisms develop, thus preventing any severe memory impairments during lithium treatment.[24]

At plasma levels of lithium above 2.0 mEq/L, more severe side effects include fatigue, muscle weakness, slurred speech, and worsening tremors. Thyroid gland function becomes depressed, and the thyroid gland may enlarge further, resulting in goiter. Muscle fasciculations, increased reflexes, abnormal motor movements, and even seizures, psychosis, and stupor may occur. At yet higher concentrations (levels exceeding 2.5 mEq/L), toxic effects include muscle rigidity, coma, renal failure, cardiac arrhythmias, and death.

Treatment of poisoning or overdosage is nonspecific; there is no antidote to lithium. Usually drug administration is halted and sodium-containing fluids are infused immediately. If toxic signs are serious, hemodialysis, gastric lavage, diuretic therapy, antiepileptic medication, and other supports may be urgently needed. Complete recovery from intoxication may be prolonged, with full renal and neurological recovery taking weeks or months.

In general, lithium is not advised during pregnancy, particularly in the first trimester, as the risk of fetal malformation involving the cardiovascular system is increased. Thus, lithium possesses a degree of teratogenic potential, especially to the heart. If mood stabilization treatment is necessary during pregnancy, other agents should be employed if possible. When a pregnant woman is on lithium therapy, the drug should be discontinued for several days before delivery, because the newborn will have difficulty excreting the drug. On the other hand, restarting lithium with 24 hours of delivery is important to reduce the risk of relapse.

Unfortunately, the alternatives to lithium (discussed later) have teratogenic potentials of their own. Therefore, the treatment of both pregnant and potentially pregnant bipolar females is difficult and must be administered with caution.[2] Silverstone and Romans (1996)[3] state:

> When discussing with the mother whether or not to stop lithium before or during pregnancy, the relatively low risk of fetal abnormality should be weighed against the increased risk of relapse of bipolar illness with all the attendant disruptions to family life. A case can be made for continuing lithium provided adequate screening tests including ultrasound and fetal echocardiography are carried out.

Noncompliance

Up to one-half of patients taking lithium stop taking the drug against medical advice. Noncompliance is associated with significant morbidity, recurrent manic episodes, and greatly increased suicide risk.[26] Indeed, the illness course after stopping lithium treatment is actually worse than would be predicted from the natural history of bipolar disease. Thus, treatment of only a few years followed by drug withdrawal is either of negligible benefit or "actually harmful to bipolar patients."[27]

Noncompliance seems to result largely from intolerance of side effects, particularly memory impairment and cognitive slowing,[28] weight gain, and the subjective feeling of reduced energy and productivity.[3] Other reasons include missing the manic "highs," feelings that the disorder has resolved and the drug is unnecessary, feelings of stigmatism, and so on. Psychological support, family therapy, and other treatments and encouragements can help the patient stay on the drug.

Baldessarini and coworkers (1996)[26] studied the rate of relapse following acute and gradual withdrawal of lithium, hoping that gradual withdrawal would reduce the high risk of early morbidity in bipolar disorder patients discontinuing successful long-term maintenance on lithium. While they concluded that gradual withdrawal reduced early relapse, the great majority of patients under either protocol did relapse, especially those classified as bipolar I (see Figure 8.3). This finding appears to reinforce the notion that once mood stabilization therapy is started, it may be a life-long necessity. Therefore, whether or not to start therapy is a major decision as discontinuation is associated with a depressingly high rate of relapse.[3] Peselow and coworkers (1994)[29] conjectured that combination therapy (lithium plus either carbamazepine or valproate) may afford greater protection against subsequent affective relapse than the initial course on lithium alone. Data supporting this claim were published in 1997 by Solomon and coworkers[30] (studying lithium plus valproate) and by Bocchetta and coworkers[31] (studying lithium plus carbamazepine). In both reports, adding a second drug to lithium improved clinical results and reduced rates of recurrence or relapse.

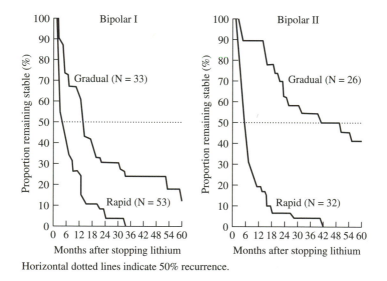

Horizontal dotted lines indicate 50% recurrence.

FIGURE 8.3 Proportion of bipolar I patients (left graph) and bipolar II patients (right graph) after stopping lithium therapy either rapidly (lower lines) or gradually (upper lines). [From R. J. Baldessarini et al. (1996).[26]]

It is disturbing to note that more than 60 percent of bipolar I patients and almost 50 percent of bipolar II patients have a history of substance abuse.[32] In some individuals substance abuse predated the first bipolar episode, and in others the abuse postdated the affective diagnosis. Perhaps in both instances, it may, at least initially, represent an attempt at self-medication for the symptoms accompanying the affective disorder. Regardless, this comorbidity of disease needs to be recognized and addressed during treatment.

Alternatives to Lithium: Carbamazepine and Valproic Acid

> Heterogeneity does exist within bipolar disorder. Persons with mania differ in family history of affective illness, their age at the onset of illness, sex, and organic cause and course of the illness.[33]

Therefore, it is not surprising that a substantial proportion of patients with bipolar disorder either are resistant to lithium treatment or develop side effects that limit its effectiveness.[34] Only about 60 to 70 percent of patients can be adequately controlled on lithium alone (for maintenance/prevention therapy), and the drug is even less effective in controlling episodes of acute or rapid cycling mania. Therefore, there is a need for alternative agents, effective in patients for whom lithium is inadequate, patients who are noncompliant with lithium therapy, and patients who are intolerant of lithium's side effects.

Carbamazepine

Studies conducted in the early 1990s (five comparison trials) indicated that *carbamazepine* (Tegretol, see Figure 8.1) is at least as effective as lithium in preventing the recurrence of mania.[35] In addition, some patients who did not respond adequately to either lithium or carbamazepine alone responded to the two drugs used together.[31,33] Also, carbamazepine was superior to lithium in correcting rapid-cycling bipolar disorder, a condition for which lithium is quite ineffective.[36]

Dardennes and coworkers (1995)[37] reviewed the comparative studies of lithium and carbamazepine and concluded that the therapeutic efficacy of carbamazepine remains questionable. This pessimistic view of carbamazepine was challenged by Silverstone and Romans (1996).[3] Current algorithms generally regard carbamazepine as a second-line, possibly a first-line, treatment for mania, especially when used in combination.[6,11]

It is important to note that patients who fail to respond to carbamazepine often have taken an amount of the drug that is inadequate in plasma. There is correlation between therapeutic effectiveness and the plasma level of the drug, with the therapeutic level of carbamazepine estimated to be between 5 and 10 micrograms per milliliter,[38] the same range used for antiepileptic effectiveness. Petit and coworkers (1991)[38] reported that blood levels of the drug can be determined from a sample of saliva rather than from a blood sample, because the amount of drug in saliva correlates well with the amount of drug in blood.

Adverse effects of carbamazepine include gastrointestinal upset, sedation, ataxia, visual disturbances, and dermatological reactions. Carbamazepine may also have slight detrimental effects on cognitive functioning, but any negative effect on higher-order cognitive functioning is rather limited.[39] Nevertheless, some patients may be particularly sensitive to the cognitive side effects of the drug. More serious reactions involve the blood, ranging from a relatively benign reduction in white blood cell count (leukopenia) to, on rare occasions, severe aplastic anemia. For this reason blood should be analyzed periodically.

Drug interactions involving carbamazepine are common and result from drug-induced stimulation of drug-metabolizing enzymes in the liver. As a result, tolerance to the drug develops and more drug is needed to maintain a therapeutic blood level; this tolerance also extends to other drugs metabolized by the same enzymes.

Because carbamazepine is potentially teratogenic (it produces a neural tube defect in 1 percent of offspring),[40] it should not be administered during pregnancy if possible. It is thought that supplemental administration of folic acid may reduce this risk in mothers who decide to continue carbamazepine during pregnancy.

Valproic Acid (Valproate, Divalproex)

As discussed in Chapter 2, valproate (see Figure 8.1) is an antiepileptic drug that acts by augmenting the postsynaptic action of GABA at its receptors. Motohashi (1992)[41] postulated that valproate (as well as lithium) may exert its mood stabilization action through an action on $GABA_B$ receptors in the hippocampus. About the same time that carbamazepine was being investigated for treating mania, valproate was also being examined. Today there is increasing interest in valproate as an antimanic drug, particularly effective in the treatment of acute mania, mixed states, schizo-affective disorder, and rapid-cycling bipolar disorder.[42-44] It may also be as effective as and less toxic than lithium when used in low doses as an alternative to lithium in the treatment of cyclothymia.[45] It is also more effective than lithium in patients with comorbid depression.[46]

In acute mania in treatment-resistant patients (nonresponders to lithium therapy), positive response rates of up to 71 percent have been reported.[47] Other reports[30,48] suggest that the therapeutic combination of valproate and lithium may provide an effective treatment for both bipolar I and rapid-cycling bipolar disorders. Therapeutic blood levels of valproate appear to be in the range of 50 to 100 micrograms per milliliter. In 1997, valproate (as Depacon) became available in a parenteral formulation intended for intravenous use to control epileptic seizures. It will be interesting to see if this formulation is used to achieve more rapid control of severe, acute episodes of mania, episodes that currently require use of anxiolytics or antipsychotics.

Side effects associated with valproate include gastrointestinal upset, sedation, lethargy, hand tremor, alopecia (loss of hair), and some metabolic changes in the liver. Valproate may be slightly more detrimental to cognitive function than carbamazepine.[49] Like lithium and carbamazepine, valproate can be teratogenic, and caution must be exercised in using this agent in women who might become pregnant during drug therapy.[2,3]

In addition to its uses as an antiepileptic and an antimanic drug, valproate has been used in the treatment of borderline personality disorder[50] and disorders associated with behavioral dyscontrol (agitation, aggression, temper outbursts).[51,52] Here, instead of attempting to alleviate individual symptoms through the use of psychological therapies, pharmacologic therapy is utilized in an attempt to provide general mood stabilization. In a report by Stein and coworkers (1995),[50] a small group (11 individuals) with borderline personality disorder were treated with valproate for 8 weeks. Improvement was noted in 50 percent, and the study concluded that valproate was "modestly helpful for mood and irritability, as well as for anger, rejection sensitivity, and impulsivity." No placebo controls were utilized.

Other Agents of Use in Bipolar Disorder

Chapter 9 discusses the pharmacology of *antipsychotic drugs*. Here, we note the use of these drugs as adjunctive agents in the management of acute manic episodes, especially in highly agitated or psychotic individuals.[5] The antipsychotics have a more rapid onset of action than do mood stabilizers and may be therapeutically effective while waiting for the effects of the mood stabilizer to become apparent.

Little objective evidence exists to support routine use of antipsychotic drugs as a maintenance treatment for bipolar disorder,[5] although up to 60 percent of patients with acute mania are now treated with antipsychotic drugs,[53,54] despite their potential for inducing extrapyramidal side effects (see Chapter 9). As Figure 8.2 illustrates, antipsychotic drugs (listed as "neuroleptic," "risperidone," and "clozapine") are still included in treatment algorithms. They "may be necessary in those patients whose psychotic symptoms have inadequately responded to standard mood-stabilizing agents."[5]

In Chapter 4 the pharmacology of the *benzodiazepines* was presented. Two such drugs (*clonazepam* and *lorazepam*) are used to treat acute mania. These two drugs seem to be most effective when combined with lithium in the treatment of lithium-resistant bipolar disorder and acute attacks of mania "in sedating the acutely agitated manic patient while waiting for the effects of other mood-stabilizing agents to become evident."[5] In reviewing the effectiveness of lorazepam and clonazepam in treating acute mania, Gerner (1993)[55] refers to these drugs as "adjunctive nonspecific antimanic agents."

The pharmacology of *antidepressant drugs* is presented in Chapter 7. Some bipolar patients with recurrent depressive episodes may require continuous treatment with one of these agents.[3,5,56] However, therapy with antidepressants is undertaken with the knowledge that antidepressants may precipitate a manic episode.[55,56] The practice guidelines of the American Psychiatric Association (1994)[5] state:

> As some bipolar patients continue to develop depression despite optimal use of mood stabilizers, antidepressants are often necessary for acute and/or prophylactic treatment. Patients who require antidepressant treatment should receive the lowest effective dose for the shortest time necessary.

Because lithium interferes with membrane ion function, *verapamil* and other *calcium channel blockers* have been tried in the treatment of bipolar disorder. To date, despite early reports of impressive improvements, the effectiveness of verapamil remains controversial; any benefits obtained appear to be limited or short-lived.[8] Thus, early enthusiasm (in the early 1990s) for these agents appears to be lessening.

Clonidine is an antihypertensive drug that has been tried in treatment-refractory patients with bipolar disorder. Because clonidine decreases the release of norepinephrine, it was hypothesized that such action might lead to a reduction in manic episodes. Despite initial positive results, effectiveness remains unproven.[55] There are no reports of any potential effectiveness of the combination of clonidine and lithium in patients who do not respond to lithium alone.

Dubovsky and Buzan (1997)[57] review the efficacy of novel alternative medications in treating bipolar disease.

Psychotherapeutic and Psychosocial Treatments

A combination of drug therapy and psychotherapeutic interventions is the most effective treatment modality for bipolar illness today.

> Patients with bipolar disorder suffer from the psychosocial consequences of past episodes, the ongoing vulnerability to future episodes, and the burdens of adhering to a long-term treatment plan that may involve some unpleasant side effects. In addition, many patients have clinically significant mood instability between episodes.[5]

Goals of psychotherapeutic treatments are to reduce distress and improve functioning between episodes and to decrease the frequency and intensity of future episodes. Successful treatment involves a social network primed to recognize the early symptoms of an episode, to seek help for individuals who lack insight into their condition, and to assist with recognition of side effects and toxicities, thus aiding in compliance with therapy. Issues of importance:

- Emotional consequences of periods of major mood disorder and diagnosis of a chronic mental illness
- Developmental deviations and delays caused by past episodes
- Problems associated with stigmatization
- Problems regulating self-esteem
- Fears of recurrence and consequent inhibition of normal psychosocial functioning
- Interpersonal difficulties
- Marriage, family, childbearing, and parenting issues
- Academic and occupational problems
- Other legal, social, and emotional problems that arise from reckless, violent, withdrawn, or bizarre behavior that may occur during episodes

It is also important to ensure that the manic state is not being caused by medications, such as antidepressants and behavioral stimulants (including illegal drugs such as cocaine), corticosteroids (cortisone), anabolic steroids, caffeine, antiparkinsonian drugs, over-the-counter cough and cold preparations, and diet aids. One must also rule out diseases known to cause or exacerbate mania—notably thyroid disease, because mania secondary to thyroid hyperactivity is common.

Psychotherapy interventions used with pharmacotherapy include cognitive-behavioral therapy, psychodynamically oriented therapy, family therapy, couples therapy, interpersonal psychotherapy, and self-help groups. For complete treatment, a practitioner well versed in the pharmacological management of poorly responsive bipolar patients is necessary. Other personnel are required to monitor the effectiveness of treatment, side effects, other causative factors, and compliance with therapy. The American Psychiatric Association guidelines[5] and the text by Janicak and coworkers (1993)[4] review the efficacy of specific psychosocial and psychotherapeutic modalities.

NOTES

1. American Medical Association, "Drugs Used in Mood Disorders," in *Drug Evaluations, Annual 1993* (Chicago: American Medical Association, 1993), 278.
2. INTERCOM, "The Experts Converse: Practical Considerations in the Use of Mood Stabilizers," *Journal of Clinical Psychiatry* (March 1997): 1–12.
3. T. Silverstone and S. Romans, "Long Term Treatment of Bipolar Disorder," *Drugs* 51 (1996): 367–382.
4. P. G. Janicak, J. M. Davis, S. H. Preskorn, and F. J. Ayd, Jr., *Principles and Practice of Psychopharmacotherapy* (Baltimore: Williams & Wilkins, 1993), 337.
5. American Psychiatric Association, "Practice Guidelines for the Treatment of Patients with Bipolar Disorder," *American Journal of Psychiatry* 151, no. 12, suppl. (December 1994). Reprinted in *Practice Guidelines* (Washington, D.C.: American Psychiatric Association, 1996).
6. Expert Consensus Panel, "Treatment of Bipolar Disorder," *Journal of Clinical Psychiatry* 57, Suppl. 12A (1996): 1–85.
7. Work Group on Quality Issues, W. Ayres and J. Dunne, chairs, American Academy of Child and Adolescent Psychiatry, "Practice Parameters for the Assessment and Treatment of Children and Adolescents with Bipolar Disorder," *Journal of the American Academy of Child and Adolescent Psychiatry* 36 (1997): 138–157.
8. R. J. Baldessarini, "Drugs and the Treatment of Psychiatric Disorders: Depression and Mania," in J. G. Hardman, L. E. Limbird, P. B. Molinoff, R. W. Ruddon, and A. G. Gilman, eds., *Goodman and Gilman's The Pharmacological Basis of Therapeutics*, 9th ed. (New York: McGraw-Hill, 1995), 446–450.
9. G. Winokur, W. Coryell, M. Keller, et al., "A Prospective Follow-up of Patients with Bipolar and Primary Unipolar Affective Disorder," *Archives of General Psychiatry* 50 (1993): 457–465.
10. R. Guscott and L. Taylor, "Lithium Prophylaxis in Recurrent Affective Illness: Efficacy, Effectiveness, and Efficiency," *British Journal of Psychiatry* 164 (1994): 741–746.

11. INTERCOM, "The Experts Converse: An Algorithmic Approach to the Pharmacologic Treatment of Acute Mania," *Journal of Clinical Psychiatry* (September 1996): 1–12.

12. G. Sachs, P. Renshaw, B. Lafer, et al., "Variability of Brain Lithium Levels During Maintenance Treatment: A Magnetic Resonance Spectroscopy Study," *Biological Psychiatry* 38 (1995): 422–428.

13. J. A. Roth, "Antidepressants—Drugs Used in the Treatment of Mood Disorders," in C. M. Smith and A. M. Reynard, eds., *Textbook of Pharmacology* (Philadelphia: Saunders, 1992), 318.

14. R. M. Post, S. R. Weiss, and D. M. Chuang, "Mechanisms of Action of Anticonvulsants in Affective Disorders: Comparisons with Lithium," *Journal of Clinical Psychopharmacology* 12, Suppl. 1 (1992): 23S–35S.

15. E. D. Risby, J. K. Hsiao, H. K. Manji, et al., "The Mechanisms of Action of Lithium: II. Effects on Adenylate Cyclase Activity and Beta-Adrenergic Receptor Binding in Normal Subjects," *Archives of General Psychiatry* 48 (1991): 513.

16. H. K. Manji, J. K. Hsiao, E. D. Risby, et al., "The Mechanisms of Action of Lithium: I. Effects on Serotoninergic and Noradrenergic Systems in Normal Subjects," *Archives of General Psychiatry* 48 (1991): 505–512.

17. Y. Okamoto, A. Kagaya, N. Motohashi, and S. Yamawaki, "Inhibitory Effects of Lithium Ion on Intracellular Ca^{++} Mobilization in the Rat Hippocampal Slices," *Neurochemistry International* 26 (1995): 233–238.

18. H. K. Manji, G. Chen, H. Shimon, et al., "Guanine Nucleotide-Binding Proteins in Bipolar Affective Disorder," *Archives of General Psychiatry* 52 (1995): 135–144.

19. P. P. Li, L. T. Young, Y. K. Tam, et al., "Effects of Chronic Lithium and Carbamazepine Treatment on G-Protein Subunit Expression in Rat Cerebral Cortex," *Biological Psychiatry* 34(1993): 162–170.

20. R. H. Lenox, R. K. McNamara, J. M. Watterson, and D. G. Watson, "Myristoylated Alanine-Rich C Kinase Substrate (MARCKS): A Molecular Target for the Therapeutic Action of Mood Stabilizers in the Brain?," *Journal of Clinical Psychiatry* 57, Suppl. 13 (1996): 23–31.

21. H. K. Manji, G. Chen, J. K. Hsiao, E. D. Risby, et al., "Regulation of Signal Transduction Pathways by Mood-Stabilizing Agents: Implications for the Delayed Onset of Therapeutic Efficacy," *Journal of Clinical Psychiatry* 57, Suppl. 13 (1996): 34–46.

22. M. M. Rasenick, K. A. Chaney, and J. Chen, "G Protein–Mediated Signal Transduction as a Target of Antidepressants and Antibipolar Drug Action: Evidence from Model Systems," *Journal of Clinical Psychiatry* 57, Suppl. 13 (1996): 49–55.

23. J. H. Kocis, E. S. Shaw, P. E. Stokes, et al., "Neuropsychological Effects of Lithium Discontinuation," *Journal of Clinical Psychopharmacology* 13 (1993): 268–275.

24. G. Richter-Leven, H. Markram, and M. Segal, "Spontaneous Recovery of Deficits in Spatial Memory and Cholinergic Potentiation of NMDA in CA-1 Neurons During Chronic Lithium Treatment," *Hippocampus* 2 (1992): 279–286.

25. H. K. Manji, R. Etcheberrigaray, G. Chen, and J. L. Olds, "Lithium Decreases Membrane-Associated Protein Kinase C in Hippocampus: Selectivity for the Alpha Isozyme," *Journal of Neurochemistry* 61 (1993): 2303–2310.

26. R. J. Baldessarini, L. Tondo, G. L. Faedda, et al., "Effects of the Rate of Discontinuing Lithium Maintenance Treatment in Bipolar Disorders," *Journal of Clinical Psychiatry* 57 (1996): 441–448.

27. G. Goodwin, "Recurrence of Mania After Lithium Withdrawal," *British Journal of Psychiatry* 164 (1994): 149–152.

28. J. R. Calabrese and M. J. Woyshville, "Lithium Therapy: Limitations and Alternatives in the Treatment of Bipolar Disorders," *Annals of Clinical Psychiatry* 7 (1995): 103–122.

29. E. D. Peselow, R. R. Fieve, C. Difiglia, and M. P. Sanfilipo, "Lithium Prophylaxis of Bipolar Illness: The Value of Combination Treatment," *British Journal of Psychiatry* 164 (1994): 208–214.

30. D. A. Solomon, C. E. Ryan, G. I. Keitner, et al., "A Pilot Study of Lithium Carbonate Plus Divalproex Sodium for the Continuation of Maintenance Treatment of Patients with Bipolar I Disorder," *Journal of Clinical Psychiatry* 58 (1997): 95–99.

31. A. Bocchetta, C. Chillotti, G. Severio, et al., "Carbamazepine Augmentation in Lithium-Refractory Bipolar Patients: A Prospective Study on Long-term Prophylactic Effectiveness," *Journal of Clinical Psychopharmacology* 17 (1997): 92–96.

32. J. A. Feinman and D. L. Dunner, "The Effect of Alcohol and Substance Abuse on the Course of Bipolar Affective Disorder," *Journal of Affective Disorders* 37 (1996): 43–49.

33. B. L. Cook and G. Winokur, "Perspectives on Bipolar Illness," *Comprehensive Therapy* 16 (1990): 18–23.

34. R. T. Joffe, "Valproate in Bipolar Disorder: The Canadian Perspective," *Canadian Journal of Psychiatry* 38, Suppl. 2 (1993): S46–S50.

35. J. G. Small, M. H. Klapper, V. Milstein, et al., "Carbamazepine Compared with Lithium in the Treatment of Mania," *Archives of General Psychiatry* 48 (1991): 915–921.

36. E. DiCostanzo and F. Schifano, "Lithium Alone or in Combination with Carbamazepine for the Treatment of Rapid-Cycling Bipolar Affective Disorder," *Acta Psychiatrica Scandinavica* 83 (1991): 456–459.

37. R. Dardennes, C. Even, F. Bange, and A. Heim, "Comparison of Carbamazepine and Lithium in the Prophylaxis of Bipolar Disorders. A Meta-Analysis," *British Journal of Psychiatry* 166 (1995): 378–381.

38. P. Petit, R. Lonjon, M. Cociglio, et al., "Carbamazepine and Its 10,11-Epoxide Metabolite in Acute Mania: Clinical and Pharmacokinetic Correlates," *European Journal of Clinical Pharmacology* 41 (1991): 541–546.

39. A. P. Aldenkamp, W. C. J. Alpherts, G. Blennow, et al., "Withdrawal of Antiepileptic Medication in Children—Effects on Cognitive Function: The Multicenter Holmfrid Study," *Neurology* 43 (1993): 41–50.

40. F. W. Rosa, "Spina Bifida in Infants of Women Treated with Carbamazepine During Pregnancy," *New England Journal of Medicine* 324 (1991): 674–677.

41. N. Motohashi, "GABA Receptor Alterations After Chronic Lithium Administration: Comparison with Carbamazepine and Sodium Valproate," *Progress in Neuro-Psychopharmacology and Biological Psychiatry* 16 (1992): 571–579.
42. C. L. Bowden, A. M. Brugger, A. C. Swann, et al., "Efficacy of Divalproex Versus Lithium and Placebo in the Treatment of Mania," *Journal of the American Medical Association* 271 (1994): 918–924.
43. J. R. Calabrese, S. H. Fatemim, and M. J. Woyshville, "Predictors of Response to Mood Stabilizers," *Journal of Clinical Psychopharmacology* 16 (1996): 24–31.
44. P. E. Keck and S. L. McElroy, "Outcome in the Pharmacologic Treatment of Bipolar Disorder," *Clinical Psychopharmacology* 16 (1996): 15–23.
45. F. M. Jacobsen, "Low-Dose Valproate: A New Treatment for Cyclothymia, Mild Rapid Cycling Disorders, and Premenstrual Syndrome," *Journal of Clinical Psychiatry* 54 (1993): 229–234.
46. A. C. Swann, C. L. Bowden, D. Morris, et al., "Depression During Mania: Treatment Response to Lithium or Divalproex," *Archives of General Psychiatry* 54 (1997): 37–42.
47. L. McCoy, N. A. Votolato, S. B. Schwarzkopf, and H. A. Nasrallah, "Clinical Correlates of Valproate Augmentation in Refractory Bipolar Disorder," *Annals of Clinical Psychiatry* 5 (1993): 29–33.
48. V. Sharma, E. Persad, D. Mazmanian, and K. Karunaratne, "Treatment of Rapid Cycling Bipolar Disorder with Combination Therapy of Valproate and Lithium," *Canadian Journal of Psychiatry* 38 (1993): 137–139.
49. P. R. Bittencourt, M. J. Mader, M. M. Bigarella, et al., "Cognitive Functions, Epileptic Syndromes, and Antiepileptic Drugs," *Arquivos de Neuro-Psiquiatria* 50 (1992): 24–30.
50. D. J. Stein, D. Simeon, M. Frenkel, M. N. Islam and E. Hollander, "An Open Trial of Valproate in Borderline Personality Disorder," *Journal of Clinical Psychiatry* 56 (1995): 506–510.
51. D. R. Guay, "The Emerging Role of Valproate in Bipolar Disorder and Other Psychiatric Disorders," *Pharmacotherapy* 15 (1995): 631–647.
52. S. J. Donovan, E. S. Susser, E. V. Nunes, et al., "Divalproex Treatment of Disruptive Adolescents: A Report of 10 Cases," *Journal of Clinical Psychiatry* 58 (1997): 12–15.
53. A. J. Gelenberg and H. S. Hopkins, "Antipsychotics in Bipolar Disorder," *Journal of Clinical Psychiatry* 57, Suppl. 9 (1996): 49–52.
54. M. Tohen, C. A. Zarate, F. Centorrino, et al., "Risperidone in the Treatment of Mania," *Journal of Clinical Psychiatry* 57 (1996): 249–253.
55. R. H. Gerner, "Treatment of Acute Mania," *Psychiatric Clinics of North America* 16 (1993): 448.
56. G. L. Zornberg and H. G. Pope, Jr. "Treatment of Depression in Bipolar Disorder: New Directions for Research," *Journal of Clinical Psychopharmacology* 13 (1993): 397–408.
57. S. L. Dubovsky and R. D. Buzon, "Novel Alternatives and Supplements to Lithium and Anticonvulsants for Bipolar Affective Disorder," *Journal of Clinical Psychiatry* 58 (1997): 224–242.

Chapter 9

ANTIPSYCHOTIC DRUGS: CONVENTIONAL AND NEW-GENERATION AGENTS

Schizophrenia is one of the most severe and debilitating of psychiatric illnesses, usually beginning in late adolescence or early adulthood.[1] The disorder is associated with marked social or occupational dysfunction, and its course and outcome vary greatly. In some individuals, the disorder is persistent, others have remissions and exacerbations, but full recovery occurs in only a small minority.[1] Schizophrenia is also a common disorder, with approximately 1 in every 100 persons developing it during his or her lifetime.[2] Approximately 1.2 million people have schizophrenia in the United States at the present time,[3] and more than 100,000 new cases are diagnosed each year.[4] A majority of affected individuals are unemployed, and family costs (e.g., lost work time and treatment expenses) may range from $410 to $15,000 per year per patient.[2] Like the affective disorders, schizophrenia is associated with an increased risk of suicide. Approximately 10 to 15 percent of individuals with schizophrenia take their own lives, usually within the first 10 years of developing the disorder.

Several organizations are developing clinical practice guidelines intended to summarize data to inform mental/behavioral health workers about the care of patients diagnosed with various mental and/or behavioral disorders. Relevant to the later discussion of the pharmacology of antipsychotic drugs, in April 1997 the American Psychiatric Association published their *Practice Guideline for the Treatment of Patients with Schizophrenia.*[85] This guideline is recommended reading for all mental/behavioral health personnel who work with individuals diagnosed as schizophrenic.

Classically, the symptoms of schizophrenia have been classified as "positive" and "negative." The positive symptoms are those typical of psychosis and include delusions and hallucinations, bizarre behaviors, dissociated or fragmented thoughts, incoherence, and illogicality. The negative symptoms include blunted affect, impaired emotional responsiveness, apathy, loss of motivation and interest, and social withdrawal. This differentiation of symptomatology is of importance in the pharmacology of antipsychotic drugs because the classic agents affect primarily the positive symptoms, while the "second-generation" antipsychotic drugs relieve both the positive and the negative symptoms.

The early 1990s status of treatment for schizophrenia was summarized in a 1992 congressional report[3]:

> Currently, there is no way to prevent or cure schizophrenia; however, treatments that control some of its symptoms are available. The optimal treatment generally integrates antipsychotic drugs and supportive psychosocial treatment. Individuals acutely ill with schizophrenia may require hospitalization. Furthermore, rehabilitation is generally necessary to enhance social and occupational outcomes.

By 1996 this status had been remarkably modified, summarized by Gerlach and Casey (1996)[5] as follows:

> The 1990s promise to be an interesting decade in both the clinical and preclinical development of new antipsychotic medicines. It will be a decade with many new antipsychotics showing significantly divergent characteristics, including effects upon negative symptoms and a low level of extrapyramidal side effects. It will also be a decade where the receptors' molecular structures and interactions with antipsychotics are better understood, where new animal models are developed and where brain imaging techniques play a natural role in the analysis of the method of action of new antipsychotics.

In addition:

> Until recently, antipsychotics have been reserved for seriously ill patients because of the numerous adverse effects associated with their use. The recent development of new agents, however, has opened a new era in antipsychotic drug use.[6]

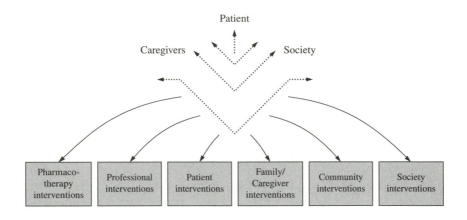

FIGURE 9.1 A comprehensive model of interdisciplinary interventions between patient, caregivers, and the community.

With the introduction of several new atypical antipsychotic agents (and several more to come shortly), there is now hope of raising patients' functioning to levels that truly can facilitate reintegration into the community. In the late 1990s, pharmacologic breakthroughs occurred that offered patients a real chance of leading more normal lives. This revolution, however, occurred in an atmosphere of reduced social services and support. Indeed, the challenge of the new millennium will be not to discover superior agents to improve functional levels, but to prepare social services, family, and counselors to help patients develop their newly found skills and abilities. Only through multilevel interventions can patients with severe and persistent mental illness successfully reintegrate into the community (see Figure 9.1).

Etiology of Schizophrenia

Today, it is thought that schizophrenia is a genetically influenced, developmental brain disorder.[7,8] Figure 9.2 illustrates the risk that relatives of affected individuals will develop schizophrenia. In addition, the schizoaffective and schizotypal personality disorders also appear to have a genetic component.[7] However, nongenetic factors also play important roles, and the exact genetic factor remains unknown. Indeed, interplay between genetic and environmental factors seems to be important in the pathogenesis of schizophrenia.

For many years, scientific evidence favored a dopamine theory of schizophrenia, according to which the disorder arises from dysregulation

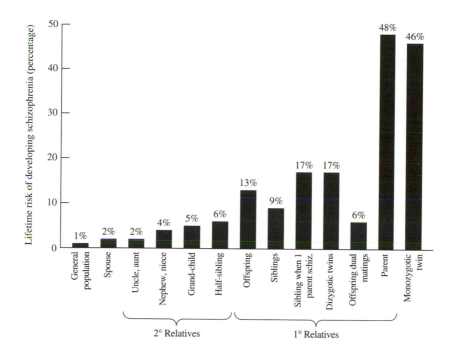

FIGURE 9.2 Lifetime risks of developing schizophrenia among relatives of an affected individual. Data from about 40 European family and twin studies conducted between 1920 and 1987. [Reprinted with permission from I. I. Gottesman, *Schizophrenia Genesis* (New York: W. H. Freeman and Company, 1991).]

in certain brain regions of the dopamine system.[9] This theory was based on several facts:

- The traditional antipsychotic (neuroleptic) drugs are all potent and effective blockers of a certain subclass of dopamine receptors, the dopamine$_2$ receptor, and/or a recently cloned subclass of the dopamine$_2$ receptor, the dopamine$_3$ receptor.[9]

- Blockage of the dopamine$_2$ receptors by binding assay linearly correlates with clinical potency as antipsychotic agents (see Figure 9.3).

- Drugs such as cocaine, which potentiate the activity of dopamine (see Chapter 5), can precipitate or aggravate schizophrenia-like psychosis.

- The atypical antipsychotic drug clozapine is a blocker of a different subclass of dopamine receptors, the dopamine$_4$ receptors.

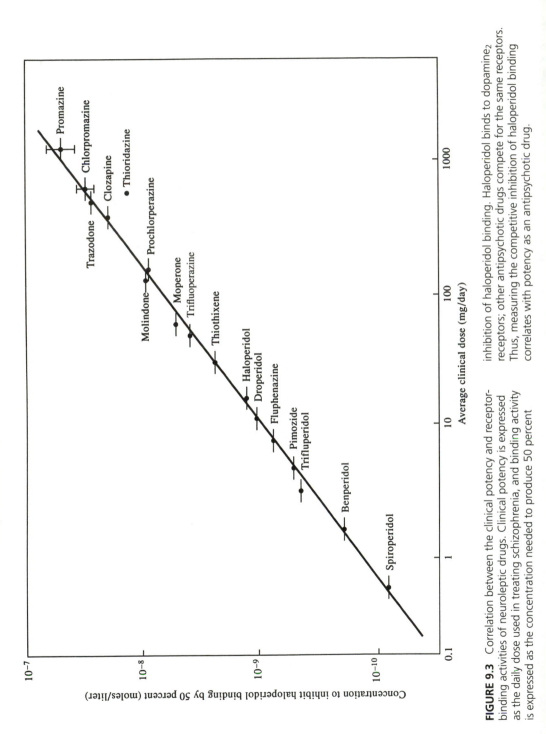

FIGURE 9.3 Correlation between the clinical potency and receptor-binding activities of neuroleptic drugs. Clinical potency is expressed as the daily dose used in treating schizophrenia, and binding activity is expressed as the concentration needed to produce 50 percent inhibition of haloperidol binding. Haloperidol binds to dopamine$_2$ receptors; other antipsychotic drugs compete for the same receptors. Thus, measuring the competitive inhibition of haloperidol binding correlates with potency as an antipsychotic drug.

- The new atypical neuroleptic, risperidone, is a blocker of both dopamine$_2$ and serotonin$_2$ receptors.

- Studies have shown increased densities of dopamine$_3$ receptors in the brains of deceased, nondrug-treated schizophrenics compared with deceased, drug-treated schizophrenics.[9]

The newer antipsychotic drugs argue against a pure dopaminergic theory, as they affect multiple transmitter systems. Despite such multiplicity of receptor actions (discussed later) with the newer antipsychotics:

> Other receptors may also be involved in the therapeutic or adverse effects of specific drugs; however, *all effective antipsychotic drugs block some type of dopamine receptor* [italics added].[4]

In addition, while a hyperdopaminergic theory of schizophrenia may partially explain psychosis, it does not account for the complex and multidimensional nature of the disease, including its diversity of clinical expression (especially the negative symptoms).

Other hallmarks of schizophrenia are the following[2]:

- Correlation of frontal lobe deficits with negative and disorganized symptoms in schizophrenia

- Abnormalities in the hippocampus relating to symptoms such as memory disturbance

- Compromised activity in the left relative to the right hemisphere as a common finding in the disorder

In the 1990s, disturbances of brain development during the prenatal period in genetically predisposed individuals were proposed as causative factors of schizophrenia.[10] This led to a "neurodevelopmental theory" of schizophrenia. In support of this hypothesis, Akbarian and coworkers (1993)[11,12] identified disturbances in normal patterns of cellular development and migration, which are thought to occur during the second trimester of pregnancy; these altered cellular patterns have serious consequences for the establishment of a normal pattern of cortical connections leading to a potential breakdown of frontal lobe function in schizophrenics. Their similar findings in the hippocampus[13] indicated that there may be a more global developmental defect that leads to both the positive (limbic system) and the negative (prefrontal cortex) symptoms of schizophrenia.

Bloom (1993)[14] suggested that an unidentified mechanism might alter neuronal development, such as "premature switching off of genes responsible for trophic factors or their receptors in response to an unidentified external or prenatal insult." In 1995 Akbarian and coworkers[15] extended their work, reporting that a gene responsible for the production of the enzyme *glutamic acid decarboxylase*, the key enzyme responsible for GABA synthesis in the brain, was expressed at lower levels in the prefrontal cortex of schizophrenics. They hypothesized that GABA neurotransmission is altered in the prefrontal cortex, suggesting that this impairment is the consequence of reduced GABA biosynthesis in the inhibitory local circuit neurons of the prefrontal cortex.[16] Lee and Tobin (1995)[17] relate the reduction in GABA neurotransmission in the prefrontal cortex to the positive and negative symptomatology of schizophrenia:

> The positive symptoms of schizophrenia, for example, may result from dopaminergic overactivity in the basal ganglia, which could be secondary to the dorsal lateral-prefrontal cortical (DLPFC) GABA deficits and a corresponding alteration in the input to subcortical nuclei. In contrast, negative symptoms may result from altered DLPFC projections to either brain region, involving nondopaminergic systems, thereby explaining the limited spectrum of action of current neuroleptics. A tantalizing hypothesis is that DLPFC GABA deficits result in alterations in function of other cortical regions, as opposed to subcortical regions, resulting in complex cognitive deficits.

Conversely, in the same year, Olney and Farber[18] studied the dysfunction of dopaminergic and N-methyl D-aspartate-glutamate receptors:

> A unified hypothesis pertaining to combined dysfunction of dopamine and N-methyl-D-aspartate-glutamate receptors that highlights N-methyl-D-aspartate-glutamate receptor hypofunction as a key mechanism that can help explain major clinical and pathophysiological aspects of schizophrenia. . . . We propose that since N-methyl-D-aspartate-glutamate receptor hypofunction can cause psychosis in humans and corticolimbic neurodegenerative changes in the rat brain, and since these changes are prevented by certain antipsychotic drugs, including atypical neuroleptic agents (clozapine, olanzapine, fluperlapine), a better understanding of the N-methyl-D-aspartate-glutamate receptor hypofunction and ways of preventing its neurodegenerative consequences in the rat brain may lead to improved pharmacotherapy in schizophrenia.[18]

Similarly, Bachus and Kleinman (1996)[19] reviewed the neuropathology of schizophrenia and concluded:

> Increasingly, focus is shifting to a role for glutaminergic dysfunction in schizophrenia, opening the possibility that drugs that act upon glutamate function, either directly or indirectly via co-modulators of glutamate transmission, could potentially be developed as adjunctive or primary novel pharmacotherapeutic strategies. . . . Although there are a number of drugs that can regulate the psychotic symptoms associated with the sub-cortical dopamine system, there are essentially no drugs to date that successfully target the cortical glutamate system and cognitive deficits.

The cause of such neurodevelopmental dysfunction in the genetic expression of an enzyme (or enzymes) responsible for neurotransmitter synthesis (GABA, NMDA, or otherwise) is unknown. Several recent reports explore such prenatal etiologies as Rh incompatibility,[20] prenatal nutritional deficiency,[21] or other intrauterine insults.

To summarize, the neurodevelopmental model of schizophrenia appears to imply a two-hit etiology of the disorder; individuals at risk because of genetic factors and having been exposed to a prenatal insult[22] show an increased incidence of the disease. As a result, prefrontal cortical neuronal development is affected, neurotransmitter synthesis is altered, and both positive and negative symptomatology follow as a result of the important connections between the prefrontal cortex and other brain structures.[8,17]

Overview of Antipsychotic Drugs

Mechanism of Action

The clinical efficacy of antipsychotic drugs (both "traditional" and "new-generation") is, in general, highly correlated with their ability to competitively block dopamine receptors.[1] While it is now also clear that, with the new-generation agents, other receptors are involved in the therapeutic effects of specific antipsychotics, all effective antipsychotic drugs block some type of dopamine receptor.[23]

The extent of binding to dopamine$_2$ receptors predicts efficacy, daily dosage, and likelihood of causing extrapyramidal side effects.[24] Studies demonstrate that "the therapeutic effects of neuroleptics,*

---

*The word *neuroleptic* means "to take control of the neuron." Some 40 years ago, the antipsychotic and motor (extrapyramidal) effects of classical antipsychotics (e.g., chlorpromazine) were thought to be linked and inseparable. This led to the *neuroleptic threshold concept* that held that the neuroleptic dose was gradually increased to the level that produced extrapyramidal side effects. Thus, the "right dose" was the one that caused some degree of motor side effects. In other words, classical neuroleptic drugs had a narrow therapeutic index (see Figure 9.4, left graph). New-generation antipsychotics, in general, have a better therapeutic ration, with antipsychotic effects seen at doses which do not produce motor side effects (Figure 9.4, right graph).[25]

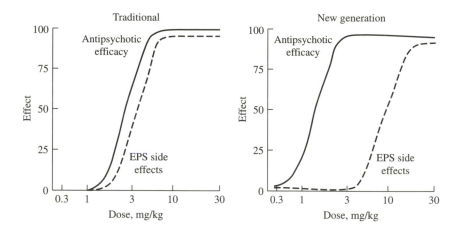

FIGURE 9.4 Dose-response curves for antipsychotic efficacy (solid lines) and extrapyramidal symptoms (dotted lines) for traditional antipsychotic neuroleptics (left graph) and new generation antipsychotics (right graph). [From D. E. Casey, "Motor and Mental Aspects of EPS," *International Journal of Psychopharmacology* 10 (1995): 105–114.]

with the exception of clozapine, are achieved beginning at about 70 percent dopamine D_2 receptor occupancy, while extrapyramidal side effects are generally seen at higher D_2 receptor occupancies."[24]

As Figure 9.4 illustrates, it is now possible to separate antipsychotic efficacy from extrapyramidal side effects. Drugs that exhibit this pattern do so through a variety of receptor mechanisms (to be discussed for each agent), but, in general, this separation is vitally important. As Casey (1996)[26] states:

> The antipsychotic compounds being developed today all have demonstrable efficacy combined with encouragingly low extrapyramidal profiles and a low liability to produce tardive dyskinesia (discussed later) at therapeutic doses.

Thus, while the terms "classical," "traditional," or "neuroleptic" antipsychotic apply to the drugs with inseparable therapeutic and extrapyramidal effects (see Figure 9.4, left graph), the term "new generation" applies to the newer agents, which do separate the two. These new-generation drugs are as revolutionary in the 1990s as chlorpromazine was in the 1950s.

Clozapine (Clozaril) was the first of the new-generation antipsychotics to become available (in the early 1990s), followed by the introduction in 1995 of *risperidone* (Risperdal). Clozapine is a relatively weak blocker of dopamine D_2 receptors, much more effectively blocking serotonin 5-HT_{2A} receptors.[27] Risperidone exhibits high levels of dopamine$_2$ receptor blockade and a very high affinity for 5-HT_{2A} receptors. These actions, as Richelson (1996)[24] states,

> mitigate against the extrapyramidal side effects. This serotonergic receptor blockade may also be the underlying mechanism for the efficacy of an atypical neuroleptic (a new-generation antipsychotic) to treat the negative symptoms of schizophrenia.

Table 9.1 lists the possible therapeutic and adverse effects that follow receptor blockade by antipsychotic drugs. At this point, focus on the blockade of dopamine D_2 and serotonin 5-HT_{2A} receptors. Others will be discussed as individual drugs are presented.

Olanzapine (Zyprexa), introduced in late 1996, acts much like clozapine, "except for a higher affinity for D_2 receptors and a slightly lower affinity for 5-HT_{2A} receptors."[27] Only about 40 percent of dopamine$_2$ receptors are blocked by either clozapine or olanzapine. A fourth new-generation agent, *sertindole* (Serlect), was introduced in 1997. It affects a variety of dopamine receptors as well as serotonin receptors.

New-generation antipsychotics thus combine dopamine$_2$ and serotonin 5-HT_{2A} blockade, explaining efficacy against both positive and negative symptoms of schizophrenia. To complicate matters further, clozapine also has affinity for dopamine$_4$ receptors, which are highly localized in both the mesolimbic system and the frontal cortex, as opposed to the dopamine$_2$ receptors, which are found primarily in the structures of the basal ganglia (see Figure 9.5).[28] Reynolds (1996)[29] discusses the possible role of dopamine D_4 receptors in the action of antipsychotic drugs, especially clozapine, questioning the importance of this newly identified receptor in the pathogenesis of schizophrenia.

Dopamine$_2$ and dopamine$_4$ receptors are located at several sites within the brain:

- Mesolimbic (nucleus accumbens, amygdala, hippocampus) and frontal cortical areas of the brain. Activation of these receptors is thought to be responsible for the therapeutic action of the drugs.
- Extrapyramidal system (the caudate nucleus and the putamen of the basal ganglia). Activation of these receptors results in the motor dysfunctions that are produced by the drugs.

TABLE 9.1 Possible therapeutic and adverse effects of receptor blockade by neuroleptics

Blockade of dopamine D_2 receptors
  Therapeutic effects
    Amelioration of the positive signs and symptoms of psychosis
  Adverse effects
    Extrapyramidal movement disorders: dystonia, parkinsonism, akathisia, tardive dyskinesia, rabbit syndrome
    Endocrine effects: prolactin elevation (galactorrhea, gynecomastia, menstrual changes, sexual dysfunction in males)
Blockade of muscarinic receptors
  Therapeutic effects
    Mitigation of extrapyramidal side effects
  Adverse effects
    Blurred vision
    Attack or exacerbation of narrow angle glaucoma
    Dry mouth
    Sinus tachycardia
    Constipation
    Urinary retention
    Memory dysfunction
Blockade of serotonin $5-HT_{2A}$ receptors
  Therapeutic effects
    Amelioration of the negative signs and symptoms of psychosis
    Mitigation of extrapyramidal side effects
  Adverse effects
    Unknown
Blockade of histamine H_1 receptors
  Therapeutic effects
    Sedation
  Adverse effects
    Sedation
    Drowsiness
    Weight gain
    Potentiation of central depressant drugs
Blockade of α_1-adrenoceptors
  Therapeutic effects
    Unknown
  Adverse effects
    Potentiation of the antihypertensive effects of prazosin, terazosin, doxazosin, and labetalol
    Postural hypotension, dizziness
    Reflex tachycardia
Blockade of α_2-adrenoceptors
  Therapeutic effects
    Unknown
  Adverse effects
    Blockade of the antihypertensive effects of clonidine and methyldopa

From Richelson (1996),[24] p. 8.

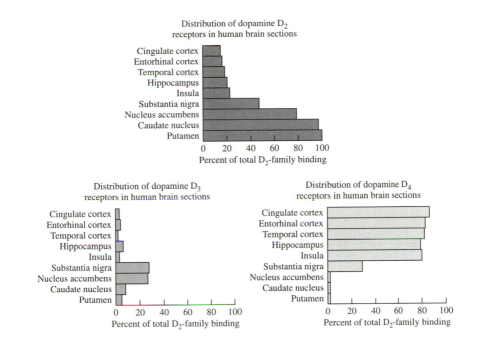

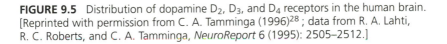

FIGURE 9.5 Distribution of dopamine D_2, D_3, and D_4 receptors in the human brain. [Reprinted with permission from C. A. Tamminga (1996)[28] ; data from R. A. Lahti, R. C. Roberts, and C. A. Tamminga, *NeuroReport* 6 (1995): 2505–2512.]

- Hypothalamic-pituitary axis. Activation of these receptors correlates with the hormonal alterations that are induced by these agents.

- Certain centers of the brain stem, especially the chemoreceptor trigger zone of the medulla. Activation of these receptors correlates with the antivomiting (antiemetic) effect of these drugs.

Table 9.2 summarizes the binding of several antipsychotic drugs to various receptors in the central nervous system (CNS).

Historical Background

Prior to 1950 effective drugs for treating psychotic patients were virtually nonexistent, and such patients were usually permanently or semipermanently hospitalized. By 1955 more than half a million psychotic persons in the United States were residing in mental hospitals, but in 1956 a dramatic and steady reversal in this trend began (see Figure 9.6). By 1983 fewer than 220,000 were institutionalized. This decline occurred despite a

TABLE 9.2 Relative in-vitro binding profiles of one traditional antipsychotic neuroleptic (haloperidol) and four new-generation antipsychotic drugs

Receptor	Sertindole	Clozapine	Haloperidol	Olanzapine	Risperidone
D_1	28.0	130.0	36.0	25.0	50.0
D_2	4.1	410.0	7.5	19.0	4.0
D_3	1.6	83.0	2.7	?	6.7
D_4	14.0	21.0	23.0	27.0	7.0
$5\text{-}HT_{2A}$	0.4	7.8	55.0	3.7	0.76
$5\text{-}HT_{2C}$	1.2	15.0	2100.0	6.1	14.0
α_1	3.4	9.2	18.0	18.0	1.7
α_2	350.0	64.0	2000.0	180.0	2.3
H_1	600.0	23.0	>1000.0	7.7	110.0
Muscarinic	2500.0	9.4	5500.0	20.0	6500.0

D_1, D_2, D_3, D_4 = dopamine receptors
$5\text{-}HT_{2A}, 5\text{-}HT_{2C}$ = serotonin receptors
α_1, α_2 = adrenergic receptors
Muscarinic = cholinergic receptor
H_1 = histamine receptor

Reprinted with permission from Tamminga (1996),[28] p. 430.

doubling in the numbers of admissions to state hospitals. Until the early 1990s, schizophrenics were routinely stabilized on medication and discharged from institutions quite rapidly.* What accounted for such a dramatic shift resided in a class of drugs called the *phenothiazines*.

In 1952 French researcher H. Laborit used *promethazine* (the first of the phenothiazines) to deepen anesthesia. Later that year, other French researchers studied a second phenothiazine, *chlorpromazine* (Thorazine). This drug was administered in a "cocktail" to patients the night before surgery to allay their fears and anxieties. Chlorpromazine (see Figure 9.7) was found to lower the amount of

---

*Although the discharge rate of schizophrenics from institutions is high, we must be concerned about their ultimate functioning in society. Many patients who were discharged on phenothiazines failed to continue their medication, and they functioned poorly as a result. It has been estimated that about 50 percent of the adult homeless population in the United States may suffer from inadequately controlled schizophrenia.

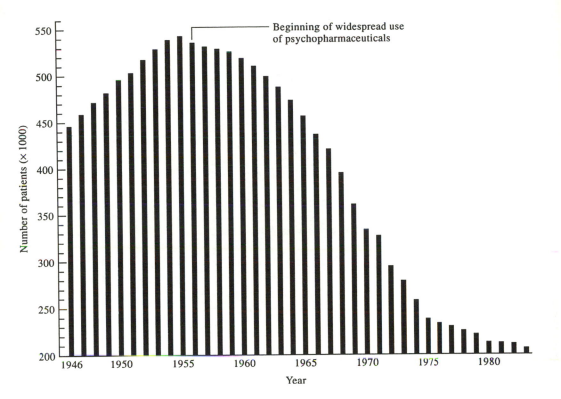

FIGURE 9.6 Numbers of resident patients in state and local government mental hospitals in the United States from 1946 through 1983. Note the dramatic change that began in 1956 with the introduction of psychoactive drugs into therapy.

anesthetic drugs that a patient needed without making the patient unconscious; instead, treatment with chlorpromazine produced a state characterized by calmness, conscious sedation, and disinterest in and detachment from external stimuli. This condition was termed a *neuroleptic state*, and chlorpromazine was the first neuroleptic drug. Because of these behavioral effects, chlorpromazine was found to be remarkably effective in alleviating the clinical manifestations of the psychotic process. Although chlorpromazine did not provide a permanent cure, its use in conjunction with supportive therapy allowed thousands of patients who otherwise would have been hospitalized permanently to return to their communities, albeit in a less than satisfactory state.

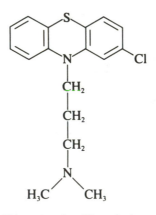

Chlorpromazine (Thorazine)

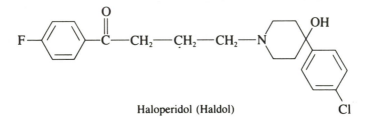

Haloperidol (Haldol)

FIGURE 9.7 Structural formulas of a phenothiazine (chlorpromazine) and a butyrophenone (haloperidol).

In the continuing search for more effective and less bothersome drugs, alternatives to the phenothiazines have been (and are continuing to be) developed. Reserpine (Serpasil) was a late 1950s alternative, but significant side effects have today rendered the drug obsolete. The second class of alternative agents was the *butyrophenones,* developed in Belgium in the mid-1960s. Two butyrophenones are currently available—*haloperidol* (Haldol; see Figure 9.7) and *droperidol* (Inapsine). Neither drug seems to have significant advantages over the phenothiazines, but haloperidol is occasionally used for patients who cannot tolerate the phenothiazines. During the 1970s other agents became available, including *loxapine* (Loxitane) and *molindone* (Moban), both of which have significant side effects (parkinsonian, involuntary, extrapyramidal motor movements).

In the late 1990s, we are in a new era of treatment goals for the schizophrenic patient. Treatment of only the positive symptoms of schizophrenia may make the patient more manageable, but it begs an important question: How do these changes actually benefit the person with schizophrenia?[2] Previously peripheral concerns, such as quality of life, are now being addressed.[2] The new-generation neuroleptics—clozapine, risperidone, olanzapine, and sertindole—are providing the means to address these vital issues. In addition, as we discussed, they are providing tools with which researchers can explore the mechanisms underlying the genesis of the illness. These new-generation drugs have vast implications for how health care is delivered to schizophrenic patients, challenging the "system" as never before.[30,31] The documented savings in hospitalization (and rehospitalization) costs associated with the new-generation drugs can occur only by committing increased funds for the new drugs as well as increased commitment to social and community services for outpatient treatment of schizophrenic patients who may "waken" from their prior incapacitation.

Major versus Minor Tranquilizers

The benzodiazepines (see Chapter 4) are often called tranquilizers because they reduce anxiety states and neurotic behavior and produce a state of calmness or tranquilization. They are, however, not effective in treating psychosis. In contrast, the antipsychotic drugs discussed in this chapter are sometimes also referred to as tranquilizers. To distinguish these two very different classes of drugs, the benzodiazepines are sometimes called "minor tranquilizers," while the antipsychotic drugs have been referred to as "major tranquilizers." Although these terms are less commonly used today, they are occasionally encountered. Thus, the terms "major tranquilizer," "neuroleptic," "antipsychotic," and "antischizophrenic" can all be used interchangeably.

Note that the word "tranquilizer" implies an agent that induces a peaceful, tranquil, calm, or pleasant state. Such a state can be produced by a minor tranquilizer, such as diazepam. However, the psychological effects produced by the major tranquilizers—the antipsychotic drugs—are seldom pleasant or euphoric. Indeed, they may cause unpleasant or dysphoric feelings, especially when administered to nonpsychotic persons. Hence, these drugs do not cause positive behavioral reinforcement and are not encountered as drugs of abuse.

Classification

As should be apparent by now, antipsychotic drugs can be broadly classified into two groups: (1) standard, classical, or traditional agents, and (2) new-generation agents. The phenothiazines are the prototypical agents of the first class, while clozapine, risperidone, olanzapine, and sertindole are the currently available agents of the second class.

With the traditional antipsychotics, it has not been possible to separate the therapeutic effects on the positive symptoms from their prominent side effects involving the extrapyramidal motor system. These side effects closely resemble the motor alterations observed in patients who have Parkinson's disease, consisting of rigidity, tremor, slowed movements, and restlessness. Some of these symptoms disappear when the medication is discontinued, but persistent or permanent motor disorders (e.g., tardive dyskinesia) also occur. The new-generation agents have two advantages: (1) They may be therapeutically effective without causing this neuroleptic syndrome, and (2) they help relieve the negative symptoms.

The Phenothiazines

The phenothiazines remain the most widely used class of drugs for treating psychosis. They are also used extensively for other purposes, such as to treat nausea and vomiting, to sedate patients before anesthesia, to delay ejaculation, to relieve severe itching, to manage the psychotic component that may accompany acute manic attacks, to treat alcoholic hallucinosis, and to manage the hallucinations caused by psychedelic agents. Table 9.3 lists the 10 phenothiazines currently available for clinical use. Our discussion focuses on the prototypical agent of this class, *chlorpromazine* (Thorazine).

Pharmacokinetics

The phenothiazines are absorbed erratically and unpredictably from the gastrointestinal tract. However, because patients usually take these drugs for long periods of time (even for a lifetime), the oral route of administration is still effective and commonly used. Intramuscular injection of phenothiazines is also quite effective; it increases the effectiveness of the drug to about 4 to 10 times that achieved with oral administration. Once these drugs are in the bloodstream, they are rapidly distributed throughout the body. The levels of phenothiazines that are found in the brain are low compared with the levels found in other body tissues; the highest concentrations are found in the lungs, liver, adrenal glands, and spleen.

The phenothiazines have half-lives of 24 to 48 hours, and they are slowly metabolized in the liver. The clinical effects of a single dose persist for at least 24 hours. Thus, taking the daily dose at bedtime will often minimize certain side effects (such as excessive sedation). The phenothiazines become extensively bound to body tissues, which partially accounts for their slow rate of elimination. Indeed, metabolites

TABLE 9.3 Antipsychotic drugs

Chemical classification	Drug name: Generic (Trade)	Dose equivalent (mg)	Sedation	Autonomic side effects[a]	Involuntary movement
Phenothiazine	Chlorpromazine (Thorazine)	100	High	High	Moderate
	Prochlorperazine (Compazine)	15	Moderate	Low	High
	Fluphenazine (Prolixin)	2	Low	Low	High
	Trifluoperazine (Stelazine)	5	Moderate	Low	High
	Perphenazine (Trilafon)	8	Low	Low	High
	Acetophenazine (Tindal)	20	Moderate	Low	High
	Carphenazine (Proketazine)	25	Moderate	Low	High
	Triflupromazine (Vesprin)	25	High	Moderate	Moderate
	Mesoridazine (Serentil)	50	High	Moderate	Low
	Thioridazine (Mellaril)	100	High	Moderate	Low
Thioxanthene	Thiothixene (Navane)	4	Low	Low	High
	Chlorprothixene (Taractan)	100	High	High	Moderate
Butyrophenone	Haloperidol (Haldol)	2	Low	Low	Very High
Miscellaneous	Loxapine (Loxitane)	10	Moderate	Low	Moderate
	Molindone (Moban)	10	Moderate	Moderate	Moderate
	Pimozide (Orap)	2	Low	Low	Moderate
New generation	Clozapine (Clozapil)	50	Moderate	Moderate	Low
	Risperidone (Risperdal)	1	Low	Low	Low-Moderate
	Olanzapine (Yprexa)	1.5	Moderate	Low	Low
	Sertindole (Serlect)	NA[b]	NA	NA	Low

[a]Autonomic side effects include dry mouth, blurred vision, constipation, urinary retention, and reduced blood pressure.

[b]Not available

of some of the phenothiazines can be detected for several months after the drug has been discontinued. Such slow elimination may also contribute to the slow rate of recurrence of psychotic episodes following the cessation of drug therapy.

To date, therapeutic drug monitoring and correlation of plasma levels of neuroleptics with clinical response and toxicity have not been widely utilized; most dosage decisions are made on a trial-and-error basis.[32] Studies have shown, however, that the plasma concentrations vary widely among patients given similar amounts of orally administered neuroleptics.[33] These differences probably result from large variations in drug absorption and metabolism. Marder and coworkers (1993)[32] summarize the circumstances in which plasma-level monitoring is useful:

- Where patients fail to respond to what is usually an adequate dose
- When it is difficult to discriminate drug side effects from symptoms of schizophrenia
- When antipsychotic drugs are combined with other drugs that may affect the antipsychotic's pharmacokinetics
- In the very young, the elderly, and the medically compromised, in whom the pharmacokinetics of neuroleptics may be altered
- If noncompliance or poor compliance is suspected

Pharmacological Effects

In addition to blocking the dopamine$_2$ receptors, the phenothiazines also block acetylcholine, serotonin, histamine, and norepinephrine receptors. The consequences of such blockade are summarized in Table 9.2. To summarize, blockade of acetylcholine receptors results in dry mouth, dilated pupils, blurred vision, constipation, urinary retention, and tachycardia; blockade of norepinephrine receptors can result in hypotension and sedation. Blockade of histamine receptors has sedating as well as antiemetic effects. Indeed, phenothiazines are widely used in medicine for their antinausea effect.

Limbic System. Dopamine-secreting neurons located in the central midbrain portion of the brain stem send axonal projections to those parts of the limbic system that regulate emotional expression as well as to the limbic forebrain areas, where thought and emotions are integrated (see Appendix IV). Indeed, an increased sensitivity of dopamine receptors in those areas may be responsible for the positive symptomatology of schizophrenia. Thus, chlorpromazine decreases paranoia, fear, hostility, and agitation; it also reduces the intensity of schizophrenic delusions and hallucinations. In addition, chlorpromazine dramatically relieves the agitation, restlessness, and hyperactivity associated with an acute schizophrenic attack. The delusions and hallucinations are particularly sensitive to treatment.

Brain Stem. Through actions on the brain stem, phenothiazines suppress the centers involved in behavioral arousal (the ascending reticular activating center) and vomiting (the chemoreceptor trigger zone). By suppressing activity in the reticular formation, the phenothiazines induce an indifference to external stimuli, reducing the inflow of sensory stimuli that would otherwise reach higher brain centers.

Basal Ganglia. Neuroleptic drugs produce two main kinds of motor disturbances, which comprise both the most bothersome and the most serious side effects associated with the use of these agents.[34,35] The two syndromes are (1) acute extrapyramidal reactions, which develop early in treatment in up to 90 percent of patients, and (2) tardive (late) dyskinesia, which occurs much later, during and even after cessation of chronic neuroleptic therapy.

The acute extrapyramidal side effects are threefold (see Table 9.4):

- Akathesia, which is a syndrome of the subjective feeling of anxiety, accompanied by restlessness, pacing, constant rocking back and forth, and other repetitive, purposeless actions
- Dystonia, which is characterized by involuntary muscle spasms and sustained abnormal, bizarre postures of the limbs, trunk, face, and tongue

TABLE 9.4 Extrapyramidal neurological syndromes associated with use of antipsychotic drugs, in relation to duration of exposure

Acute		Chronic
Early (hours to days)	Intermediate (days to weeks)	Late (months to years)
Acute dystorias	Parkinsonism Akathisia	Tardive dyskinesias

From Owens (1996),[35] Table II, p. 901.

- Neuroleptic-induced parkinsonism, which resembles idiopathic (of unknown etiology) Parkinson's disease (drugs used to treat parkinsonism are discussed in Appendix III)

Neuroleptic-induced parkinsonism is characterized by tremor at rest, rigidity of the limbs, and slowing of movement with a reduction in spontaneous activity. In idiopathic parkinsonism, these symptoms occur when the concentration of dopamine in the nuclei of the basal ganglia (caudate nucleus, putamen, and globus pallidus) decreases to about 20 percent of normal. Here neuroleptic drug-induced blockade of dopamine receptors in excess of 70 to 80 percent occupancy produces the parkinsonism-like symptoms.

Tardive dyskinesia is a much more puzzling and serious form of movement disorder. Victims exhibit involuntary hyperkinetic movements, often of the face and tongue but also of the trunk and limbs, which can be severely disabling. More characteristic are sucking and smacking of the lips, lateral jaw movements, and darting, pushing, or twisting of the tongue. Choreiform movements of the extremities are frequent. The syndrome appears a few months to several years after the beginning of neuroleptic treatment (hence the description *tardive*) and is often irreversible. The incidence of tardive dyskinesia has been estimated at more than 10 percent of patients who are treated with neuroleptic drugs, but this side effect depends greatly on the dosage, the age of the patient (it is most common in patients older than 50), and the particular drug used. Adequately controlling dyskinesia may necessitate restarting the neuroleptic medication or increasing the dosage, which is a problem if parkinsonian side effects are troublesome. Casey (1993),[34] Owens (1996),[35] and Baldessarini (1995)[36] review these effects at length.

Hypothalamus-Pituitary. Pathways of dopamine-secreting neurons extend from the hypothalamus to the pituitary gland. The hypothalamus is intimately involved in the emotions, eating and drinking, sexual behavior, and the secretion of some pituitary hormones. By suppressing the function of the hypothalamus, phenothiazines interrupt these functions. By suppressing the appetite, food intake may be reduced. By suppressing the temperature-regulating centers of the hypothalamus, body temperature will fluctuate widely with changes in room temperature. In addition, several body hormones are affected. Dopamine is likely the hormone that inhibits the release of *prolactin* in the hypothalamus. Thus, when dopamine receptors are blocked, the hormone prolactin is released, which often causes breast enlargement in males and lactation in females. Phenothiazines also reduce the release of hormones from the pituitary gland, which regulate the secretions of sex hormones. Thus, in men ejaculation may be blocked; in women libido may be decreased, ovulation may be blocked, and normal menstrual cycles may be suppressed, resulting in infertility.

Side Effects and Toxicity

The therapeutic use of the phenothiazines invariably leads to many side effects. Indeed, much of the art of managing patients with schizophrenia is in the diagnosis and management of side effects. Specific phenothiazines are chosen not so much because of differences in therapeutic efficacy but because of the relative intensities of their side effects.

In general, the "high-potency" phenothiazines (e.g., fluphenazine, trifluoperazine, and perphenazine; see Table 9.3) cause less sedation, fewer anticholinergic side effects, less postural hypotension, and more extrapyramidal side effects than the "low-potency" phenothiazines (e.g., chlorpromazine and thioridazine). Where sedation is desirable, either a low-potency phenothiazine used alone or a high-potency drug combined with a benzodiazepine has the desired therapeutic effect. Where the anticholinergic side effects limit drug compliance, a high-potency drug is desirable, and the drug-induced movement disorders can often be controlled with other medications (anticholinergic, antihistaminic, antiadrenergic, or antiparkinsonian drugs), which are discussed in Appendix III.

In patients who are at risk for developing extrapyramidal side effects, who cannot tolerate phenothiazines or who are "treatment resistant," two options are available: (1) They can be prophylactically medicated with anticholinergic, antiparkinsonian, or antiadrenergic drugs, or (2) they can receive a trial of a new-generation antipsychotic as a replacement for the phenothiazine. Kane (1996)[37] and Marder (1996)[38] discuss management of treatment-resistant patients, including its definition and alternative treatment strategies. Marder states that there are three categories of treatment-resistant patients:

> The first category includes patients who continue to demonstrate positive psychotic symptoms when they receive adequate trials of an antipsychotic. . . . The second category of poor responders consists of patients who are unable to tolerate the side effects of antipsychotics. . . . The third category includes patients who have persistent negative symptoms while they are treated with an antipsychotic.

Marder concludes this review by stating:

> There is substantial evidence that these patients will demonstrate
> improvement . . . when they receive clozapine and risperidone as
> well as newer antipsychotics including olanzapine, sertindole, and
> quetiapine.[38]

Other potentially serious, but much less common, side effects of phenothiazines include altered pigmentation of the skin, pigment deposits in the retina, permanently impaired vision, decreased pituitary function, menstrual dysfunction, and allergic (hypersensitivity) reactions, which include liver dysfunction and blood disorders.

It has long been recognized that cognitive disturbances are evident in 40 to 60 percent of schizophrenic patients.[39] Tests show deficits in attention, language, memory, problem solving, judgment, concentration, planning, concept formation, and other "executive functions."[40,41] Servan-Schreiber and coworkers (1996)[40] proposed that "a single deficit in the processing of context information* may underlie various cognitive impairments observed in schizophrenia" and that "such an impairment is associated with positive rather than negative symptoms, and that it may worsen with the course of the illness." Neurochemical assays suggest that serotonin, dopamine, and glutamate all play significant roles in schizophrenia-induced cognitive impairments.[41] Certainly these impairments impede psychosocial performance and eventual reintegration into society and are therefore especially relevant targets for new therapeutic modalities.[41]

Goldberg and Weinberger (1996)[42] reviewed the effects of traditional neuroleptics and clozapine on cognitive function and concluded that these drugs have few predictable effects on cognition. Phenothiazines with anticholinergic and/or sedative side effects may even have additional detriments. Depressingly, review of clozapine studies led Goldberg and Weinberger to conclude that few if any cognitive measures improved with this new-generation agent. Any improvements in symptom status did not translate into markedly improved quality of life, living arrangements, or occupational status:

> Taken in toto, these results suggest the need for new pharmacological agents that specifically target cognitive dysfunction in schizophrenia, i.e., *nootropics*, as neither typical nor atypical neuroleptics appear capable of normalizing key impaired cognitive functions in schizophrenia.[42]

---

*Servan-Schreiber et al. (1996)[40] define context information as "information that has to be held actively in mind in such a form that it can be used to mediate an appropriate behavioral response." It can be the "result of processing a sequence of previous stimuli, a specific previous stimulus, or even a set of task instructions. . . . It is relevant to the performance of almost all cognitive tasks."

In general, this statement applies to results reported by Tollefson (1996)[41] and Meltzer and coworkers (1996),[43] who demonstrate minor improvements in cognitive function in animal tests of cognitive function, results that will probably translate into only minimal changes in patients. However, at least the new-generation agents did not cause further impairments, as can haloperidol and the phenothiazines.

Tolerance and Dependence

One of the positive attributes of the phenothiazines is that they are not behaviorally reinforcing and so are not prone to compulsive abuse. They do not produce tolerance, physical dependence, or psychological dependence. Psychotic patients may take phenothiazines for years without increasing their dose because of tolerance; if a dose is increased, it is usually done to increase the control of psychotic episodes.

Despite the fact that discontinuation of a phenothiazine is not followed by symptoms of drug withdrawal, possibly because of the long half-lives of the antipsychotic drugs and their metabolites, the therapeutic dilemmas associated with neuroleptic withdrawal are considerable.[44] In general, since neuroleptic treatment does not cure schizophrenia and long-term use is associated with risk of serious side effects (especially tardive dyskinesia), at some point consideration is often given to reducing or discontinuing medication. Here, neuroleptic withdrawal can be followed by psychotic exacerbation or relapse, although not all patients relapse after medication withdrawal.[44] Adverse effects of withdrawal other than relapse are mild and transient. In considering drug withdrawal, "The clinician and the patient have to choose between two unwelcome risks: relapse (with drug withdrawal) and adverse effects of continued treatment."[44]

Haloperidol (Haldol)

In 1967 *haloperidol* (see Figure 9.7) was introduced to the United States as the first therapeutic alternative to the phenothiazines. A related compound, *droperidol,* was subsequently introduced. Haloperidol is used primarily for its antipsychotic effects, while droperidol is used primarily for its antinausea and antiemetic properties.

Pharmacologically, haloperidol is remarkably similar to the phenothiazines. It produces sedation and an indifference to external stimuli and reduces initiative, anxiety, and activity. It is well absorbed orally and has a moderately slow rate of metabolism and excretion. Indeed, stable blood levels can be seen for up to 3 days following discontinuation of the drug. It takes approximately 5 days for 40 percent of a single dose to be excreted by the kidneys.

The mechanism of the antipsychotic action of haloperidol is like that of the phenothiazines—it occupies and competitively blocks dopamine$_2$ receptors. Haloperidol does not produce many of the serious side effects occasionally observed in patients who are taking phenothiazines (jaundice, blood abnormalities, and so on), but it causes parkinsonian motor movements that are of the same or greater intensity as those induced by the high-potency phenothiazines. Prophylactic antiparkinsonian medication may be needed. Sedation is unusual. In general, however, haloperidol is an effective drug for treating psychotic patients, offering an alternative for patients who do not respond to the phenothiazines.

New-Generation Antipsychotics

Until recently most attempts at finding alternative agents to the phenothiazines and haloperidol met with little success. Indeed, from 1975 to 1990, not a single new antipsychotic was marketed in the United States. Two alternative medications (molindone and loxapine) were introduced before 1975. Since 1990, clozapine (1990), risperidone (1994), pimozide (1996), olanzapine (1996), and sertindole (1997) have been introduced and several new drugs (e.g., quetiapine) are on the horizon for future introduction.

Molindone

Molindone (Moban) is structurally unique as an antipsychotic medication (see Figure 9.8): it resembles the neurotransmitter serotonin. Whether this resemblance is related to its antipsychotic action is unknown. Molindone resembles other antipsychotic drugs in therapeutic efficacy, occupancy of dopamine receptors, and side effects. It produces moderate sedation, increased motor activity, and possibly euphoria. It can also lead to abnormal motor (parkinsonian) movements that resemble those observed in patients taking phenothiazines. Molindone is rapidly absorbed when it is taken orally, and it is metabolized before it is excreted. Clinical effects following a single dose of molindone persist for about 24 to 36 hours. Interestingly, it is also a blocker of the enzyme monoamine oxidase (see Chapter 8), and its use is infrequently associated with tardive dyskinesia.[45]

Loxapine

Loxapine (Loxitane) is an antipsychotic drug with a unique structure (see Figure 9.8). It resembles somewhat the tricyclic antidepressants,

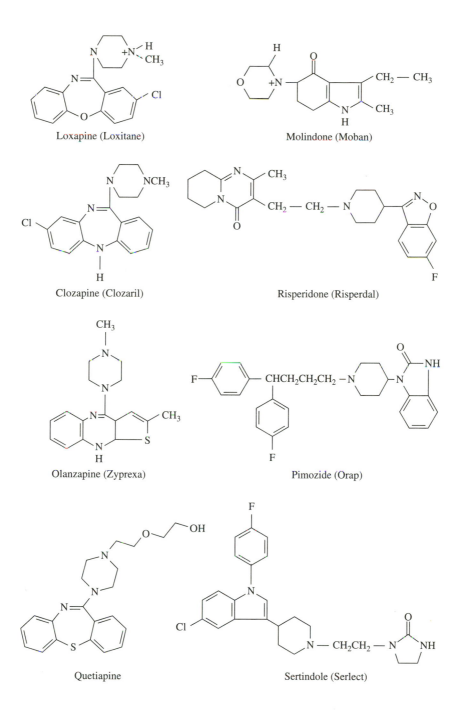

FIGURE 9.8 Structural formulas of new-generation antipsychotic drugs marketed or soon to be marketed in the United States.

especially amoxapine (see Chapter 7), but its actions differ little from those of the traditional antipsychotic drugs. It has antipsychotic, antiemetic, and sedative properties and causes abnormal motor movements. It lowers convulsive thresholds somewhat more than the phenothiazines. Taken orally, loxapine is well absorbed, and it is metabolized and excreted within about 24 hours.

Pimozide

Pimozide (Orap) is a newly available, structurally unique (see Figure 9.8) antipsychotic drug. It shares with the phenothiazines the ability to block dopamine receptors. Currently, the drug is marketed in the United States as an alternative drug for the treatment of motor and phonic tics in patients with Tourette's disorder who are unresponsive to other medications. In Europe and South America, however, pimozide is a widely used neuroleptic antipsychotic drug, which may ameliorate some of the negative symptomatology of schizophrenia.[46] Interestingly, pimozide may also have a somewhat unique role in the pharmacologic treatment of delusional disorder.[46,47]

The side effects that most limit use of pimozide (besides the usual movement disorders and tardive dyskinesia) are electrocardiographic abnormalities that, to date, have not been reported to be life-threatening.

Clozapine

Clozapine (Clozaril) is an antipsychotic drug whose structure is closely related to that of loxapine (see Figure 9.8). Clozapine is useful in treating treatment-resistant schizophrenics, relieves much of the negative symptomatology of schizophrenia, and lacks many of the extrapyramidal side effects associated with the standard neuroleptics, especially the parkinsonian-like extrapyramidal motor movements and tardive dyskinesia. Indeed, patients with primary Parkinsonism can demonstrate psychotic symptoms (such as visual hallucinations and delusions). Here, traditional neuroleptics worsen the Parkinsonism, whereas clozapine has been reported to treat the psychosis in Parkinson's patients without aggravating the movement disorder.[48]

Background. Although of intense interest only lately, clozapine is not a new drug. Synthesized in 1959, clozapine was introduced into clinical practice in Europe in the early 1970s. Its lack of extrapyramidal side effects was appreciated immediately. However, in 1975 several schizophrenic patients in Finland died of severe infectious diseases after developing agranulocytosis (loss of white cells in the blood) while taking clozapine.[32,49] As a result, clinical testing ceased, and the drug was withdrawn from unrestricted use in Europe. Later, clozapine was reexamined for two major reasons: (1) The agranulocytosis was found to be reversible when the drug was discontinued, and (2) the drug was found to be therapeutically beneficial in schizophrenic patients who failed to respond to the traditional neuroleptic compounds. In 1986 a large, multicenter trial of the drug in the United States found a 30 percent improvement among 318 severely psychotic schizophrenics who were unresponsive to other drugs; only 1 to 2 percent developed agranulocytosis. More recent studies show that the rate of improvement may approach 60 percent with longer therapy.[50]

> In some cases, the improvements in both positive and negative symptoms will result in striking changes with patients who appear hopelessly lost in a psychotic world, emerging as individuals who can be discharged from hospitals or participate meaningfully in rehabilitation programs. Some have termed this "wakenings." Other clozapine "responders" may not improve substantially in their positive symptoms but will report that their mood and sense of well-being are much improved. For these individuals the deficits associated with schizophrenia may not improve, but the quality of life is better.[32]

Meltzer (1993)[49] states that clozapine is also particularly effective against a third type of psychotic symptomatology (besides the positive and negative symptoms), which he calls *disorganization*. This set of symptoms consists of loose association, inappropriate affect, incoherence, and reduction in rational thought processes.

Thus, while agranulocytosis limits the drug's use in patients adequately controlled by traditional neuroleptics, clozapine is indicated for use in treatment-resistant schizophrenics and patients who suffer severe extrapyramidal side effects with conventional drugs, who have severe negative symptoms, and perhaps who have severe tardive dyskinesia. In addition, because the drug ameliorates both the positive and negative symptoms and users suffer fewer of the extrapyramidal side effects, compliance is better than that achieved with conventional antipsychotics; only a small percentage of patients discontinue the drug for either lack of efficacy or intolerance of side effects.[51] For example, in one study[52] 76 percent of institutionalized patients discharged on clozapine therapy were still taking the drug 12 months later, greatly reducing the likelihood of readmission.

Pharmacokinetics. The pharmacokinetics of clozapine varies significantly among patients.[42] The drug is well absorbed orally, and significant metabolism takes place as the drug reaches plasma and is carried to the liver, before it is distributed throughout the body.[53] Plasma levels of the drug peak in about 1 to 4 hours, and its distribution in the body appears to vary, with some patients sequestering significant quantities of drug. Clozapine is metabolized in the liver into two major metabolites, both of which are fairly inactive pharmacologically. The reported metabolic half-life of clozapine was 9 to 17 hours in one study[54] and 6 to 33 hours in another.[32]

Jann and coworkers (1993)[53] addressed the relationship between plasma levels of clozapine and therapeutic effectiveness. They estimated that in the treatment of patients with refractory schizophrenia, a minimum concentration of 350 micrograms per milliliter was needed.

Pharmacodynamics. Earlier in this chapter, we discussed theories regarding both the etiology of schizophrenia and the mechanisms of action of antipsychotic drugs, including clozapine. As reviewed by Brunello and coworkers (1995)[55]:

> If schizophrenia is in some way related to morphological abnormalities, it becomes hard to believe that a *curative* treatment will ever be possible. Considering this scenario, treatment of schizophrenia will be restricted to symptomatic and preventive therapy and therefore, more effective and better tolerated antipsychotics are necessary. . . . Clozapine constitutes a major advance in particular for patients not responding to conventional neuroleptics.

Clozapine has high binding affinity for dopamine$_4$, serotonin$_{1C}$, serotonin$_2$, alpha-1 (an adrenergic receptor), muscarinic (an acetylcholine receptor), and histamine receptors, but moderate affinity is also seen for many other receptor subtypes.[55,56] Brunello and coworkers (1995)[55] proposed:

> Clozapine, differently from all other conventional neuroleptics, is a mixed but weak D_1/D_2 antagonist. This observation has prompted speculation that the synergism between D_1 and D_2 receptors might allow antipsychotic effects to be achieved below the threshold for unwanted motor side effects.

Although most researchers agree that binding to the dopamine$_4$ receptor is important, Meltzer (1992)[56] stresses the critical importance of drug binding to the serotonin receptors. Regardless of the pharmacodynamics, clozapine and its derivatives provide researchers with important new tools for investigating the cellular mechanisms of the schizophrenias.

Side Effects and Toxicity. The most common side effect of clozapine is sedation, which can limit the amount of drug administered. Other bothersome side effects include hypotension, tachycardia, fever (including a rare neuroleptic malignant syndrome), increased salivation, dizziness, and weight gain. Recently, Popli and coworkers[57] reported four individuals in whom clozapine use was associated "with either a *de novo* onset or severe exacerbation of preexisting diabetes mellitus [sugar diabetes]."

As discussed, the major concern with clozapine is the 1 to 2 percent risk of developing severe, life-threatening (although reversible) agranulocytosis. White blood cell counts must be monitored at least weekly for the first 4 to 5 months of therapy and monthly thereafter, with more frequent monitoring if the white blood cell count is decreasing. Other drugs that can cause reductions in white blood cell count (most notably carbamazepine; see Chapter 8) should not be taken concomitantly.

The etiology of clozapine-induced agranulocytosis appears to involve a cellular-toxic mechanism.[58,59] In support of this concept, Eutrecht (1992)[60] reported that clozapine can be metabolized not only in the liver but also by the neutrophils (a specialized type of white blood cell) themselves! An intermediate compound in this metabolic process is reactive and is postulated to be toxic to the cell, possibly killing the cell that formed it either directly or through an immunological mechanism. The newly available, structurally related antipsychotic olanzapine does not appear to possess this propensity to be metabolized by neutrophils, and agranulocytosis has not yet been reported. Therefore, at this time, blood testing for possible olanzapine-induced neutropenia is not necessary.[61]

Cost Concerns. Clozapine therapy is much more expensive than therapy with any of the conventional antipsychotic drugs, partially because of the necessary blood monitoring. Currently, the annual cost of taking clozapine (including the costs of weekly blood monitoring) totals $6,000 to $8,000. There are an estimated 300,000 to 600,000 schizophrenics who do not respond to other neuroleptics or who cannot tolerate their side effects.[62] These people form a large potential market for clozapine, but the high costs make mental health workers reluctant to prescribe the drug more, despite the reduced rate of rehospitalization. Dichotomies like this one underlie many of the current dilemmas in the treatment of schizophrenia.

Risperidone

Risperidone (Risperdal) was introduced in 1994 as a very promising new-generation antipsychotic drug. Risperidone was first administered to schizophrenic patients in 1986; since then it has been used in Europe and its pharmacology has been studied extensively.

Risperidone acts as a potent inhibitor of both dopamine$_2$ and sero-tonin$_2$ receptors, particularly the latter receptors.[63] As discussed earlier, the serotonin antagonism can result in improved control of psychotic symptoms and alleviation of neuroleptic-induced extrapyramidal side effects.

> From the distribution of serotonin$_2$ receptors, one would expect dopaminergic transmission to be enhanced in the basal ganglia, re-sulting in diminished extrapyramidal symptoms. . . . Improved frontal cortical function results in the normalization of descending GABA and NMDA neuronal function . . . systems also implicated in the pathogenesis of positive and negative symptoms.[64]

The pharmacokinetics of risperidone have been very well stud-ied.[53,65,66] The drug is well absorbed when administered orally and is highly bound to plasma proteins. It is metabolized to an active inter-mediate (9-hydroxy-risperidone), but the rate of metabolism varies be-cause of genetic differences. The metabolic half-life in rapid metaboliz-ers is about 3 hours, 10 hours in intermediate metabolizers, and 21 hours in slow metabolizers. The half-life of the active intermediate is about 20 hours in all groups. Whether these various rates of hepatic metabolism have important clinical consequences is unclear.

Several studies and reviews have concluded that risperidone is at least as effective as haloperidol in reducing the positive symptomatol-ogy of schizophrenia without producing a high incidence of extrapyra-midal side effects (at least at low to moderate therapeutic doses).[67-69] Risperidone also appears to be efficacious in reducing the positive symptoms of schizophrenia in a subgroup of chronically hospitalized schizophrenic patients who have not responded to other neuroleptics.[70] Common side effects of risperidone include agitation, anxiety, insom-nia, headache, extrapyramidal effects (at high doses), and nausea.

According to Remington (1993),[71] risperidone can be considered a first-line agent in treating schizophrenia because of its efficacy and safety profile. This suggestion has now become a therapeutic recom-mendation, with risperidone recommended as a first-line antipsychotic when negative symptoms predominate in "first episode patients."[72]

Olanzapine

Introduced in late 1996, *olanzapine* (Zyprexa) is structurally closely re-lated to clozapine (see Figure 9.8). Olanzapine appears to display a level of *in vitro* binding between those of haloperidol and clozapine; it displays a higher affinity for dopamine D_2 receptors and a slightly lower affinity for serotonin 5-HT$_2$ receptors.[27,73] Olanzapine produces a clozapine-like image, blocking 40 to 60 percent of D_2 receptors (a blockade associated with good clinical response) and 84 percent occupancy of cortical serotonin 5-HT_2 receptors.[73] The drug is also a blocker of acetylcholine receptors (an anticholinergic), which probably contributes to its lack of extrapyramidal effects (along with the blockade of 5-HT_2 receptors).[27]

The clinical efficacy of olanzapine was documented by Beasley and coworkers (1996),[74] both in a placebo-controlled trial and in comparison with haloperidol.[75] Improvements in both positive and negative symptoms were impressive. Extrapyramidal side effects are only rarely observed.

Pharmacokinetics. Olanzapine is well absorbed orally. Peak plasma levels occur in about 5 to 8 hours. Metabolized in the liver, olanzapine has an elimination half-life in a range of 27 to 38 hours with a mean of 30 hours,[76] allowing once-a-day dosage. Only 7 percent of the drug is excreted unchanged.

Side Effects. The majority of side effects induced by olanzapine are relatively minor, consisting of weight gain, sedation, orthostatic hypotension, and dizziness. Cognitive function does not appear to be impaired by olanzapine.[41] Very importantly, in contrast to clozapine, there have been no reports of agranulocytosis or reduced white blood cell count with olanzapine.[61]

In summary, the newly released drug olanzapine is structurally and pharmacologically similar to clozapine but devoid of the white blood cell problems, eliminating the need for intermittent evaluation of blood chemistry. This is likely to improve patient compliance with therapy because the patient need not present for blood draws. Recent reviews on the pharmacology and clinical efficacy of olanzapine include that by Fulton and Goa (1997),[77] the monograph edited by Beasley (1997),[78] and *The Medical Letter on Drugs and Therapeutics* (1997).[79]

Remoxipride

Remoxipride (Roxiam) is an atypical antipsychotic agent of proven efficacy, but it probably will not become available in the United States because of an unacceptable incidence of severe blood dyscrasias. The symposium edited by Sedvall (1990)[80] discusses the pharmacology of remoxipride at length.

Sertindole

Sertindole (Serlect), introduced in 1997, is the newest of the new-generation antipsychotics. It binds (in decreasing order of affinity) to serotonin 5-HT_2, alpha 1-adrenoreceptors, and cortical dopamine D_2 receptors. It therefore possesses the dual action of D_2 and 5-HT_2 receptor blockade thought to "define" the new-generation antipsychotics. Such dual action is predicted to be therapeutically useful in ameliorating both the positive and the negative symptoms of schizophrenia, with a low incidence of extrapyramidal side effects. The metabolic half-life of sertindole varies from 24 to 200 hours, with a mean of 55 to 90 hours.[76] Time and experience will define the role of sertindole, its efficacy, and its side effects.

Among the other new-generation antipsychotic drugs that may appear on the market shortly are *quetiapine* and *ziprasidone*. The late 1990s should be most interesting as a variety of new antipsychotics becomes available. Hopefully, comparative double-blind clinical studies will be reported, allowing one-to-one comparison of efficacy, tolerability, and compliance.

Antipsychotic Drugs in the Young and the Elderly

The treatment of schizophrenia in children has received scant attention. Neuroleptics are prescribed with caution and trepidation because of the severity of side effects and the potential for inducing tardive dyskinesia, which may eventually develop in 8 to 51 percent of patients.[81] The use of clozapine in children is limited by the risk of agranulocytosis, necessitating weekly blood tests, which makes this treatment unappealing to most adolescents. Kumra and coworkers (1996)[82] reported a double-blind comparison of clozapine and haloperidol in 21 adolescents with early-onset schizophrenia. Clozapine was clearly superior to haloperidol for positive and negative symptoms. Two children had a true "awakening" from their thought disorder and psychotic symptoms. One of these children,

> who had delusions, auditory hallucinations, mutilated himself, and had other severe negative symptoms, had a complete remission of psychosis and behavioral problems after receiving clozapine and conversed in sentences for the first time in years. He now lives with his family, attends a day program regularly, and has been able to maintain friendships.

Three recent reports have addressed the use of risperidone in children and adolescents. Armenteros and coworkers (1997)[83] reported successful amelioration of both positive and negative symptoms of schizophrenia in 10 adolescents. McDougle and coworkers (1997) [84] reported efficacy in treating pervasive developmental disorders in 18 children and adolescents. Kunka and coworkers (1997),[85] however, reported that two of 13 schizophrenic adolescents treated with risperidone developed signs of drug-induced liver toxicity that reversed with cessation of risperidone.

The use of neuroleptics in the *elderly*, especially the debilitated, nursing home population, has always been both widespread and controversial. In an effort to more appropriately use these drugs in the elderly nursing home population, federal legislation was passed in 1987. This legislation was intended to block overtreatment of elderly individuals with neuroleptic medications:

> Rather than prescribe these medications for vague indications that range from agitation to restlessness to fidgeting, doctors are required to document the diagnostic indication for concurrent neuroleptic use (i.e., coexistent schizophrenia, brief reactive psychosis, or acute delirium) [see Table 9.5]. Furthermore, the continued use of such medications must be justified in an ongoing way, even if the underlying diagnosis is considered appropriate.[86]

In 1994 Semla and coworkers[87] reported that neuroleptics could be stopped or the dose lowered in up to 75 percent of chronically treated nursing home elderly. Drug-induced parkinsonism is frequently induced in these patients. Alternative pharmacologic treatments (if

---

TABLE 9.5 Guideline for the use of neuroleptic medications in nursing home patients as written in the 1987 Omnibus Budget Reconciliation Act (OBRA) regulations

---

A. Appropriate indications for neuroleptic use

- Schizophrenia
- Schizoaffective disorder
- Delusional disorder
- Psychotic mood disorder
- Acute psychotic episodes
- Brief reactive psychosis
- Schizophrenia form disorder
- Atypical psychosis
- Tourette's disorder
- Huntington's disorder
- Organic mental disorders (i.e., dementia and delirium)

B. Inappropriate indications for neuroleptic use

- Wandering
- Restlessness
- Anxiety
- Fidgeting
- Nervousness
- Uncooperativeness
- Agitation (without danger)
- Poor self-care
- Impaired memory
- Unsociability
- Indifference to surroundings
- Depression (without psychosis)
- Insomnia

From Sunderland (1996),[83] Table I, p. 54.

deemed necessary) include buspirone, diphenhydramine (Benadryl), ox-azepam, and many others. New-generation antipsychotics are currently being evaluated, although the anticholinergic side effects (with drugs such as clozapine) may impair cognition. Further research in this important area is desperately needed, especially because the demented elderly population will rapidly expand in numbers over the next 20 years.

NOTES

1. J. M. Kane, "Schizophrenia," *New England Journal of Medicine* 334 (1996): 34–41.
2. B. Jones, "Schizophrenia: Into the Next Millennium," *Canadian Journal of Psychiatry* 38, Suppl. 3 (September 1993): S67–S69.
3. U.S. Congress, Office of Technology Assessment, *The Biology of Mental Disorders* (Washington, D.C.: U.S. Government Printing Office, September 1992), 7.
4. G. D. Tollefson, "Update on New Atypical Antipsychotics," in "Academic Highlights, Advancements in CNS Drugs: Recent Advances and Considerations in the Treatment of Schizophrenia," *Journal of Clinical Psychiatry* 57 (1996): 318–319.
5. J. Gerlach and D. E. Casey, "New Antipsychotics: Preclinical and Clinical Research," *Psychopharmacology* 124 (1996): 1.
6. INTERCOM, "The Experts Converse: Antipsychotic Agents: Minimizing Side Effects to Maximize Compliance," *Journal of Clinical Psychiatry* (Oct. 1, 1996).
7. C. A. Prescott and I. I. Gottesman, "Genetically Mediated Vulnerability to Schizophrenia," *Psychiatric Clinics of North America* 16 (1993): 245–267.
8. C. A. Ross and G. D. Pearlson, "Schizophrenia, the Heteromodal Association Neocortex and Development: Potential for a Neurogenetic Approach," *Trends in Neurological Sciences* 19 (1996): 171–176.
9. E. V. Gurevich, Y. Bordelon, R. M. Shapiro, et al., "Mesolimbic Dopamine D_3 Receptors and Use of Antipsychotics in Patients with Schizophrenia," *Archives of General Psychiatry* 54 (1997): 225–232.
10. H. A. Nasrallah, "Neurodevelopmental Pathogenesis of Schizophrenia," *Psychiatric Clinics of North America* 16 (1993): 269–293.
11. S. Akbarian, W. E. Bunney, Jr., S. G. Potkin, et al., "Altered Distribution of Nicotinamide-Adenine Dinucleotide Phosphate-Diaphorase Cells in Frontal Lobe of Schizophrenics Implies Disturbances of Cortical Development," *Archives of General Psychiatry* 50 (1993): 169–177.
12. S. Akbarian, J. J. Kim, S. G. Potkin, et al., "Maldistribution of Interstitial Neurons in Prefrontal White Matter of the Brains of Schizophrenic Patients," *Archives of General Psychiatry* 53 (1996): 425–436.
13. S. Akbarian, A. Vinuela, J. J. Kim, et al., "Distorted Distribution of Nicotinamide-Adenine Dinucleotide Phosphate-Diaphorase Neurons in Temporal Lobe of Schizophrenics Implies Anomalous Cortical Development," *Archives of General Psychiatry* 50 (1993): 178–187.

14. F. E. Bloom, "Advancing a Neurodevelopmental Origin for Schizophrenia," *Archives of General Psychiatry* 50 (1993): 224–227.

15. S. Akbarian, J. J. Kim, S. G. Potkin, et al., "Gene Expression for Glutamic Acid Decarboxylase Is Reduced Without Loss of Neurons in Prefrontal Cortex of Schizophrenics," *Archives of General Psychiatry* 52 (1995): 258–266.

16. D. A. Lewis, "Neural Circuitry of the Prefrontal Cortex in Schizophrenia," *Archives of General Psychiatry* 52 (1995): 269–273.

17. D. E. Lee and A. J. Tobin, "Reduced Inhibitory Capacity in Prefrontal Cortex of Schizophrenics," *Archives of General Psychiatry* 52 (1995): 267–268.

18. J. W. Olney and N. B. Farber, "Glutamate Receptor Dysfunction and Schizophrenia," *Archives of General Psychiatry* 52 (1995): 998–1007.

19. S. E. Bachus and J. E. Kleinman, "The Neuropathology of Schizophrenia," *Journal of Clinical Psychiatry* 57, Suppl. 11 (1996): 72–83.

20. J. M. Hollister, P. Laing, and S. A. Mednick, "Rhesus Incompatibility as a Risk Factor for Schizophrenia in Male Adults," *Archives of General Psychiatry* 53 (1996): 19–24.

21. E. Susser, R. Neugebauer, H. W. Hoek, et al., "Schizophrenia After Prenatal Famine," *Archives of General Psychiatry* 53 (1996): 25–31.

22. R. J. Wyatt, "Neurodevelopmental Abnormalities and Schizophrenia: A Family Affair," *Archives of General Psychiatry* 53 (1996): 11–15.

23. P. Seemam, "Dopamine Receptor Sequences: Therapeutic Levels of Neuroleptics Occupy D_2 Receptors, Clozapine Occupies D_4," *Neuropsychopharmacology* 7 (1992): 261–284.

24. E. Richelson, "Preclinical Pharmacology of Neuroleptics: Focus on New Generation Compounds," *Journal of Clinical Psychiatry* 57, Suppl. 11 (1996): 4–11.

25. D. E. Casey, "Extrapyramidal Symptoms in Old and New Antipsychotics" (433–436), in J. M. Kane, chairperson, "Choosing Among Old and New Antipsychotics," *Journal of Clinical Psychiatry* 57 (1996): 427–438.

26. D. E. Casey, "Movement Disorders," *Journal of Clinical Psychiatry* 57 (1996): 316–317.

27. R. Kerwin, "Imaging Studies of Neuroleptic Occupancy," *Journal of Clinical Psychiatry* 57 (1996): 315–316.

28. C. A. Tamminga, "Pharmacodynamic Mechanisms of Antipsychotic Drug Actions" (428–431), in J. M. Kane, chairperson, "Choosing Among Old and New Antipsychotics," *Journal of Clinical Psychiatry* 57 (1996): 427–438.

29. G. P. Reynolds, "The Importance of Dopamine D_4 Receptors in the Action and Development of Antipsychotic Agents," *Drugs* 51 (1996): 7–11.

30. P. Weiden, R. Aquila and J. Standard, "Atypical Antipsychotic Drugs and Long-Term Outcome in Schizophrenia," *Journal of Clinical Psychiatry* 57, Suppl. 11 (1996): 53–60.

31. P. S. Albright, S. Livingstone, D. L. Keegan, et al., "Reduction of Healthcare Resource Utilization and Costs Following the Use of Risperidone for Patients with Schizophrenia Previously Treated with Standard Antipsychotic Therapy," *Clinical Drug Investigation* 11 (1996): 289–299.

32. S. R. Marder, D. Ames, W. C. Wirshing, and T. VanPutten, "Schizophrenia," *Psychiatric Clinics of North America* 16 (1993): 568–570.
33. S. H. Preskorn, M. J. Burke, and G. A. Fast, "Therapeutic Drug Monitoring," *Psychiatric Clinics of North America* 16 (1993): 611–641.
34. D. E. Casey, "Neuroleptic-Induced Acute Extrapyramidal Syndromes and Tardive Dyskinesia," *Psychiatric Clinics of North America* 16 (1993): 589–610.
35. D. G. Cunningham Owens, "Adverse Effects of Antipsychotic Agents: Do Newer Agents Offer Advantages?," *Drugs* 51 (1996): 895–930.
36. R. J. Baldessarini, "Drugs and the Treatment of Psychiatric Disorders: Psychosis and Anxiety," in J. G. Hardman, L. E. Limbird, P. B. Molinoff, R. W. Ruddon, and A. G. Gilman, eds. *Goodman and Gilman's The Pharmacological Basis of Therapeutics*, 9th ed. (New York: McGraw-Hill, 1995), 399–430.
37. J. M. Kane, "Treatment-Resistant Schizophrenic Patients," *Journal of Clinical Psychiatry* 57, Suppl. 9 (1996): 35–40.
38. S. R. Marder, "Management of Treatment-Resistant Patients With Schizophrenia," *Journal of Clinical Psychiatry* 57, Suppl. 11 (1996): 26–30.
39. T. E. Goldberg, J. R. Kelsoe, D. R. Weinberger, et al., "Performance of Schizophrenic Patients on Putative Neuropsychological Tests of Frontal Lobe Function," *International Journal of Neurosciences* 42 (1988): 51–58.
40. D. Servan-Schreiber, J. D. Cohen, and S. Steingard, "Schizophrenic Deficits in the Processing of Context: A Test of a Theoretical Model," *Archives of General Psychiatry* 53 (1996): 1105–1112.
41. G. D. Tollefson, "Cognitive Function in Schizophrenic Patients," *Journal of Clinical Psychiatry* 57, Suppl. 11 (1996): 31–39.
42. T. E. Goldberg and D. R. Weinberger, "Effects of Neuroleptic Medications on the Cognition of Patients With Schizophrenia: A Review of Recent Studies," *Journal of Clinical Psychiatry* 57, Suppl. 9 (1996): 62–65.
43. H. Y. Meltzer, P. A. Thompson, M. A. Lee, et al., "Neuropsychologic Deficits in Schizophrenia: Relation to Function and Effects of Antipsychotic Drug-Treatment," *Neuropsychopharmacology* 14 (1996): S27–S33.
44. P. L. Gilbert, M. J. Harris, L. A. McAdams, and D. V. Jeste, "Neuroleptic Withdrawal in Schizophrenic Patients," *Archives of General Psychiatry* 52 (1995): 173–188.
45. R. R. Owen, Jr., and J. O. Cole, "Molindone Hydrochloride: A Review of Laboratory and Clinical Findings," *Journal of Clinical Psychopharmacology* 9 (1989): 268–276.
46. L. A. Opler, D. M. Klahr, and P. M. Ramirez, "Pharmacologic Treatment of Delusions," *Psychiatric Clinics of North America* 18 (1995): 379–391.
47. M. J. Tueth and J. A. Cheong, "Clinical Uses of Pimozide," *Southern Medical Journal* 86 (1993): 344–349.
48. W. S. Musser and M. Akil, "Clozapine as a Treatment for Psychosis in Parkinson's Disease," *Journal of Neuropsychiatry and Clinical Neurosciences* 8 (1996): 1–9.
49. H. Y. Meltzer, "New Drugs for the Treatment of Schizophrenia," *Psychiatric Clinics of North America* 16 (1993): 365–385.

50. A. Breier, R. W. Buchanan, D. Irish, and W. T. Carpenter, Jr., "Clozapine Treatment of Outpatients with Schizophrenia: Outcome and Long-term Response Patterns," *Hospital and Community Psychiatry* 44 (1993): 1145–1149.

51. N. R. Schooler, "Clozapine and Risperidone: Recent Findings in Two New Drugs (431–433), in J. M. Kane, chairperson, "Choosing Among Old and New Antipsychotics," *Journal of Clinical Psychiatry* 57 (1996): 427–438.

52. S. M. Essock, W. A. Hargreaves, F. A. Dohm, et al., "Clozapine Eligibility Among State Hospital Patients," *Schizophrenia Bulletin* 22 (1996): 15–25.

53. M. J. Byerly and C. L. DeVane, "Pharmacokinetics of Clozapine and Risperidone: A Review of Recent Literature," *Journal of Clinical Psychopharmacology* 16 (1996): 177–187.

54. M. W. Jann, S. R. Grimsley, E. C. Gray, and W. H. Chang, "Pharmacokinetics and Pharmacodynamics of Clozapine," *Clinical Pharmacokinetics* 24 (1993): 161–176.

55. N. Brunello, C. Masotto, L. Steardo, R. Markstein, and G. Racagni, "New Insights into the Biology of Schizophrenia Through the Mechanism of Action of Clozapine," *Neuropsychopharmacology* 13 (1995): 177–213.

56. H. Y. Meltzer, "The Importance of Serotonin-Dopamine Interactions in the Action of Clozapine," *British Journal of Psychiatry* 17, suppl. (May 1992): 22–29.

57. A. P. Popli, P. E. Konicki, G. J. Jurjus, et al., "Clozapine and Associated Diabetes Mellitus," *Journal of Clinical Psychiatry* 58 (1997): 108–111.

58. S. L. Gerson and H. Meltzer, "Mechanisms of Clozapine-Induced Agranulocytosis," *Drug Safety* 7, Suppl. 1 (1992): 17–25.

59. A. V. Pisciotta, S. A. Konings, L. L. Ciesemier, et al., "On the Possible Mechanisms and Predictability of Clozapine-Induced Agranulocytosis," *Drug Safety* 7, Suppl. 1 (1992): 33–44.

60. J. P. Eutrecht, "Metabolism of Clozapine by Neutrophils: Possible Implications for Clozapine-Induced Agranulocytosis," *Drug Safety* 7, Suppl. 1 (1992): 51–56.

61. D. E. Casey, "Side Effect Profiles of New Antipsychotic Agents," *Journal of Clinical Psychiatry* 57, Suppl. 11 (1996): 40–45.

62. H. Y. Meltzer, "Clozapine: A Major Advance in the Treatment of Schizophrenia," *The Harvard Mental Health Letter* 10 (August 1993): 4–6.

63. R. W. Kerwin, G. F. Busatto, and L. S. Pilowsky, "Dopamine D_2 Receptor Occupancy in Vivo and Response to the New Antipsychotic Risperidone," *British Journal of Psychiatry* 163 (1993): 833–834.

64. A. Megens, F. Awouters, S. Schotte, et al., "Survey on the Pharmacodynamics of the New Antipsychotic Risperidone," *Psychopharmacology* 114 (1994): 9–23.

65. G. Mannens, M.-L. Huang, W. Meuldermans, et al., "Absorption, Metabolism, and Excretion of Risperidone in Humans," *Drug Metabolism and Disposition* 21 (1993): 1134–1141.

66. M. Huang, A. Van Peer, R. Woestenborghs, et al., "Pharmacokinetics of the Novel Antipsychotic Agent Risperidone and the Prolactin Response in Healthy Subjects," *Clinical Pharmacology and Therapeutics* 54 (1993): 257–268.

67. S. R. Marder and R. C. Meibach, "Risperidone in the Treatment of Schizophrenia," *American Journal of Psychiatry* 151 (1994): 825–835.

68. A. A. Cardoni, "Risperidone: Review and Assessment of Its Role in the Treatment of Schizophrenia," *Annals of Pharmacotherapy* 29 (1995): 610–618.

69. S. R. Marder, "Clinical Experience With Risperidone," *Journal of Clinical Psychiatry* 57, Suppl. 9 (1996): 57–61.

70. R. C. Smith, J. W. Cua, B. Lipetsker, and A. Bhattacharyya, "Efficacy of Risperidone in Reducing Positive and Negative Symptoms in Medication-Refractory Schizophrenia: An Open Prospective Study," *Journal of Clinical Psychiatry* 57 (1996): 460–466.

71. G. J. Remington, "Clinical Considerations in the Use of Risperidone," *Canadian Journal of Psychiatry* 38, Suppl. 3 (1993): S96–S100.

72. A. Francis, J. P. Docherty, and D. A. Kahn, "Treatment of Schizophrenia," *Journal of Clinical Psychiatry* 57, Suppl. 12B (1996): 1–58.

73. L. S. Pilowsky, G. F. Busatto, M. Taylor, et al., "Dopamine D_2 Receptor Occupancy *in vivo* by *de novo* Atypical Antipsychotic Olanzapine: A ^{123}I IBZM Single Photon Emission Tomography (SPECT) Study," *Journal of Psychopharmacology* 124 (1996): 148–153.

74. C. M. Beasley, Jr., T. Sanger, W. Satterlee, et al., "Olanzapine HGAP Study Group. Olanzapine Versus Placebo: Results of a Double-Blind, Fixed-Dose Olanzapine Trial," *Psychopharmacology* 124 (1996): 159–167.

75. C. M. Beasley, Jr., G. Tollefson, P. Tran, et al., "The Olanzapine HGAP Study Group: Olanzapine Versus Placebo and Haloperidol. Acute Phase of the North American Double-Blind Olanzapine Trial," *Neuropsychopharmacology* 14 (1996): 111–123.

76. L. Ereshefsky, "Pharmacokinetics and Drug Interactions: Update for New Antipsychotics," *Journal of Clinical Psychiatry* 57, Suppl. 11 (1996): 12–25.

77. B. Fulton and K. L. Goa, "Olanzapine: A Review of Its Pharmacological Properties and Therapeutic Efficacy in the Management of Schizophrenia," *Drugs* 53 (1997): 281–298.

78. C. M. Beasley, ed., "Practical Issues in Using Olanzapine," *Journal of Clinical Psychiatry* Monograph series, no. 15 (February 1997): 1–39.

79. M. Abramowicz, ed., "Olanzapine for Schizophrenia," *The Medical Letter on Drugs and Therapeutics* 38 (Jan. 17, 1997): 5–6.

80. G. Sedvall, "Development of a New Antipsychotic, Remoxipride," *Acta Psychiatrica Scandinavica* 82, Suppl. 358 (1990).

81. R. L. Findling, S. J. Grcevich, I. Lopez, and S. C. Schulz, "Antipsychotic Medications in Children and Adolescents," *Journal of Clinical Psychiatry* 57, Suppl. 9 (1996): 19–23.

82. S. Kumra, J. A. Frazier, L. K. Jacobsen, et al., "Childhood-Onset Schizophrenia: A Double-Blind Clozapine-Haloperidol Comparison," *Archives of General Psychiatry* 53 (1996): 1090–1097.

83. J. L. Armenteros, A. H. Whitaker, M. Welikson, et al., "Risperidone in Adolescents with Schizophrenia: An Open Pilot Study," *Journal of the American Acaademy of Child and Adolescent Psychiatry* 36 (1997): 697–700.

84. C. J. McDougle, J. P. Holmes, M. R. Bronson, et al., "Risperidone Treatment of Children and Adolescents with Pervasive Developmental Disorders: A Prospective, Open-Label Study," *Journal of the American Academy of Child and Adolescent Psychiatry* 36 (1997): 685–693.

85. S. Kumra, D. Herion, L. K. Jacobsen, et al., "Case Study: Risperidone-Induced Hepatotoxicity in Pediatric Patients," *Journal of the American Academy of Child and Adolescent Psychiatry* 36 (1997): 701–705.

86. T. Sunderland, "Treatment of the Elderly Suffering from Psychosis and Dementia," *Journal of Clinical Psychiatry* 57, Suppl. 9 1996): 53–56.

87. T. Semla, K. Palla, B. Poddig, et al., "Effect of the Omnibus Reconciliation Act 1987 on Antipsychotic Prescribing in Nursing Home Residents," *Journal of the American Geriatrics Society* 42 (1994): 648–652.

88. Work Group on Schizophrenia, M. I. Herz, chair, American Psychiatric Association Practice Guidelines, "Practice Guideline for the Treatment of Patients with Schizophrenia," *American Journal of Psychiatry* 154, no. 4, suppl. (1997): 1–63.

Chapter 10

OPIOID ANALGESICS

Pain is caused by the activation of small-diameter sensory (afferent) fibers of peripheral nerves. These pain-sensing (*nociceptive*) sensory neurons originate in peripheral tissues, such as skin, muscle, and abdominal viscera, and are activated by various mechanical, thermal, chemical, and injury stimuli. Because these neurons are activated by noxious (painful) stimuli, their receptors are called *nociceptors* (see Figure 10.1). The action potentials (electrical discharge) in these neurons are conducted to their synaptic terminals, which are located in the dorsal horn of the spinal cord and where (in its simplest concept) a chemical transmitter called *substance P* is released.

Substance P, which is a neuropeptide (11 amino acids in length) present in pain-transmitting afferent neurons, thus plays a role in the transmission of nociceptive information from the site of injury to the spinal cord, and its release in the dorsal horn of the spinal cord is regulated intrinsically by endogenous *endorphins* (discussed later) and extrinsically by any drug of a class called the *opioids* (or morphine-like drugs). Indeed, endorphins and opioids exert at least part of their analgesic (pain-relieving) action by acting directly on substance P neurons (presynaptically) to inhibit substance P release.[1,2] In other words, opioids and endorphins exert presynaptic inhibition on the terminals of afferent sensory neurons to inhibit substance P release, an analgesic action.

When it is released, substance P activates other spinal cord neurons, which in turn transmit information about noxious stimuli to the brain by means of two specialized afferent pathways (from the spinal

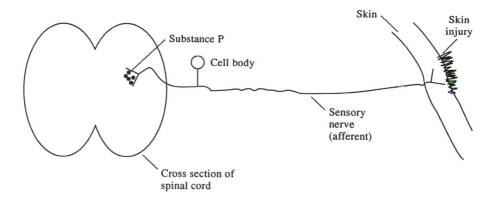

FIGURE 10.1 Activation of peripheral nociceptive (pain) fibers results in the release of substance P from nerve terminals in the dorsal horn of the spinal cord. The cell body for the nerve is located in the dorsal root ganglion.

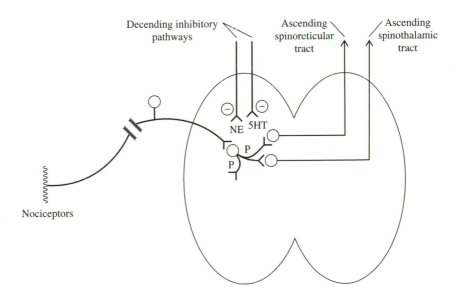

FIGURE 10.2 Release of substance P in the dorsal horn of the spinal cord with transmission of secondary relay pathways to higher centers. Descending inhibitory pathways (–) are also shown (expanded in Figure 10.3). NE = norepinephrine; 5HT = serotonin.

cord to the brain)—the spinothalamic tract and the spinoreticular tract (see Figure 10.2). Thus, pain is first "perceived" by activation of nociceptive receptors (in the skin and other parts of the body) and is carried to the spinal cord by afferent nerve fibers, which release substance P. This perception is relayed to the brain stem and the thalamus and, eventually, to higher centers in the brain (such as the limbic system and the somatosensory cortex) for interpretation. In addition to the dorsal horn of the spinal cord, the thalamus, brain stem, and limbic system are also rich in opioid receptors, on which both the opioids and endorphins act. These centers in the brain are all important sites of action for opioids.

As Figure 10.3 illustrates, two descending pathways, which originate in the lower brain stem, modulate the transmission of pain impulses by activating descending pain-inhibitory systems. Activation of either of these pathways, which consist of descending (brain stem to spinal cord) norepinephrine- and serotonin-releasing neurons, activates endorphin neurons in the dorsal horn of the spinal cord, which, in turn, exerts an analgesic action by further inhibiting substance P release from the primary afferent nociceptive neurons. Indeed, it is these descending pathways on which the antidepressants act to exert their own analgesic actions (see Chapter 7). As Satoh and Minami (1995)[2] state:

> Microinjections of morphine into the gigantocellular reticular nucleus, lateral paragigantocellular nucleus, raphe magnus nucleus, and PAG [periaqueductal gray] produced analgesic effects in much lower doses than systemic injections, suggesting that the cells specific to the supraspinal mechanisms for analgesic effects of opiates [opioids] exist in these brain regions.

The *affective component* of pain is the component that determines our emotional response by reducing the distress associated with the pain. The affective component of pain may be the underlying factor in the mechanism of chronic pain for which no objective cause can be identified.[3] States of chronic pain may arise from deficits in the central processing of nociceptive afferent actions, whereby input that might be innocuous in some persons debilitates others. In such persons, treatment with opioids is not very effective (and sometimes even harmful because dependence can develop). For these persons treatment is focused on behavior modification, cognitive-behavioral therapy, or self-management approaches that include biopsychosocial models of therapy. Drug therapy for these individuals relies on the use of antidepressants (see Chapter 7) and nonopioid analgesics (see Appendix II).

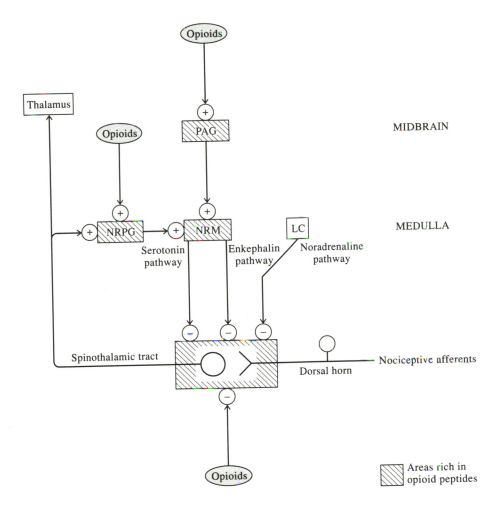

FIGURE 10.3 Sites of action of opioids on pain transmission. Opioids excite neurons in the periaqueductal gray matter (PAG) and in the midbrain and medulla. From there, serotoninergic and enkephalinergic neurons run to the dorsal horn and exert an inhibitory influence on transmission. Opioids also act directly on the dorsal horn. The locus coeruleus (LC) sends noradrenergic neurons to the dorsal horn, which also inhibits transmission. The pathways shown in this diagram represent a considerable oversimplification, but they depict the general organization of the supraspinal control mechanisms.

History

Opium has been used for thousands of years to produce euphoria, analgesia, sleep, and relief from diarrhea. The earliest descriptions of the effects of opium were written about 300 B.C., although references have been found dating to about 3000 B.C. Opium was used primarily for its constipating effect and later for its sleep-inducing properties (noted by writers such as Homer, Virgil, and Ovid). Opium was also used to treat a wide variety of medical problems, and recreational abuse and addiction were quite common.

From the early Greek and Roman days through the sixteenth and seventeenth centuries, the medicinal and recreational uses of opium were well established, with a bustling trade in opium existing between the East and the West. Indeed, control of opium was a central issue during the wars in China in 1839. Until the nineteenth century, the opioids that were used medicinally and recreationally consisted of crude opium, which is the extract of the exudate from the opium poppy. It was not until the early 1800s that morphine was isolated from opium, and since then morphine (rather than crude opium) has been used throughout the world as the premier agent for treating severe pain.

In the United States, morphine and opium were widely used during the nineteenth century. They were freely available from physicians, drugstores, and general stores, by mail order, and in patent medicines sold through a variety of channels. It was not until after the Civil War (when opioid addiction was referred to as "soldier's disease") and the invention of the hypodermic needle in 1856 that a new type of drug user appeared in the United States—one who self-administered opioids by injection.

By the early part of the twentieth century, concern began to mount about the dangers of opioids and the dependence they could induce. In 1914 the Harrison Narcotic Act was passed, and the use of most opioid products was strictly controlled. Nonmedical uses of opioids were banned.

The use of opioids is deeply entrenched in society; it is widespread and impossible to stop. Opioids exert pleasurable effects, produce tolerance and physiological dependence, and have a potential for compulsive misuse, all liabilities that are likely to resist any efforts at legal control. Also, the opioids will continue to be used in medicine because they are irreplaceable as pain-relieving agents. Goldstein (1994)[4] writes of the opioids: "They dramatically relieve emotional as well as physical pain. This property contributes to making them extremely seductive for self-administration."

Terminology

Before discussing drugs used in the treatment of severe pain, some terms should be introduced. The terminology of opioids can be confusing. *Opioid* is a generic, all-inclusive term that applies to any agonist drug with morphine-like activity. Conversely, an *opioid antagonist* is any drug that antagonizes the effects of morphine. The term "opioid" applies to naturally occurring as well as to semisynthetic and synthetic compounds.

Opiate refers specifically to any drug derived from the juice of the opium poppy *Papaver somniferum*; here, the two opiates of interest are *morphine* and *codeine*. Thus, morphine is an opiate, but methadone, which is a synthetic drug, is not, although both are classified as opioids.

Endorphin is a generic, all-inclusive term that applies to any "endogenous substance" (i.e., one naturally formed in the living animal) that exhibits pharmacological properties of morphine.[5] There are three "families" of endogenous opioid peptides—*enkephalins, dynorphins*, and *beta-endorphins*[6]—which will be discussed later.

The term *narcotic* is derived from the Greek word *narke*, meaning numbness or stupor. Originally referring to any drug that induced sleep, the term later became associated with opioids, such as morphine and heroin. Today, it is an imprecise and pejorative term,[7] increasingly used in a legal context to refer to a wide variety of abused substances that includes nonopioids, such as cocaine and marijuana. The term is not useful in a pharmacological context, and its use with reference to opioids is discouraged. It will not be used here.

Opioids are agonists at highly specific receptor sites, and there is general agreement on the existence of at least three types of opioid receptors: *mu, kappa*, and *delta*. Each of the three major receptor types has recently been cloned, sequenced, and well studied.

It should be noted that opioids occur in nature in two places: in the juice of the opium poppy (morphine and codeine) and within our own bodies as any of the endorphins. All other drugs (opioid analgesics) that bind to opioid receptors are prepared either from morphine (*semisynthetic opioids*) or are synthesized from other precursor compounds (*synthetic opioids*).

Clinically, opioids can be classified according to their receptor interactions (*agonist, partial agonist, mixed agonist-antagonist*, or *pure antagonist*), the pain intensity (moderate or severe) for which they are conventionally used, their half-lives (short or long), or the specific opioid receptors (mu, delta, or kappa) with which a specific drug interacts.[7] Table 10.1 shows the putative effects mediated by an agonist opioid acting on the three main opioid receptors. The "strong" opioids, such as morphine, primarily act upon mu receptors, and their pharmacological effects include analgesia, respiratory depression, miosis (pinpoint pupils), euphoria, and constipation. Morphine is therefore a "pure" mu agonist. Other agents will be discussed later.

Opioid Receptors

Opioid receptors are widely distributed throughout the gray matter of the brain, the brain stem, and the spinal cord. It has been known for more than 20 years that the three types—mu, delta, and kappa—each have unique pharmacological profiles, anatomical distributions, and functions. For example:

> The dynorphins and enkephalins (two specific families of endorphins) appear to be the endogenous ligands for kappa and delta receptors, respectively, although whether beta-endorphin or even morphine itself is the endogenous ligand for the mu receptors remains speculative.[8]

Despite this knowledge about receptor subtypes and endorphins, it was not until the 1990s that the opioid receptors were isolated, purified, cloned, sequenced, and the three-dimensional structures modeled, first in animals and then in humans.[1,2,9,10] Studies have revealed that all opioid receptors belong to a superfamily of "G-protein-coupled receptors," all of which possess seven membrane-spanning regions (see Figure 10.4). Each opioid receptor type (mu, kappa, delta) arises from its own gene[8] and is expressed through a specific messenger RNA (mRNA).

Each receptor is a chain of approximately 400 amino acids (like a long string of pearls, each "pearl" an amino acid linked to another, usually different, amino acid on either side). Overall, the amino acid sequences of the receptors are about 60 percent identical to one another; highest identicalities are found in the seven transmembrane regions (about 75 percent identical) and intracellular regions (about 65 percent identical). Conversely, the extracellular regions are considerably divergent with only 35 to 40 percent identicality between receptor types (see Figure 10.4)[1,2]

It is likely that such extracellular diversity is responsible for the specific "fit" of an endogenous endorphin or an exogenous opioid to a specific receptor.[11] Such a fit for a fentanyl derivative for a mu receptor is illustrated in Figure 10.5. In this figure, note that the "flat" drawing of the receptor shown in Figure 10.4 is now depicted more realistically as a three-dimensional receptor with seven helical coils embedded in the membrane and three amino acid "loops" and a terminal chain (located in the extracellular, synaptic space) forming a fit with lofentanyl, a potent opioid agonist. Here, in the 400-amino-acid-long chain that comprises the mu receptor, aspartic acid at position 147, asparagine at 150, threonine at 294, and histidine at 297 form the recognition site for the drug and bind the opioid to this mu receptor.[11]

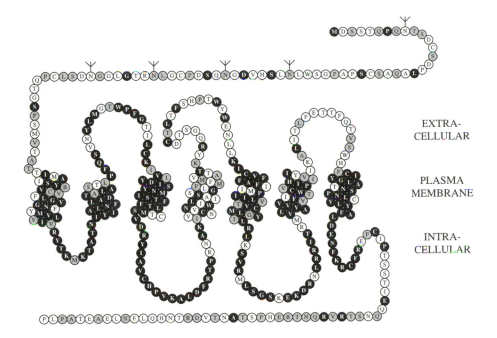

FIGURE 10.4 Two-dimensional model of the rat mu-opioid receptor. The receptor is a chain of about 390 amino acids (the letter in each circle is the first letter of the individual amino acid), with 7 transmembrane coils, and a terminal chain both intracellular (linked to a G-protein, not illustrated) and extracellular (binds the transmitter). Amino acids conserved in mu, delta, and kappa receptors are shown in black; amino acids conserved in mu and *either* delta or kappa receptors are shown in gray; amino acids preset only in this mu receptor (not in delta or kappa) are shown in white circles. [From Minami and Satoh (1995),[1] p. 124.]

For those interested in this aspect of biology, the question is "So what?" What is the consequence of the binding of an opioid agonist (e.g., lofentanyl in Figure 10.5) to the mu receptor? To answer this, we delve a bit deeper into the function of the opioid receptors. In recent years it has become clear that the primary effect of opioid receptor activation (by either an endorphin or an opioid) is *reduction in* or *inhibition of neurotransmission*.[10] Such inhibition occurs largely through opioid-induced presynaptic inhibition of neurotransmitter release (see Figure 10.6):

> The intracellular biochemical events of opioid receptor occupancy are now reasonably well established and it appears that it is increased potassium conductance (leading to hyperpolarization), calcium channel inactivation, or both, that produce an immediate reduction in neurotransmitter release.[8]

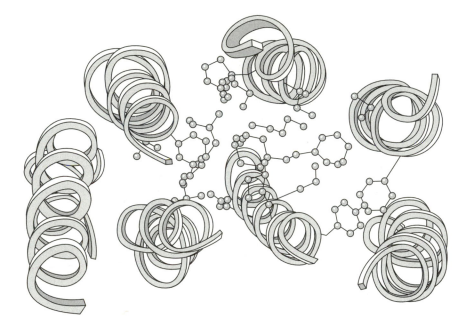

FIGURE 10.5 Speculative three-dimensional depiction of interaction of the mu-opioid receptor with the potent pure mu-agonist lofentanyl. Transmembrane helices are depicted by coils. The cell membrane within which the coils reside is not illustrated. Lofentanyl structure is shown by the connected small circles, which represent carbon molecules of the drug. Specific side chains of amino acids on the receptor helices bind with specific portions of the lofentanyl molecule. [Modified from Uhl, Childers, and Pasternak (1994),[11] figure 3. Original details by H. Moereels, L. M. Kaymans, J. Leysen, and P. Janssen (Janssen Research Foundation, Beerse, Belgium).]

Thus, activation of opioid receptors reduces neuronal excitability through inhibition of calcium channels and activation of potassium channels.[1]

> The hyperpolarization of the membrane potential by potassium current activation and the limiting of calcium ion entry by suppression of calcium ion currents are both tenable mechanisms for explaining opioid blockade of neurotransmitter release and pain transmission in varying neuronal pathways.[8]

These actions follow from a *coupling* of the intracellular loops and the terminal amino acid chain of the receptor protein (Figure 10.4) to the inhibitory system of *adenylate cyclase* enzyme through release of an

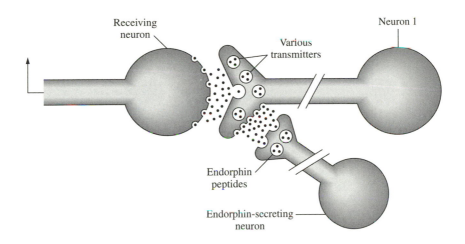

FIGURE 10.6 Cartoon illustration to demonstrate the presynaptic inhibition (exerted by an endorphin-secreting neuron) on neuron 1, inhibiting its release of transmitter. In the spinal cord, neuron 1 would be a primary afferent (sensory pain neuron), with enkephalin inhibiting substance P release. In the ventral tegmentum, neuron 1 might be a GABA-secreting neuron, with an endorphin inhibiting GABA release, "disinhibiting" a dopaminergic neuron, a mechanism of opioid-induced "reward."

intermediate inhibitory protein (termed "G_o" in the literature; see Figure 10.7).[1,2] As Burkle et al. (1996)[12] state:

> The analgesic effect is mediated through coupling to a guanine nucleotide-binding protein (G-protein), which concomitantly results presynaptically in an inhibition of excitatory neurotransmitter release and postsynaptically in an inhibition of cyclic adenosine monophosphate, suppression of voltage-sensitive calcium channels, and hyperpolarization of the postsynaptic membrane through increased potassium conductance.

Grudt and Williams (1995)[14] discuss this opioid-activated inhibition of adenylate cyclase, which is linked to the modulation of ion channel activity (see Figure 10.7), and conclude that, in the whole animal, the situation is actually even more complex:

> It is now clear that opioid actions extend beyond the G_i/G_o-linked activation of potassium conductance, decrease in calcium conductance, and inhibition of adenylate cyclase. The ability of one or more opioid receptor subtypes on a single cell to mediate multiple effects suggests that opioids can initiate a whole cascade of events.[13]

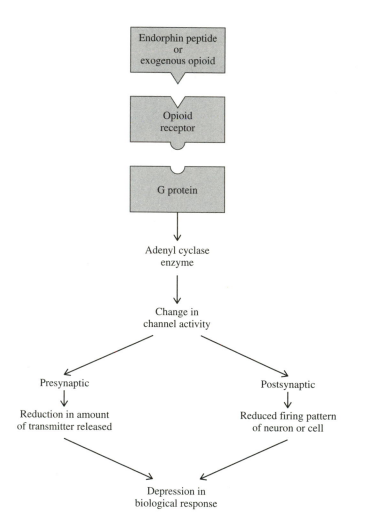

FIGURE 10.7 Sequence of steps involved in opioid- or endorphin-induced cellular alterations. "Change in channel activity" involves increased potassium ion conductance and reduced calcium ion conductance, both serving to depress cellular activity.

Regardless, for the present the cellular inhibitory ability of opioids can be explained by the three actions of G-protein–linked inhibition of adenylate cyclase, decrease in calcium conductance, and activation of potassium conductance.

Mu Receptors

Mu opioid receptors (and the messenger RNA that expresses the receptor protein) are present in all structures in the brain and spinal cord involved in morphine-induced analgesia. Such structures include the periaquaductal gray, spinal trigeminal nucleus, caudate and geniculate nuclei, thalamus, and spinal cord (dorsal horn). Mu receptors are also present in brain stem nuclei involved in control of respiration and in morphine's depression of respiration; in brain stem structures involved in initiation of nausea and vomiting, and in the nucleus accumbens, an area involved in the compulsive abuse of opioids, behavioral stimulants, and other drugs subject to compulsive abuse. Few or no mu receptors (or its mRNA) are found in the cerebral cortex or cerebellum.

Kappa Receptors

Kappa receptors (and the mRNA that expresses the receptor protein) are found in high concentrations in the basal ganglia, nucleus accumbens, ventral tegmentum, deep layers of cerebral cortex, hypothalamus, periaquaductal grey, dorsal horn of spinal cord, and other areas. Satoh and Minami (1995)[2] hypothesize: "Kappa-opioid receptor is synthesized and transported to the terminals of dopaminergic neurons and there it reduces the release of dopamine."

Kappa receptors therefore seem to be involved in analgesia, dysphoria (as opposed to mu-receptor-induced euphoria, possibly because of the blockade of dopamine release), psychotomimetic effects (disori-

TABLE 10.1 Responses mediated by opioid receptors

Receptor	Response on activation
μ (mu)	Analgesia, respiratory depression, miosis, euphoria, reduced gastrointestinal motility
κ (kappa)	Analgesia, dysphoria, psychotomimetic effects, miosis, and respiratory depression

From Cherny (1996),[7] p. 715.

entation, depersonalization feelings), and mild respiratory depression (Table 10.1). The mixed agonist-antagonist drugs, such as *pentazocine* (Talwin), are agonists at the kappa receptors. Dynorphin is the endorphin with the greatest affinity for the kappa receptor.

Delta Receptors

As stated, the enkephalins are the endogenous endorphins for the delta receptors. These receptors are involved in analgesia at both the spinal and brain levels, but further pharmacologic characterization is open to investigation.[1] Delta receptors are also found in the nucleus accumbens and limbic system, possibly playing a role in the emotional responses to opioids.

Classification of Opioid Analgesics

Using this knowledge of opioid receptors, we can classify the opioid analgesics. First, we can tabulate the activity of each drug at each type of receptor and indicate whether it activates (agonistic action) or inhibits (antagonistic action) the function of any of the three specific opioid receptors. We can thus categorize each drug as a pure agonist (at a given receptor), a pure antagonist, a partial agonist, or a mixed agonist-antagonist (Table 10.2).

Pure Agonists

As discussed in Chapter 1, an agonist is a drug that has an affinity for (binds to) cell receptors to induce changes in the cell characteristic of the natural ligand (for example, here, an endorphin) for that receptor. Thus, an agonist action can be either excitatory or inhibitory to the cell, depending upon the biological function of that receptor and its ligand. *Morphine*, which is our prototype opioid analgesic (Table 10.2), *methadone*, an orally active, long-acting opioid used to treat heroin dependency, and *fentanyl*, a short-acting opioid with clinical use in anesthesia and a very high potential for abuse, bind specifically to mu receptors (Table 10.3).[14] As Reisine and Bell (1993)[14] state: "These findings indicate that opioid drugs used clinically (and with a high potential for abuse) predominantly interact with mu receptors."

Pure Antagonists

Pure antagonists have affinity for a receptor (here, one of the three types of opioid receptors, but primarily the mu receptor because most clinically useful opioids are mu agonists), but after attaching they elicit

TABLE 10.2 Classification of opioid analgesics by analgesic properties

Pure agonists	Mixed agonist/Antagonists	Pure antagonists	Partial Agonists
Morphine	Nalbuphine (Nubain)	Naloxone (Narcan)	Buprenorphene (Buprene)
Codeine	Butorphanol (Stadol)	Naltrexone (Trexan)	Tramadol (Ultram)[a]
Heroin	Pentazocine (Talwin)	Nalmefene (Revex)	
Meperidine (Demerol)	Dezocine (Dalgan)		
Methadone (Dolophine)			
Oxymorphone (Numorphan)			
Hydromorphone (Dilaudid)			
Fentanyl (Sublimaze)			

[a] Tramadol also blocks reuptake of norepinephrine and serotonin.

TABLE 10.3 Classification of opioid analgesics by actions at opioid receptors.

Compound	Receptor types[a]		
	Mu	**Kappa**	**Delta**
Morphine	+++	+	+
Naloxone	–	–	–
Pentazocine	+/0	+	NA
Butorphanol	+/0	+	NA
Nalbuphine	–	+	NA
Buprenorphine	++	+	+
Fentanyl	+++	+	+
Dezocine	+	+	+

[a] The mu receptor is thought to mediate supraspinal analgesia, respiratory depression, euphoria, and physical dependence; the kappa receptor, spinal analgesia, miosis, and sedation. Categorizations are based on best inferences about actions in humans. See text for further explanation. Agonists are indicated by one or more plus signs, antagonists by a minus sign, and agents that have no significant action at the receptor by zero. NA, data not available.

no change in cellular functioning. They do, however, block access of both endogenous ligands (here, endorphins) or an exogenous drug (e.g., morphine) either present in the body (precipitating withdrawal) or administered with or after the antagonist (resulting in no effect of the agonist). An example of the latter is the clinical use of an opioid antagonist (e.g., *naltrexone*) in treatment programs for heroin addicts, where heroin taken after naltrexone elicits no analgesic or euphoric effects.

Mixed Agonist-Antagonists

A mixed agonist-antagonist drug produces an agonist effect at one receptor and an antagonistic effect at another. Clinically useful mixed drugs are kappa agonists and weak mu antagonists (they bind to both kappa and mu receptors, but only the kappa receptor is activated). In contrast to a pure agonist, a mixed agonist-antagonist usually displays a "ceiling effect" for analgesia;[7] in other words, it has decreased efficacy compared to a pure agonist and usually will not be as effective in treating severe pain. Also, when a mixed agonist-antagonist is administered to an opioid-dependent person, the antagonist effect at a mu receptor precipitates an acute withdrawal syndrome. *Pentazocine* (Talwin) is the prototype agonist-antagonist (it and several related drugs are discussed later).

Partial Agonists

A partial agonist binds to opioid receptors but has a low intrinsic activity (low efficacy). It therefore exerts an analgesic effect, but such effect has a ceiling at less than the maximal effect produced by a pure agonist. *Buprenorphine* (Buprenex) is the prototype partial agonist opioid. When administered to a "naive" individual, analgesia is observed; when administered to an addict, however, blockade of the pure agonist can occur and withdrawal can be precipitated. Compared to a mixed agonist-antagonist, the partial agonist buprenorphine binds to all three types of opioid receptors,[14] albeit with lower efficacy. Its potential for producing respiratory depression (discussed below) is also reduced, compared to that produced by morphine.

Morphine

Of the two analgesics (morphine and codeine) found in the opium poppy, morphine (see Figure 10.8) is the more effective analgesic and represents about 10 percent of the crude exudate. Codeine is much less potent, less efficacious, and constitutes only 0.5 percent of the crude exudate. Despite decades of research, no other drug has been found that exceeds morphine's effectiveness as an analgesic. Indeed, morphine is our prototype opioid, and no other drug is clinically superior for treating severe pain.

Pharmacokinetics

Morphine is administered orally, rectally, or by injection. In general, absorption of morphine from the gastrointestinal tract (oral or rectal) is slow and incomplete compared to absorption following injection. Blood levels reach only about half of that achieved when the drug is administered by injection. Absorption through the rectum is adequate, and several opioids (morphine, hydromorphone, and oxymorphone) are available in suppository form. Such preparations might be indicated in patients suffering from muscle-wasting diseases (such as in patients with terminal cancer) who cannot tolerate other routes of administration.

Highly fat-soluble opioids, such as fentanyl, are also readily absorbed from the oral mucosa and through the skin. The former route of administration is utilized (in a fentanyl "lollipop") as a route of analgesic drug delivery to treat surgical pain in children. Fentanyl is also available in a skin patch, from which the fentanyl diffuses slowly across the skin into plasma, providing a steady and reasonably consistent blood level over a period of about 24 hours.[15] Such a preparation

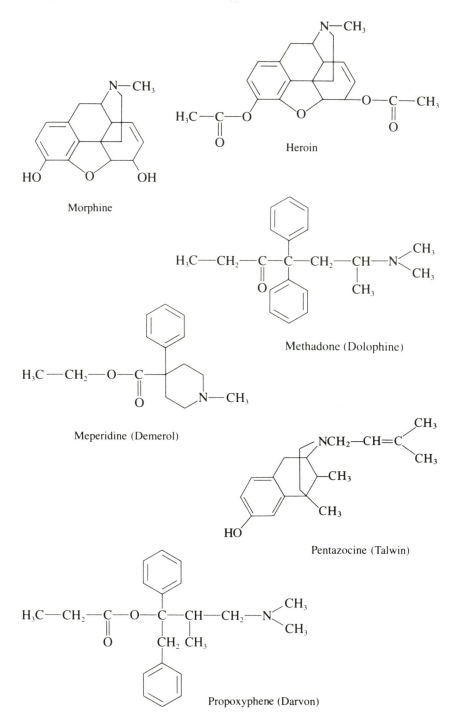

FIGURE 10.8 Structure formulas of morphine, heroin, and four synthetic narcotic analgesics.

is useful for patients with chronic pain who want to avoid the peaks and valleys associated with intermittent administration of drug.

Earlier discussion of opioid action in the dorsal horn of the spinal cord leads us to discussion of the use of morphine and other opioids administered directly into the spinal canal (through small catheters) to control the pain of obstetric labor and delivery, to treat postoperative pain, and (for long-term use) to relieve otherwise intractable pain associated with terminal cancer. The technology is revolutionizing the treatment of terminally ill patients who are suffering from severe pain. No individual today should have to suffer severe, unremitting pain as his or her life ends.

Morphine is usually administered by intramuscular, subcutaneous, or intravenous injection. The problems and limitations of the injection of drugs (see Chapter 1) include death from accidental overdose, rapid onset of adverse drug reactions, the necessity of using sterile techniques, and the inability to retrieve the drug if too much is administered.

As is known from the history of opium smoking in Asian cultures, the opioids may be administered by inhalation, most commonly by inhaling the smoke from burning crude opium. The rapidity of onset of drug action rivals that following intravenous injection.

Opioids achieve significant levels in the brain within seconds to minutes after an intravenous injection. The more water-soluble (lipid-insoluble) opioids, such as morphine, penetrate the blood-brain barrier somewhat more slowly than the more lipid-soluble opioids. Thus, morphine exists in the bloodstream in a relatively lipid-insoluble form, which does not cross the blood-brain barrier easily. Only small amounts of morphine (20 percent) ever penetrate the brain. In contrast, heroin (discussed later in this chapter) crosses the blood-brain barrier easily. This difference may explain why the "flash" or "rush" following intravenous injection of heroin is so much more intense than that perceived after injecting morphine. The opioids also reach all body tissues, including the fetus; infants born of addicted mothers are physically dependent on opioids and exhibit withdrawal symptoms that require intensive therapy.

Morphine is metabolized by the liver, and one of its metabolites (morphine-6-glucuronide) is actually ten- to twentyfold more potent as an analgesic than morphine. Indeed, most of the analgesic action of morphine is mediated by this active metabolite.[16-18] The half-lives of morphine and morphine-6-glucuronide are both 3 to 4 hours. Patients with impaired kidney function tend to accumulate the metabolite and thus may be more sensitive to morphine administration.[18] Metabolite accumulation would also tend to prolong the analgesic actions of drug and metabolite.

Urine-screening tests to determine whether a person has used narcotics detect codeine and morphine as well as their metabolites. Because heroin is metabolized to morphine, and because street heroin also contains acetylcodeine (which is metabolized to codeine), heroin use is suspected when both morphine and codeine are present in a patient's urine. However, such tests cannot accurately determine which specific drug (heroin, codeine, or morphine) has been used. Furthermore, codeine is widely available in cough syrups and analgesic preparations, and even poppy seeds contain small amounts of morphine. Thus, depending on the drug that was taken, morphine and codeine metabolites may be detected in a patient's urine for 2 to 4 days.

Pharmacological Effects

Morphine exerts its major effects on mu receptors, producing a syndrome characterized by analgesia, relaxed euphoria, sedation, a sense of tranquility, reduced apprehension and concern, respiratory depression, suppression of the cough reflex, and pupillary constriction.

Analgesia. Morphine produces intense analgesia and indifference to pain, reducing the intensity of pain and thus reducing the associated distress by altering the central processing of pain (at the level of the thalamus, limbic system, and cerebral cortex).[18] Morphine analgesia occurs without loss of consciousness and without affecting other sensory modalities. Indeed, the pain may persist as a sensation, but patients "feel more comfortable."[6] In other words, the perception of the pain is significantly altered. An injection of naloxone (Narcan) displaces morphine from the mu receptors and blocks the analgesic effect.

Euphoria. Morphine produces a pleasant euphoric state, which includes a strong feeling of contentment, well-being, and lack of concern. Indeed, this is part of the affective, or reinforcing, response of the drug.

> Opioids, like cocaine, are used for their positive effects. Use of exogenous opioids gives the addict access to the reinforcement system . . . in the locus coeruleus and elsewhere. This positive reward system, normally reserved to reward the performance of species-specific survival behaviors, once reached by exogenous self-administration of drugs of abuse, provides the user with an experience that the brain equates with profoundly important events like eating, drinking, and sex. Opioid use becomes an acquired drive state that permeates all as-

pects of human life. Withdrawal from opioid use is mediated by separate neural pathways that cause withdrawal events to be perceived as life-threatening, and the subsequent physiologic reactions often lead to renewed opioid consumption.[19]

Regular users and those who are psychologically attracted to morphine describe the effects of intravenous injection in ecstatic and often sexual terms, but the euphoric effect becomes progressively less intense after repeated use. At this point, users inject the drug for one or more of several possible reasons: to try to reexperience the extreme euphoria experienced after the first few injections, to maintain a state of pleasure and well-being, to prevent mental discomfort that may be associated with reality, or to prevent withdrawal symptoms.

Because morphine exerts powerful effects on pain and emotion, we might ask what role the endorphins play as "natural" analgesics or euphoriants. The answer is unknown, since naloxone (when it is injected intravenously) does not precipitate feelings of pain, dysphoria, or any other major response. In marathon runners, however, it has been reported that endorphin levels in plasma increase fourfold;[20] these natural analgesics reduce depression and provide an overall feeling of well-being (a "runner's high"). Endorphins may therefore be part of a natural euphoric reward system and a determinant of our mood.

The mechanism of morphine's positive reinforcing and euphoria-producing action probably involves more than mu receptors, especially the dopaminergic.[21,22] Opioids activate mu receptors within the mesolimbic dopamine reward system by means of the ventral tegmental–nucleus accumbens pathway that we saw to be involved in the rewarding effects of cocaine, the benzodiazepines, and alcohol.[23,24] This receptor action is illustrated in Figures 10.6 and 10.9. Simonato (1996)[21] summarizes the complexity of this action:

> In the ventral tegmental area, morphine inhibits GABA neurons via mu-opioid receptors, thus disinhibiting dopaminergic neurons and increasing dopamine input in the nucleus accumbens and in other areas; this phenomenon may be involved in the mechanism of reward, i.e., the positive reinforcer to opioid addiction.

Sedation and Anxiolysis. Morphine produces anxiolysis, sedation, and drowsiness, but the level of sedation is not as deep as that produced by the central nervous system (CNS) depressants. Although persons who are taking morphine will doze, they can usually be awakened readily. During this state, "mental clouding" is prominent, which is accompanied by a lack of concentration, apathy, complacency, lethargy, reduced mentation, and a sense of tranquility. Obviously, in

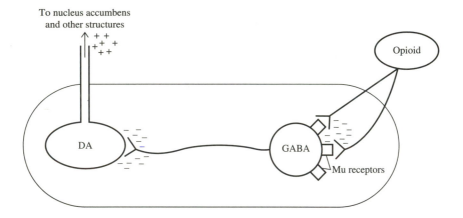

FIGURE 10.9 Schematic illustration of how dopamine-secreting neurons in the ventral tegmental area are excited by opioids. Dopamine-containing neurons are hyperpolarized by GABA acting at GABA_A receptors. GABA-containing neurons are hyperpolarized by opioids acting at mu receptors. Thus, opioids reduce the inhibition exerted by GABA on dopamine neurons. DA = dopamine.

such a state, cognitive impairment results. These anxiolytic actions of opioids likely follow from mu receptor inhibition of neuronal activity in the locus coeruleus, the principal clustering of norepinephrine neurons in the brain.[25]

Depression of Respiration. Morphine causes a profound depression of respiration by decreasing the respiratory center's sensitivity to higher levels of carbon dioxide in the blood. The respiratory rate is reduced even at therapeutic doses; at higher doses the rate slows even further, respiratory volume decreases, breathing patterns become shallow and irregular, and, at sufficiently high levels, breathing ceases. Respiratory depression is the single most important acute side effect of morphine and is the cause of death from acute opioid overdosage. The combination of morphine (or other opioid) with alcohol or other sedatives can be especially dangerous.

Suppression of Cough. Opioids suppress the "cough center," which is also located in the brain stem. Thus, opioid narcotics have historically been used as cough suppressants, codeine being particularly popular for this purpose. Today, however, less addicting drugs are used as cough suppressants; opioids are inappropriate choices for treating persistent cough.

Pupillary Constriction. Morphine (as well as other mu and kappa agonists) causes pupillary constriction (miosis). Indeed, pupillary constriction in the presence of analgesia is characteristic of narcotic ingestion.

Nausea and Vomiting. Morphine stimulates receptors in an area of the medulla that is called the chemoreceptor trigger zone. Stimulation of this area produces nausea and vomiting, which are the most characteristic and unpleasant but not life-threatening side effects of morphine and other opioids.

Gastrointestinal Symptoms. Morphine and the other opioids relieve diarrhea as a result of their direct actions on the intestine, the most important action of morphine outside the CNS. Opioids cause intestinal tone to increase, motility to decrease, feces to dehydrate, and intestinal spasm (and cramping) to occur. This combination of a decreased propulsion, an increased intestinal tone, a decrease in the rate of movement of food, and dehydration harden the stool and further retard the advance of fecal material. All these effects contribute to the constipating effect of opioids. Because tolerance to the constipating effects of the opioids does not develop, drug-dependent individuals have long-term problems with constipation. Similarly, drug withdrawal is characterized by severe abdominal cramping and diarrhea, as intestinal tone returns to normal.

Nothing more effective than the opioids has yet been developed for treating severe diarrhea. In recent years two opioids have been developed that only very minimally cross the blood-brain barrier into the CNS. The first is *diphenoxylate* (the primary active ingredient in Lomotil), and the second is *loperamide* (Imodium). These drugs are exceedingly effective opioid antidiarrheals but are not analgesics, nor are they prone to compulsive abuse, because they do not reach the CNS.

Other Effects. Morphine can release histamine from its storage sites in mast cells in the blood. This can result in localized itching or more severe allergic reactions, including bronchoconstriction (an asthma-like constriction of the bronchi of the lungs). Opioids also affect white blood cell function, perhaps producing alterations in the immune system that are as yet poorly defined. The science of psychoneuroimmunology (PNI) has been actively investigating this area of opioid action.

Tolerance and Dependence

The development of tolerance and dependence with repeated use is a characteristic feature of all opioid drugs, including morphine.[6] Indeed, use of opioids is limited because of the development of *tolerance,* the presence of uncomfortable side effects, and their potential for compulsive abuse. Of these, the development of tolerance is a major limitation to their clinical usefulness.

The molecular basis of tolerance is not known. Reisine and Bell (1993)[14] suggest that it could involve opioid receptor desensitization, resulting from uncoupling of the opioid receptor from its intercellular interactions with G-proteins and adenylate cyclase enzyme. Alternatively, Reisine and Pasternak (1996)[6] implicate involvement of glutamate receptors and a substance called nitric oxide in morphine tolerance.

The rate at which tolerance develops varies widely. When morphine or other opioid narcotics are used only intermittently, little, if any, tolerance develops. Thus, when a person's sprees of drug use are separated by prolonged periods without using drugs, the opioids retain their initial efficacy. When administration is repeated, tolerance may become so marked that massive doses have to be administered to either maintain a degree of euphoria or prevent withdrawal discomfort (avoidance of discomfort is more common). The degree of tolerance is illustrated by the fact that the dose of morphine can be increased from clinical doses (i.e., 50 to 60 milligrams per day) to 500 milligrams per day over as short a period as 10 days.[25]

Tolerance to one opioid leads to cross tolerance to all other natural and synthetic opioids, even if they are chemically dissimilar. Cross tolerance, however, does not develop between the opioids and the sedative hypnotics. In other words, a person who has developed a tolerance for morphine will also have a tolerance for heroin but not for alcohol or barbiturates.

In Chapter 1, we described *physical dependence* as an altered state of biology induced by a drug, whereby withdrawal of a drug is followed by a complex set of biological events typical for that class of drugs. Acute withdrawal from opioids has been well studied, since it can be easily precipitated in drug-dependent individuals by injecting the opioid antagonist naloxone (Narcan). Withdrawal results in a profound reduction in the release of dopamine in the nucleus accumbens,[21] a reduction in the level of dynorphin in the nucleus accumbens,[26] and a large (300 percent) increase in the release of norepinephrine in various structures, including the hippocampus,[27] nucleus accumbens,[28] and locus coeruleus.[29] As stated by Simonato (1996)[21]:

> The firing rate of the locus coeruleus is actively inhibited by morphine, returns to baseline levels with tolerance, and rises dramatically during withdrawal; these phenomena may be involved in the mechanism of dependence, i.e., the negative reinforcer to opioid addiction.

Immediate symptoms of withdrawal include restlessness, drug craving, sweating, extreme anxiety, depression, irritability, dysphoria, fever, chills, violent retching and vomiting, increased respiratory rate (panting), cramping, insomnia, explosive diarrhea, and intense aches and pains. The magnitude of these acute withdrawal symptoms depends on the dose of opioid, the frequency of previous drug administration, and the duration of drug dependence. Acute opioid withdrawal is not considered to be life-threatening, although it can seem unbearable to the person experiencing it.

To help alleviate the symptoms of acute withdrawal, several approaches have been tried. One extremely rapid method is termed *rapid opioid detoxification* or, perhaps more appropriately, *rapid anesthesia-aided detoxification* (RAAD).[27] A pure opioid antagonist, such as naloxone or naltrexone (discussed later), is administered intravenously to the addict while he or she is asleep under general anesthesia; the procedure goes on for several hours. After the procedure, the patient is maintained on orally administered naltrexone, allegedly to reduce opioid craving, and undergoes psychotherapy for relapse prevention. The technique is controversial, in part because it is expensive, it involves the risks of anesthesia, and it is rather elaborate. Simon[27] addresses these criticisms.

Other techniques to alleviate withdrawal symptoms include the use of clonidine (an adrenergic agent that decreases the severity of withdrawal), or a switch to the partial agonist buprenorphine[28] (discussed later), and, experimentally, the use of a cannabinoid (marijuana-like) agonist[29] (see Chapter 11). Obviously, much more will be forthcoming in this area of therapeutics.

Following acute withdrawal, focus is directed toward the so-called *protracted abstinence syndrome*,[25] beginning when the acute phase of opioid withdrawal ends and persisting for up to six months. Symptoms of this syndrome include depression, abnormal responses to stressful situations, drug hunger, decreased self-esteem, anxiety, and other psychological disturbances. Complicating the diagnosis of prolonged abstinence syndrome is the high prevalence of other psychiatric disorders (e.g., affective and personality disorders) in opioid-dependent individuals. As reported by Brooner and coworkers (1997),[30] psychiatric comorbidity was documented in 47 percent of 716 treatment-seeking opioid abusers, with antisocial personality disorder (25 percent) and major depression (15 percent) being the most common diagnoses. Older studies reported comorbidity rates as high as 80 percent. Thus, recurrence or expression of underlying personality problems that drug use may have masked should be expected, diagnosed, and treated appropriately.

Several behavioral theories have been posited to account for continued opioid use[25]:

- Continued use avoids the distress and dysphoria associated with withdrawal (a negative reinforcing effect).

- The euphoria produced by the opioids leads to their continued use (a positive reinforcing effect).

- Preexisting dysphoric or painful affective states are alleviated. This presumes that the opioids were initially used as a type of self-medication to treat these symptoms, and dependence gradually developed.

- The euphoric response is an atypical response to opioids that occurs in individuals with preexistent psychopathology.

- Preexisting psychopathology may be the basis for initial experimentation and euphoria, but repeated use is prompted by the desire to avoid withdrawal.

- Some individuals have deficient endorphin systems that are corrected by the use of opioids.

- Repeated use of opioids leads to permanent dysfunction in the endorphin system to the point that normal function requires the continued use of exogenous opioids.

- Drug effects and drug withdrawal can become linked through environmental cues and internal mood states. Here, emotions and external cues recall the distress of withdrawal or the memory of opioid euphoria or opioid reduction of dysphoria or painful affective states.

To varying degrees, all of these theories are probably involved in a given individual's use of opioids. Opioid tolerance and dependence lies not merely in a few predisposed individuals, because these can develop in anyone who uses the drugs repeatedly, and such is not necessarily associated with a propensity toward abuse. A patient in the chronic pain of terminal illness should not be denied opioids, despite the inevitable development of tolerance and dependence, a condition that can be controlled with even small amounts of drug.[6]

Other Pure Agonist Opioids

Heroin (diacetylmorphine, diamorphine) is three times more potent than morphine and is produced from morphine by a slight modification of chemical structure (Figure 10.8). The increased lipid solubility of heroin leads to faster penetration of the blood-brain barrier, producing an intense rush when it is either smoked or injected intravenously. Heroin is metabolized to monoacetylmorphine and morphine, the latter being eventually metabolized and excreted. Heroin is legally available in Great Britain and Canada.[7] where it can be used clinically. The drug is not legal in the United States. When heroin is smoked together with crack cocaine, euphoria is intensified, the anxiety and paranoia associated with cocaine are tempered, and the depression that follows after the effects of cocaine wear off is reduced. Unfortunately, this combination creates a multidrug addiction that is extremely difficult to treat.

Codeine, along with morphine, occurs naturally in opium. It is only about one-tenth as potent as morphine, but it is absorbed better than morphine when taken orally. Used for the management of mild to moderate pain, codeine is often combined with aspirin or acetaminophen (Tylenol) in oral tablets. The plasma half-life and duration of action is about 3 to 4 hours.

Hydromorphone (Dilaudid) and *oxymorphone* (Numorphan) are both structurally related to morphine. Both of these drugs are as effective as morphine; they are 6 to 10 times more potent than morphine. Somewhat less sedation but equal respiratory depression is observed.

Meperidine (Demerol) is a synthetic opioid whose structure differs from that of morphine (Figure 10.8). Because of this structural difference, meperidine was originally thought to be free of many of the undesirable properties of the opioids. However, meperidine is addictive and can be substituted for morphine or heroin in addicts and is widely prescribed medically. It is one-tenth as potent as morphine, produces a similar type of euphoria, and is equally likely to cause dependence. Meperidine's side effects differ from morphine's and include tremors, delirium, hyperreflexia, and convulsions. These effects are produced by a metabolite of meperidine (normeperidine) that has no analgesic action but can cause CNS excitation. Meperidine and normeperidine can accumulate in individuals who have kidney dysfunction or who use only meperidine for their opioid addiction.

Methadone (Dolophine) is a synthetic mu agonist opioid, the pharmacological activity of which is very similar to that of morphine. The outstanding properties of methadone are its effective analgesic activity, its efficacy by the oral route, its extended duration of action in suppressing withdrawal symptoms in physically dependent individuals, and its tendency to show persistent effects with repeated administration.[6] Its half-life is about 24 hours. To control opioid withdrawal, oral methadone is substituted for the injected opioid to which the patient is addicted. Later, the dependent individual can be withdrawn slowly from the methadone, or the methadone can be continued indefinitely.

LAAM (levo-alpha-acetylmethadol) is related to methadone and is an oral opioid analgesic that was approved in mid-1993 (after many years of delay) for the clinical management of opioid dependence in heroin addicts. LAAM is well absorbed from the gastrointestinal tract. It has a slow onset and a long duration of action (about 72 hours). It is metabolized to compounds that are also active as opioid agonists. Its primary advantage over methadone is its long duration of action; in maintenance therapy it is administered by mouth three times a week. Its use in the treatment of opioid dependence is discussed later in this chapter.

Propoxyphene (Darvon) is an analgesic compound that is structurally similar to methadone (Figure 10.8). As an analgesic for treating mild to moderate pain, it is less potent than codeine but more potent than aspirin. When propoxyphene is taken in large doses, opioid-like effects are seen; when it is used intravenously, it is recognized by addicts as a narcotic. Taken orally, propoxyphene does not have much potential for abuse. Some cases of drug dependence have been reported, but to date they have not been of major concern. Because commercial intravenous preparations of propoxyphene are not available, intravenous abuse is encountered only when persons attempt to inject solutions of the powder that is contained in capsules, which are intended for oral use.

Fentanyl (Sublimaze) and three related compounds, sufentanil (Sufenta), alfentanil (Alfenta), and remifentanil (Ultiva) are short-acting, intravenously administered, agonist opioids that are structurally related to meperidine. These four compounds are intended to be used during and after surgery to relieve surgical pain. As discussed earlier, fentanyl is now available in a skin patch and an oral lozenge on a stick (a "lollipop"). The transdermal route of drug delivery offers prolonged, rather steady levels of drug in blood; the lollipop is used for the short-term treatment of surgical pain in children.

Fentanyl and its three derivatives are 80 to 500 times as potent as morphine as analgesics and profoundly depress respiration. Death from these agents is invariably caused by respiratory failure. In illicit use, fentanyl is known as "China white." Numerous derivatives (such as methylfentanyl) can be manufactured illegally; they emerge periodically and have been responsible for multiple fatalities.*

---

*To control the manufacture and distribution of illicit derivatives of fentanyl, the federal Drug Enforcement Agency (DEA) has been authorized to declare any drug a Schedule I narcotic substance if it poses an immediate public health hazard. Within the past 10 years, dozens of analogue drugs have been placed under Schedule I control, including MMDA (see Chapter 12) and certain meperidine (Demerol) derivatives, especially MPPP and MPTP. Both MPPP and MPTP are neurotoxic by-products of meperidine, and both induce a severe, irreversible, and progressive parkinsonian disease state. Such control was first invoked for the fentanyl analogue 3-methylfentanyl in 1985. Since then many other fentanyl analogues have been placed under control. Newer legislation makes it illegal to engage in any drug activities using these illicit analogues, regardless of whether the drug has been duly scheduled under the DEA's Controlled Substance Act.

New in 1997 was *remifentanyl,* the shortest half-life opioid yet available. Its half-life is only 9 to 11 minutes, the drug being rapidly metabolized by specific enzymes (esterases) present in blood.[12,31] Little drug remains to be metabolized in the liver. Remifentanyl is intended to be used to control brief, intense pain during surgery. For longer duration of effect, the drug must be given by continuous intravenous infusion.

Partial Agonist Opioids

Buprenorphine (Buprenex) is a newer, semisynthetic, partial agonist opioid whose action is characterized by a limited stimulation of mu receptors, which is responsible for its analgesic properties. As a partial agonist, however, there is a ceiling to its analgesic effectiveness as well as to its potential for inducing euphoria and respiratory depression. Buprenorphine has a very long duration of action (about 24 hours), because it binds very strongly to mu receptors, limiting its reversibility by naloxone when reversal is considered necessary. The drug can be given by oral, parenteral, or sublingual routes. At low doses, buprenorphine can substitute for morphine (in morphine-dependent individuals) and it is analgesic (in nontolerant individuals). However, higher doses do not substitute well for morphine, and they can precipitate withdrawal symptoms. As discussed earlier, buprenorphine is being evaluated as an alternative, or subsequent step, to methadone for narcotic detoxification and maintenance programs.[32]

Tramadol (Ultram), available in Europe for many years, became available for use as an analgesic in the United States in 1995.[33] The drug is claimed to have a "dual" analgesic action, as a partial agonist at mu receptors as well as blocking the presynaptic reuptake of norepinephrine and serotonin. In the United States the drug is available only for oral use. Well absorbed orally, the drug undergoes a two-step metabolism, and the first metabolite (mono-demethyl tramadol) is as active or more active than the parent compound.[34] As a partial agonist, the drug exhibits a ceiling effect on analgesia (but not as analgesic as morphine), which limits respiratory depression and abuse potential. Side effects are considerable and include drowsiness and vertigo, nausea, constipation, and headache. Additive sedation with CNS depressants is observed. The place of this drug over other analgesics remains unclear.

Mixed Agonist-Antagonist Opioids

Four drugs that bind with varying affinity to the mu and kappa receptors are *pentazocine* (Talwin), *butorphanol* (Stadol), *nalbuphine* (Nubain), and *dezocine* (Dalgan) (see Figure 10.10). These four drugs

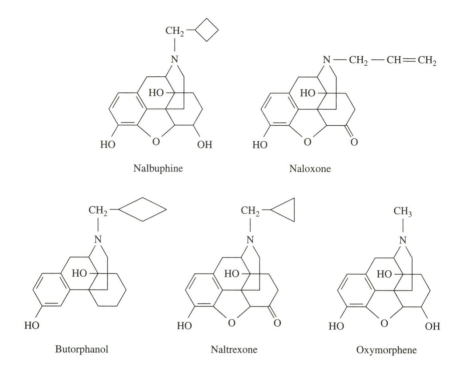

FIGURE 10.10 Structural formulas of oxymorphone and four analogues. Oxymorphone is a pure mu agonist. Nalbuphine and butorphanol have mixed agonistic/antagonistic properties, while naloxone and naltrexone are pure antagonists.

are weak mu agonists; most of their analgesic effectiveness (which is quite limited) results from their stimulation of kappa receptors (see Table 10.3). Low doses cause moderate analgesia; higher doses produce little additional analgesia. In opioid-dependent individuals, these drugs precipitate withdrawal. A high incidence of adverse psychotomimetic side effects (dysphoria, anxiety reactions, hallucinations, and so on), most prominent with pentazocine, are associated with the use of these agents, limiting their use.

Pentazocine and butorphanol are prototypical mixed agonist-antagonists. Neither of these drugs has much potential for producing respiratory depression or physical dependence. In 1993 butorphanol, previously available only for use by injection, became available as a nasal spray, the first analgesic so formulated. After spraying into the nostrils, peak plasma levels (and maximal effect) are achieved in about an hour, with a duration of 4 to 5 hours.[7]

In recent years abuse of pentazocine has been increasing, particularly in combination with tripelennamine, an antihistamine. This combination of drugs, called "Ts and blues," has caused serious medical complications, including seizures, psychotic episodes, skin ulcerations, abscesses, and muscle wasting. (The latter three effects are caused by the repeated injections rather than by the drugs themselves.)

Nalbuphine is primarily a kappa agonist of limited analgesic effectiveness. Because it is also a mu antagonist, it is not likely to produce either respiratory depression or patterns of abuse.

Dezocine, the newest of the mixed agonist-antagonist opioids, was introduced in 1990. As a moderate mu agonist and a weak delta and kappa agonist, dezocine can substitute for morphine. Its clinical efficacy and potential for abuse appear limited.

Opioid Antagonists

Three clinically available drugs, *naloxone* (Narcan), *naltrexone* (Trexan), and *nalmefene* (Revex) are structural derivatives of oxymorphone, a pure opioid agonist (see Figure 10.10), and have an affinity for opioid receptors (especially mu receptors), but after binding they exert no agonist effects of their own. Therefore, they antagonize the effects of agonist opioids and are termed *pure opioid antagonists*.

Naloxone is the prototype antagonist. It has little or no effect when injected into nonopioid-dependent persons, but it rapidly precipitates withdrawal when injected into opioid-dependent persons. Naloxone is neither analgesic nor subject to abuse. Because naloxone is not absorbed from the gastrointestinal tract, it must be given by injection. Furthermore, its duration of action is very brief, in the range of 15 to 30 minutes. Thus, for continued opioid antagonism, it must be reinjected at short intervals to avoid "renarcotization." Naloxone is used to reverse the respiratory depression that follows acute narcotic intoxication (overdoses) and to reverse narcotic-induced respiratory depression in newborns born of opioid-dependent mothers. The limitations of naloxone include its short duration of action and its parenteral route of administration.

Naltrexone became clinically available in 1985 as the first orally absorbed, pure narcotic antagonist. Its actions resemble those of naloxone, but naltrexone is well absorbed orally and has a long duration of action, necessitating only a single daily dose of about 40 to 80 milligrams. Naltrexone is used clinically in narcotic treatment programs when it is desirable to maintain a person on chronic therapy with a narcotic antagonist. In such persons who take naltrexone daily, any injection of a pure opioid agonist will be ineffective.

As discussed in Chapter 3, naltrexone has been approved for use in the treatment of alcoholism, reducing the cravings for alcohol during the maintenance period of treatment.[35] It is likely that such action follows from the antagonism of endorphin action (which would be expected to reduce dopaminergic activity in the ventral tegmental–nucleus accumbens reward system discussed earlier). Naltrexone also appears to reduce the cravings for heroin and other opioids.[36]

Naltrexone has also been reported to have some efficacy in the treatment of autism[37–38] and self-injurious behaviors,[39] disorders where some evidence points to a role of the endogenous opioid system. While naltrexone does not treat any core etiology of autism, it can reduce the hyperactivity, irritability, and self-injurious behaviors. Self-injurious behavior can be used to maintain a high level of endogenous opioids, either to prevent decreases in endorphins or to experience the euphoric effect of opioid stimulation following injury.[40] In the study by Roth and coworkers (1996),[39] six of seven female patients with self-injurious behavior ceased such behavior entirely during naltrexone therapy, with resumption of injurious behavior when the drug was withdrawn. If replicated, this may prove to be a most interesting use of the drug.

Nalmefene, introduced in 1996, is an injectable pure antagonist with a half-life of about 10 hours, in contrast to the short half-life of naloxone. The drug is useful by injection for the treatment of acute opioid-induced respiratory depression caused by overdosage. With its long half-life, the incidence of "renarcotization" is greatly reduced. If administered to an addict, however, the precipitation of withdrawal can be prolonged and require additional medical treatment.

Pharmacotherapy of Opioid Dependence

The neurochemistry of opioid addiction in the brain is unknown, as are the cellular mechanisms underlying drug withdrawal and craving. Simonato (1996)[21] discusses a *theory of complexity*:

> A system composed of separate elements is determined by its organization, which will limit the potential of individual parts, but new properties will emerge that are not characteristic of the parts. Therefore, a perturbation applied to a subset of parts (direct morphine effects on neurons expressing opioid receptors) will induce complex changes in the system (brain) that, in turn, will depend on organization of the interconnections between the parts (anatomy).

The complex interactive mechanisms of addiction are a step beyond the more acute and direct effects of morphine, effects that can lead to the development of tolerance and dependency.

Hypotheses to account for continued opioid use despite its life-threatening consequences are listed earlier in this chapter. As with all behavior-reinforcing drug addictions, an opioid-dependent individual goes for therapy for any of a number of reasons. These range from referral for negative legal, family, social, or job consequences to a personal desire to be free of opioid use and the drug-oriented lifestyle. As with the abuse of alcohol (see Chapter 3) and stimulants (see Chapter 6), therapy is aimed at clearing the offending drug from the body, managing withdrawal, diagnosing and treating coexisting psychopathology, and preventing relapse. With the opioids, however, the situation has an important difference.

First, cocaine and the amphetamines are "power drugs," while opioids promote a state of tranquility, analgesia, and sedation. *Opioid intoxication* is characterized by sedation, mental quieting, and tranquility. Crime associated with opioid use is usually performed when the user is not intoxicated or is in (or fears) withdrawal. If an adequate amount of the drug is supplied (usually at little cost), violent acts and crime are minimized. Therefore, maintaining an opioid-dependent person (e.g., a heroin addict) on opioid is an entirely different situation from attempting to maintain a stimulant-dependent person (e.g., a cocaine addict) on a behavioral stimulant.

Therefore, total abstinence from all opioids need not be an objective for all addicts. Goals, however, must include prevention of relapse to the use of illicitly obtained, injectable opioids (such as heroin). Continuing, medically managed opioid therapy may be necessary for many addicts, and such an approach follows medical models of illness.[42] For example, a diabetic may require insulin for the remainder of his or her life, a patient with high blood pressure may require antihypertensive medication for a lifetime, and a patient with bipolar disorder might require long-term lithium therapy for mood stabilization. Similarly, an opioid addict may require ongoing opioid therapy, perhaps for a lifetime.

We must carefully distinguish between physical dependence and addiction. The former implies drug intake to block a set of biological reactions that occur when the drug is not taken. The latter includes not only dependence but a total life-style oriented to obtaining and using a drug in the face of severe adverse consequences. A patient with terminal cancer may have pain that can be relieved only by the use of opioids. This person is likely to become physically dependent on the opioid and experience withdrawal if the drug is withheld. Concern over whether the patient is addicted becomes secondary to the humane management of pain in the terminally ill patient. The pain associated with terminal illness requires aggressive management, and the development of physical dependence is a minor concern.

In contrast, the drug dependence that develops as a result of using opioids for nonmedical use has been treated very differently. Until very recently, the objective has been medically managed withdrawal to an opioid-free state. Withdrawal, often followed by naltrexone maintenance, can be successful in patients who are highly motivated to remain opioid-free. Examples include addicted physicians and other medical personnel whose continued licensure to practice their profession is contingent on completely abstaining from opioids. The supervised ingestion of naltrexone (about three to four times per week) implies that any other opioid will be ineffective. In many (if not most) addicts, however, naltrexone therapy is unacceptable, and continued opioid therapy is needed:

> Opioid maintenance therapy remains the primary pharmacological approach for the treatment of opioid dependence. The benefits of maintenance therapy, including significant reductions in illicit opioid use, increases in treatment retention, and improved psychosocial functioning, have been clearly demonstrated within the methadone maintenance model.[32]

Despite these benefits, methadone maintenance (methadone being a pure opioid agonist) is considered undesirable pharmacotherapy by a significant number of addicts and communities.[32] Thus, effective alternatives need to be identified. LAAM (discussed earlier) is one such alternative but it is similar to methadone. Another alternative that has been proposed is buprenorphine maintenance, where this partial mu agonist replaces both the illicit opioid and methadone:

> It is our confident belief . . . that buprenorphine will, in due course, be declared a safe and effective drug for maintenance treatment of heroin addicts.[32]

If it is felt that buprenorphine should be stopped:

> Patients transferred to buprenorphine experience little or no withdrawal and craving is generally suppressed. Buprenorphine can then be discontinued or naltrexone treatment can be initiated.[25]

Currently, however, most opioid addicts are withdrawn from narcotic use by being switched to methadone and then either being eventually withdrawn from methadone or put on long-term methadone maintenance. With methadone maintenance, addicts are stabilized on methadone and remain in their communities without withdrawing from the orally administered opioid. After one or two years, many former heroin addicts can be withdrawn from the methadone over a period of several weeks. The withdrawal discomforts are relatively minor, and some patients can complete the withdrawal process and not relapse to the use of heroin or other illicit opioid. Others later return to using heroin. Still others discontinue the withdrawal process and remain on methadone maintenance. The opioid, however, must be combined with intensive psychological counseling, and the patient must adopt a productive lifestyle.

Goldstein (1994)[42] reviews more than 20 years of administering methadone maintenance therapy to 1,000 heroin addicts in New Mexico. More than half of the patients were traced and analyzed. Of these, more than one-third are now dead; causes include violence, overdosage, and alcoholism. About one-quarter are still enmeshed in the criminal justice system. Another one-quarter go on and off methadone maintenance, indicating that opioid dependence, whether on heroin or on methadone, is a lifelong condition for a considerable fraction of the addict population. With half of the treated population of 1,000 addicts unaccounted for, the data are obviously incomplete. It is likely that many of these unaccounted-for former addicts are either drug-free or are stabilized on an opioid and remain functional in their communities. The successful graduates of therapy are the most difficult to track, usually preferring to remain anonymous in their communities.

Regardless, treatment of opioid dependence leads to a productive life-style in only a minority of cases. The most interesting data now support lifelong opioid maintenance (e.g., methadone) as a treatment possibility, with buprenorphine maintenance or naltrexone treatment as options when necessary. When opioid-withdrawn individuals relapse, they must be readmitted to methadone (or LAAM) maintenance immediately. Unfortunately, many people still see physical dependence on an opioid as "bad" in and of itself. These attitudes must be changed before widespread attempts at long-term opioid maintenance can be fully evaluated. Stein and Kosten (1997)[43] edit a review of current treatments of opioid dependency.

NOTES

1. M. Minami and M. Satoh, "Molecular Biology of the Opioid Receptors: Structures, Functions, and Distributions," *Neuroscience Research* 23 (1995): 121–145.
2. M. Satoh and M. Minami, "Molecular Pharmacology of the Opioid Receptors," *Pharmacology and Therapeutics* 68 (1995): 343–364.

3. R. W. Hansen and K. E. Gerber, *Coping with Chronic Pain: A Guide to Patient Management* (New York: Guilford, 1990).

4. A. Goldstein, *Addiction: From Biology to Drug Policy* (New York: W. H. Freeman and Company, 1994), 138.

5. J. R. Cooper, F. E. Bloom, and R. H. Roth, *The Biochemical Basis of Neuropharmacology*, 7th ed. (New York: Oxford University Press, 1995), 431.

6. T. Reisine and G. Pasternak, "Opioid Analgesics and Antagonists," in J. G. Hardman, L. E. Limbird, P. B. Molinoff, R. W. Ruddon, and A. G. Gilman, eds., *Goodman & Gilman's The Pharmacological Basis of Therapeutics*, 9th ed. (New York: McGraw-Hill, 1996), 521.

7. N. I. Cherny, "Opioid Analgesics: Comparative Features and Prescribing Guidelines," *Drugs* 51 (1996): 713–737.

8. R. Atcheson and D. G. Lambert, "Update on Opioid Receptors," *British Journal of Anaesthesia* 73 (1994): 132–134.

9. R. C. Thompson, A. Mansour, H. Akil, and S. J. Watson, "Cloning and Pharmacological Characterization of a Rat mu Opioid Receptor," *Neuron* 11 (1993): 903–913.

10. R. J. Knapp, E. Malatynska, N. Collins, et al., "Molecular Biology and Pharmacology of Cloned Opioid Receptors," *Federation of the American Society for Experimental Biology (FASEB) Journal* 9 (1995): 516–525.

11. G. R. Uhl, S. Childers, and G. Pasternak, "An Opiate-Receptor Gene Family Reunion," *Trends in Neurological Sciences* 17 (1994): 89–93.

12. H. Burkle, S. Dunbar, and H. Van Aken, "Remifentanil: A Novel, Short-Acting, mu-Opioid," *Anesthesia and Analgesia* 83 (1996): 646–651.

13. T. J. Grudt and J. T. Williams, "Opioid Receptors and the Regulation of Ion Conductances," *Reviews in the Neurosciences* 6 (1995): 279–286.

14. T. Reisine and G. I. Bell, "Molecular Biology of Opioid Receptors," *Trends in Neurological Sciences* 16 (1993): 506–510.

15. W. Jeal and P. Benfield, "Transdermal Fentanyl: A Review of Its Pharmacological Properties and Therapeutic Efficacy in Pain Control," *Drugs* 53 (1997): 109–138.

16. H. J. McQuay, D. Carroll, C. C. Faura, et al., "Oral Morphine in Cancer Pain: Influences on Morphine and Metabolite Concentration," *Clinical Pharmacology and Therapeutics* 48 (1992): 236–244.

17. R. Osborne, P. Thompson, S. Joel, et al., "The Analgesic Activity of Morphine-6-Glucuronide," *British Journal of Clinical Pharmacology* 34 (1992): 130–138.

18. R. K. Portenoy, H. T. Thaler, C. E. Inturrisi, et al., "The Metabolite Morphine-6-Glucuronide Contributes to the Analgesia Produced by Morphine Infusion in Patients with Pain and Normal Renal Function," *Clinical Pharmacology and Therapeutics* 51 (1992): 422–431.

19. M. S. Gold, "Opiate Addiction and the Locus Coeruleus: The Clinical Utility of Clonidine, Naltrexone, Methadone, and Buprenorphine," *Psychiatric Clinics of North America* 16 (1993): 65.

20. D. A. Mahler, L. N. Cunningham, G. S. Skrinar, W. J. Kraemer, and G. L. Colice, "Beta-Endorphin Activity and Hypercapnic Ventilatory Responsiveness After Marathon Running," *Journal of Applied Physiology* 66 (1989): 2431–2436.

21. M. Simonato, "The Neurochemistry of Morphine Addiction in the Neocortex," *Trends in Pharmacological Sciences* 17 (1996): 410–415.

22. T. S. Shippenberg, R. Bals-Kubik, and A. Herz, "Examination of the Neuro-chemical Substrates Mediating the Motivational Effects of Opioids: Role of the Mesolimbic Dopamine System and D-1 Versus D-2 Dopamine Receptors," *Journal of Pharmacology and Experimental Therapeutics* 265 (1993): 53–59.

23. X. R. Yuan, S. Madamba, and G. R. Siggins, "Opioid Peptides Reduce Synaptic Transmission in the Nucleus Accumbens," *Neuroscience Letters* 134 (1992): 223–228.

24. P. Leone, D. Pocock, and R. A. Wise, "Morphine-Dopamine Interaction: Ventral Tegmental Morphine Increases Nucleus Accumbens Dopamine Release," *Pharmacology, Biochemistry, and Behavior* 39 (1991): 469–472.

25. J. H. Jaffe, "Opiates: Clinical Aspects," in J. H. Lowinson, P. Ruiz, R. B. Millman, and J. G. Langrod, eds., *Substance Abuse: A Comprehensive Textbook*, 2nd ed. (Baltimore: Williams & Wilkins, 1993), 186–194.

26. R. Y. Yukhananov, Q. Z. Zhai, S. Persson, C. Post, and F. Nyberg, "Chronic Administration of Morphine Decreases Level of Dynorphin A in the Rat Nucleus Accumbens," *Neuropharmacology* 32 (1993): 703–709.

27. D. L. Simon, "Rapid Opioid Detoxification Using Opioid Antagonists: History, Theory, and the State of the Art," *Journal of Addictive Diseases* 16 (1997): 103–122.

28. K. J. Schuh, S. L. Walsh, G. E. Bigelow, et al., "Buprenorphine, Morphine and Naloxone Effects During Ascending Morphine Maintenance in Humans," *Journal of Pharmacology and Experimental Therapeutics* 278 (1996): 836–846.

29. M. J. Christie, J. T. Williams, P. B. Osborne, and C. E. Bellchambers, "Where's the Locus in Opioid Withdrawal?" *Trends in Pharmacological Sciences* 18 (1997): 134–140.

30. R. K. Brooner, V. L. King, M. Kidorf, et al., "Psychiatric and Substance Abuse Comorbidity Among Treatment-Seeking Opioid Abusers," *Archives of General Psychiatry* 54 (1997): 71–80.

31. S. S. Patel and C. M. Spencer, "Remifentanil," *Drugs* 52 (1996): 417–427.

32. W. Ling, D. R. Wesson, C. Charuvastra, and C. J. Klett, "A Controlled Trial Comparing Buprenorphine and Methadone Maintenance in Opioid Dependence," *Archives of General Psychiatry* 53 (1996): 401–407.

33. "Tramadol—A New Oral Analgesic," *The Medical Letter on Drugs and Therapeutics*, 37 (July 7, 1995): 59–60.

34. L. L. Norton and M. J. Ferrill, "Tramadol: Establishing a Place in Therapy," *American Journal of Pain Management* 6 (1996): 42–50.

35. R. M. Weinreib and C. P. O'Brien, "Naltrexone in the Treatment of Alcoholism," *Annual Review of Medicine* 48 (1997): 477–487.

36. G. Gerra, A. Marcato, and R. Caccacari, "Clonidine and Opiate Receptor Antagonists in the Treatment of Heroin Addiction," *Journal of Substance Abuse Treatment* 12 (1995): 35–41.

37. M. Campbell, "Resolved: Autistic Children Should Have a Trial of Naltrexone," *Journal of the American Academy of Child and Adolescent Psychiatry* 35 (1996): 246–250.

38. S. H. Willemsen-Swinkels, J. K. Buitelaar, F. G. Weijnen, and H. Van Engeland, "Placebo-Controlled Acute Dosage Naltrexone Study in Young Autistic Children," *Psychiatry Research* 58 (1995): 203–215.

39. A. S. Roth, R. B. Ostroff, and R. E. Hoffman, "Naltrexone as a Treatment for Repetitive Self-Injurious Behavior: An Open-Label Trial," *Journal of Clinical Psychiatry* 57 (1996): 233–237.

40. J. T. Gillman and R. F. Tuchman, "Autism and Associated Behavioral Disorders: Pharmacotherapeutic Intervention," *Annals of Pharmacotherapy* 29 (1995): 47–56.

41. A. Goldstein, "Heroin Addiction: Neurobiology, Pharmacology, and Policy," *Journal of Psychoactive Drugs* 23 (1991): 123–133.

42. A. Goldstein, *Addiction: From Biology to Drug Policy* (New York: W. H. Freeman and Company, 1994), 142–154.

43. E. M. Stine and T. R. Kosten, eds., *New Treatments for Opiate Dependence* (New York: Guilford, 1997).

Chapter 11

MARIJUANA: A UNIQUE SEDATIVE-EUPHORIANT-PSYCHEDELIC DRUG

The hemp plant *Cannabis sativa*, the source for marijuana, grows throughout the world and flourishes in most temperate and tropical regions. It is one of humanity's oldest cultivated nonfood plants. The major psychoactive ingredient of the marijuana plant is *delta-9-tetrahydrocannabinol* (THC). THC and other natural and synthetic *cannabinoids* produce the characteristic motor, cognitive, psychedelic, and analgesic effects that are described in this chapter. THC is most concentrated in the resin from the flowers of the female plant.

Names for *Cannabis* products include *marijuana, hashish, charas, bhang, ganja,* and *sinsemilla*. Hashish and charas, which consist of the dried resinous exudate of the female flowers, are the most potent preparations, with a THC content averaging between 10 and 20 percent. Ganja and sinsemilla refer to the dried material found in the tops of the female plants, where the THC content averages about 5 to 8 percent. Bhang and marijuana are lower-grade preparations taken from the dried remainder of the plant, and their THC content varies between 2 to 5 percent.

Until recently marijuana was classified according to its behavioral effects, usually as a mild sedative-hypnotic agent, with clinical effects similar to those of alcohol and the antianxiety agents. Unlike the sedative-hypnotic compounds, however, higher doses of THC may also produce

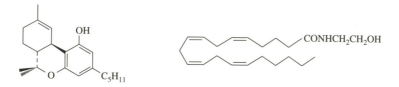

FIGURE 11.1   Structures of delta-9-tetrahydrocannabinol (THC) and anandamide, the endogenous ligand (neurotransmitter) of the cannabinoid receptor.

relaxed euphoria, hallucinations, and heightened sensations—effects that are similar to a mild LSD experience. Very high doses of THC do not depress respiration and are not lethal. Also, little cross tolerance occurs between THC and the sedative-hypnotics. THC also produces a unique spectrum of pharmacologic effects, including disruption in attentive mechanisms, impairment of short-term memory, altered sensory awareness, analgesia, altered control of motor movements and postural control, and (on the immune system) a possible immunosuppressive action.[1] This spectrum of action has led to possible uses (discussed later) in the treatment of various symptoms associated with disorders ranging from multiple sclerosis to AIDS to terminal cancer.

The chemical structure of THC is unique, resembling that of neither the sedatives nor the psychedelics (see Figure 11.1, left). It was once thought that THC might act like a general anesthetic, affecting neuronal membranes to increase membrane fluidity (an action that has not been correlated with psychedelic action). This has now been dismissed as a mechanism of action. There have, however, been new and truly exciting developments during the 1990s in several areas of *Cannabis* and cannabinoid research, including substantial strides in our understanding of pharmacological, biochemical, and behavioral mechanisms of action for the cannabinoid compounds and of the smoked material.[2]

History

The use of *Cannabis sativa* dates from about 2700 B.C.,[3] primarily as a mild intoxicant. For such use, marijuana was considered to be somewhat milder than alcohol and much less useful for religious and psychedelic experiences than the naturally occurring psychedelic drugs (because *Cannabis* produces much less sensory distortion). Over the years, products from *Cannabis sativa* have been claimed to have a wide variety of medical uses, although few persist in native cultures.

Cannabis sativa is rather new to Western culture. Marijuana—at least until the beginning of the twentieth century—was not widely used in the United States. Its psychoactive properties had certainly been discovered but had not attracted much attention. During the early 1920s, marijuana was portrayed as being evil, part of underground activities, and a menace. Claiming that an association existed between marijuana and crime, laws were passed, first in Louisiana and then throughout the country, to outlaw its use. By the mid-1930s, marijuana was looked upon on as a narcotic and as a drug responsible for crimes of violence. By 1940 the public was convinced that marijuana was a "killer drug" and a potent narcotic that (1) induced people to commit crimes of violence, (2) led to heroin addiction, and (3) was a great social menace.

The emotional campaign against marijuana continued through the 1950s, but in the 1950s and early 1960s, marijuana became extremely popular among youths, and its popularity continued thereafter. By 1972 at least 2 million Americans used marijuana daily, and marijuana use exceeded the use of alcohol among many young adults. Surveys taken through 1986 revealed that the percentage of high school seniors who smoked marijuana daily declined from a peak of 11 percent in 1978 to less than 4 percent. Disquieting, however, were the observations that the number of students who smoked cigarettes had not declined, use of alcohol had continued unabated, and use of cocaine had increased and remained persistent. Marijuana was (and still is) rarely used by persons over the age of 50. In 1990 an estimated 6 to 10 million Americans smoked marijuana at least once every week.

A 1993 survey revealed that the apparent decline in marijuana use had ceased, and a small resurgence was occurring. Alcohol and tobacco use also continued unabated. Among high school seniors, 26 percent had used marijuana in the previous year (up from 22 percent in 1992) and 19 percent smoked tobacco cigarettes daily. Among eighth-grade students, 8 percent had used marijuana within the past year and 14 percent smoked cigarettes daily. These figures did not include significant numbers of school dropouts, who traditionally exhibit a much higher incidence of drug use. In 1996 approximately 35 percent of U.S. high school seniors reported having used marijuana at least once in the preceding 12 months, with daily use estimated at 4.6 percent of high school seniors.[4]

In November 1996 voters in Arizona and California approved ballot initiatives to permit the legal use of marijuana for purported medical purposes. Approval of these initiatives signaled the first time since the repeal of Prohibition some 50 years ago that the public has approved a pullback on the "war on drugs." Certainly, medical efficacy of marijuana is controversial; no double-blind studies have compared the relative efficacies of marijuana to any drug of proven efficacy. Whether or not these two initiatives are the first steps toward legalization is unknown; certainly the 1998 state elections in which marijuana initiatives are bound to appear will be most interesting.

Mechanism of Action: The Cannabinoid Receptor

Evidence gathered up to the mid-1980s led to the hypothesis that THC and other cannabinoids act via a pharmacologically distinct set of receptors. In 1986 Howlett and coworkers[5] demonstrated that THC inhibited the intracellular enzyme adenylate cyclase and that such inhibition required the presence of a G-protein complex, similar to the opioid receptors discussed in Chapter 10. THC does not directly inhibit the enzyme;[6,7] rather, it acts on a specific receptor in such a way that the enzyme is ultimately inhibited.

In 1990 Matsuda and coworkers[8] isolated and cloned from rat cerebral cortex a specific G-protein–coupled receptor that both inhibited adenylate cyclase and bound cannabinoids. Today, we know that this *cannabinoid receptor* inhibits calcium ion flux and facilitates potassium channels,[9] just as the opioids do on their receptors (see Chapter 10). Thus, there should be little surprise that the cannabinoid receptor is structurally similar to the opioid receptor.

The cannabinoid receptor is a chain of 473 amino acids with seven hydrophobic domains that extend through the cell membrane (see Figures 11.2 and 11.3); each region (or cylinder) is composed of one hydrophobic domain.[10,11] As shown by Deadwyler, Hampson, and Childers (1995),[1] when THC binds to the outer portion of the receptor, the "cyclic nucleotide second-messenger system" is activated to inhibit adenylate cyclase and, ultimately, to regulate potassium (and calcium) ion currents (see Figures 11.4 and 11.5). This sequence of actions is also discussed by Musty and coworkers (1995)[12] and by Shen and coworkers (1996).[13]

Thus, the cannabinoid receptor had been isolated and cloned, its transmembrane and three-dimensional structures proposed, and its cellular transduction mechanisms delineated. The identification of a naturally occurring "ligand" that binds to the cannabinoid receptor and thus might function as a "natural THC" remained to be demonstrated. In the search for this ligand, Devane and coworkers[14] in 1992 isolated from porcine brain an arachidonic acid derivative named *anandamide* (see Figure 11.1), which was shown to bind to the cannabinoid receptor and produce cannabinoid-like pharmacological

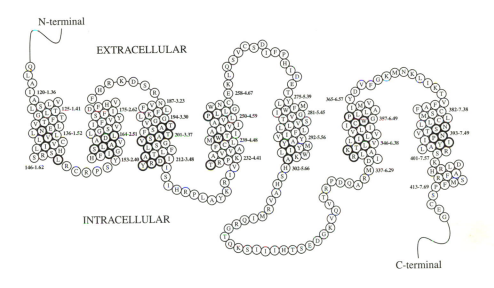

FIGURE 11.2 Two-dimensional representation of the anandamide receptor, which is a protein consisting of a chain of more than 450 amino acids (the first letter of each individual amino acid is shown). Like the opioid receptors, the anandamide receptor is a G-protein linked, seven-membrane spanning structure with three extracellular loops. [Model from R. D. Bramblett et al. (1995).[11]]

effects. Many more reports between 1993 and 1995 demonstrated that anandamide produces behavioral, hypothermic, and analgesic effects that parallel those caused by psychotropic cannabinoids. Indeed, anandamide exhibits the essential criteria required to be classified as the *endogenous ligand* at cannabinoid receptors (see R. G. Pertwee (1995)[2] for a detailed discussion).

As can be seen from Figure 11.1, anandamide is structurally dissimilar to THC. Thomas and coworkers (1996)[15] constructed three-dimensional pharmacologic models of THC and anandamide and demonstrated that in such conformation the molecules are in actuality quite similar (see Figure 11.6) and would be predicted to interact with the same receptor.

Cadas and coworkers (1996)[16] studied the biosynthesis of anandamide and determined that it is synthesized within neurons from a precursor phospholipid, under the regulation of calcium ions and cyclic adenosine monophosphate. Similarly, Derkinderen and coworkers (1996)[17] demonstrated a role for anandamide in modulating synap-

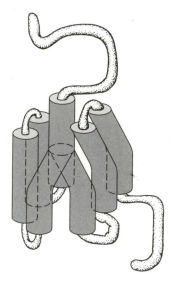

FIGURE 11.3 Predicted tertiary structure of the cannabinoid receptor. The primary structure comprises seven relatively hydrophobic domains (depicted as cylinders) that extend through the plasma membrane. The N-terminal extracellular (above) and C-terminal intracellular (below) extensions and intervening loops are depicted as stippled regions. [From Howlett et al. (1991).[10]]

tic plasticity in rat hippocampus, an effect that may be important in learning and memory processes. Shen and coworkers (1996)[13] also studied rat hippocampus and demonstrated that anandamide, THC, and other anandamide-receptor agonists inhibit the presynaptic release of the excitatory neurotransmitter glutamate via an inhibitory G-protein, as illustrated in Figure 11.5. These data were consistent with marijuana-induced detrimental effects on cognitive functioning.

In the late 1980s it was hypothesized that the hippocampus, cerebral cortex, cerebellum, and basal ganglia were the loci of action of THC because these structures are involved in cognition and memory, mood, and higher intellectual functions, as well as motor functions, all of which are affected by THC.[6] Herkenham and coworkers (1991, 1992)[18,19] delineated the unique pattern of localization of cannabinoid receptors in the brain (see Figures 11.7 and 11.8). First, large numbers of receptors found in the basal ganglia and cerebellum are involved in many forms of movement and postural control that are affected by smoking marijuana. Second, the cerebral cortex, especially the frontal cortex, is rich in cannabinoid receptors. Binding of THC here likely

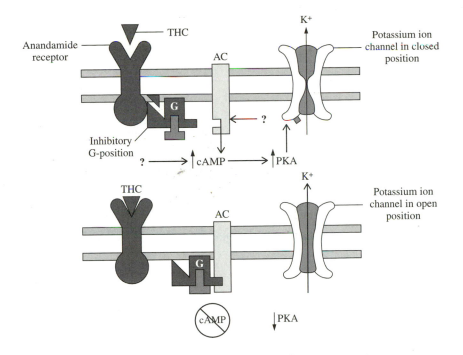

FIGURE 11.4 Proposed interaction of the anandamide receptor with a potassium ion channel. In the top panel, the anandamide receptor is depicted in the unoccupied state with the inhibitory G-protein inactivated. Here, moderate levels of adenylate cyclase (AC) enzyme-stimulated cyclic AMP (cAMP) activate an enzyme (protein kinase, PK), which leads to changes in potassium channel proteins, producing a narrower channel and decreased potassium conductance. In the bottom panel, THC binds to the anandamide receptor, which releases the inhibitor G-protein, which binds to and inhibits adenylate cyclase. cAMP is not activated and the protein kinase remains inactive. Potassium channel proteins remain inactive and the potassium channel remains open. Potassium ions (K+) can exit the neuron, and, ultimately, the release of other neurotransmitters (such as glutamate) is inhibited.[Modified from Deadwyler, Hampson, and Childers (1995).[1]]

mediates at least some of the psychoactive effects of the drug, including the drug-induced "high"; the characteristic distortions of the sense of time, sound, color, and taste; alterations in the ability to concentrate; and production of a dreamlike state.[18] Cannabinoid receptors are also dense in the hippocampus; this fact may account for THC-induced disruption of memory, memory storage, and coding of sensory input. Because brain stem structures do not bind cannabinoids, THC

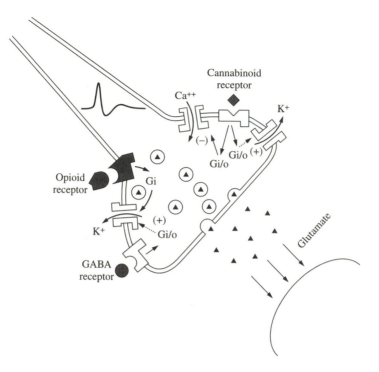

FIGURE 11.5 Schematic diagram illustrating involvement of anandamide (cannabinoid) receptors, GABA receptors, and opioid receptors to regulate potassium ion (K+) efflux and neurotransmitter (here, glutamate) release, inhibiting neuronal function. These receptors are pharmacologically distinct and may couple to their own inhibitor G proteins, but share common adenylate cyclase catalytic units. [Modified from Deadwyler, Hampson, and Childers (1995).[1]]

does not affect basal body functions, including respiration. The lack of cannabinoid-anandamide receptors in the brain stem explains the relative nonlethality of THC.

In 1994 Lynn and Herkenham[20] studied the peripheral effects of cannabinoids, reporting that, outside the brain, cannabinoid receptors are found only in specific components of the immune system (confined to beta-lymphocyte-enriched areas such as the spleen), indicating that the immunosuppressive activity of THC may be cannabinoid receptor-mediated. Nonspecific binding of cannabinoids was found in several areas, including the heart, lungs, endocrine system, and reproductive organs.

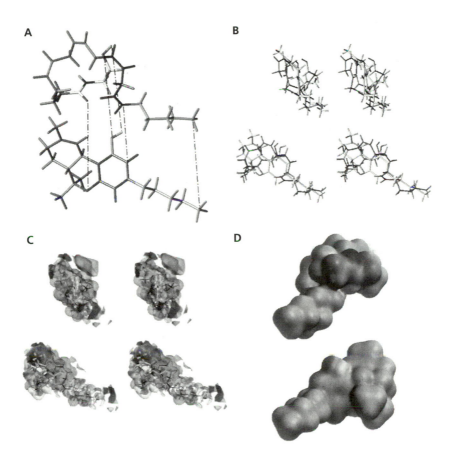

FIGURE 11.6 Several structural comparisons of anandamide and THC. (**A**) Stick model showing alignment of the two molecules with dashed lines signifying the five atoms used for superpositioning. (**B**) Views of the overlaid structures that predict three-dimensional similarity and thus affinity for the same receptor. (**C**) Stereoviews of overlaid structures show nonoverlapping molecular volumes. (**D**) Another view of the steric shape and bulk of anandamide (top) and THC (bottom). [From Thomas et al. (1996).[15]]

Pharmacokinetics

Most marijuana available in the United States has a THC content that rarely exceeds 8 percent and usually averages 4 to 5 percent. In the United States, THC is usually administered in the form of a hand-rolled marijuana cigarette (the average marijuana cigarette contains

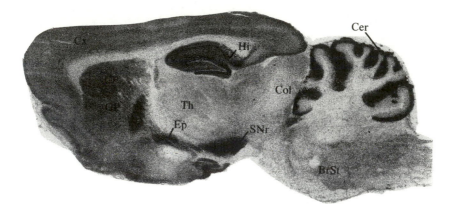

FIGURE 11.7 Autoradiographic binding of a potent cannabinoid to cannabinoid receptors in the rat brain. BrSt = brain stem; Cer = cerebellum; Col = colliculi; CP = caudate-putamen; Cx = cerebral cortex; Ep = entopeduncular nucleus; GP = globus pallidus; Hi = hippocampus; SNr = substantia nigra; Th = thalamus.

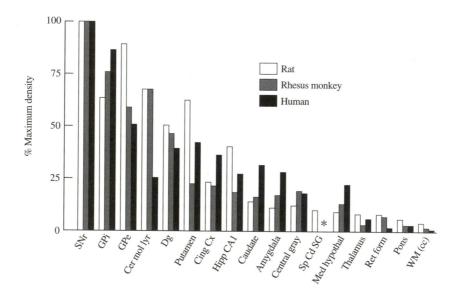

FIGURE 11.8 Relative densities of cannabinoid receptors across brain structures in rat, rhesus monkey, and human. Cer mol lyr = cerebellum, molecular layer; Cing Cx = cingulate cortex; Dg = dentate gyrus; GPe = external globus pallidus; GPi = internal globus pallidus; Hipp CA1 = hippocampal field CA1; Med hypothal = medial hypothalamus; Ret form = reticular formation; Sp Cd SG = substantia gelatinosa of spinal cord (*only rat measured); WM (cc) = white matter of corpus callosum.

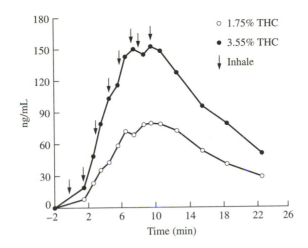

FIGURE 11.9 Mean plasma concentrations of total THC for smoked marijuana and infused THC on days 1 and 22. One marijuana cigarette was smoked from 0 to 15 minutes and was followed by intravenous infusion from 15 to 65 minutes, as indicated by arrows. Results from day 22 were obtained after daily smoking of marijuana and suggest that tolerance failed to develop. [From Perez-Reyes et al. (1991).[21]]

between 0.5 and 1 gram of plant material). Thus, if a marijuana cigarette contains 1 gram of plant material with a THC content of about 5 percent, the cigarette contains approximately 50 milligrams of THC. In general, about one-fourth to one-half of the THC present in a marijuana cigarette is actually available in the smoke. Thus, if a cigarette contains 50 milligrams of THC, about 12 to 25 milligrams are available in the smoke. In practice, the amount of THC absorbed into the bloodstream as a result of the social smoking of one marijuana cigarette is probably in the range of 0.4 to 10 milligrams.

As discussed in Chapter 1, the absorption of inhaled drugs is rapid and complete. The onset of behavioral effects of THC in smoked marijuana occurs almost immediately after smoking begins and corresponds with the rapid attainment of peak concentrations in plasma (see Figure 11.9).[21] Unless more is smoked, the effects seldom last longer than 3 to 4 hours (see Figure 11.10). Huestis and coworkers (1992),[22] in a study of the pharmacokinetics of marijuana smoking, noted peak blood levels of THC of 80 and 150 nanograms of drug per milliliter of plasma (ng/mL) occurring 10 minutes after initiation of smoking cigarettes containing 1.75 percent and 3.55 percent THC, respectively. Within 2 hours, levels were below 5 ng/mL but remained

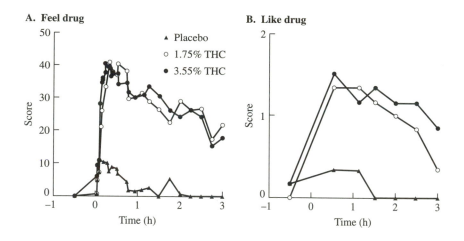

FIGURE 11.10 Mean ratings of "high" from the combination of smoked marijuana and infused THC on days 1 and 22. As in Figure 11.9, the lack of development of tolerance is apparent.

detectable for up to 12 hours after smoking a single cigarette. Heart rate and blood pressure both increased, while skin temperature decreased. The subjective "high" was of rapid onset and persisted for more than 12 hours, indicating either persistence of drug in the central nervous system (CNS) or a threshold of about 5 ng/mL, above which the "high" is perceived.

THC is also absorbed when it is administered orally, but the absorption is slow and incomplete. The onset of action usually takes 30 to 60 minutes, with peak effects occurring 2 to 3 hours after ingestion. THC is approximately three times more effective when it is smoked than when it is taken orally.

Once THC is absorbed, it is distributed to the various organs of the body, especially those that have significant concentrations of fatty material. Thus, THC readily penetrates the brain; the blood-brain barrier does not appear to hinder its passage. Similarly, THC readily crosses the placental barrier and reaches the fetus. It is almost completely metabolized by liver enzymes to a pharmacologically active metabolite (11-hydroxy-delta-9-THC) that is subsequently converted to inactive metabolites, which are then excreted.[23] The metabolism of THC is quite slow; an elimination half-life of about 30 hours is generally accepted, although some researchers report a half-life of about 4 days.[24] Therefore, THC can persist in the body for several days to several weeks. Such a delay tends to prolong and intensify the activity of subsequently smoked marijuana.

Because only minute quantities of THC are found in the urine of persons who use the drug, tests for THC focus primarily on isolating its metabolites. Although acute or occasional use is detected for about 1 to 3 days, chronic smokers (even if they smoke only two to three times weekly) have persistently positive urine tests for THC metabolites. A heavy smoker who stops smoking may show positive urine tests for about a month after cessation. Thus, a positive urinalysis can indicate either recent use or use that occurred several weeks earlier. Multiple sampling may be necessary to differentiate the results. A single positive urine test does not necessarily mean that a person was under the influence of marijuana at the time the urine specimen was collected.

Pharmacological Effects in Animals

THC and other cannabinoids produce a unique syndrome of behavioral effects in a wide variety of animal species. At low doses, they produce a mixture of depressant and stimulatory effects, and at higher doses, predominantly CNS depression. THC and anandamide (THC's endogenous ligand) are sedative and analgesic (at both spinal and brain stem levels),[25,26] decrease spontaneous motor activity,[27,28] decrease body temperature, calm aggressive behavior, potentiate the effects of barbiturates and other sedatives, block convulsions, and depress reflexes. In primates, specifically, THC decreases aggression, decreases the ability to perform complex behavioral tasks, seems to induce hallucinations, and appears to cause temporal distortions. THC causes monkeys to increase the frequency of their social interactions. High doses can depress ovarian function, lower the concentration of female sex hormones,[29] decrease ovulation, and possibly decrease sperm production.

Pharmacological Effects in Humans

In humans, THC primarily affects the functioning of the CNS, the cardiovascular system, and the immune system.

Central Nervous System

The central nervous system (CNS) effects of THC in humans vary with dose, route of administration, experience of the user, vulnerability to psychoactive effects, and setting of use.[30] In general, all the senses may be enhanced, and the perception of time is usually altered. Users report an increased sense of well-being, mild euphoria, relaxation, and relief from anxiety. "The subjective effects include dissociation of ideas. Illusions and hallucinations occur infrequently."[31]

> During this time [of intoxication] there is impairment of cognitive functions, perception, reaction time, learning, and memory. Impairment of coordination and tracking behavior has been reported to persist for several hours beyond the perception of the high. These impairments have obvious implications for the operation of a motor vehicle, and performance in the workplace or at school.[30]

At higher doses of THC, the user experiences an intensification of emotional responses and alterations in sensation that resemble mild sensory distortions and even mild hallucinations. Few persons who smoke marijuana socially are seeking these effects. Only a small percentage of persons who smoke marijuana use it to induce a pronounced state of sensory distortion.

At very high doses, acute depressive reactions, acute panic reactions, or mild paranoia have been observed,[31] probably brought on by the alterations in perception produced by THC; some panic responses may follow the feeling of a loss of mental control. Several surveys indicate that 50 to 60 percent of marijuana users have reported at least one anxiety experience.[30] Only at psychotoxic doses of THC do delusions, paranoia, hallucinations, confusion and disorientation, depersonalization, altered sensory perception, and loss of insight occur, and these reactions are unusual and generally short lasting. Common predisposing factors include preexisting personality disturbances or schizophrenia. Thomas (1993)[32] reviews the psychiatric symptoms seen in *Cannabis* users:

> The usual phenomena of cannabis intoxication includes experiences which in a nonintoxicated state would be considered as psychiatric symptoms. These can be distinguished from adverse reactions to cannabis, the commonest of which is an acute anxiety state. Acute psychotic episodes can also follow ingestion of the drug but are infrequent. These can be classified as acute confusional states and episodes occurring in clear consciousness. . . . The evidence that cannabis has a causative role in chronic psychotic or affective disorders is not convincing, although the drug may modify the course of an already established illness.

The effects of marijuana on cognition, learning, memory, and attention have been the focus of increasing study; these effects may be the major adverse effects of THC. Acute use certainly impairs the ability to perform complex functions requiring attention and mental coordination (e.g., driving), although simple reflex activities are less affected. Solowij and coworkers (1991)[33] concluded that chronic users

> have difficulty in setting up an accurate focus of attention and in filtering out irrelevant information. The data suggest a dysfunction in the allocation of attentional resources and stimulus evaluation strategies. These results imply that long-term cannabis use may impair the ability to efficiently process information.

The authors of the study were unable to assess to what extent this deficit might be due to chronic buildup of THC and whether functioning would return to normal upon prolonged discontinuation of use. An obvious question is to what extent the smoking of marijuana might affect attention deficit disorders of either childhood or early adulthood.

Block and coworkers (1992)[34] studied the acute effects of marijuana smoking on cognition, reporting significant impairment in learning, associative processes, and psychomotor performance. Notably, marijuana altered associative processes, encouraging more uncommon associations. A freer, less logically controlled flow of thought followed smoking. Abstraction and vocabulary were less affected. Other reported cognitive deficits following marijuana use include impaired memory and deficits in concept formation, learning, attention, and signal detection.

Pope and Yurgelun-Todd (1996)[35] studied heavy marijuana users over a 20-hour drug-free period. Initially, these users displayed impairments of attention and executive functions that persisted during the short withdrawal period. Lundqvist (1995)[36,37] and Solowij (1995)[38] describe a marijuana-induced impaired ability to focus attention and filter out irrelevant information. Users demonstrate weakness in attention and synthetic skills, difficulty making subtle distinctions in relevance and memory, decreased psychospatial skills, poor mental representations of the environment, and poor routines of daily life.[37] These impairments are associated with feelings of alienation and that life is not under their control and lacks meaning. During therapy users "begin to show improvement in cognitive functioning within 14 days of abstinence combined with therapy, and function normally at the end of 6 weeks of therapy."[36]

In 1996 Fletcher and coworkers[39] studied two cohorts of long-term *Cannabis* users and nonusers in Costa Rican men over a 20-year period. The cohorts were compared with younger, shorter-term users and nonusers. As expected, older users demonstrated greater impairment in complex learning tasks of memory and recall, selective attention, and divided attention. To place these detrimental effects of marijuana in perspective, the Fletcher study concludes:

> The deficiencies observed . . . are subtle. The older long-term users are largely functional and employable, and they do not demonstrate the types of dementia and amnesic syndromes associated with alcohol use of comparable magnitude. The health of the subjects continues to be adequate over time, and no evidence exists for the severity of health risks associated with the use of other drugs, such as alcohol. Nevertheless, the risks of long-term use of even smaller amounts of cannabis are likely magnified in a more technological society. . . . Certain occupations may carry particular risk because of safety issues and effects on productivity and learning. . . . The findings suggest a need to focus efforts on the prevention of cannabis use through balanced educational programs for children and their parents. It is clear that the younger cohort and, to a lesser extent, the older cohort began to move toward polydrug use, a pattern consistent with studies of North American subjects. This pattern underscores the need for preventive efforts to reduce the risk of consumption of drugs by young people.

Kouri and coworkers (1995)[40] studied cohorts of heavy versus occasional marijuana smokers in a college population. By objective measurement of psychiatric functioning (diagnosed DSM disorders), the two groups were indistinguishable. They differed, however, in the level of use of other drugs, with one-third of heavy marijuana users displaying a history of some form of substance abuse or dependence (Tables 11.1 and 11.2).

In order to understand the behavioral attractiveness of marijuana, Gardner and Lowinson (1991)[41] reviewed marijuana's interactions with brain reward systems, particularly in the dopamine-mediated, medial forebrain bundle projection. They stated:

> Acute enhancement of brain reward mechanisms appears to be the single essential commonality of abuse prone drugs, and the hypothesis that recreational and abused drugs act on these brain mechanisms to produce the subjective reward that constitutes the "high" or "rush" or "hit" sought by drug users is, at present, the most compelling hypothesis available on the neurobiology of recreational drug use and abuse.

Also involved are synaptic interconnections of opioid and many other neurotransmitters. Indeed, Gardner and Lowinson argue that THC acts on this system as do other abused drugs, inducing the release of

TABLE 11.1 Lifetime substance use among heavy versus occasional marijuana smokers

	Heavy smokers (n = 45)	Occasional smokers (n = 44)
	n (%)	n (%)
SUBJECTS WHO HAD EVER USED		
Hallucinogens	44 (98)	23 (42)[c]
Hallucinogens > 10 times	36 (80)	5 (11)[c]
Cocaine	32 (71)	8 (18)[c]
Cocaine > 10 times	20 (44)	0[c]
Inhalants	11 (24)	3 (7)[a]
Stimulants	14 (31)	7 (16)
Sedative-hypnotics	27 (60)	7 (16)[c]
Opioids	12 (27)	1 (2)[b]
Any of the above	45 (100)	26 (59)[c]
SUBJECTS CURRENTLY USING		
Cigarettes ≥ 1 pack/day	17 (38)	5 (11)[b]
Alcohol > 10 drinks/week	17 (38)	9 (20)

Significance of differences between groups = [a]$p < .05$; [b]$p < 01$; [c]$p < .001$.

From Kouri et al. (1995).[40]

dopamine in reward loci including the basal ganglia, the nucleus accumbens, and the prefrontal cortex.[41]

An "amotivational" syndrome has long been associated with chronic marijuana use; it compels users to "drop out" because of a loss of interest in goal-oriented endeavors. The etiology of this syndrome is unclear, although Musty and Kaback (1995)[42] report that between 40 and 50 percent of adolescents admitted to a treatment program were found to have depressive symptoms at admission (indicating comorbidity of substance abuse with depression). They summarized:

> Both light and heavy users with symptoms of depression had significantly lower scores than those without depressive symptoms, on the overall Orientation to Life questionnaire and on each subscale measuring Meaningfulness, Manageability and Comprehensibility. These data suggest that amotivational symptoms observed in heavy marijuana users in treatment are due to depression.

TABLE 11.2 Lifetime diagnoses of substance abuse and dependence in heavy versus occasional marijuana smokers

	Heavy smokers (n = 45)	Occasional smokers (n = 44)
	n(%)	n(%)
SUBSTANCE		
Cannabis	45 (100)	0
Alcohol	11 (24)	5 (11)
Cocaine	6 (13)	0
Hallucinogens	3 (7)	0
Sedative-hypnotics	1 (2)	0
Polysubstance	2 (4)	0
ANY SUBSTANCE OTHER THAN CANNABIS[a]	15 (33)	5 (11)

[a]Total for heavy users is less than the sum of the individual diagnoses because some subjects reported more than one form of substance abuse or dependence.
Significance of differences: cannabis, $p < .001$; cocaine $p = .03$; any substance other than cannabis, $p = .01$.

From Kouri et al. (1995).[40]

It is interesting to speculate that, at least in many users, marijuana may have been first tried (and subsequently used) as self-medication for their affective disorder (over and above the drive for stimulation of dopaminergic reward mechanisms). This issue has not yet been addressed.

Of note, because many marijuana smokers may suffer from depression, Wilens, Biederman, and Spencer (1997)[43] reported several cases of transient cognitive changes, delirium, and tachycardia in adolescents who were medicated with tricyclic antidepressants and smoked marijuana. If verified by others, this would be a drug interaction of potential importance in children and adolescents taking antidepressants for attention deficit hyperactivity disorder (ADHD), depression, or other affective disorders.

Cardiovascular System

As described by Huestis and coworkers (1992),[22] an increase in heart rate and blood pressure are commonly observed physiological effects of THC. Blood vessels of the cornea can dilate, which results in bloodshot eyes that can be observed in persons who have just smoked marijuana. THC users frequently report increased appetite, dry mouth, occasional dizziness, and slight nausea. Respiratory depression is not observed.

Although the increased heart rate could be a problem for people with cardiovascular disease, dangerous physical reactions to marijuana are almost unknown. No human being is known to have died of overdosage. By extrapolation from animal experiments, the ratio of lethal to effective (intoxicating) dose is estimated to be on the order of thousands to one.[3]

Pulmonary System

The gaseous and particulate components of both marijuana and tobacco smoke provide some insights into the potential for marijuana to cause pulmonary damage. In a classic study, Hoffman and coworkers (1975)[44] performed such an analysis (see Table 11.3) and noted that, with the exception of the presence of THC in marijuana and nicotine in tobacco, both inhalants are remarkably similar, with marijuana smoke containing more tars and many of the same carcinogenic compounds identified in tobacco smoke.

Reports of altered lung function due to smoking marijuana show evidence of bronchial irritation and inflammation. Tashkin and coworkers (1995)[45,46] note changes in heavy marijuana smokers consistent with tobacco-induced lung injury, although a 1997 study by the same researchers[47] noted that tobacco smoking but not marijuana smoking is associated with a decline in lung function:

> These findings do not support an association between regular marijuana smoking and chronic COPD [chronic obstructive pulmonary disease] but do not exclude the possibility of other adverse respiratory effects.

Aside from its irritant effects, the obvious question is whether marijuana smoke causes lung cancer. No direct evidence shows that chronic marijuana smoking causes lung cancer, but we may be in a prodromal phase of *Cannabis*-induced lung cancer. Certainly, no scientist would state with absolute certainty that chronic smoking of marijuana is safe to pulmonary tissue; it seems extremely unlikely that the pulmonary toxicities seen with cigarettes will not be seen to some degree in heavy marijuana smokers.

TABLE 11.3 Gases and particulates in marijuana and tobacco smoke

	Marijuana cigarette	Tobacco cigarette
GAS PHASE ANALYSIS		
Carbon monoxide (vol %)	3.99	4.58
(mg)	17.6	20.2
Carbon dioxide (vol %)	8.27	9.38
(mg)	57.3	65.0
Ammonia (μg)	228	178
HCN (μg)	532	498
Isoprene (μg)	83	310
Acetaldehyde (μg)	1200	980
Acetone (μg)	443	578
Acrolein (μg)	92	85
Acetonitrile (μg)	132	123
Benzene (μg)	76	67
Toluene (μg)	112	108
Dimethylnitrosamine (ng)	75	84
Methylethylnitrosamine (ng)	27	30
PARTICULATE MATTER ANALYSIS		
Phenol (μg)	76.8	138.5
o-cresol (μg)	76.8	24
m-, p-cresol (μg)	54.4	65
2,4- and 2,5-dimethylphenol (μg)	6.8	14.4
Cannabidiol (μg)	190	——
Delta-9-tetracannabinol (μg)	820	——
Nicotine	——	2850
Naphthalene (ng)	3000	1200
1-methylnaphthalene (ng)	6100	3650
2-methylnaphthalene (ng)	3600	1400
Benzo(a)anthracene (ng)	75	43
Benzo(a)pyrene (ng)	31	22.1

From D. Hoffman, K. D. Brunemann, G. B. Gori, and E. L. Wynder.[44]

Immune System

As noted earlier, outside the CNS, specific cannabinoid receptors are found primarily in the immune system. Long-term marijuana use is associated with a degree of immunosuppression, which might render the smoker susceptible to infections or disease. Although data in this area are controversial and implications have not been proven, marijuana smoking, in some circumstances, can partially suppress immunity. The clinical significance of this occurrence is not known, but it should be noted that other depressant drugs, such as alcohol, barbiturates, benzodiazepines, and anticonvulsants, share this immunosuppressive action.

Because both the spleen and the lymphocytes (white blood cells) are important to the body's immune response, they have been investigated to determine how they are affected by cannabinoids. Kaminski and coworkers (1992)[48] identified protein-binding cannabinoid receptors in the membranes of spleen cells. When activated by THC, these receptors inhibit the intracellular adenylate cyclase second-messenger system and thereby reduce the ability of these spleen cells to function adequately in the immune response. Diaz, Specter, and Coffey (1993)[49] reported similar effects on lymphocytes. Cabral and coworkers (1995)[50] reported that both THC and anandamide inhibit the function of specialized tumor-killing cells. The implications of such actions and the physiological role of anandamide in immunomodulation are unknown.

To put the immunosuppressive action of marijuana in perspective, in humans, marijuana-induced immune suppression is subtle and in many cases insignificant. There is, at this time, little evidence for cannabinoid-induced immunosuppression as a causative agent in disease.

Reproductive System

Evidence of THC-induced suppression of sexual function and reproduction is being gathered. The chronic use of marijuana by males can reduce levels of the hormone testosterone and sperm formation. Reductions in male fertility and sexual potency, however, have not been reported. In females, the levels of the hormones FSH (follicle-stimulating hormone) and LH (luteinizing hormone) are reduced by the use of marijuana. Menstrual cycles can be affected and anovulatory cycles have been reported. All these actions are reversible when drug use is discontinued.[51]

Marijuana freely crosses the placenta, and so its use probably should be avoided during pregnancy. Fried (1995)[52] has been evaluating the effects of maternal marijuana use on offspring and notes a relative lack of effect in children aged 1 to 3 years. At 4 years, however, children displayed "increased behavioral problems and decreased performance on visual perceptual tasks, language comprehension, sustained attention and memory." Prenatal marijuana exposure may affect "executive functioning—goal-directed behavior that included planning, organized search, and impulse control." Fried concludes: "Such an interpretation would be consistent with the literature . . . suggesting that chronic marijuana use may impact prefrontal lobe functioning."

Side Effects

The major side effects associated with acute marijuana use are dose-related extensions of its recreational uses: sedation, altered motor coordination (resulting from intoxication), impaired cognition, and reduced short-term memory. Marijuana impairs a person's ability to drive an automobile safely, much as alcohol does. During marijuana intoxication, however, "the impairment persists for 4 to 8 hours, well beyond the time that the subjective effects of the drug have dissipated. The impairment is apparent to trained observers: 94 percent of subjects fail roadside sobriety tests 90 minutes after smoking marijuana; 60 percent still fail after 150 minutes."[53]

In a study of trauma injuries (67 percent involving motor vehicle accidents), marijuana was detected in 35 percent of subjects, and alcohol was present in 33 percent. A combination of both marijuana and alcohol was present in 16.5 percent of victims and neither drug was present in 49 percent.[54]

Similarly, Brookoff and coworkers (1994)[55] studied reckless drivers who tested negative for alcohol use. Of 150 such individuals who submitted urine samples, 20 (13 percent) tested positive for cocaine, 50 (33 percent) tested positive for marijuana, and an additional 18 (12 percent) tested positive for both cocaine and marijuana. Ninety-four of the 150 drivers were considered intoxicated (to trained observers) and 80 of those (85 percent) tested positive for cocaine or marijuana. Intoxicated drivers testing positive for alcohol were not tested for the coexistence of marijuana, although one would predict that the number of positives would be significant.

There is persistent concern that *Cannabis* use might precipitate or exacerbate psychotic episodes. Linszen and coworkers (1994)[56] noted in young schizophrenic patients that marijuana use was associated with significantly more and earlier psychotic relapses or exacerbations of symptoms. The results support the concept that heavy *Cannabis* misuse is at least a stressor for psychotic relapse in young schizophrenics. Thomas (1993)[32] argues, "There has not emerged over the past few decades any convincing evidence that moderate cannabis use leads to any persistent psychiatric disorder, a similar conclusion to that reached by the Indian Hemp Commission (1894) 100 years ago." Zimmer and Morgan (1997)[57] address 20 "myths" about marijuana's adverse effects, objectively discussing the literature behind each supposed misconception and, in general, dismissing the emotional arguments behind the presumed harmful effects of marijuana.

Tolerance and Dependence

Tolerance to *Cannabis* occurs and is thought to result from an adaptation of the brain to the continuous presence of the drug. Tolerance develops rapidly, but it seems to disappear rapidly, too. In animals, much greater degrees of tolerance develop and can persist for long periods. The relevance of this observation to marijuana use in humans is unclear.

Until recently, it was generally thought that physical dependence on THC did not develop. As stated by O'Brien (1995),[30] "Compulsive or regular marijuana users do not appear to be motivated by fear of withdrawal symptoms." Withdrawal symptoms, however, do occur and consist of restlessness, irritability, mild agitation, insomnia, sleep disturbances, nausea, cramping, and drug craving.[4,30] Overall, the withdrawal syndrome is considered to be relatively mild, beginning within a few hours after cessation of drug administration and lasting about four to six days.

Duffy and Milin (1996)[4] describe three cases in adolescents indicating that the withdrawal syndrome may be more serious than is generally appreciated and that drug craving contributes to the persistent use of *Cannabis* in adolescents despite motivation to stop. They conclude:

> The importance of gaining an appreciation for cannabis withdrawal in adolescent users is underscored by the high prevalence of cannabis use among adolescents, the association of cannabis use with the subsequent use of hard drugs, and the serious psychosocial sequelae associated with chronic cannabis use. Systematic study is warranted to understand better the magnitude of the problem of cannabis dependence in adolescents. We need to ask about withdrawal symptoms in adolescent cannabis users to identify significant symptoms and intervene as required, perhaps necessitating brief admission, extended care, and/or pharmacotherapy.

Animals tend not to self-administer THC-containing products, and THC does not substitute for drugs with strong reinforcing properties. According to Abood and Martin (1992)[31]: This observation suggests limited potential for development of physical dependence, as well as limited psychological dependence due to the weak reinforcing properties of delta-9-THC.

As with other psychoactive drugs, marijuana dependence is determined by three critical elements:

1. Preoccupation with the acquisition of the drug
2. Compulsive use of the drug
3. Relapse to, or recurrent use of, the drug

To date, these elements have not been major problems with marijuana used alone, although the report by Duffy and Milin (1996)[4] is disconcerting. The criteria are far more commonly met in multidrug dependence. Therefore, few treatment programs are oriented solely toward marijuana abuse, as both multidrug dependence and comorbid disease are invariably present. Treatments such as psychotherapy can be appropriate for frequent users of marijuana, but this is not therapy for marijuana abuse. Instead, it is therapy for an underlying psychopathology (such as depression), one symptom of which is the abuse of *Cannabis*. Grinspoon and Bakalar (1992)[3] write:

> Being attached to cannabis is not so much a function of any inherent psychopharmacologic property of the drug as it is emotionally driven by the underlying psychopathology. Success in curtailing cannabis use requires dealing with that pathology.

Therapeutic Uses

Currently, there are one approved and several possible therapeutic uses for THC and its various derivatives. *Dronabinol* (Marinol), which is synthetic THC formulated in sesame oil, has been available for more than 10 years for use as an appetite stimulant in patients with AIDS and for use in the treatment of nausea and vomiting associated with chemotherapy in cancer patients. Schwartz, Voth, and Sheridan (1997)[58] reviewed the use of smoked marijuana and oral dronabinol in this population of patients and compared the use of THC-containing products with physician-prescribed antiemetic (antivomiting) compounds; the latter had superior efficacy in treating chemotherapy-induced nausea and vomiting. Other uses of dronabinol are to reduce the muscle spasms and pain in multiple sclerosis and reduce the intraocular pressure in glaucoma. Antidepressant and analgesic effects are also claimed.

The recent passage of initiatives legalizing the use of marijuana for medicinal uses in Arizona and California has reopened this issue of therapeutics. Is marijuana "snake oil," or does it have true therapeutic efficacy, equal to or greater than those of existing agents? The answer is far from clear and is probably somewhere between yes and no.

To date, marijuana (or THC) has never been tested in any sort of double-blind study against any other agent of known efficacy. Such studies are certainly needed. Also, the prominent effects already discussed (perhaps desirable effects by many people) would tend to limit marijuana use as a "pure" therapeutic agent. In other words, marijuana itself would be unlikely to achieve analgesic or antiemetic efficacy without concomitant sedation, euphoria, motor dysfunction, impaired cognition, and so on. If, however, one desired such combination of effects, its use might then be unique and appropriate. In a 1997 editorial in the *New England Journal of Medicine*, Kassirer[59] stated:

> I believe that a federal policy that prohibits physicians from alleviating suffering by prescribing marijuana for seriously ill patients is misguided, heavy-handed, and inhumane. Federal authorities should rescind their prohibition of the medical use of marijuana for seriously ill patients and allow physicians to decide which patients to treat. The government should change marijuana's status from that of a Schedule 1 drug [considered to be potentially addictive and with no current medical use] to that of a Schedule 2 drug [potentially addictive but with some accepted medical use] and regulate it accordingly.

Currently, much effort is being expended to identify derivatives of delta-9-THC to identify compounds of varying affinity and efficacy at anandamide (cannabinoid) receptors. Progress in this area is slow, because until recently all cannabinoid receptors in the CNS were thought to be of one type and had not been subdivided, as had many other receptors. The cannabinoid receptors were all referred to as CB_1 receptors (those in the periphery are known to be somewhat different and are called CB_2 receptors).[2] Rinaldi-Carmona and coworkers (1996)[60] have characterized a CB_{1A} receptor subtype, and experimental compounds have been identified that differentially bind to CB_1 and CB_{1A} receptor types. Thus, in the future it may be possible to separate claimed therapeutic efficacy from what traditional medicine would call "side effects." For example, Abrahamov and coworkers (1995)[61] studied delta-8-THC as an antiemetic in children who were being treated for various cancers. The drug was an effective antinauseant and side effects were stated to be minimal. As additional derivatives are studied, some of the current confusion about therapeutic efficacy may become clearer.

Also of note is the fact that several anandamide receptor antagonists have been identified.[2] Since agonists (like THC) impair learning and memory, an antagonist might have the opposite effect and be useful in treating such diseases as dementia, obviously without THC-like CNS effects.

The future of cannabinoid research into therapeutic applications of THC derivatives will be interesting, controversial, and yet filled with potential for significant advances in the treatment of various disorders (see *Newsweek*, Feb. 3, 1997, pp. 20–27).

Marijuana and Public Safety

The first reports that causally linked the use of marijuana to aggression, violence, and crime appeared during the 1930s. Governmental commissions over the past 100 years (the first being the Indian Hemp Commission Report of 1894) have all concluded that marijuana is not the demon that it is often perceived to be. Nevertheless, the laws against marijuana are often excessively harsh, with a marked discrepancy between the true danger to society and perceived danger.

Today, only the unsophisticated believe that marijuana leads to violence and crime.[3] Indeed, marijuana is much less likely than alcohol to precipitate aggressive behavior. Instead of inciting criminal behavior, *Cannabis* induces a mild lethargy that is not conducive to the commission of crimes. The release of inhibitions results in fantasy and verbal (rather than behavioral) expression. During the "high," marijuana users may say and think things they would not ordinarily say and think, but they generally do not do things that are foreign to their nature.[3]

To date, the reports of all governmental commissions that have investigated marijuana have not opposed legally restricting *Cannabis*, nor do they suggest that *Cannabis* is a safe drug for general use.[51] They do, however, question the severity of punishment when the perceived danger to society is far greater than the actual dangers to either society or the individual. Recent controversies over the medical availability and prescription of *Cannabis* are only the latest in a long string of federal responses to perceived danger.

What, then, should society do about the harshness of existing legal penalties? Two conservative actions might be (1) to decriminalize possession of small amounts of marijuana for personal use, keeping marijuana possessed in public contraband and subject to summary seizure and forfeiture, and (2) to change the legal status of marijuana from Schedule 1 to Schedule 2 (cocaine and morphine are Schedule 2 drugs because they have an approved medical use), allowing physicians to prescribe the drug when they feel that is an appropriate action. Marijuana used under a physician's prescription would not be subject to seizure and forfeiture.

A plea of marijuana intoxication should not be a defense for any criminal act committed when a person was under its influence, and proof of marijuana intoxication should not constitute a negation of specific intent. Given the fact that marijuana use produces sedation, interferes with motor coordination, and impairs frontal lobe "executive" functioning, driving with measurable amounts of marijuana in the blood should be punishable. Similarly, employers should be able to establish antimarijuana policies just as they establish antialcohol policies for drug use in the workplace.

Although marijuana is not a "killer weed," it is not an innocuous substance that is devoid of toxicity. The legal statutes should protect individuals who use the drug for medical reasons, modest-dosage recreational users, nonusers who might be affected by intoxicated users (i.e., hit by an intoxicated driver), and juveniles who might not be able to make rational decisions concerning the risks and benefits of the drug. Society appears to be moving toward the acceptance of marijuana as a therapeutic drug for the seriously ill (with less movement toward its use as a recreational drug), but legal guidelines are still far from decided. Perhaps its medical availability should be a medical, rather than a legal, decision.

NOTES

1. S. A. Deadwyler, R. E. Hampson, and S. R. Childers, "Functional Significance of Cannabinoid Receptors in Brain," in R. G. Pertwee, ed., *Cannabinoid Receptors* (London: Academic Press, 1995), 205–231.
2. R. G. Pertwee, ed., *Cannabinoid Receptors* (London: Academic Press, 1995).
3. L. Grinspoon and J. B. Bakalar, "Marijuana," in J. H. Lowinson, P. Ruiz, R. B. Millman, and J. G. Langrod, eds., *Substance Abuse: A Comprehensive Textbook*, 2nd ed., (Baltimore: Williams & Wilkins, 1992), 236–246.
4. A. Duffy and R. Milin, "Case Study: Withdrawal Syndrome in Adolescent Chronic Cannabis Users," *Journal of the American Academy of Child and Adolescent Psychiatry* 35 (1996): 1618–1621.
5. A. C. Howlett, J. M. Qualy, and L. L. Khachatrian, "Involvement of G_i in the Inhibition of Adenylate Cyclase by Cannabimimetic Drugs," *Molecular Pharmacology* 29 (1986): 307–313.
6. M. Bidaut-Russell, W. A. Devane, and A. C. Howlett, "Cannabinoid Receptors and Modulation of Cyclic AMP Accumulation in the Rat Brain," *Journal of Neurochemistry* 55 (1990): 21–26.
7. C. A. Audette, S. H. Burstein, S. A. Doyle, and S. A. Hunter, "G-Protein Mediation of Cannabinoid-Induced Phospholipase Activation," *Pharmacology, Biochemistry, and Behavior* 40 (1991): 559–563.
8. L. A. Matsuda, S. J. Lolait, M. J. Brownstein, et al., "Structure of a Cannabinoid Receptor and Functional Expression of the Cloned cDNA," *Nature* 346 (1990): 561–564.

9. R. G. Pertwee, "Pharmacological, Physiological and Clinical Implications of the Discovery of Cannabinoid Receptors: An Overview," in R. G. Pertwee, ed., *Cannabinoid Receptors* (London: Academic Press, 1995), 1–34.

10. A. C. Howlett, T. M. Champion-Dorow, L. L. McMahon, and T. M. Westlake, "The Cannabinoid Receptor: Biochemical and Cellular Properties in Neuroblastoma Cells," *Pharmacology, Biochemistry, and Behavior* 40 (1991): 565–569.

11. R. D. Bramblett, A. M. Panu, J. A. Ballesteros, and P. H. Reggio, "Construction of a 3D Model of the Cannabinoid CB1 Receptor: Determination of Helix Ends and Helix Orientation," *Life Sciences* 56 (1995): 1971–1982.

12. R. E. Musty, P. Reggio, and P. Consroe, "A Review of Recent Advances in Cannabinoid Research and the 1994 International Symposium on Cannabis and the Cannabinoids," *Life Sciences* 56 (1995): 1933–1940.

13. M. Shen, T. M. Piser, V. S. Seybold, and S. A. Thayer, "Cannabinoid Receptor Agonists Inhibit Glutamatergic Synaptic Transmission in Rat Hippocampal Cultures," *Journal of Neuroscience* 16 (1996): 4322–4334.

14. W. A. Devane, L. Hanus, A. Breuer, et al., "Isolation and Structure of a Brain Constituent that Binds to the Cannabinoid Receptor," *Science* 258 (1992): 1946–1949.

15. B. F. Thomas, I. B. Adams, W. Mascarella, et al., "Structure-Activity Analysis of Anandamide Analogs: Relationship to a Cannabinoid Pharmacophore," *Journal of Medicinal Chemistry* 39 (1996): 471–479.

16. H. Cadas, S. Gaillet, M. Beltramo, et al., "Biosynthesis of an Endogenous Cannabinoid Precursor in Neurons and Its Control by Calcium and cAMP," *Journal of Neuroscience* 16 (1996): 3934–3942.

17. P. Derkinderen, M. Toutant, F. Burgaya, et al., "Regulation of a Neuronal Form of Focal Adhesion Kinase by Anandamide," *Science* 273 (1996): 1719–1722.

18. M. Herkenham, A. B. Lynn, M. R. Johnson, et al., "Characterization and Localization of Cannabinoid Receptors in Rat Brain: A Quantitative in Vitro Autoradiographic Study," *Journal of Neuroscience* 11 (1991): 563–583.

19. M. Herkenham, "Cannabinoid Receptor Localization in Brain: Relationship to Motor and Reward Systems," *Annals of the New York Academy of Sciences* 654 (1992): 19–32.

20. A. B. Lynn and M. Herkenham, "Localization of Cannabinoid Receptors and Nonsaturable High-Density Cannabinoid Binding Sites in Peripheral Tissues of the Rat: Implications for Receptor-Mediated Immune Modulation by Cannabinoids," *Journal of Pharmacology and Experimental Therapeutics* 268 (1994): 1612–1623.

21. M. Perez-Reyes, W. R. White, S. A. McDonald, et al., "The Pharmacological Effects of Daily Marijuana Smoking in Humans," *Pharmacology, Biochemistry, and Behavior* 40 (1991): 691–694.

22. M. A. Huestis, A. H. Sampson, B. J. Holicky, et al., "Characterization of the Absorption Phase of Marijuana Smoking," *Clinical Pharmacology and Therapeutics* 52 (1992): 31–41.

23. T. Matsunaga, Y. Yasuyuki, K. Watanabe, et al., "Metabolism of Delta^9-Tetrahydrocannabinol by Cytochrome P450 Isozymes Purified from Hepatic Microsomes of Monkeys," *Life Sciences* 56 (1995): 2089–2095.

24. E. Johansson, M. M. Hardin, S. Agurell, and L. E. Hollister, "Terminal Elimination Plasma Half-Life of Delta-1-Tetrahydrocannabinol in Heavy Users of Marijuana," *European Journal of Clinical Pharmacology* 37 (1989): 273–277.

25. W. J. Martin, S. L. Patrick, P. O. Coffin, K. Tsou, and J. M. Walker, "An Examination of the Central Sites of Action of Cannabinoid-Induced Antinociception in the Rat," *Life Sciences* 56 (1995): 2103–2109.

26. A. G. Hohmann, W. J. Martin, K. Tsou, and J. M. Walker, "Inhibition of Noxious Stimulus-Evoked Activity of Spinal Cord Dorsal Horn Neurons by the Cannabinoid WIN-55,212-2," *Life Sciences* 56 (1995): 2111–2118.

27. J. Romero, L. Garcia, M. Cebeira, et al., "The Endogenous Cannabinoid Receptor Ligand, Anandamide, Inhibits the Motor Behavior: Role of Nigrostriatal Dopaminergic Neurons," *Life Sciences* 56 (1995): 2033–2040.

28. J. Romero, E. Garcia-Palomero, S. Y. Lin, et al., "Extrapyramidal Effects of Methanandamide, an Analog of Anandamide, the Endogenous CB$_1$ Receptor Ligand," *Life Sciences* 56 (1995): 1249–1257.

29. T. Wenger, B. E. Toth, and B. R. Martin, "Effects of Anandamide (Endogen Cannabinoid) on Anterior Pituitary Hormone Secretion in Adult Ovariectomized Rats," *Life Sciences* 56 (1995): 2057–2063.

30. C. P. O'Brien, "Drug Addiction and Drug Abuse," in J. G. Hardman, L. E. Limbird, P. B. Molinoff, R. W. Ruddon, and A. G. Gilman, eds., *Goodman and Gilman's The Pharmacological Basis of Therapeutics*, 9th ed. (New York: Macmillan, 1995), 572–573.

31. M. E. Abood and B. R. Martin, "Neurobiology of Marijuana Abuse," *Trends in Pharmacological Sciences* 13 (1992): 201.

32. H. Thomas, "Psychiatric Symptoms in Cannabis Users," *British Journal of Psychiatry* 163 (1993): 141–149.

33. N. Solowij, P. T. Michie, and A. M. Fox, "Effects of Long-Term Cannabis Use on Selective Attention: An Event-Related Potential Study," *Pharmacology, Biochemistry, and Behavior* 40 (1991): 683.

34. R. I. Block, R. Farinpour, and K. Braverman, "Acute Effects of Marijuana on Cognition: Relationships to Chronic Effects and Smoking Techniques," *Pharmacology, Biochemistry, and Behavior* 40 (1992): 907–917.

35. H. G. Pope and D. Yurgelun-Todd, "The Residual Cognitive Effects of Heavy Marijuana Use in College Students," *Journal of the American Medical Association* 275 (1996): 521–527.

36. T. Lundqvist, "Specific Thought Patterns in Chronic Cannabis Smokers Observed During Treatment," *Life Sciences* 56 (1995): 2141–2144.

37. T. Lundqvist, "Chronic Cannabis Use and the Sense of Coherence," *Life Sciences* 56 (1995): 2145–2150.

38. N. Solowij, "Do Cognitive Impairments Recover Following Cessation of Cannabis Use?," *Life Sciences* 56 (1995): 2119–2126.

39. J. M. Fletcher, J. B. Page, D. J. Francis, et al., "Cognitive Correlates of Long-Term Cannabis Use in Costa Rican Men," *Archives of General Psychiatry* 53 (1996): 1051–1057.

40. E. Kouri, H. G. Pope, D. Yurgelun-Todd, and S. Gruber, "Attributes of Heavy versus Occasional Marijuana Smokers in a College Population," *Biological Psychiatry* 38 (1995): 475–481.

41. E. L. Gardner and J. H. Lowinson, "Marijuana's Interaction with Brain Reward Systems: Update 1991," *Pharmacology, Biochemistry, and Behavior* 40 (1991): 571.

42. R. E. Musty and L. Kaback, "Relationships Between Motivation and Depression in Chronic Marijuana Users," *Life Sciences* 56 (1995): 2151–2158.

43. T. E. Wilens, J. Biederman, and T. J. Spencer, "Case Study: Adverse Effects of Smoking Marijuana While Receiving Tricyclic Antidepressants," *Journal of the American Academy of Child and Adolescent Psychiatry* 36 (1997): 45–48.

44. D. I. Hoffman, K. D. Brunemann, G. B. Gori, and E. L. Wynder, "On the Carcinogenicity of Marijuana Smoke," *Recent Advances in Phytochemistry* 9 (1975): 63–81.

45. E. Gil, B. Chen, E. Kleerup, M. Webber, and D. P. Tashkin, "Acute and Chronic Effects of Marijuana Smoking on Pulmonary Alveolar Permeability," *Life Sciences* 56 (1995): 2193–2199.

46. M. P. Sherman, E. E. Aeberhard, V. Z. Wong, M. S. Simmons, M. D. Roth, and D. P. Tashkin, "Effects of Smoking Marijuana, Tobacco, or Cocaine Alone or in Combination on DNA Damage in Human Alveolar Macrophages," *Life Sciences* 56 (1995): 2201–2207.

47. D. P. Tashkin, M. S. Simmons, D. L. Sherrill, and A. H. Coulson, "Heavy Habitual Marijuana Smoking Does Not Cause an Accelerated Decline in FEV_1 with Age," *American Journal of Respiratory and Critical Care Medicine* 155 (1997): 141–148.

48. N. E. Kaminski, M. E. Abood, F. K. Kessler, et al., "Identification of a Functionally Relevant Cannabinoid Receptor on Mouse Spleen Cells That Is Involved in Cannabinoid-Mediated Immune Modulation," *Molecular Pharmacology* 42 (1992): 736–742.

49. S. Diaz, S. Specter, and R. G. Coffey, "Suppression of Lymphocyte Adenosine 3':5'-Cyclic Monophosphate (cAMP) by Delta-9-Tetrahydrocannabinol," *International Journal of Immunopharmacology* 15 (1993): 523–532.

50. G. A. Cabral, D. M. Toney, K. Fischer-Stenger, et al., "Anandamide Inhibits Macrophage-Mediated Killing of Tumor Necrosis Factor-Sensitive Cells," *Life Sciences* 56 (1995): 2065–2072.

51. A. Goldstein, *Addiction: From Biology to Drug Policy* (New York: W. H. Freeman and Company, 1994), 174–176.

52. P. A. Fried, "The Ottawa Prenatal Prospective Study (OPPS): Methodological Issues and Findings—It's Easy to Throw the Baby Out with the Bath Water," *Life Sciences* 56 (1995): 2159–2168.

53. J. W. Jaffe, "Drug Addiction and Drug Abuse," in A. G. Gilman, T. W. Rall, A. S. Nies, and P. Taylor, eds., *Goodman and Gilman's The Pharmacological Basis of Therapeutics,* 8th ed. (New York: Pergamon, 1990), 551.

54. C. A. Soderstrom, A. L. Trifillis, B. S. Shanker, and W. E. Clark, "Marijuana and Alcohol Use Among 1,023 Trauma Patients: A Prospective Study," *Archives of Surgery* 123 (1988): 733–737.

55. D. Brookoff, C. S. Cook, C. Williams, and C. S. Mann, "Testing Reckless Drivers for Cocaine and Marijuana," *New England Journal of Medicine* 331 (1994): 518–522.

56. D. H. Linszen, P. M. Dingemans, and M. E. Lenior, "Cannabis Abuse and the Course of Recent-Onset Schizophrenic Disorders," *Archives of General Psychiatry* 51 (1994): 273.

57. L. Zimmer and J. P. Morgan, *Marijuana Myths, Marijuana Facts* (New York: Lindesmith Center, 1997).

58. R. H. Schwartz, E. A. Voth, and M. J. Sheridan, "Marijuana to Prevent Nausea and Vomiting in Cancer Patients: A Survey of Clinical Oncologists," *Southern Medical Journal* 90 (1997): 167–172.

59. J. P. Kassirer, "Federal Foolishness and Marijuana," *New England Journal of Medicine* 336 (1997): 366–367.

60. M. Rinaldi-Carmona, B. Calandra, D. Shire, et al., "Characterization of Two Cloned Human CB1 Cannabinoid Receptor Isoforms," *Journal of Pharmacology and Experimental Therapeutics* 278 (1996): 871–878.

61. A. Abrahamov, A. Abrahamov, and R. Mechoulam, "An Efficient New Cannabinoid Antiemetic in Pediatric Oncology," *Life Sciences* 56 (1995): 2097–2102.

Chapter 12

PSYCHEDELIC DRUGS: MESCALINE, LSD, PHENCYCLIDINE, AND OTHER HALLUCINOGENS

Psychedelic drugs are a group of heterogeneous compounds that induce visual and auditory hallucinations, separating the persons who use them from reality. These agents may disturb cognition and perception and, in some instances, produce behavior that is similar to that observed in psychotic patients. Because of this wide range of psychological effects, what single term might best be used to classify these agents has long been debated.[1]

The term "hallucinogen" has been widely used, because these agents can induce hallucinations in high enough doses. However, that term is somewhat inappropriate because hallucinations are unusual at normally encountered doses, at which illusory phenomena and perceptual distortions are more common. Thus, the term "illusionogenic" has been used. The term "psychotomimetic" has also been used because of the alleged ability of these drugs to mimic psychoses or induce psychotic states. However, the effects of most of these drugs do not produce the same behavioral patterns that are observed in persons who experience psychotic episodes. Thus, because no one of these terms characterizes the pharmacology of these drugs, we must rely on a descriptive term, such as "phantasticum" (proposed by Lewin in 1924) or

---

TABLE 12.1 Classification of psychedelic drugs

ANTICHOLINERGIC PSYCHEDELIC DRUG
Scopolamine

CATECHOLAMINE-LIKE PSYCHEDELIC DRUGS
Mescaline
DOM, MDA, DMA, MDMA, TMA, MDE
Myristin, elemicin

SEROTONIN-LIKE PSYCHEDELIC DRUGS
Lysergic acid diethylamide (LSD)
Dimethyltryptamine (DMT)
Psilocybin, psilocin, bufotenine
Ololiuqui (morning glory seeds)
Harmine

PSYCHEDELIC ANESTHETIC DRUGS
Phencyclidine (Sernyl)
Ketamine (Ketalar)

"psychedelic" (proposed by Osmond in 1957), to imply that these agents all have the ability to alter sensory perception.

Many psychedelic agents occur in nature; others are synthetically produced in laboratories, many of which are clandestine. Naturally occurring psychedelic drugs have been used for thousands of years, primarily for their effects on sensory perception. For some individuals, these drugs have magical or mystical properties. Prior to the 1960s, the compounds were restricted primarily to religious rituals, and most persons were barely aware of their existence. During the late 1960s and 1970s, however, some people advocated their use to enhance perception, expand reality, promote personal awareness, and stimulate or induce comprehension of the spiritual or supernatural. These drugs heighten awareness of sensory input, often accompanied by an enhanced sense of clarity but a diminished control over what is experienced. Frequently, there is a feeling that one part of the self seems to be a passive observer, while another part of the self participates and receives the vivid and unusual sensory experiences. In this state, the slightest sensation may take on profound meaning.

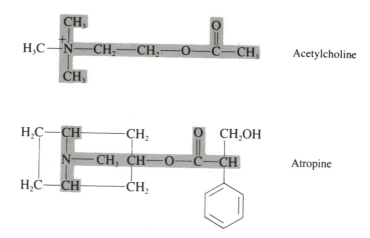

FIGURE 12.1 Structural formulas of acetylcholine (a chemical transmitter) and the anticholinergic psychedelic scopolamine, which acts by blocking acetylcholine receptors The shaded portion of each molecule illustrates structural similarities, which presumably contribute to receptor "fit."

Most psychedelic drugs structurally resemble one of four neurotransmitters: acetylcholine, two catecholamines (norepinephrine and dopamine), and serotonin. These structural similarities lead to three classes for categorizing psychedelic drugs (see Table 12.1): *anticholinergic, catecholamine-like, or serotonin-like*. Table 12.1 includes a fourth class of psychedelic drugs, the *psychedelic anesthetics*, which exert their psychedelic actions by affecting a specific subclass of glutamate receptors, the NMDA receptors (see Appendix IV).

Anticholinergic Psychedelic Drugs

Scopolamine, an acetylcholine receptor antagonist, is the classic example of an anticholinergic psychedelic drug (see Figure 12.1). Having receptor affinity but devoid of intrinsic activity, scopolamine blocks the access of acetylcholine to its receptors—hence the term "anticholinergic."

Historical Background

The history of scopolamine is long and colorful. The drug is distributed widely in nature, found in especially high concentrations in the plant *Atropa belladonna* (belladonna or deadly nightshade), in *Datura stramonium* (Jamestown weed, jimsonweed, stinkweed, thorn apple, or devil's apple), and in *Mandragora officinarum* (mandrake). Both professional and amateur poisoners of the Middle Ages frequently used deadly nightshade as a source of poison. In fact, the plant's name, *Atropa belladonna*, is derived from Atropos, the Greek goddess who supposedly cuts the thread of life. Belladonna means "beautiful woman," which refers to its ability to dilate the pupils when it is applied topically to the eyes (eyes with widely dilated pupils were presumably a mark of beauty).

Plants that contain *atropine* (another drug found in scopolamine-containing plants) and scopolamine have been used and misused for centuries. For example, the delirium caused by these substances may have persuaded certain persons that they could fly—and that they were witches. Marijuana and opium preparations from the Far East were once fortified with material from *Datura stramonium*. Today, cigarettes made from the leaves of *Datura stramonium* and *Atropa belladonna* are smoked occasionally to induce intoxication. Throughout the world, leaves of plants that contain atropine or scopolamine are still used to prepare intoxicating beverages.

Pharmacological Effects

Scopolamine and atropine act on the peripheral nervous system to depress salivation (causing dry mouth), reduce sweating, increase body temperature, dilate the pupils, blur vision, and markedly increase heart rate.[2] Atropine is a poor psychedelic because it only very poorly crosses the blood-brain barrier and therefore does not readily enter the central nervous system (CNS). Of the two drugs, scopolamine is the primary CNS-active intoxicant. Within the CNS, low doses of scopolamine produce drowsiness, mild euphoria, profound amnesia, fatigue, delirium, mental confusion, dreamless sleep, and loss of attention. Rather than expanding consciousness, awareness, and insight, scopolamine clouds consciousness and produces amnesia; it does not expand sensory perception.

In higher doses, a behavioral state that resembles a toxic psychosis occurs. Delirium, mental confusion, sedation, and amnesia dominate CNS effects; superimposed on these effects are peripheral actions, such as tachycardia, blurred vision, urinary retention, and dry mouth. All these effects can convey a sense of excitement and loss of control to the user. However, the clouding of consciousness and the reduction in memory of the episode render scopolamine rather unattractive as a psychedelic drug. Indeed, it is more appropriate to refer to it as a somewhat dangerous intoxicant, amnestic, and deliriant.

Catecholamine-like Psychedelic Drugs

Norepinephrine and dopamine receptors are important sites of action for a large group of psychedelic drugs that are structurally similar to both catecholamine neurotransmitters, as well as to the amphetamines (see Figure 12.2). Structurally, the catecholamine psychedelics differ from norepinephrine, dopamine, and the amphetamines by the addition of one or more methoxy (OCH_3) groups to the carboxy ring structure. Methylation seems to confer psychedelic properties on top of the behavioral stimulant properties.[3] Methoxylated amphetamine derivatives include mescaline, DOM (also called STP), MDA, MDMA ("ecstasy"), MMDA, DMA, and certain drugs that are obtained from nutmeg (myristin and elemicin).

Despite these catecholamine-like actions, however, their psychedelic actions are probably ultimately exerted by augmentation of serotonin neurotransmission, which results in LSD-like effects,[4] and by release of dopamine, which accounts for the stimulant and reinforcement.[5] Thus, we should first expand on the mechanism of action of these drugs.

As early as the late 1960s, most psychedelics were known to produce a remarkably similar set of effects. These included sensory-perceptual distortion; altered perceptions of colors, sounds, and shapes; complex hallucinations and synesthesia; dreamlike feelings; depersonalization; altered affect (depression or elation); and somatic effects (tingling skin, weakness, tremor, and so on). During the mid- and late 1980s, it was noted that psychedelic drugs produce marked alterations in brain serotonin.[6] As serotonin receptors were characterized in the early 1990s, it became clear that LSD was a serotonin receptor agonist and that the catecholamine-like psychedelics functioned ultimately as indirectly acting serotonin agonists.[5] Krebs and Geyer (1994)[6] state that "the effects of LSD . . . reflect a combination of 5-HT_{1A} and 5-HT_2 effects and support the view that there is an interaction between 5-HT_{1A} and 5-HT_2 receptors."[6] In slight contrast, the catecholamine-like psychedelics exhibit more selectivity for the 5-HT_2 receptor[6] and activate dopaminergic systems, including that in the nucleus accumbens.[5] Which subclasses of serotonin receptors are involved in psychedelic actions is still being debated. Serotonin 5-HT_{2A} and 5-HT_{2C},[7] 5-HT_{1A-1D} and 5-HT_2,[8] the interactive 5-HT_{1A} and 5-HT_2 discussed earlier,[6] have all been implicated. For the present, we can safely classify these psychedelics as serotonin agonists (the serotonin-like psychedelics as *direct-acting agonists*, and the catecholamine-like psychedelics as *indirect-acting agonists*), with 5-HT_2 receptors certainly involved. For the catecholamine-like psychedelics:

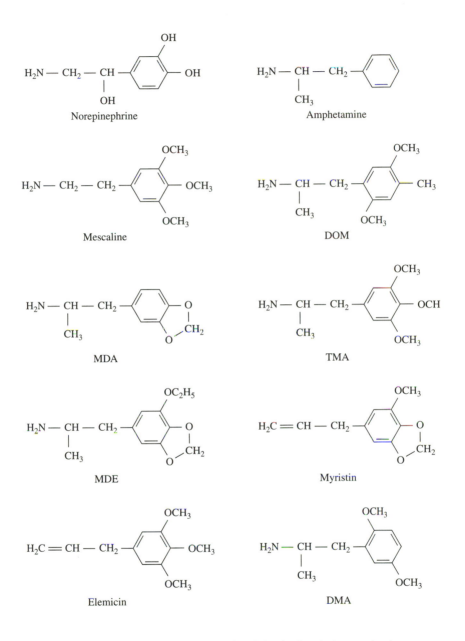

FIGURE 12.2 Structural formulas of norepinephrine (a chemical transmitter), amphetamine, and eight catecholamine-like psychedelic drugs. These eight drugs are structurally related to norepinephrine and are thought to exert their psychedelic actions by altering the transmission of nerve impulses at norepinephrine and serotonin synapses in the brain.

Our working hypothesis is that the human psychopharmacology of MDMA (one such agent) is the result of a combined action . . . in both serotonergic and catecholamine pathways.[5]

Mescaline

Peyote (Lophophora williamsii) is a common plant in the southwestern United States and in Mexico. It is a spineless cactus that has a small crown, or "button," and a long root. When the plant is used for psychedelic purposes, the crown is cut from the cactus and dried into a hard brown disk. This disk, which is frequently referred to as a "mescal button," may later be softened in a person's mouth and swallowed. The psychedelic chemical in the button is mescaline.

Historical Background. The use of peyote extends back to pre-Columbian times, when the cactus was used in the religious rites of the Aztecs and other Mexican Indians. Currently, peyote is legally available for use in the religious practice of the Native American Church of North America—an organization that claims some 250,000 members from Indian tribes throughout North America. Members of the Native American Church regard peyote as sacramental. The use of peyote for religious purposes is not considered to be abuse, and peyote is seldom abused by members of the Native American Church. Today, the federal government and 23 states permit its sacramental use.

Pharmacological Effects. Early research on the peyote cactus led in 1896 to the identification of mescaline as its pharmacologically active ingredient. After the chemical structure of mescaline was elucidated in 1918, the compound was produced synthetically. Because of its structural resemblance to norepinephrine, a wide variety of synthetic mescaline derivatives has now been synthesized, and all have methoxy (OCH_3) groups or similar additions on their benzene rings (see Figure 12.2). Why methoxylation of the benzene ring adds psychedelic properties to the drug is not clear, but it likely confers affinity for the serotonin receptors.

When taken orally, mescaline is rapidly and completely absorbed, and significant concentrations are usually achieved in the brain within 30 to 90 minutes. The effects of a single dose of mescaline persist for approximately 10 hours. The drug does not appear to be metabolized before it is excreted.

Interest in mescaline centers on the fact that it produces unusual psychic effects and visual hallucinations. The usual oral dose (5 mg/kg) in the average normal subject causes anxiety, sympathomimetic effects, hyperreflexia of the limbs, tremors, and visual hallucinations that consist of brightly colored lights, geometric designs, animals and occasionally people; color and space perception is often concomitantly impaired, but otherwise the sensorium is normal and insight is retained.

Hermle and coworkers (1992)[9] administered mescaline orally to 12 normal male volunteers and evaluated the effects. They describe an acute psychotic state 3.5 to 4 hours after the drug is taken:

> The psychotic effects were mainly concerned with the dissolution of ego-boundaries, visual hallucinations, and dimensions of "oceanic boundlessness," often mixed with anxious passivity experiences.

Brain imaging studies revealed that mescaline increased blood flow to the frontal lobes, the right side more "hyperfrontal" than the left.

Synthetic Amphetamine Derivatives

DOM, MDA, DMA, MDE, TMA, and MDMA are structurally related to mescaline and methamphetamine and, as might be expected, produce similar effects. They have moderate behavioral-stimulant effects at low doses, but like LSD, psychedelic effects dominate as doses increase. These derivatives are considerably more potent and more toxic than mescaline.

DOM (*d*i-meth*o*xy-*m*ethamphetamine) has effects that are similar to those of mescaline; doses of 1 to 6 milligrams produce euphoria, which is followed by a 6- to 8-hour period of hallucinations. DOM is 100 times more potent than mescaline but much less potent than LSD. The use of DOM is associated with a high incidence of overdose (because it is potent and street doses are poorly controlled). Acute toxic reactions are common; they consist of tremors that may eventually lead to convulsive movements, prostration, and even death. Because toxic reactions are common, the use of DOM is not widespread.

MDA (*m*ethylene-*d*ioxy-*a*mphetamine), *DMA* (*d*imethoxy-*m*ethylamphetamine), *MDE* (*m*ethylene-*d*ioxy-*e*thylamphetamine, or "Eve"), *TMA* (*tri*methoxy-*a*mphetamine), and other structural variations of amphetamine are encountered as "designer psychedelics." MDA is also a metabolite of MDMA,[10] and much of MDMA's effect may be due to the presence of MDA. In general, the pharmacological effects of these drugs resemble those of mescaline and LSD; they reflect the mix of catecholamine and serotonin interactions. Side effects and toxicities (including fatalities) are similar to those discussed below for MDMA.

MDMA (*m*ethylene-*d*ioxy-*m*ethamphetamine, also called "ecstasy" or "Adam") resembles MDA in structure but may be less hallucinogenic, inducing a less extreme sense of disembodiment and visual distortion.[11]

As stated, it is metabolized to an active intermediate, MDA. In experiments, MDMA has been shown to release serotonin and cause acute depletion of serotonin from most axon terminals in the forebrain, as well as produce irreversible destruction of serotonin neurons in laboratory animals.[12] Ricaurte and coworkers (1990)[13] argue for a similar toxic action in humans. Thus, MDMA is potentially too dangerous for human use. Despite this, abuse of MDMA appears to be increasing, with concomitant increases in reports of severe toxicities, including fatalities. Severe toxicities appear to follow the ingestion of MDMA during periods of intense activity, such as skiing[14] and dancing at "rave parties."[10,15] Symptoms include hyperthermia, tachycardia, disorientation, dilated pupils, convulsions, rigidity, and breakdown of skeletal muscle with kidney failure.[10,15,16] Despite the risks and the more common side effects of depersonalization, paranoia, anxiety, panic, suicidal ideation, and so on, the "intense euphoric high" promotes continued use.[15] The serious, potentially fatal complications associated with the destruction of serotonin neurons and the "malignant" hyperthermic response will no doubt result in continuing fatalities.[16]

Myristicin and Elemicin

Nutmeg and mace are common household spices sometimes abused for their hallucinogenic properties.[17] *Myristin* and *elemicin*, the pharmacologically active ingredients in nutmeg and mace, are responsible for this psychedelic action. Ingestion of large amounts (between 1 and 2 teaspoons, usually brewed in tea) may, after a delay of 2 to 5 hours, induce euphoria, visual hallucinations, acute psychotic reactions, and feelings of impending doom, depersonalization, and unreality. Considering the close structural resemblance of myristin and elemicin to mescaline (see Figure 12.2), these psychedelic actions are not unexpected. However, both drugs produce many unpleasant side effects, including vomiting, nausea, and tremors. After nutmeg or mace has been taken to produce its psychedelic action, the side effects usually dissuade users from trying these agents a second time.

Serotonin-like Psychedelic Drugs

The serotonin-like psychedelic drugs include lysergic acid diethylamide (LSD), psilocybin and psilocin (both from the mushroom *Psilocybe mexicana*), dimethyltryptamine (DMT), and bufotenine (see Figure 12.3). Because of their structural resemblance to each other and to serotonin, it has long been presumed that these agents somehow exerted their effects through interactions at serotonin synapses.

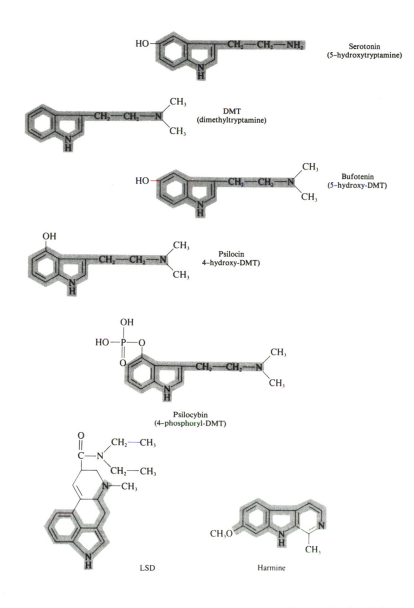

FIGURE 12.3 Structural formulas of serotonin (a chemical transmitter) and six serotonin-like psychedelic drugs. These six drugs are structurally related to serotonin (as indicated by the shading) and are thought to exert their psychedelic actions through alterations of serotonin synapses in the brain. Although LSD is structurally much more complex than serotonin, the basic similarity of the two molecules is apparent.

Almaula and coworkers (1996)[18] mapped the binding site for LSD on the 5-HT$_{2A}$ receptor and correlated the binding with receptor activation. In contrast, Penington and Fox (1994)[19] review literature claiming that LSD exerts a spectrum of agonist-antagonist effects on a variety of 5-HT receptor subtypes, but they think that the best candidate appears to be agonist actions on 5-HT$_{1C}$ receptors. They further demonstrate that LSD-induced 5-HT$_{1C}$ activation decreases serotonin neurotransmission as a result of presynaptic increases in potassium ion conductance and reduced calcium ion influx in neurons of the dorsal raphe nucleus. This action results in an inhibition of serotonin release throughout the brain.[19] Eventually these actions result in the psychedelic syndrome that is characteristic of all these drugs.

> One speculation about the process by which hallucinogens manifest their impressive alterations of mood, perception, and thought is that the *pontine (dorsal) raphe*, a major center of serotonin activity [see Appendix IV], serves as a filtering station for incoming sensory stimuli. It screens the flood of sensations and perceptions, eliminating those that are unimportant, irrelevant, or commonplace. A drug like LSD may disrupt the sorting process, allowing a surge of sensory data and an overload of brain circuits. Dehabituation, in which the familiar becomes novel, is noted under LSD. It may also be caused by lowering the sensory gates by inhibition of the raphe activity.[4]

Lysergic Acid Diethylamide (LSD)

During the 1960s and early 1970s, *lysergic acid diethylamide* (LSD) became one of the most remarkable and controversial drugs known. LSD, in doses that are so small that they might even be considered infinitesimal, is capable of inducing remarkable psychological change in a person, enhancing self-awareness and altering internal reality, while causing relatively few alterations in the general physiology of the body.

Historical Background. LSD was first synthesized in 1938 by Albert Hofmann, a Swiss chemist, as part of an organized research program to investigate possible therapeutic uses of compounds obtained from ergot.[20] Ergot is a natural product derived from a fungus (*Claviceps purpurea*), which grows as a parasite on rye in the grain fields of Europe and North America. The active products that are extracted from ergot are derivatives of lysergic acid. The pharmacological actions of these derivatives do not usually include hallucinations, but they do include constriction of blood vessels and increased contractions of the uterus. Therapeutically, ergot alkaloids are used to treat migraine headaches and to control postpartum hemorrhaging.

Early pharmacological studies of LSD in animals failed to reveal anything unusual; the psychedelic action was neither sought nor expected. Thus, LSD remained unnoticed until 1943, when Doctor Hofmann had an unusual experience:

> In the afternoon of 16 April, 1943, . . . I was seized by a peculiar sensation of vertigo and restlessness. Objects, as well as the shape of my associates in the laboratory, appeared to undergo optical changes. I was unable to concentrate on my work. In a dreamlike state I left for home, where an irresistible urge to lie down overcame me. I drew the curtains and immediately fell into a peculiar state similar to drunkenness, characterized by an exaggerated imagination. With my eyes closed, fantastic pictures of extraordinary plasticity and intensive color seemed to surge toward me. After two hours this state gradually wore off.[21]

Hofmann correctly hypothesized that his experience resulted from the accidental ingestion of LSD. To further characterize the experience, Hofmann self-administered what seemed to be a minuscule oral dose (only 0.25 milligram).[20] We now know, however, that this dose is about 10 times the dose required to induce psychedelic effects in most persons. As a result of this miscalculation, his response was quite spectacular:

> After 40 minutes, I noted the following symptoms in my laboratory journal: slight giddiness, restlessness, difficulty in concentration, visual disturbances, laughing. . . . Later, I lost all count of time. I noticed with dismay that my environment was undergoing progressive changes. My visual field wavered and everything appeared deformed as in a faulty mirror. Space and time became more and more disorganized and I was overcome by a fear that I was going out of my mind. The worst part of it being that I was clearly aware of my condition. My power of observation was unimpaired. . . . Occasionally, I felt as if I were out of my body. I thought I had died. My ego seemed suspended somewhere in space, from where I saw my dead body lying on the sofa. . . . It was particularly striking how acoustic perceptions, such as the noise of water gushing from a tap or the spoken word, were transformed into optical illusions. I then fell asleep and awakened the next morning somewhat tired but otherwise feeling perfectly well.[21]

In 1949 the first North American study of LSD in humans was conducted, and during the 1950s large quantities of LSD were distributed to scientists for research purposes. A significant impetus to research was the notion that the effects of LSD might constitute a model for psychosis, which would provide some insight into the biochemical and physiological processes of mental illness and its treatment. Some therapists tried LSD as an adjunct to psychotherapy to help patients verbalize their problems and gain some insight into the underlying causes, but this has not proven to be an effective treatment.[22] This early work with LSD on human volunteers introduced the LSD experience to college campuses and, from there, to a wider audience. The drug reached its peak in popularity during the late 1960s, after which its use decreased and stabilized.[23] Considering the history of other psychedelic drugs, it is unlikely that the recreational use of LSD will ever disappear.

Pharmacokinetics. LSD is usually taken orally, and it is rapidly absorbed by that route. Usual doses range from about 25 micrograms to more than 300 micrograms. Because such amounts are so small, LSD is often added to other substances, such as squares of paper, the backs of stamps, or sugar cubes, which can be handled more easily.[23] LSD is absorbed within about 60 minutes, reaching peak blood levels in about three hours. It is distributed rapidly and efficiently throughout the body; it diffuses easily into the brain and readily crosses the placenta. The largest amounts of LSD in the body are found in the liver, where the drug is metabolized before it is excreted. The usual duration of action is 6 to 8 hours.

Because of its extreme potency, only minuscule amounts can be detected in urine. Thus, conventional urine-screening tests are inadequate to detect LSD. When the use of LSD is suspected, urine is collected (up to 30 hours after ingestion) and an ultrasensitive radioimmunoassay is performed to verify the presence of the drug.

Physiological Effects. Although the LSD experience is characterized by its psychological effects, subtle physiological changes also occur. Persons who take LSD may experience a slight increase in body temperature, dilatation of the pupils, slightly increased heart rate and blood pressure, increased levels of glucose in the blood, and dizziness, drowsiness, nausea, and other effects that, although noticeable, seldom interfere with the psychedelic experience.

LSD is known to possess a low level of toxicity. Gable (1993)[24] estimates for LSD an effective dose of 50 micrograms and a lethal dose of 14,000 micrograms. These figures provide a therapeutic ratio of 280, making the drug a remarkably nonlethal compound. This calculation does not include any fatal accidents or suicides that occur when persons are intoxicated by LSD. Indeed, most deaths attributed to LSD result from accidents, homicides, or suicide.[23] The use of LSD during pregnancy is certainly unwise, although a distinct fetal LSD syndrome has not been described.

Psychological Effects. The psychological effects of LSD are quite intense. At doses of 25 to 50 micrograms, pupillary dilation and a glassy-eyed appearance may be noticed. These effects are accompanied by alterations in perception, thinking, emotion, arousal, and self-image. Time is slowed or distorted; sensory input intensifies. Cognitive alterations include enhanced power to visualize previously seen or imagined objects and decreased vigilance and logical thought. Visual alterations are the most characteristic phenomenon; they typically include colored lights, distorted images, and vivid and fascinating images and shapes. Colors can be heard and sounds may be seen. The loss of boundaries and the fear of fragmentation create a need for a structuring or supporting environment and experienced companions. During the "trip," thoughts and memories can emerge under self-guidance, sometimes to the user's distress. Mood may be labile, shifting from depression to gaiety, from elation to fear. Tension and anxiety may mount and reach panic proportions.

The LSD-induced psychedelic experience typically occurs in phases[3]:

1. The *somatic phase* occurs after absorption of the drug and consists of CNS stimulation and autonomic changes that are predominantly sympathomimetic in nature.
2. The *sensory* (or perceptual) *phase* is characterized by sensory distortions and pseudohallucinations, which are the effects desired by the drug user.
3. The *psychic phase* signals a maximum drug effect, with changes in mood, disruption of thought processes, altered perception of time, depersonalization, true hallucinations, and psychotic episodes. Experiencing this phase is considered a "bad trip."

In contrast to naturally occurring psychoses, auditory hallucinations are rare in LSD-induced psychosis. Synesthesias, the overflow from one sensory modality to another, may occur, but it is rare.

Tolerance and Dependence. Tolerance of both the psychological and physiological alterations that are induced by LSD readily and rapidly develops, and cross tolerance occurs between LSD and other psychedelics. This tolerance is lost within several days after the user stops taking the drug.

Physical dependence on LSD does not develop, even when the drug is used repeatedly for a prolonged period of time. In fact, most heavy users of the drug say that they ceased using LSD because they tired of it, had no further need for it, or had enough. Even when the drug is discontinued because of concern about bad trips or about physical or mental harm, few withdrawal signs are exhibited. Laboratory animals do not self-administer LSD.

Adverse Reactions and Toxicity. The adverse reactions attributed to LSD generally fall into five categories:

1. Chronic or intermittent psychotic states

2. Persistent or recurrent major affective disorder (i.e., depression)

3. Exacerbation of preexisting psychiatric illness

4. Disruption of personality or chronic brain syndrome, known as "burnout"

5. Post-hallucinogenic perceptual disorder (i.e., flashbacks character- ized by the periodic hallucinogenic imagery months or even years after the immediate effect of LSD has worn off.)[23]

Dimijian (1984)[25] wrote:

> Unpleasant experiences with LSD are relatively frequent and may in- volve an uncontrollable drift into confusion, dissociative reactions, acute panic reactions, a reliving of earlier traumatic experiences, or an acute psychotic hospitalization. Prolonged nonpsychotic reactions have included dissociative reactions, time and space distortion, body image changes, and a residue of fear or depression stemming from morbid or terrifying experiences under the drug. . . . With the failure of usual defense mechanisms, the onslaught of repressed material overwhelms the integrative capacity of the ego, and a psychotic reac- tion results. It appears that this [LSD-induced] disruption of long- established patterns of adapting may be a lasting or semipermanent effect of the drug.

LSD reduces a person's normal ability to control emotional reac- tions, and drug-induced alterations in perception can become so in- tense that they overwhelm one's ability to cope. There is also the pos- sible problem of persistent flashbacks, which may occur weeks or even months after the last use of the drug. Rang and Dale (1991)[26] elaborate:

There has been much concern over reports that LSD and other psychotomimetic drugs, as well as causing potentially dangerous "bad trips," can lead to more persistent mental disorders. There are recorded instances in which altered perception and hallucinations have lasted for up to three weeks following a single dose of LSD, and also reports of a persistent state resembling paranoid schizophrenia, which responds to antipsychotic drugs but may recur later. It is not at all clear whether this is due to a long-term effect of LSD, or whether LSD-taking is more likely in subjects destined to develop schizophrenia. The cautious view must be that LSD is causative. This, coupled with the fact that the occasional "bad trip" can result in severe injury through violent behavior, means that LSD and other psychotomimetics must be regarded as highly dangerous drugs.

Other Serotonin-Like Hallucinogens

DMT. DMT (*dim*ethyl *t*ryptamine) is a short-acting, naturally occurring psychedelic compound that is structurally related to serotonin. DMT can produce LSD-like effects in the user, and, like LSD, it has been shown to bind to serotonin 5-HT_2 receptors. Widely used throughout much of the world, DMT is an active ingredient (along with bufotenine, discussed next) of various types of South American snuffs. Unlike LSD, DMT is not absorbed when it is taken orally; it must be smoked or sniffed to be effective. DMT appears to be largely metabolized by the enzyme monoamine oxidase (MAO); no reports are available on the potential adverse effects of DMT taken by individuals treated with MAO inhibitors (see Chapter 7).

In 1994 Strassman, Qualls, and coworkers[27,28] conducted controlled investigations of DMT in "highly motivated," experienced hallucinogen users. Administered intravenously (0.04 mg/kg to 0.4 mg/kg body weight), onset of action occurred within 2 minutes and was negligible at 30 minutes. DMT elevated blood pressure, heart rate, and temperature, dilated pupils, and increased body endorphin and hormone levels. The psychedelic threshold dose was 0.2 mg/kg body weight, with lower doses primarily being "affective and somaesthetic."[28] Hallucinogenic effects included

a rapidly moving, brightly colored visual display of images. Auditory effects were less common. "Loss of control," associated with a brief, but overwhelming "rush," led to a dissociated state, where euphoria alternated or coexisted with anxiety. These effects completely replaced subjects' previously ongoing mental experience and were more vivid and compelling than dreams or waking awareness.[28]

Strassman et al.[28] present a new psychological testing instrument (the Hallucinogen Rating Scale) for evaluating effects of such drugs.

Bufotenine. *Bufotenine* (5-hydroxy DMT), like LSD and DMT, is a potent serotonin agonist hallucinogen with an affinity for several types of serotonin receptors. The name "bufotenine" comes from the name for a toad of the genus *bufo*, whose skin secretions supposedly produce hallucinogenic effects when ingested. Fuller and coworkers (1995)[30] studied the pharmacokinetics of bufotenine administered to rats. After subcutaneous injection, the half-life is about 2 hours with MAO responsible for metabolism (as it is for DMT).

In humans, research in the 1960s attempted to correlate the presence of bufotenine in urine (in humans bufotenine is formed from an unusual metabolic pathway for the metabolism of serotonin) with various psychiatric disorders. In the late 1990s, there is increasing interest in this correlation. Takeda (1994)[31] reviews the breakdown of serotonin (summarized in Figure 12.4), noting that the pathway to bufotenine is an abnormal metabolic pathway and "is an unusual route that is associated with the production of venoms or hallucinogens and is not associated with normal homeostasis in animals." Takeda and coworkers (1995)[32] studied urine specimens obtained from controls and from inpatients on a psychiatry ward. All patients were Japanese. Only two of 200 control urine specimens were positive for bufotenine; in 18 autistic patients with mental retardation and epilepsy, urine was positive in all; in autistic patients with mental retardation (no epilepsy), 32 of 47 were positive; in 18 patients with depression, urine was positive in 15; 13 of 15 schizophrenic patients tested positive for bufotenine. They concluded that the presence of bufotenine in urine may serve as a marker for some psychiatric disorders.

Karkkainen and coworkers (1995)[33] studied the urinary excretion of bufotenine in 112 Finnish male violent offenders. Suspiciousness was positively correlated, and socialization was negatively correlated with urinary bufotenine excretion. This and other results indicated that violent offenders with paranoid personality traits have higher urinary levels of bufotenine than other violent offenders.

These intriguing reports raise important questions about the role of altered metabolic pathways of serotonin (producing methylated derivatives) in the etiology of human psychiatric disorders such as autism and paranoia.

Psilocybin and Psilocin. *Psilocybin* (4-phosphoryl-DMT) and *psilocin* (4-hydroxy-DMT) are two psychedelic agents that are found in many

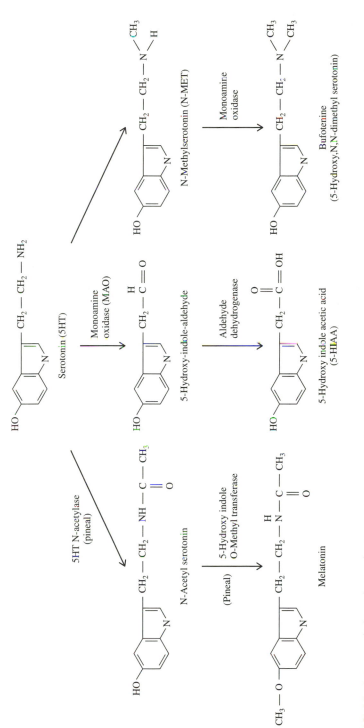

FIGURE 12.4   Metabolic pathways for serotonin (5-HT). The major pathway (shown in the center) leads to production of 5-HIAA, which is excreted by the kidneys. The pathway shown on the left occurs in the pineal gland and leads to the production of the neurohormone mela-tonin. The pathway on the right is an abnormal metabolic pathway leading to methylation of the terminal nitrogen group, and ultimately to the formation of bufotenine, a putative psychogenic substance. See text for discussion.

species of mushrooms that belong to the genera *Psilocybe, Panaeolus, Copelandia,* and *Conocybe.* These mushrooms grow throughout much of the world, including Thailand,[34] the Venezuelan Andes,[35] Central America, and the northwestern portion of the United States.[36]

Psilocin and psilocybin are approximately 1/200 as potent as LSD, and their effects last about 6 to 10 hours. Unlike DMT, psilocin and psilocybin are absorbed effectively when taken orally; the mushrooms are eaten raw to induce psychedelic effects. There is great variation in the concentration of psilocybin and psilocin among the different species of mushrooms, as well as significant differences among mushrooms of the same species. For example, the usual oral dose of *Psilocybe semilanceata* ("liberty caps") may consist of 10 to 40 mushrooms, while the dose for *Psilocybe cyanescens* may be only 2 to 5 mushrooms. Also, some extremely toxic species of mushrooms are not psychoactive, but they bear a superficial resemblance to the mushrooms that contain psilocybin and psilocin. Thus, to avoid unpleasant experiences, one must be familiar with all hallucinogenic and poisonous species of mushrooms. Because the effects of psilocybin so closely resemble those produced by LSD, the "psilocybin" sold illicitly may be LSD, and ordinary mushrooms laced with LSD may be sold as "magic mushrooms."[37]

As Figure 12.3 shows, the only difference between psilocybin and psilocin is that psilocybin contains a molecule of phosphoric acid. After the mushroom has been ingested, phosphoric acid is enzymatically removed from psilocybin, thus producing psilocin, the active psychedelic agent.

Although the psychedelic effects of *Psilocybe mexicana* have long been part of Indian folklore, *Psilocybe* intoxication was not described until 1955, when Gordon Wasson, a New York banker, traveled through Mexico. He mingled with native tribes and was allowed to participate in a *Psilocybe* ceremony, in which he consumed the magic mushroom. Wasson said:

> It permits you to travel backward and forward in time, to enter other planes of existence, even to know God. . . . Your body lies in the darkness, heavy as lead, but your spirit seems to soar and leave the hut, and with the speed of thought to travel where it listeth, in time and space, accompanied by the shaman's singing. . . . At least you know what the ineffable is, and what ecstasy means. Ecstasy! The mind harks back to the origin of that word. For the Greeks, ekstasis meant the flight of the soul from the body. Can you find a better word to describe this state?[38]

As might be predicted, the hallucinations and distortions of time and space that are caused by psilocybin resemble those produced by LSD. Weil (1980)[39] narrates his experiences with psilocybin mushrooms.

Ololiuqui. *Ololiuqui* (in morning glory seeds) is a naturally occurring hallucinogen that is used by Central and South American natives both as an intoxicant and as a hallucinogen. The drug is used ritually for spiritual communication, as are extracts of most plants that contain psychedelic drugs. The use of ololiuqui seeds in Central and South America was first described by the Spaniard Hernandez, who stated, "When the priests wanted to commune with their Gods . . . [they ate ololiuqui seeds and] a thousand visions and satanic hallucinations appeared to them."[40]

The seeds were analyzed in Europe by Albert Hofmann (the discoverer of LSD), who identified several ingredients, one being lysergic acid amide (not lysergic acid diethylamide, LSD). The lysergic acid amide that Hofmann identified is approximately one-tenth as active as LSD as a psychoactive agent. However, considering the extreme potency of LSD, lysergic acid amide is still quite potent.

Side effects of ololiuqui include nausea, vomiting, headache, increased blood pressure, dilated pupils, sleepiness, and so on. These side effects are usually quite intense and serve to limit the recreational use of ololiuqui. Ingestion of 100 or more seeds produces sleepiness, distorted perception, hallucinations, and confusion. Flashbacks have been reported, but they are infrequent.

Harmine. *Harmine* is a psychedelic agent that is obtained from the seeds of *Peganum harmala,* a plant native to the Middle East. These seeds have been used as intoxicants for centuries. Intoxication by harmine is usually accompanied by nausea and vomiting, sedation, and finally sleep. The psychic excitement that users experience consists of visual distortions that are similar to those induced by LSD. A psychedelic agent structurally similar to harmine, *ibogaine,* is discussed as an anticraving drug in Chapter 14.

Grob and coworkers (1996)[41] and Dobkin de Rios (1996)[42] describe a hallucinogenic concoction of potent psychoactive plants indigenous to the Brazilian and Peruvian Amazon. The active hallucinogen, termed *hoasca* or *ayahuasca,* contains harmine and two closely related compounds, harmaline and tetrahydroharmine. Less potent and longer-acting than DMT, hoasca is incorporated into native religious ceremonies as a legal, psychoactive sacrament, similar to the situation with peyote (discussed earlier) in the United States.

Phencyclidine: A Psychedelic Anesthetic

Phencyclidine (PCP, or "angel dust") and a related compound, *ketamine,* are referred to as psychedelic anesthetics. Their structures are illustrated in Figure 12.5. These two drugs are structurally unrelated to the other psychedelic agents, and their psychedelic effects are not thought to involve action on serotonin neurons.[43]

Phencyclidine was developed in 1956 as a potent analgesic-amnestic-anesthetic agent. It was briefly used as an anesthetic in humans before being abandoned because of a high incidence of bizarre and serious psychiatric reactions, including agitation, excitement, delirium, disorientation, and hallucinatory phenomena (considered undesirable in the surgical patient!). The altered perception, disorganized thought, suspiciousness, confusion, and lack of cooperation that were exhibited resembled a schizophrenic state[44,45] that consisted of both positive and negative symptoms.[46] Phencyclidine is still used as a veterinary anesthetic, primarily as an immobilizing agent.*

Small amounts of illicit phencyclidine became available in the mid-1960s, when it was referred to as the "peace pill" (PCP). Today, illicit phencyclidine still persists, with periodic resurgences in popularity. Phencyclidine has appeared in the form of powders, tablets, leaf mixtures, and 1-gram "rock" crystals. It is commonly sold as "crystal," "angel dust," "hog," "PCP," "THC," "cannabinol," or "mescaline." When phencyclidine is sold as crystal or angel dust (terms also used for methamphetamine), the drug is usually in concentrations that vary between 50 and 90 percent. When it is purchased under other names or in concoctions, the amount of phencyclidine falls to between 10 and 30 percent, with the typical street dose being about 5 milligrams.[43] Phencyclidine can be eaten, snorted, or injected, but it is most often smoked, sprinkled on tobacco, parsley, or marijuana.[2]

Pharmacokinetics

PCP is well absorbed whether taken orally or smoked. When it is smoked, peak effects occur in about 15 minutes, when about 40 percent of the dose appears in the user's bloodstream. Oral absorption is slower; maximum blood levels are not reached until about 2 hours after the drug has been taken. Following absorption and distribution, the drug persists in the body, mainly through a process termed *enterohepatic recirculation*, where the drug in plasma is secreted into the

---

*Ketamine induces a phencyclidine-like anesthetic state in low doses with only a moderate incidence of the bothersome psychiatric side effects. Ketamine is occasionally used in humans to provide anesthesia in patients who cannot tolerate the cardiovascular depressant effects of other anesthetics.

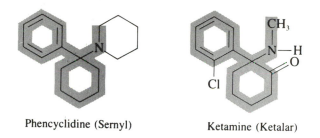

Phencyclidine (Sernyl)   Ketamine (Ketalar)

FIGURE 12.5 Structural formals of the psychedelic anesthetic drugs phencyclidine and ketamine.

stomach for later reabsorption, with the process continuing until the liver metabolizes the drug.[47] The elimination half-life is about 18 hours but ranges from about 11 to 51 hours. Cook and coworkers (1982)[47,48] describe the metabolism and excretion of phencyclidine after intravenous, oral, and smoked administration. A positive urine assay for PCP is assumed to indicate that PCP was used within the previous week. Because false-positive test results are common, a positive assay requires secondary confirmation.

Mechanism of Action

In 1979 experiments in rats demonstrated that phencyclidine binds to specific receptors in the brain. Within the next few years the binding sites were found to include the anterior forebrain (neocortex and olfactory structures), dentate gyrus, hippocampus, and the dorsal horns of the spinal cord. By 1990 it was concluded that these PCP receptors are located postsynaptically rather than presynaptically.[49]

Phencyclidine attaches to a binding site located within the channel of a specific receptor called the N-methyl-D-aspartate (NMDA) receptor, and phencyclidine is classified pharmacologically as an NMDA receptor antagonist, because it physically occludes the central pore and blocks the flow of calcium ions through the pore (see Appendix IV). The NMDA receptor is one of several types of receptors on which glutamate acts as the endogenous neurotransmitter (the other types of glutamate receptors are collectively called non-NMDA receptors):

> Glutamate receptors play a fundamental role in the function and dysfunction of the brain. These receptors are classified in two major classes according to their physiological and pharmacological properties: the NMDA and the non-NMDA receptors. NMDA receptors are

highly permeable to calcium and are considered crucial for induction of synaptic plasticity and neurotoxicity. NMDA receptors, in contrast to non-NMDA receptors, are targets of potent psychotropic agents such as the dissociative anesthetic phencyclidine, and the anticonvulsant and anxiolytic dizolcipine, collectively known as noncompetitive NMDA antagonists. PCP is an open channel blocker of the NMDA receptor, transiently occluding the pore. It . . . has . . . a promising strategy to prevent glutamate-mediated neuronal cell death and associated disorders such as stroke, epilepsy, and Huntington's disease.[50]

NMDA receptors are also involved in synaptic plasticity and in long-term enhancement of synaptic efficacy (i.e., long-term potentiation), thought to be the basis of processes involved in learning and memory. Indeed, NMDA blockers such as phencyclidine are among the best amnestic drugs known. NMDA antagonists have also been proposed as potentially advantageous as neuroprotective agents, potentially useful for the treatment of CNS ischemia and head trauma.[51] No NMDA agonists have been identified, although such agents might be of interest as potential cognitive enhancers. (They might also be convulsant and/or neurotoxic!) The action as a noncompetitive antagonist of the NMDA-glutamate receptor mediates the analgesic, psychotomimetic, and amnesic effects of phencyclidine.*

Orser, Pennefather, and MacDonald (1997)[53] investigated the mechanism of action of ketamine and concluded that it inhibits NMDA receptors by two mechanisms: (1) blockade of the open channel by occupying a site within the channel in the receptor protein (as discussed earlier for phencyclidine), and (2) reduction in the frequency of NMDA channel opening by drug binding to a second attachment site on the outside of the receptor protein. Phencyclidine probably shares this duality of action.

Psychological Effects

Phencyclidine dissociates individuals from themselves and their environment. It induces an unresponsive state with intense analgesia and amnesia, although the patient's eyes remain open (with a blank stare),

---

*Ikin and coworkers (1990)[52] isolated and analyzed the NMDA/PCP receptor complex. The receptor has a molecular weight of 203,000 and is composed of four membrane-spanning polypeptides (molecular weights of 67,000, 57,000, 46,000, and 33,000), which cluster together to form an ion channel that resembles the benzodiazepine-GABA receptor. Here, however, the drug-binding site (the PCP receptor) is located within the lumen of the ion channel. Attachment of PCP to the receptor occludes the channel and inhibits calcium ion influx when the transmitter (glutamate) attaches to its receptor on the outer surface.

and he or she may even appear to be awake. When not used under controlled conditions, phencyclidine in low doses produces mild agitation, euphoria, disinhibition, or excitement in a person who appears to be grossly drunk and exhibits a blank stare. The subject may be rigid and unable to speak. In many cases, however, the patient is communicative, although he or she does not respond to pain.

> PCP acutely induces a psychotic state in which subjects become withdrawn, autistic, negativistic, and unable to maintain a cognitive set, and manifest concrete, impoverished, idiosyncratic, and bizarre responses to proverbs and projective testing. Some subjects show catatonic posturing. These schizophrenic-like alterations in brain functioning went beyond the symptom level. . . . Any person under the influence of even a small amount of PCP . . . will have profound alterations of higher emotional functions affecting judgment and cognition.[54]

High doses of phencyclidine induce a state of coma or stupor. However, abusers tend to "titrate" their dose to maximize the intoxicant effect while attempting to avoid unconsciousness. Blood pressure usually becomes elevated, but respiration does not become depressed. The patient may recover from this state within 2 to 4 hours, although a state of confusion may last for 8 to 72 hours. The disruption of sensory input by PCP causes unpredictable exaggerated, distorted, or violent reactions to environmental stimuli. Such reactions are augmented by PCP-induced analgesia and amnesia.

Massive oral overdoses, involving up to 1 gram of street-purchased phencyclidine, result in prolonged periods of stupor or coma. This state may last for several days and may be marked by intense seizure activity, increased blood pressure, and a depression of respiration that is potentially lethal. Following this stupor, a prolonged recovery phase, marked by confusion and delusions, may last as long as 2 weeks. In some persons, this state of confusion may be followed by a psychosis that lasts from several weeks to a few months.

Side Effects and Toxicity

The course of recovery from a PCP-induced schizophrenic-like psychotic state is variable for reasons that are poorly understood. Flashbacks from phencyclidine may represent recurrence of psychosis. The intoxicated state may lead to severe anxiety, aggression, panic, paranoia, and rage. A user can also display violent reactions to sensory input, leading to such problems as falls, drowning, burns, driving accidents, and aggressive behavior. Self-inflicted injuries and injuries sustained while physical restraints are applied are frequent, and the potent analgesic action certainly contributes to the lack of response to pain. Respiratory depression, generalized seizure activity, and pulmonary edema have all been reported.

Tolerance, Dependence, and Abuse

PCP is the only psychedelic drug self-administered by monkeys. In man, this pattern of compulsive abuse is also seen. By inference, therefore, phencyclidine seems to stimulate brain reward areas and therefore places the user at risk of compulsive abuse despite negative health consequences. This probably is true, because there is an interaction between dopaminergic and glutaminergic neurons;[55,56] phencyclidine indirectly increases extracellular concentrations of dopamine.[57,58]

Tolerance to phencyclidine develops in laboratory animals, and twofold dose increases have been observed. Physiological dependence in humans is characterized by drug craving, anxiousness, tremor, gastrointestinal upset, and "cold sweats."[2]

Therapy for PCP intoxication is aimed at reducing the systemic level of the drug, keeping the individual calm and sedated, and preventing any of several severe adverse medical effects and involves:

- Minimization of sensory inputs by placing the intoxicated individual in a quiet environment
- Oral administration of activated charcoal, which can bind any PCP present in the stomach and intestine and prevent its reabsorption
- Precautionary physical restraint to prevent self-injury
- Sedation with either a benzodiazepine (such as lorazepam) for agitation or an antipsychotic (such as haloperidol, clozapine, or olanzapine) for psychosis

Hyperthermia, hypertension, convulsions, renal failure, and other medical consequences should be treated as necessary by medical experts. PCP-induced psychotic states may be long-lasting (even for several weeks), especially in individuals with schizophrenia.

NOTES

1. J. T. Ungerleider and R. N. Pechnick, "Hallucinogens," in J. H. Lowinson, P. Ruiz, R. B. Millman, and J. G. Langrod, eds., *Substance Abuse: A Comprehensive Textbook,* 2nd ed. (Baltimore: Williams & Wilkins, 1992), 280–289.

2. J. C. M. Brust, "Other Agents: Phencyclidine, Marijuana, Hallucinogens, Inhalants, and Anticholinergics," *Neurologic Clinics* 11 (1993): 555–561.

3. H. W. Hitner, "Psychotomimetic Drugs," in J. R. DiPalma and G. J. DiGregorio, eds., *Basic Pharmacology in Medicine*, 3rd ed. (New York: McGraw-Hill, 1990), 242–244.

4. S. Cohen, *The Chemical Brain: The Neurochemistry of Addictive Disorders* (Irvine, Calif.: Care Institute, 1988), 66–67.

5. D. Marona-Lewicka, G. Rhee, J. E. Sprague, and D. E. Nichols, "Reinforcing Effects of Certain Serotonin-Releasing Amphetamine Derivatives," *Pharmacology, Biochemistry, and Behavior* 53 (1996): 99–105.

6. K. M. Krebs and M. A. Geyer, "Cross-Tolerance Studies of Serotonin Receptors Involved in Behavioral Effects of LSD in Rats," *Psychopharmacology* 113 (1994): 429–437.

7. D. Fiorella, S. Helsley, D. S. Lorrain, et al., "The Role of 5-HT$_{2A}$ and 5-HT$_{2C}$ Receptors in the Stimulus Effects of Hallucinogenic Drugs. III: The Mechanistic Basis for Supersensitivity of the LSD Stimulus Following Serotonin Depletion," *Psychopharmacology* 121 (1995): 364–372.

8. N. Zec, J. J. Filiano, A. Panigrahy, et al., "Developmental Changes in [^{3}H] Lysergic Acid Diethylamide [^{3}H-LSD] Binding to Serotonin Receptors in the Human Brainstem," *Journal of Neuropathology and Experimental Neurology* 55 (1996): 114–126.

9. L. Hermle, M. Funfgeld, G. Oepen, et al., "Mescaline-Induced Psychopathological, Neuropsychological, and Neurometabolic Effects in Normal Subjects: Experimental Psychosis as a Tool for Psychiatric Research," *Biological Psychiatry* 32 (1992): 976–991.

10. J. R. Coore, "A Fatal Trip with Ecstasy: A Case of 3,4-Methylene-Dioxymethampetamine/3,4-Methylenedioxy-Amphetamine Toxicity," *Journal of the Royal Society of Medicine* 89 (1996): 51P-52P.

11. A. Goldstein, *Addiction: From Biology to Drug Policy* (New York: W. H. Freeman and Company, 1994), 197.

12. M. E. Molliver, U. V. Berger, L. A. Mamounas, et al., "Neurotoxicity of MDMA and Related Compounds: Anatomic Studies," *Annals of the New York Academy of Sciences* 600 (1990): 640–661.

13. G. A. Ricaurte, K. T. Finnegan, I. Irwin, and J. W. Langston, "Aminergic Metabolites in Cerebrospinal Fluid of Humans Previously Exposed to MDMA: Preliminary Observations," *Annals of the New York Academy of Sciences* 600 (1990): 699–708.

14. M. Demirkiran, J. Jankovic, and J. M. Dean, "Ecstasy Intoxication: An Overlap Between Serotonin Syndrome and Neuroleptic Malignant Syndrome," *Clinical Neuropharmacology* 19 (1996): 157–164.

15. R. S. Cohen, "Adverse Symptomatology and Suicide Associated with the Use of Methylenedioxymethamphetamine (MDMA; 'Ecstasy')," *Biological Psychiatry* 39 (1996): 819–820.

16. J. E. Malberg, K. E. Sabol, and L. S. Seiden, "Co-administration of MDMA with Drugs that Protect Against MDMA Neurotoxicity Produces Different Effects on Body Temperature in the Rat," *Journal of Pharmacology and Experimental Therapeutics* 278 (1996): 258–267.

17. M. K. Abernethy and L. B. Becker, "Acute Nutmeg Intoxication," *American Journal of Emergency Medicine* 10 (1992): 429–430.

18. N. Almaula, B. J. Ebersole, D. Zhang, et al., "Mapping the Binding Site Pocket of the Serotonin 5-Hydroxytryptamine$_{2A}$ Receptor," *Journal of Biological Chemistry* 271 (1996): 14672–14675.

19. N. J. Penington and A. P. Fox, "Effects of LSD on Ca^{++} Currents in Central 5-HT-Containing Neurons: 5-HT$_{1A}$ Receptors May Play a Role in Hallucinogenesis," *Journal of Pharmacology and Experimental Therapeutics* 269 (1994): 1160–1165.

20. A. Hofmann, "Notes and Documents Concerning the Discovery of LSD," *Agents and Actions* 43 (1994): 79–81.

21. *Interim Drug Report of the Commission of Inquiry into the Nonmedical Use of Drugs* (Ottawa: Information Canada, 1970), 58–59.

22. A. Goldstein, *Addiction: From Biology to Drug Policy* (New York: W. H. Freeman and Company, 1994), 202.

23. R. H. Schwartz, "LSD: Its Rise, Fall, and Renewed Popularity Among High School Students," *Pediatric Clinics of North America* 42 (1995): 403–413.

24. R. S. Gable, "Toward a Comparative Overview of Dependence Potential and Acute Toxicity of Psychoactive Substances Used Nonmedically," *American Journal of Drug and Alcohol Abuse* 19 (1993): 263–281.

25. G. G. Dimijian, "Contemporary Drug Abuse," in A. Goth, ed., *Medical Pharmacology*, 11th ed. (St. Louis: Mosby, 1984), 156.

26. H. P. Rang and M. M. Dale, *Pharmacology*, 2nd ed. (Edinburgh: Churchill Livingstone, 1991), 743–744.

27. R. J. Strassman and C. R. Qualls, "Dose-Response Study of N,N-Dimethyltryptamine in Humans. I. Neuroendocrine, Autonomic, and Cardiovascular Effects," *Archives of General Psychiatry* 51 (1994): 85–97.

28. R. J. Strassman, C. R. Qualls, E. H. Uhlenhuth, and R. Kellner, "Dose-Response Study of N,N-Dimethyltryptamine in Humans. II. Subjective Effects and Preliminary Results of a New Rating Scale," *Archives of General Psychiatry* 51 (1994): 98–108.

29. T. Lyttle, "Misuse and Legend in the 'Toad Licking' Phenomenon," *International Journal of the Addictions* 28 (1993): 521–538.

30. R. W. Fuller, H. D. Snoddy, and K. W. Perry, "Tissue Distribution, Metabolism, and Effects of Bufotenine Administered to Rats," *Neuropharmacology* 34 (1995): 799–804.

31. N. Takeda, "Serotonin-Degradative Pathways in the Toad (*Bufo bufo japonicus*) Brain: Clues to the Pharmacological Analysis of Human Psychiatric Disorders," *Comparative Biochemistry and Physiology. Pharmacology, Toxicology and Endocrinology* 107(1994): 275–281.

32. N. Takeda, R. Ikeda, K. Ohba and M. Kondo, "Bufotenine Reconsidered as a Diagnostic Indicator of Psychiatric Disorders," *NeuroReport* 6 (1995): 2378–2380.

33. J. Karkkainen, M. Raisanen, M. O. Huttunen, et al., "Urinary Excretion of Bufotenin (N,N-dimethyl-5-hydroxytryptamine) Is Increased in Suspicious Violent Offenders: A Confirmatory Study," *Psychiatry Research* 58 (1995): 145–152.

34. J. Gartz, J. W. Allen, and M. D. Merlin, "Ethnomycology, Biochemistry, and Cultivation of Psilocybe samuiensis Guzman, Bandala and Allen, A New Psychoactive Fungus from Koh Samui, Thailand," *Journal of Ethnopharmacology* 43 (1994): 73–80.

35. V. Marcano, A. Mendez, F. Castellano, et al., "Occurrence of Psilocybin and Psilocin in Psilocybe pseudobullacea (Petch) Pegler from the Venezuelan Andes," *Journal of Ethnopharmacology* 43 (1994): 157–159.

36. J. Ott, *Hallucinogenic Plants of North America* (Berkeley, Calif.: Wingbow Press, 1979).

37. A. Goldstein, *Addiction: From Biology to Drug Policy* (New York: W. H. Freeman and Company, 1994), 195.

38. M. E. Crahan, "God's Flesh and Other Pre-Columbian Phantastica," *Bulletin of the Los Angeles County Medical Association* 99 (1969): 17.

39. A. Weil, *The Marriage of the Sun and the Moon* (Boston: Houghton Mifflin, 1980), 73–79.

40. E. M. Brecher and Consumer Reports Editors, *Licit and Illicit Drugs* (Mt. Vernon, N.Y: Consumers Union, 1972), 345.

41. C. S. Grob, D. J. McKenna, J. C. Callaway, et al., "Human Psychopharmacology of Hoasca, A Plant Hallucinogen Used in Ritual Context in Brazil," *Journal of Nervous and Mental Disease* 184 (1996): 86–94.

42. M. Dobkin de Rios, "On 'Human Pharmacology of Hoasca': A Medical Anthropology Perspective," *Journal of Nervous and Mental Disease* 184 (1996): 95–98.

43. S. R. Zukin and R. S. Zukin, "Phencyclidine," in J. H. Lowinson, P. Ruiz, R. B. Millman, and J. G. Langrod, eds., *Substance Abuse: A Comprehensive Textbook,* 2nd ed. (Baltimore: Williams & Wilkins, 1992), 290–302.

44. A. L. Halberstadt, "The Phencyclidine-Glutamate Model of Schizophrenia," *Clinical Neuropharmacology* 18 (1995): 237–249.

45. S. A. Thornberg and S. R. Saklad, "A Review of NMDA Receptors and the Phencyclidine Model of Schizophrenia," *Pharmacotherapy* 16 (1996): 82–93.

46. M. O. Krebs, "Glutamatergic Hypothesis of Schizophrenia: Psychoses Induced by Phencyclidine and Cortical-Subcortical Imbalance," *Encephale* 21 (1995): 581–588.

47. C. E. Cook, D. R. Brine, A. R. Jeffcoat, et al., "Phencyclidine Disposition after Intravenous and Oral Doses," *Clinical Pharmacology and Therapeutics* 31 (1982): 625–634.

48. C. E. Cook, D. R. Brine, G. D. Quin, et al., "Phencyclidine and Phenylcyclohexene Disposition after Smoking Phencyclidine," *Clinical Pharmacology and Therapeutics* 31 (1982): 635–641.

49. J. W. Bekenstein, J. P. Bennett, Jr., G. F. Wooten, and E. W. Lothman, "Autoradiographic Evidence that NMDA Receptor-Coupled Channels Are Located Postsynaptically and Not Presynaptically in the Perforant Path-Dentate Granule Cell System of the Rat Hippocampal Formation," *Brain Research* 514 (1990): 334–342.

50. A. V. Ferrer-Montiel, W. Sun, and M. Montal, "Molecular Design of the N-methyl-d-aspartate Receptor Binding Site for Phencyclidine and Dizol-

cipine," *Proceedings of the National Academy of Science, USA* 92 (1995): 8021–8025.

51. B. Ault, M. S. Miller, M. D. Kelly, et al., "WIN 63480, A Hydrophilic TCP-Site Ligand, Has Reduced Agonist-Independent NMDA Ion Channel Access Compared to MK-801 and Phencyclidine," *Neuropharmacology* 34 (1995): 1597–1606.

52. A. F. Ikin, Y. Kloog and M. Sokolovsky, "N-Methyl-D-Aspartate/Phencyclidine Receptor Complex of Rat Forebrain: Purification and Biochemical Characterization," *Biochemistry* 29 (1990): 2290.

53. B. A. Orser, P. S. Pennefather, and J. F. MacDonald, "Multiple Mechanisms of Ketamine Blockade of N-methyl-D-aspartate Receptors," *Anesthesiology* 86 (1997): 903–917.

54. S. R. Zukin and R. S. Zukin, "Phencyclidine," in J. H. Lowinson, P. Ruiz, R. B. Millman, and J. G. Langrod, eds., *Substance Abuse: A Comprehensive Textbook*, 2nd ed. (Baltimore: Williams & Wilkins, 1992), 296.

55. I. M. White, G. S. Flory, K. C. Hooper, et al., "Phencyclidine-Induced Increases in Striatal Neuron Firing in Behaving Rats: Reversal by Haloperidol and Clozapine," *Journal of Neural Transmission*, General Section, 102 (1995): 99–112.

56. W. A. Carlezon, Jr., and R. A. Wise, "Rewarding Actions of Phencyclidine and Related Drugs in Nucleus Accumbens Shell and Frontal Cortex," *Journal of Neuroscience* 16 (1996): 3112–3122.

57. G. R. Hanson, L. P. Midgley, L. G. Bush, and J. W. Gibb, "Response of Extrapyramidal and Limbic Neurotensin Systems to Phencyclidine Treatment," *European Journal of Pharmacology* 278 (1995): 167–173.

58. E. D. French, "Phencyclidine and the Midbrain Dopamine System: Electrophysiology and Behavior," *Neurotoxicology and Teratology* 16 (1994): 355–362.

Chapter 13

ANABOLIC-ANDROGENIC STEROIDS

Neurons interact with one another through the release of chemical neurotransmitters, which are appropriately called *neurohormones*. A hormone is a substance that is released by one cell and then exerts its effect on a different organ. Neurotransmitters travel only a short distance from their site of release to their site of action (across a synaptic cleft). Other hormones (compounds such as estrogen, insulin, thyroid hormone, growth hormone, and testosterone) are released into the bloodstream and are transported to target organs that are a distance away.

In several cases, in response to low levels of circulating body hormones, the hypothalamus responds by emitting a "releasing factor" (usually a small protein) into the blood, in which it is carried to the pituitary gland, where it induces the synthesis and release of a second hormone or hormones (see Figure 13.1). The pituitary hormones are released from cells within the pituitary gland into the bloodstream and travel to distant sites in the body where they act on target organs to affect their functioning (see Figure 13.2). Pertinent to the present discussion is an understanding of the regulation of the release of one hypothalamic-releasing factor (*gonadotropin-releasing hormone, or GRF*) and two pituitary hormones (*follicle-stimulating hormone, or FSH, and luteinizing hormone, or LH*).

When the plasma level of a body hormone, such as *testosterone* (the primary male sex hormone), falls, cells in the hypothalamus (which have receptors sensitive to the circulating amount of testosterone) sense the decrease and begin producing its releasing factor

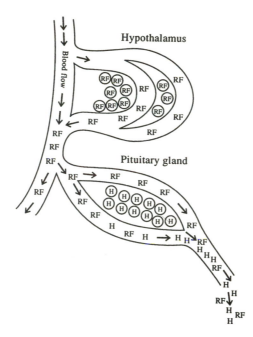

FIGURE 13.1 Blood flow enters the hypothalamus, carrying gonadotropin-releasing factors (RF) as it leaves the structure. This releasing factor induces the release of the pituitary hormones (H), FSH, and LH, which are released into the blood that leaves the gland.

(here, GRF). GRF is released and stimulates the pituitary gland to produce and release FSH and LH. In turn, FSH and LH act on the testes to induce both spermatogenesis (the production of sperm) and the synthesis and release of testosterone. (A similar process in the female regulates fertility, discussed in Appendix I.)

As testosterone levels in blood increase, the hypothalamus decreases its production of GRF; the pituitary gland decreases production of FSH and LH; the testes decrease production of testosterone (and decrease sperm production); and the process repeats. In the male, this is an ongoing process rather than a cyclic one, as it is in the female. Administering exogenous testosterone or testosterone-like drugs, called *anabolic-androgenic steroids*, overwhelms this system; abnormally high blood levels of testosterone shut off production of all these hormones (GRF, FSH, LH, and testosterone), decreasing spermatogenesis (see Figure 13.2).

Two examples of this process are pertinent to the topics of drug education and drug misuse. The first example is the regulation of female fer-

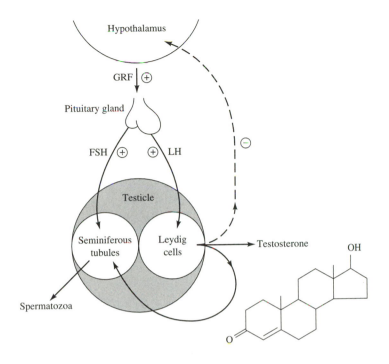

FIGURE 13.2 Hormonal regulation of male fertility. The brain (hypothalamus and pituitary gland) is involved in the control of fertility. However, fertility in the male is not subject to periodic cycling as it is in the female. The structure of naturally occurring testosterone is shown. GRF-gonadotropin-releasing factor; FSH = follicle stimulating hormone; LH = luteinizing hormone. Solid arrows = stimulation; dashed arrows = inhibition.

tility by estrogen and progesterone, two reproductive hormones that can be suppressed or increased by drugs. Contraceptive drugs suppress the release of fertility-inducing hormones from the hypothalamus and pituitary gland and therefore suppress fertility and decrease the possibility of pregnancy; drugs that increase fertility perform in the opposite way. The hormonal regulation of female fertility is discussed in Appendix I.

The second example involves the endogenous anabolic-androgenic steroid testosterone and its synthetic derivatives. These compounds (1) block the normal process that regulates testosterone, male fertility, and spermatogenesis, and (2) exert peripheral hormonal actions to increase muscle mass, enhance physical appearance and athletic performance, build muscles, and increase aggression. In recent years, the abuse of the anabolic-androgenic steroids by both men and women has become a topic of increasing concern.

Mechanism of Action and Effects

The anabolic-androgenic steroids (A-ASs) are a group of drugs that include the male sex hormone testosterone and several synthetically produced structural derivatives of testosterone. The term *anabolic-androgenic steroids* arises because these substances have both body-building (anabolic) and masculinizing (androgenic) effects.[1] In the past few years, A-ASs have become increasingly controversial because they are widely used illicitly by both men and women to promote athletic performance and to improve physical appearance. Indeed, public concern rose to the point where Congress passed the Anabolic Steroids Act of 1990 to control the distribution and sale of the drugs. This act added these drugs to Schedule III of the Controlled Substances Act of 1990, classifying them as drugs with abuse potential that may lead to dependence.

Figure 13.3 illustrates the chemical structures of testosterone and several available derivatives. These differ from each other not so much in structure but primarily in their individual resistance to metabolic degradation by liver enzymes. After oral administration, testosterone is effectively absorbed from the intestine. Following absorption, it is rapidly transported in the blood to the liver, where it is immediately metabolized. As a result, little testosterone reaches the systemic circulation.[2] Administered by injection, some of this "first-pass metabolism" is blunted, and it is the metabolic product, androstanolone, that is most active as an anabolic substance.[2] Structural modification of the testosterone molecule can reduce metabolic degradation and thus improve the effectiveness of both oral and intramuscular administration.

Not all these drugs are illicit substances. Eight synthetic A-AS substances (see Table 13.1) are approved in the United States for therapeutic uses, including testosterone replacement in hypogonadal males, the treatment of certain blood anemias and severe muscle loss following trauma, and, in females, the treatment of endometriosis and fibrocystic disease of the breast.[3]

Mechanism of Action

The mechanism of action of testosterone and other A-AS drugs is quite well understood. The natural hormone is synthesized principally in a specialized type of cell (the Leydig cell) of the testes (see Figure 13.2). This occurs under the influence of GRF released from the hypothalamus, which stimulates the synthesis and release of LH from the pituitary gland; LH acts on the Leydig cells to stimulate testosterone production.

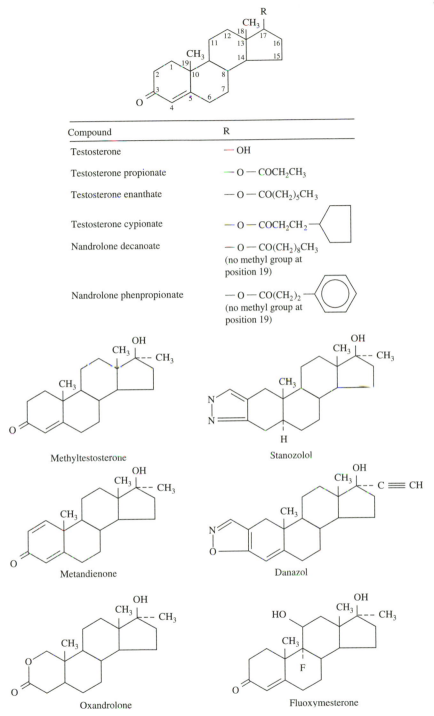

FIGURE 13.3 Structures of some common parenteral (left) and oral (right) anabolic-androgenic steroids. [Reproduced from S. E. Lucas (1993).[2]]

TABLE 13.1 Anabolic-androgenic steroids

Name	Route	Brand name
U.S. APPROVED		
Testosterone cypionate	im	Depo-Testosterone, Virilon
Nandrolone phenpropionate	im	Durabolin
Nandrolone decanoate	im	Deca-Duraboli
Danazol	po	Danocrine
Fluoxymesterone	po	Halotestin
Methyltestosterone	po	Android, Metandren, Testred, Virilon
Oxymetholone	po	Anadrol-50
Slanozolol	po	Winstrol
OUTSIDE U.S.		
Testosterone enanthate	im	Delatestryl
Testosterone propionate	im	Testex, Oreton propionate
Methenolone enanthate	im	Primobolan Depot
Ethylestrenol	po	Maxibolan
Mesterolone	po	
Methandrostenolone	po	Dianabol
Methenolone	po	Primobolan
Norethandrolone	po	
Oxandrolone	po	Anavar
Oxymesterone	po	Oranabol
VETERINARY		
Bolasterone	im	Finiject 30
Boldenone undecylenate	im	Equipoise
Stanozolol	im	Winstrol
Mibolerone	po	

Reproduced with permission from K. B. Kashkin (1992).[3]
Note: im, intramuscular; po, oral.

Once in the bloodstream, testosterone (or an exogenous A-AS) passes through the cell walls of its target tissues and attaches to steroid receptors in the cytoplasm of the cell[2] (see Figure 13.4). This hormone-receptor complex is translocated into the nucleus of the cell and attaches to the nuclear material (the DNA). A process of genetic transcription follows, and new messenger RNA is produced. Translation of this RNA results in the production of specific new pro-

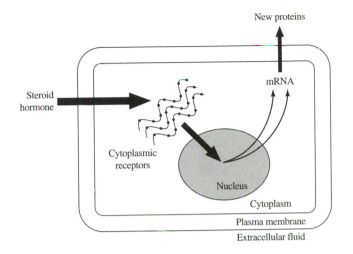

FIGURE 13.4 Mechanism of action of steroid hormones on cells. The hormone passes through the cell wall of its target tissue and binds to steroid receptors in the cytoplasm. The hormone-receptor complex moves into the nucleus and binds to sites on the chromatin, which is transcribed to give specific messenger RNA (mRNA). The mRNA is translated into specific new proteins that mediate the function of the hormone. [Reproduced with permission from S. E. Lucas (1993).[2]]

teins that leave the cell and mediate the biological functions of the hormone. Thus, the effects of A-AS on target cells are mediated by intracellular receptors and the synthesis of new proteins. The increased levels of circulating testosterone (or other A-AS drugs) exert a negative feedback effect on the hypothalamus, inhibiting further stimulation of testosterone release.

Effects on Athletic Performance

A-ASs are widely abused by athletes, recreational body builders, and nonathletes because these drugs increase muscle mass and strength and produce a more masculine appearance. The assumption that this is what happens has been around a long time, but the report by Bhasin and coworkers (1996)[4] was the first to demonstrate that supraphysiologic doses of testosterone, with or without strength training, increase fat-free mass, muscle size, and strength in normal men. As shown in Figure 13.5, exercise alone or testosterone alone produced increases in strength, triceps and quadriceps size, and fat-free mass. The combination of testosterone and exercise produced additive increases. Despite these beneficial effects of testosterone, the authors concluded:

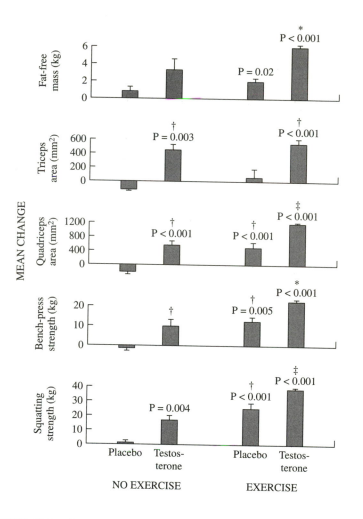

FIGURE 13.5 Changes from base line in mean (±SE) fat-free mass, triceps, and quadriceps cross-sectional areas, and muscle strength in the bench-press and squatting exercises over the 10 weeks of treatment. The P values shown are for the comparison between the change indicated and a change of zero. The asterisks indicate P < 0.05 for the comparison between the change indicated and that in either no-exercise group; the daggers, P < 0.05 for the comparison between the change indicated and that in the group assigned to placebo with no exercise; and the double daggers, P < 0.05 for the comparison between the change indicated and the changes in all three other groups. [Reproduced with permission from S. Bhasin et al. (1996).[4]]

Our results in no way justify the use of anabolic-androgenic steroids in sports, because, with extended use, such drugs have potentially serious adverse effects on the cardiovascular system, prostate, lipid metabolism, and insulin sensitivity. Moreover, the use of any performance-enhancing agent in sports raises serious ethical issues.

Thus, A-ASs can increase both the size and the strength of the athlete and thereby improve performance in athletic activities that require size and strength. Anabolic steroids have no positive effects on aerobic performance of the athlete.[5]

A-ASs induce size and strength gains through *anticatabolic, anabolic*, and *motivational effects* on the athlete. Table 13.2 summarizes the constellation of effects and side effects. The anticatabolic effect means that the A-ASs block the action of natural cortisone, which normally functions to increase energy stores during periods of stress and training. Cortisone makes energy stores available by breaking down proteins into their constituent amino acids. Carried to excess, muscle wasting can occur. This action is blocked by the A-ASs. Indeed, the anticatabolic action may be the major mechanism by which these drugs ultimately increase body mass.[5]

The anabolic effects follow and induce the synthesis of new protein in muscle cells. Effects also follow from A-AS–induced release of endogenous growth hormone, which has anabolic effects as well.[5] It is important to note, however, that the doses commonly used by athletes are 10 to 200 times the therapeutic dosage for testosterone deficiency. This often involves the "stacking" or "pyramiding" of multiple drugs, even combining oral and injectable substances through cycles of several weeks' duration.[3] According to Bower (1993)[1]: "There is near, but incomplete, scientific consensus that A-ASs do increase muscle strength and lean body mass when combined with intensive training and a proper diet." Kashkin (1992)[3] summarizes:

> It is known that androgens can increase the rate of RNA transcription above that found with exercise alone and that androgens can induce the formation of new myofilaments (the contractile filaments in muscle) and cause enlarging myofibrils (muscle cells) to divide.

The motivational effects are profound, and athletes taking A-ASs often develop very aggressive personalities, a condition nicknamed "roid rage." This effect can be reproduced in animals fed large doses of these drugs. Lucas (1993)[2] notes: "For some sports, such as football, these steroids may serve the dual purpose of increasing strength and performance as well as enhancing combativeness."

In the female athlete, A-AS drugs exert the same anabolic and anticatabolic effects found in male athletes. However, these drugs also induce in females masculinizing and other effects, including increases in facial and body hair, lowered voice, enlarged clitoris, coarser skin, and menstrual cycle cessation or irregularity. Cessation of steroid use results in a variable and often incomplete return of the altered functions.

TABLE 13.2 Effects of anabolic-androgenic steroids

Positive effects
  Transient increase in muscular size and strength
  Treatment of catabolic states
    Trauma
    Surgery
Adverse effects
  Cardiovascular
    Increase in cardiac risk factors
      Hypertension
      Altered lipoprotein fractions
      Increase in LDL/HDL ratio
    Reported strokes/myocardial infarctions
  Hepatic effects associated with oral compounds
    Elevated liver enzymes
    Peliosis hepatis (greater than 6 months' use)
    Liver tumors
      Benign
      Malignant (greater than 24 months' use)
  Reproductive system effects
    In males
      Decreased testosterone production
        Abnormal spermatogenesis
        Transient infertility
        Testicular atrophy
    In females
      Altered menstruation
  Endocrine effects
    Decreased thyroid function
  Immunologic effects
    Decreased immunoglobulins IgM/IgA/IgC
  Musculoskeletal effects
    Premature closure of bony growth centers
    Tendon degeneration
      Increased risk of tendon tears
  Cosmetic
    In males
      Gynecomastia
      Testicular atrophy
      Acne
      Acceleration of male pattern baldness
    In females
      Clittoral enlargement
      Acne
      Increased facial/body hair
      Coarsening of the skin
      Male pattern baldness
      Deepened voice
  Psychologic
    Risk of habituation
    Severe mood swings
    Aggressive tendencies
    Psychotic episodes
    Depression
    Reports of suicide
  Legislation
    Classified as Schedule III controlled substance

Reproduced with permission from H. A. Haupt (1995).[5]

These drugs are also widely used (and abused) by young male (usually noncompetitive) athletes who take them to develop the muscular physique considered fashionable. Haupt (1993)[5] estimates that about 6 percent of male high school seniors under age 18 have used or currently use A-ASs. This figure represents between 250,000 and 500,000 young adult males. It should be noted, however, that the prevalence of A-As abuse is notoriously difficult to estimate. Drewnowski and coworkers (1995)[6] report, in a study of Michigan high school seniors, an incidence of use of only 0.6 percent. DuRant and coworkers (1995),[7] in a much more thorough study, report that 4 percent of high school males and 1.2 percent of high school females used A-ASs, with the highest prevalence in the southern United States. A-AS use was associated with the use of other illegal drugs, tobacco, and alcohol and with a self-perception of poor academic performance. Middleman and DuRant (1996)[8] note that between 4 percent and 11 percent of male adolescents and 0.5 percent and 2.9 percent of female adolescents in the United States report ever having used anabolic steroids. Nilsson (1995),[9] in a study from Sweden, reports that 5.8 percent of male teenagers report having used these agents. Among recreational adult weightlifters, A-AS use ranges from 12 to 44 percent. An estimated 80 percent of professional football linebackers and linemen use these drugs.[10] Thus, regardless of the exact number, a significant number of teenagers and young adults, primarily male, use supraphysiologic doses of A-ASs to give them more muscle strength and a more powerful, masculine appearance.

In nonathletes, males use A-ASs primarily to improve physique and physical appearance. Unlike competitive athletes who may choose to terminate drug use when competition ends, nonathlete youths may continue to take A-ASs in order to maintain the cosmetic effect. As stated by Schwerin and coworkers (1996)[10]:

> Physique and physical appearance are ever important in how people are viewed in their social environment. With these come the spoils: social acceptance, admiration, and opportunity. To a certain extent, an attractive physique is related to enhanced self-esteem and perceived social competence. . . . Sometimes the drive reaches an unhealthy extreme . . . taking the form of anorexia, bulimia, and anabolic steroid use.

Furthermore:

> A-AS users present an appearance of healthfulness, strength, "sex appeal," and physical attractiveness. Other illicit drugs do not present such an image of healthfulness. . . . It may be this contradiction of

increased A-AS use leading to increased appearance of healthfulness and physical attractiveness which may allow the seriousness of A-AS use to remain underappreciated. . . . A-ASs are the only addictive substance over the short to middle term that enhances a user's physical appearance and whose purpose is to allow the user to work harder and longer (though stimulants share this latter characteristic).

Endocrine Effects

Males taking A-ASs experience a hypogonadal state, which is characterized by atrophy of the testicles, impaired production of sperm, and infertility, causing reduced libido and impotence.[11,12] These effects are usually reversible within a few months after cessation of drug use. However, as stated by Bickelman and coworkers (1995)[12]:

> Even when gonadal dysfunction occurs, persons often continue using the anabolic steroids, in part because of the neuropsychiatric effects, which include psychotic symptoms, affective syndromes, increased aggression, and psychological dependence.

In addition, gynecomastia (enlargement of the breasts in males) may occur. Many users are quite sophisticated in their drug use, using such information sources as the "Underground Steroid Handbook" to guide therapy, which includes "the use of human chorionic gonadotropin, clomiphene citrate, and tamoxifen citrate, to counter the side effects of gynecomastia and reduced testicular volume."[12] The gynecomastia apparently results from some of the A-ASs being metabolized to the female hormone estradiol.[13]

Cardiovascular Effects

Adverse effects on the cardiovascular system have been of concern, and two reports of fatal myocardial infarctions (heart attacks) occurring in users of A-ASs have been published. Atherosclerosis-induced coronary artery disease was implicated in these deaths. Thus, analysis of the potential correlation between A-ASs and atherosclerosis is important. The effect of these steroids on blood cholesterol as a predisposing factor to atherosclerotic coronary artery disease must be considered. Cholesterol is of two types: "bad" cholesterol (low-density lipoprotein cholesterol, or LDL) and "good" cholesterol (high-density lipoprotein cholesterol, or HDL). Decreasing HDL and increasing LDL are strongly correlated with an increased risk of coronary artery disease.

All A-ASs induce a reduction in serum HDL cholesterol and an elevation in LDL cholesterol. This suggests that individuals taking these drugs are at greater risk of suffering coronary artery disease. This condition can be expressed as myocardial infarctions, thromboembolic disease (blood clots and emboli), strokes, and hypertension. The actual risk of cardiovascular disease is unknown at this time, largely due to the young age of users, their relatively lean or muscular physiques, and the intermittent pattern of drug use. We may have to wait until these users are adults to determine whether they have been harmed by using A-ASs during their earlier years. Melchert and Welder (1995)[14] review these adverse cardiovascular effects of the A-ASs and propose several models to explain this toxicity.

Effects on the Liver

The use of oral A-AS preparations has been associated with a risk of liver disorders, especially jaundice and tumors.[2] Increases in the blood levels of liver enzymes, indicative of possible liver dysfunction, are quite common among users of A-ASs.[3] Hepatitis is also not uncommon. In addition, several dozen cases of liver carcinomas of unusual types have been reported.[15] The incidence of developing these potentially fatal carcinomas is estimated to be 1 to 3 percent within 2 to 8 years of exposure to drugs.

Psychological Effects

A-ASs are centrally acting drugs, involved in the regulation of sexuality, aggression, cognition, emotion, and personality.[16] Thus, drug-induced increases in aggression, competitiveness, and combativeness can be predicted in individuals using large doses of these drugs.[17] It is now well established that areas of the brain that influence mood and judgment contain steroid receptors and that sharp fluctuations in the levels of steroid hormones have profound psychological effects.[3] Steroid receptors are widely distributed in the central nervous system (CNS), especially in the hypothalamus and the limbic regions. In the hypothalamus, they autoregulate their own reproductive actions (through the negative feedback system discussed earlier). Hypothalamic actions also modulate other vegetative systems of the body, a matter of importance during steroid withdrawal. The limbic receptors appear to account for the effects of steroids on mood.

Thus, A-ASs administered in regular large doses are indeed mood-altering chemicals. They do, however, have a delayed onset of effect. This delay occurs because their mechanism of synthesizing new proteins takes days or weeks. Because their effects are not immediate, they may not be perceived as being a consequence of drug ingestion. Questions have been raised about immediate effects on opioid, GABA, and other receptors, but these effects are little understood.[3] Haupt (1993)[5] summarizes:

> There are significant adverse psychological effects associated with the use of anabolic steroids although the effects are not easily measured by current psychological inventories. Athletes taking anabolic steroids suffer some degree of personality change that may range from simple mood swings to a psychosis requiring hospitalization for treatment. A Jekyll-and-Hyde personality is common, where even the slightest provocation can cause an exaggerated, violent, and often uncontrolled response. The users of anabolic steroids often suffer disturbed personality relationships that may include separations from family and friends and even divorce. Arrest records are not uncommon. Fortunately these psychological effects are reversible when the steroids are discontinued, but the social scars may be permanent.

Kashkin (1992)[3] reviews these psychological effects at length, adding that about half of a small population of interviewed weightlifters experienced depression and an even higher percentage experienced paranoid thoughts and some psychotic features.

Health Risk Behaviors

The use of anabolic steroids has been linked to other high risk behaviors. Used in combination with alcohol and cocaine, additive increases in aggressive behavior may be observed.[18] In addition:

> The frequency of anabolic steroid use was significantly associated with the frequency of use of cocaine, the use of other drugs such as amphetamines and heroin, tobacco smoking, and alcohol use. . . . Students with self-perceived below-average academic performances and students reporting injected drug use also reported higher anabolic steroid use.[7]

Porcerelli and Sandler (1995)[19] administered psychological tests to 16 steroid-using weightlifters and body builders and 20 similar individuals who did not use steroids. They reported that steroid users had significantly higher scores on dimensions of pathological narcissism and significantly lower scores on clinical ratings of empathy. They were unable to assess whether narcissistic personality traits contributed to the initiation of steroid use or were the result of their use. McBride and coworkers (1996)[20] note an increase (in England) in the concomitant abuse of the mixed agonist-antagonist opioid nalbuphine (see Chapter 10).

Physical Dependence

Physical dependence is characterized by withdrawal symptoms when the drug is removed. Withdrawal from large doses of A-ASs can be accompanied by psychological depression, fatigue, restlessness, insomnia, loss of appetite, and decreased libido. Other withdrawal symptoms that have been reported include drug craving, headache, dissatisfaction with body image, and (rarely) suicidal ideation. Despite these observations, no defined psychiatric withdrawal syndrome has been described; withdrawal psychosis or bipolar illness has not been reported, although depression is commonplace.

As with all other psychoactive drugs, treatment of A-AS dependence first requires drug abstinence, treatment of any signs of withdrawal, and maintenance of abstinence. Behavioral and cognitive approaches are possible treatment tools.[8] Supportive therapy, including reassurance, education, and counseling, remains the mainstay of treatment.[1] Antidepressants may be indicated when dependency is complicated by major depression. A physician trained in endocrinology can best prescribe other therapies for hormonal alterations.

Abuse and Treatment

The use of A-AS drugs for athletic or cosmetic purposes constitutes drug abuse, because the doses used far exceed those needed for medical indications. Such use persists despite recognized, unavoidable side effects and negative consequences for the physical and psychological health of the user. The mechanisms responsible for dependence are largely unknown and may be psychological and/or physiological.

> Testosterone is the most potent hormonal determinant of physical and behavioral masculinization. It has been implicated for decades in the stimulation of sexual behavior, as well as in the activation of dominance and aggressive behaviors in male primates, including humans.[21]

Thus, the attraction to the use of supraphysiologic doses of testosterone derivatives is strong, with significant numbers (3 to 5 percent of adolescent males) succumbing to their attractiveness.

One societal response to the use of A-ASs has been to ban their use in athletics.

> Since the beginning of organized competition, athletes have tried to gain every possible advantage over their competitors. Sometimes this competitive edge is gained fairly by training harder or developing new and improved methods. Sometimes, however, athletes seek an

advantage by using substances that affect the body in ways that can improve athletic performance.[22]

The National Collegiate Athletic Association (NCAA) and the United States Olympic Committee (USOC) have declared the use of anabolic steroids illegal, not only because of their ability to artificially increase muscle mass and competitiveness, but also because of their serious and sometimes permanent side effects.[22] Olivier (1996)[23] argues in favor of the ban, stating that these drugs not only harm the user but create a climate of subtle coercion toward their use by others, as well as placing others (e.g., partners of steroid users) at risk of violence from users while they are on the drug (see also Choi and Pope [1994][24]). Olivier concludes:

> I have argued that prohibition of harmful practices is justified by potential harm to others (rather than just to one's self). One must bear in mind the powerful effects of subtle coercion and influence and the consequent limitations placed on choice. So, on the grounds that it is wrong to harm others or to coerce them into potentially harmful situations, this paper takes issue with sports libertarians who claim that banning performance-enhancing substances is an unjustified paternalistic action that violates the principle of autonomy.[23]

Education has to be the primary mainstay of A-AS abuse prevention, especially since the drugs (initially) promote a more healthy, masculine appearance as well as increasing muscle mass and strength. In a series of articles, Goldberg, Elliott, and coworkers (1996)[25-27] have designed and tested a team-based, educational interventional program created to reduce the intent of adolescent athletes to use A-ASs. Conducted with 702 football players in 31 high schools in Portland, Oregon, seven weekly classroom sessions, seven weekly weight-room sessions, and one evening parent session led to

> increased understanding of AAS effects, greater belief in personal vulnerability to the adverse consequences of AAS, improved drug refusal skills, less belief in AAS-promoting media messages, increased belief in the team as an information source, improved perception of athletic abilities and strength-training self-efficacy, improved nutritional and exercise behaviors, and reduced intentions to use AAS.[25]

The education program utilized by Goldberg and coworkers is discussed further in Chapter 14.*

---

*The title of the program is *The ATLAS Program.* It is available from its publisher, Jones & Bartlett, 40 Tall Pine Drive, Sudbury, MA 01776 (800-832-0034).

The abuse of A-ASs by athletes, body builders, and body-conscious individuals poses a special challenge to society in general. Perhaps the desire of adolescents and young adults to take A-ASs has been fostered largely by our societal fixations on winning and on physical appearance. Thus, successful intervention must go beyond education, counseling, law enforcement, and drug testing. Ultimately, a social environment that subtly encourages steroid abuse may have to be changed.

Dehydroepiandrosterone (DHEA)

DHEA is a hormone secreted by the adrenal glands. Widely sold as a "food supplement" in health food stores, DHEA is a precursor of both estrogen and testosterone.[28] Secretion of the hormone peaks at 20 to 25 years of age and declines by about 90 percent by age 70. Low levels of DHEA have been associated with increased incidence of cardiovascular disease and death in middle-aged men but not in women.[29] Recently, DHEA has been promoted to prevent heart disease, cancer, diabetes, obesity, dementia, aging, multiple sclerosis, and lupus; it increases feelings of physical and psychological well-being. There probably is some truth and much exaggeration in the multiple claims of efficacy for this "miracle drug." Until more is known, the compound's safety should be evaluated in order to measure its potential for causing harm.

DHEA can be classified as an androgen, because one of its metabolites is testosterone. Therefore, it is not surprising to see its use accompanied by the side effects characteristic of androgens: acne, male-pattern baldness, hirsutism, voice changes, and so on. More serious effects include the potential for causing breast or prostate cancer and liver damage. At present, as concluded in *The Medical Letter on Drugs and Therapeutics* (1996)[29]:

> DHEA, an adrenal steroid sold in health food stores, can have androgenic effects in women, including some that may be irreversible. In men, it could stimulate the growth of prostate cancer. There is no convincing evidence that DHEA has any beneficial effect on aging or any disease. Patients would be well advised not to take it.

NOTES

1. K. J. Bower, "Anabolic Steroids," *Psychiatric Clinics of North America* 16 (1993): 97–103.
2. S. E. Lucas, "Current Perspectives on Anabolic-Androgenic Steroid Abuse," *Trends in Pharmacological Sciences* 14 (1993): 61–68.

3. K. B. Kashkin, "Anabolic Steroids," in J. H. Lowinson, P. Ruiz, R. B. Millman, and J. G. Langrod, eds., *Substance Abuse: A Comprehensive Textbook*, 2nd ed. (Baltimore: Williams & Wilkins, 1992), 380–395.

4. S. Bhasin, T. W. Storer, N. Berman, et al., "The Effects of Supraphysiologic Doses of Testosterone on Muscle Size and Strength in Normal Men," *New England Journal of Medicine* 335 (1996): 1–7.

5. H. A. Haupt, "Anabolic Steroids and Growth Hormone," *American Journal of Sports Medicine* 21 (1993): 468–474.

6. A. Drewnowski, C. L. Kurth, and D. D. Krahn, "Effects of Body Image on Dieting, Exercise, and Anabolic Steroid Use in Adolescent Males," *International Journal of Eating Disorders* 17 (1995): 381–386.

7. R. H. DuRant, L. G. Escobedo, and G. W. Heath, "Anabolic-Steroid Use, Strength Training, and Multiple Drug Use Among Adolescents in the United States," *Pediatrics* 96 (1995): 23–28.

8. A. B. Middleman and R. H. DuRant, "Anabolic Steroid Use and Associated Health Risk Behaviors," *Sports Medicine* 21 (1996): 251–255.

9. S. Nilsson, "Androgenic Anabolic Steroid Use Among Male Adolescents in Falkenberg," *European Journal of Clinical Pharmacology* 48 (1995): 9–11.

10. M. J. Schwerin, K. J. Corcoran, L. Fisher, et al., "Social Physique Anxiety, Body Esteem, and Social Anxiety in Bodybuilders and Self-Reported Anabolic Steroid Users," *Addictive Behaviors* 21 (1996): 1–8.

11. I. Apakama and D. E. Neal, "Anabolic Steroid Abuse and Male Fertility," *British Journal of Urology* 76 (1995): 802–803.

12. C. Bickelman, L. Ferries, and R. P. Eaton, "Impotence Related to Anabolic Steroid Use in a Body Builder: Response to Clomiphene Citrate," *Western Medical Journal* 162 (1995): 158–160.

13. W. Schanzer, "Metabolism of Anabolic Androgenic Steroids," *Clinical Chemistry* 42 (1996): 1001–1020.

14. R. B. Melchert and A. A. Welder, "Cardiovascular Effects of Androgenic-Anabolic Steroids," *Medicine and Science in Sports and Exercise* 27 (1995): 1252–1262.

15. A. Kosaka, H. Takahashi, Y. Yajima, et al., "Hepatocellular Carcinoma Associated with Anabolic Steroid Therapy: Report of a Case and Review of the Japanese Literature," *Journal of Gastroenterology* 31 (1996): 450–454.

16. D. R. Rubinow and P. J. Schmidt, "Androgens, Brain, and Behavior," *American Journal of Psychiatry* 153 (1996): 974–984.

17. E. M. Kouri, S. E. Lukas, H. G. Pope, Jr., and P. S. Oliva, "Increased Aggressive Responding in Male Volunteers Following the Administration of Gradually Increasing Doses of Testosterone Cypionate," *Drug and Alcohol Dependence* 40 (1995): 73–79.

18. S. E. Lukas, "CNS Effects and Abuse Liability of Anabolic-Androgenic Steroids," *Annual Review of Pharmacology and Toxicology* 36 (1996): 333–357.

19. J. H. Porcerelli and B. A. Sandler, "Narcissism and Empathy in Steroid Users," *American Journal of Psychiatry* 152 (1995): 1672–1674.

20. A. J. McBride, K. Williamson, and T. Petersen, "Three Cases of Nalbuphine Hydrochloride Dependence Associated with Anabolic Steroid Use," *British Journal of Sports Medicine* 30 (1996): 69–70.

21. B. Schaal, R. E. Tremblay, R. Soussignan, and E. J. Susman, "Male Testosterone Linked to High Social Dominance but Low Physical Aggression in Early Adolescence," *Journal of the American Academy of Child and Adolescent Psychiatry* 34 (1996): 1322–1330.

22. United States Pharmacopeial Convention, Inc., "Athletes Precautions," *USP DI Update* 1 (1996): 83–86.

23. S. Olivier, "Drugs in Sport: Justifying Paternalism on the Grounds of Harm," *American Journal of Sports Medicine* 24 (1996): S43–S45.

24. F. Y. L. Choi and H. E. Pope, "Violence Towards Women and Illicit Anabolic-Androgenic Steroid Use in Strength Athletes," *Journal of Sports Science* 12 (1994): 184–185.

25. L. Goldberg, D. Elliot, G. N. Clarke, et al., "Effects of a Multidimensional Anabolic Steroid Prevention Intervention: The Adolescents Training and Learning to Avoid Steroids (ATLAS) Program," *Journal of the American Medical Association* 276 (1996): 1555–1562.

26. L. Goldberg, D. Elliot, G. N. Clarke, et al., "The Adolescents Training and Learning to Avoid Steroids (ATLAS) Prevention Program: Background and Results of a Model Intervention," *Archives of Pediatrics and Adolescent Medicine* 150 (1996): 713–721.

27. D. Elliott and L. Goldberg, "Intervention and Prevention of Steroid Use in Adolescents," *American Journal of Sports Medicine* 24 (1996): S46–S47.

28. C. L. Williams and G. M. Stancel, "Estrogens and Progestins," in J. G. Hardman, L. E. Limbird, P. B. Molinoff, R. W. Ruddon, and A. G. Gilman, eds., *Goodman and Gilman's The Pharmacological Basis of Therapeutics*, 9th ed. (New York: McGraw-Hill, 1996), 1413.

29. M. Abramowicz, ed., "Dehydroepiandrosterone (DHEA)," *The Medical Letter on Drugs and Therapeutics* 38 (1996): 91–92.

Chapter 14

DRUGS AND SOCIETY: PRIORITIES AND ALTERNATIVES

The first 13 chapters of this book discuss the pharmacology of drugs that act on the central nervous system. Some of these drugs are used primarily for the therapeutic treatment of psychiatric, neurologic, and/or behavioral disorders; some are primarily drugs of recreation use or compulsive abuse; and some fall into both categories, having value for therapeutic use but possessing characteristics that make them prone to abuse. The opioid analgesics are an example of the last category, because they relieve severe pain and are compulsively abused by some individuals, leading to narcotic addiction in many abusers.

This chapter and Chapter 15 address more directly the two issues of therapeutic use and drug abuse, presenting a few ideas and concepts that, hopefully, will be useful for readers who are, know, or treat individuals with either substance abuse problems (this chapter) or psychological disorders that are treated with a combination of pharmacotherapy and psychological therapies (Chapter 15).

Historical Perspective

As far back as recorded history, every society has used drugs to produce alterations in mood, thought, feeling, or behavior. Moreover, there have always been some people within societies who digressed from custom with respect to the time, the amount, and the situation in which these drugs were used. Abuse of psychoactive drugs has always produced problems for the individual taking the drug, for those in direct contact with the user, and for society at large.

Alcohol is the classic psychoactive drug used throughout history primarily for recreational purposes, but it is not the only such agent. Every culture has used naturally occurring substances to alleviate anxiety, produce relaxation, provide relief from boredom, alleviate pain, increase strength or work tolerance, or provide temporary distortion of reality. In most cultures, only very few naturally occurring substances were available, and their use was closely monitored, so just a relatively small minority of individuals "abused" them. Today, these patterns of abuse differ considerably from the traditional pattern:

- We have available at one time most of the naturally occurring psychoactive drugs ever identified.

- In most cases, the pharmacologically active ingredient in each natural product has been isolated, identified, and made available to those who desire the drug.

- Organic chemistry has provided us with synthetic derivatives of naturally occurring drugs. In many cases, the synthetic derivatives magnify the psychoactive potency of the natural substance 100 times or more.

- Users have devised new methods of drug delivery, starting with the invention of the hypodermic syringe in the 1860s, and "new drugs," the most recent of which are "crack" cocaine, "ICE" methamphetamine, and "designer" derivatives of fentanyl and mescaline. These developments have markedly increased the delivered dose, decreased the time to onset of drug action, and increased both the potency and the toxicity of these agents compared with their naturally occurring counterparts.[1]

As in past decades, caffeine, nicotine, and ethyl alcohol are by far the addictive drugs used by the vast majority of people. As Figure 14.1 shows, caffeine use is nearly universal, with 90 percent of Americans over the age of 11 using the drug at least once weekly. Thankfully, little harm seems to follow. Nicotine and alcohol are the next most widely used and abused addictive drugs. They have little therapeutic use but exact enormous costs from the individual and society. The probability that an American living today has a drug abuse or dependence disorder is 36 percent for nicotine, 14 percent for alcohol, and 4 percent for marijuana.[2]

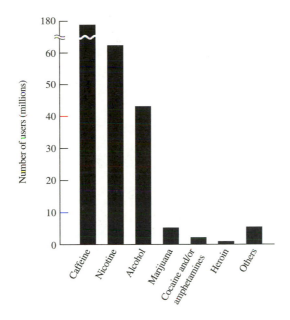

FIGURE 14.1 Use of addictive drugs in the United States in 1991. Numbers include people who used each drug at least weekly (heroin use at least once in the past year). "Others" includes inhalants and hallucinogens. [From Goldstein (1994),[2] figure 1.1, p. 6. Data from *National Household Survey on Drug Abuse,* U.S. Department of Health and Human Services, Public Health Service, Alcohol, Drug Abuse, and Mental Health Administration, DHHS Publication No. (ADM) 92-1887 (Washington, D.C., 1992).]

A 1996 survey[3] notes that 11.7 million Americans had used an illicit drug during the month prior to the survey. "Hard-core" cocaine users now number close to 500,000. "Regular" marijuana users (weekly or more frequent use) number over 5 million. One study in California[4] demonstrated that the yearly cost of treating 150,000 substance abusers was $200 million, but the financial benefits of treatment for these individuals was established at $1.5 billion, mostly as a function of reductions in crime. Thus, psychosocial treatments for drug abuse seem to yield substantial financial benefits and, hopefully, an increased quality of life for the abuser if treatment is long-term (6 months to a year).[3] While on the topic of treatment, several important points need be remembered:

- Substantial heterogeneity exists among substance abusers in the nature and severity of their addiction-related problem.

- The majority of individuals with substance abuse problems have co-morbid psychiatric disorders that require additional services,* such as pharmacotherapy or psychological therapies.[5]

- Self-medication with potent psychoactive drugs in an attempt to, at least initially, treat underlying psychiatric symptoms may have led to the substance abuse disorder.

- The potent behavior-reinforcing properties of certain psychoactive drugs sustain the attractiveness of and the need for these drugs, in addition to the ability of the drug to ameliorate the underlying psychological symptoms.

- Drug "craving" following withdrawal may represent the unmasking or worsening of preexisting psychiatric symptomatology, receptor dysfunction (now unmasked by drug removal), or any other unidentified causes, whether physiological, psychological, genetic, or environmental.

Additional treatment issues will be addressed later in this chapter.

Psychoactive Drugs as Behavioral Reinforcers

Drugs that are prone to compulsive abuse activate brain mechanisms involved in reward and positive reinforcement. The systems and structures involved include (1) dopamine, serotonin, opioid, GABA, and cannabinoid neurons and/or receptors, and (2) the median forebrain bundle, ventral tegmentum, hippocampus, frontal cortex, and nucleus accumbens. Here we attempt to describe a neuroanatomical system that underlies the behavioral reinforcing actions of all these drugs.[7] Because conditioning and learning processes are of central importance in drug addiction, one can visualize drug-seeking behavior as an amalgam of positive reinforcement, discriminative effects, aversive effects, and stimuli associated with drug use.

---

*Kessler and coworkers (1997)[6] reported that the lifetime and 12-month prevalences of alcohol abuse were 9.4 percent and 2.5 percent, respectively, while the lifetime and 12-month prevalences of alcohol dependence were 14.1 percent and 4.4 percent, respectively. Among people with either alcohol abuse or alcohol dependence, 78 percent of men and 86 percent of women had at least one other psychiatric disorder, such as conduct disorder, drug dependency, anxiety disorder, or affective disorder (depression, dysthymia, or mania).

Lessons from the Laboratory

Laboratory animals self-administer psychoactive drugs, and the degree to which an animal self-administers a particular drug closely parallels the degree of abuse exhibited by human users of a particular drug.[8] Indeed, if a drug is to maintain drug-seeking behavior, it must serve as a positive reinforcer.[9] For example, cocaine is self-administered to excess by every species of animal that has been tested, including rats, squirrels, monkeys, rhesus monkeys, pigtail macaques, baboons, dogs, and humans. The self-administration of strongly reinforcing drugs by several species also dispels the notion that the drug abuser (compared to a casual user or a nonuser) has some kind of inherent pathological condition (for example, a preexisting psychopathology) that creates a propensity for abusing drugs. Thus, we must examine briefly the reinforcing properties of the major psychoactive drugs.

Cocaine and the amphetamines are the most powerful reinforcing drugs.[10] The reinforcing property of these potent behavioral stimulants is probably the most important factor in their compulsive abuse by humans, and it plays a major role in the drug's appeal to users.

Morphine, heroin, and other opioids are readily self-administered by animals, but they tend to gradually raise the daily dose over a period of weeks, then self-administer the drug at a steady rate that avoids gross toxicity and withdrawal symptoms. The initial increase in dose probably reflects the development of drug tolerance. The subsequent stabilization in dosage probably reflects a reduction in the pleasurable effect of the drug over time, with drug use being continued primarily to avoid withdrawal symptoms. Simon (1997)[11] critically reviewed the withdrawal process and subsequent treatment of opioid dependency in humans, focusing on the new RAAD (rapid, anesthesia-aided detoxification) method (see Chapter 10).

Nicotine is not initially self-administered by animals. Over time the rate of self-administration increases, but it decreases rapidly when saline is substituted for the drug. Miller and Gold (1993)[12] state that "nicotine also has been found . . . to be a positive reinforcer, although not to the same extent as cocaine."

Caffeine is generally thought to be a relatively weak behavioral reinforcer. Some positive reinforcing effects are seen at low doses, but aversive effects are seen at higher doses. Both animals and humans demonstrate a preference for caffeine, but this preference decreases as the work required to obtain caffeine increases.[13]

Ethanol (ethyl alcohol) is an effective behavioral reinforcer, although animals usually do not self-administer the drug without prior exposure to it. Miller and Gold (1993)[12] postulate that the two-step metabolism of ethanol (by aldehyde dehydrogenase) induces a shift in the metabolism of the dopamine to form a tetrahydroisoquinoline called tetrahydropaperoline (THP). THP, in turn, is postulated to stimulate opioid and GABA receptors, which affect dopamine neurons and the nucleus accumbens.[7]

The cannabinoids (marijuana) and the psychedelics (such as PCP and LSD) are often but not always considered to be behavioral reinforcers; behavioral reinforcement effects of these drugs are difficult to demonstrate. As stated by Herkenham (1995),[14] "The abuse potential associated with marijuana smoking . . . suggests a reward mechanism." Herkenham also states, however, that evidence indicates that any drug-induced behavioral reward caused by marijuana is not exerted through action on the reward system. Certainly this is an area that requires additional research.

Mechanism of Reinforcement Action

In recent years, it has become apparent that there are specific circuits in the brain dedicated to the neural mediation of reward and pleasure.[7] The activation of this reward mechanism seems to be the single feature shared by most if not all abusable substances. Drugs subject to compulsive abuse "act on these brain mechanisms to produce the subjective reward that constitutes the reinforcing 'high', 'rush', or 'hit' sought by substance abusers."[7] Specifically, abusable drugs ultimately stimulate the nucleus accumbens dopaminergic system that runs through the medial forebrain bundle. Drugs that have negative-reward effects (such as the phenothiazines) inhibit activity in or increase the thresholds of the same system.

Exactly what is this brain reward system, and how is it influenced by drugs of such varying classes and neurotransmitter actions? First, there are two major dopaminergic (dopamine-releasing) neuronal systems in the midbrain (see Figure 14.2). A primary, or first-stage, system comprises descending (or caudally projecting) fibers of dopaminergic neurons whose cell bodies are located in the nucleus accumbens and several limbic structures. These fibers run within the medial forebrain bundle and synapse onto second-stage dopaminergic neurons whose cell bodies are located in the ventral tegmental area (VTA) of the midbrain. The second-stage fibers are the axons of these VTA cells, and they ascend (travel rostrally) in the medial forebrain bundle and project into neurons of the forebrain, largely in the nucleus accumbens, frontal cortex, amygdala, and septal area. In essence, this two-neuron system is a dopaminergic loop between the forebrain and the ventral tegmentum.[7,8]

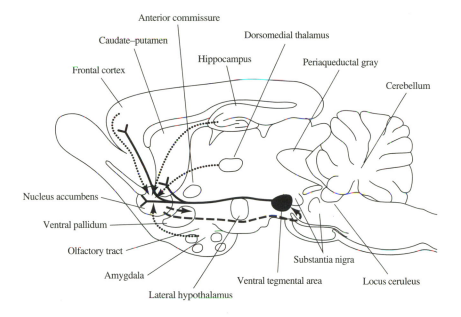

FIGURE 14.2 Sagittal rat brain section illustrating a cocaine and amphetamine neural reward circuit that includes a limbic-extrapyramidal motor interface. Dotted arrows indicate limbic afferents to the nucleus accumbens and dashed arrows represent efferents from the nucleus accumbens thought to be involved in psychomotor stimulant reward. Solid arrows indicate projections of the mesocorticolimbic dopamine system thought to be a critical substrate for psychomotor stimulant reward. This system originates in the ventral tegmental area and projects to the olfactory tubercle of the nucleus accumbens and the ventral striatal domains of the caudate-putamen. [Adapted from Koob (1992),[8] figure 1, p. 178.]

Cocaine and the amphetamines act on both the first- and the second-stage neuronal terminals. Here, the drugs mimic the effects of direct electrical stimulation of these areas. Other behavior-reinforcing drugs act only on the second-stage neurons, probably through action on the endogenous opioid circuitry:

Cell bodies, axons, and synaptic terminals of enkephalinergic and endorphinergic neurons are found in profusion throughout the extent of the reward-relevant mesotelencephalic dopamine circuitry. . . . Endogenous opioid peptide neurons synapse directly onto mesotelencephalic dopamine axon terminals, forming precisely the type of axo-axonic synapses one would expect of a system designed to modulate the flow of reward-relevant neural signals through the dopamine circuitry.[7]

Furthermore:

> The drug-sensitive dopamine "second stage" component of the reward circuitry is under the modulatory control of a wide variety of other neural systems, including the enkephalinergic mechanisms alluded to above, but also including GABAergic, seritonergic, noradrenergic, and neuropeptide neurotransmitter and neuromodulatory mechanisms.[7]

Koob (1992)[8] states:

> Dopamine forms a critical link for all reward, including opiates and sedative/hypnotics. While open to multiple neurotransmitter inputs and outputs, this view still holds a centrist position for dopamine in all reward. An emphasis on multiple independent neurochemical elements, . . . places the focus on the nucleus accumbens and its circuitry as an important, perhaps critical, substrate for drug reward.

It is important to recognize that enhancement of brain reward mechanisms explains only a portion of the motivation for compulsive abuse of drugs. Stolerman (1992)[9] reviews the complementary mechanisms that underlie drug-seeking behavior. As shown in Figure 14.3, a drug's ability to serve as a positive reinforcer is the minimum requirement for a drug to maintain drug-seeking behavior. Such positive reinforcement is maintained by three influences:

1. The neural mechanisms previously discussed

2. Behavioral mechanisms, including drug-induced euphoria, relief from anxiety or depression, functional enhancement, and relief from withdrawal

3. Multiple modulating variables, including the social context in which the drug is used, genetic factors, attitudes, expectations, and the history of previous reinforcement and reward

Cadoret and coworkers (1995)[15] studied the genetic pathways involved in the genesis of drug abuse and drug dependence in biological offspring who were separated at birth (eliminating social/environmental influences):

> Data . . . showed evidence of two genetic pathways to drug abuse/dependency. One pathway went directly from a biologic parent's alcoholism to drug abuse/dependency. The second pathway was more circuitous, and started with antisocial personality disorder in the

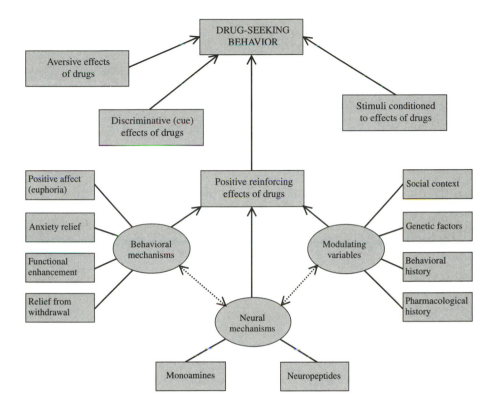

FIGURE 14.3 A psychopharmacological model of addiction as drug-seeking behavior controlled by four main processes: positive reinforcing and discriminative effects of drugs and of stimuli associated with them (which facilitate drug seeking), and aversive effects of drugs (which weaken the behavior). These four processes are common to drugs of many classes. A more detailed framework for analyzing positive reinforcing effects is shown (similar analyses could be made for discriminative and aversive effects); at this level it is envisaged that the relative importance of the different factors shown in the diagram will vary considerably between classes of drugs. [From Stolerman (1992),[9] figure 1, p. 171.]

biologic parent and proceeded through intervening variables of adoptee aggressivity, conduct disorder, antisocial personality disorder, and, eventually, ended in drug abuse/dependency. Environmental factors defined by psychiatric conditions in adoptive families independently predicted increased antisocial personality disorder in the adoptee. Adoptees born of alcohol-abusing mothers showed evidence of fetal alcohol syndrome, but controlling for this did not diminish the evidence for the direct genetic effect between an alcohol-abusing biologic parent and drug abuse/dependency in offspring.

Discriminative (cue) effects of drugs also contribute to drug-seeking behavior (Figure 14.3). Here, drug-seeking behavior is associated with its perceived effects. This factor contributes to drug relapse and withdrawal, possibly as an anxiogenic stimulus. These effects "have the potential to cue the appearance of drug-seeking behavior."[8] Aversive effects of drugs tend to reduce drug-seeking behavior by means of negative-reward and punishment mechanisms. These mechanisms "may set an upper limit to the amount of drugs that may be sought."[9]

Environmental stimuli can become associated with drug-seeking behavior through classical conditioning responses. These stimuli strengthen behavior to a level greater than that obtained by the drug effect alone. For example, in cigarette dependency, the sight of other smokers and the taste and smell of cigarette smoke may be powerful reinforcers, over and above the physiological effects of nicotine.

Drug Abuse

Over the years, laws have been passed to limit the availability of drugs and to punish drug users deemed dangerous to themselves or to society. When these laws are strictly enforced, they can reduce drug use by persons who fear reprisal, but aggressive legislation does not control a person's craving for mind-altering drugs. Moreover, legislation failed to address the legal drugs that cause the greatest amount of harm to individuals and society—ethanol and nicotine. In recent years, however, the U.S. Food and Drug Administration and President Bill Clinton have moved toward a more adamant stand against the cigarette industry. Legalization of currently illegal drugs is not likely to solve drug abuse problems, and it certainly is politically unlikely. Jonas (1992)[16] states:

> Simple legalization of the currently illegal drugs, if properly implemented, could solve much of the drug traffic-related crime problem. However, it would do nothing to solve the substance abuse problem, especially that major part of it caused by tobacco and alcohol.

Besides legislation, other traditional techniques for reducing drug abuse include education and developing negative attitudes toward drugs in both users and potential users. Such efforts have brought limited results, although the antianabolic steroid intervention (ATLAS program) described in Chapter 13 is encouraging.

As the twentieth century comes to a close, perhaps it is time to take a public health approach to the problem of drug abuse, an approach that attempts to minimize danger to the individual and society. As advocated by Jonas (1992),[16] the primary goal of this approach is to "reduce the use and abuse of all the recreational mood-altering drugs to provide for their safe, pleasurable use, consistent with centuries' old human experience, while minimizing to the greatest degree possible their harmful effects in individuals, the family, and society as a whole." Given a historical perspective of man's use of psychological drugs,[17] this is a reasonable social goal, but achievement of this goal involves multiple steps. Perhaps we might start by working toward the following:

- Elimination of cigarettes as a cause of drug-induced death, disease, and disability.
- Enforcement of existing legislation pertinent to driving a motor vehicle while under the influence of alcohol, combined with alcohol education of drivers, with a goal of the user making wiser decisions.
- Reduction of the promotion, attractiveness, and availability of cigarettes, alcohol, and illicit drugs to youths.
- Reduction of the harm that drugs inflict on youths, in both the short and the long term.

Currently, our society is in a debate over making marijuana available for somewhat vaguely described medical uses. This may or may not be a step toward legalization of the recreational use of the drug.* Hopefully, marijuana legalization will happen only when we become responsible users of alcohol and have the courage to restrict tobacco use only to those already dependent on nicotine.

Clearly, both the family and the community are vital in the effort to prevent drug abuse. Parents must set examples, show concern, exert influence, clarify values, provide open communication, and teach individual responsibility. Parents should certainly abstain from cigarettes, drink alcohol in moderation, and avoid driving after drinking. Parents can be positive educators if they act as good role models, provide accurate information, and show alternatives to the drug experience. Similarly, peer programs and peer influence can be effective in building a sense of self-worth and thus in reducing the attractiveness of drugs.

---

*I certainly agree with the call to reclassify marijuana as a Schedule II rather than a Schedule I "narcotic" so that physicians may prescribe the drug in situations considered to be appropriate (see Chapter 11). It makes no pharmacologic sense to classify marijuana as a more "dangerous" drug than cocaine. However, until we become responsible users (or nonusers) of alcohol and cigarettes, I remain unconvinced that we can "handle" an additional psychoactive drug that, although pleasurable, carries its own side effects and toxicities.

Shedler and Block (1990)[18] expanded on this concept of values and upbringing as a factor in drug abuse. Adolescents who are frequent abusers of drugs had significant behavioral maladjustments before they began to use drugs. Drug use is therefore a symptom, not a cause, of personal and social maladjustment. These authors emphasized that drug use and abuse can be understood only in the context of an individual's personality structure and developmental history. Drug abuse is only part of a broad psychological syndrome that is not adequately explained in terms of peer influences. Social policy should not try to eliminate drug experimentation by adolescents. Indeed, adolescents with a history of drug experimentation but who are not frequent users of drugs can be quite stable and well adjusted. Instead, social policies should try to foster sensitive and empathic parenting, self-esteem, interpersonal relationships, and meaningful goals in life.

Drug Education

Drug education and dependency-treatment programs must consider the extent of a person's behavioral and physiological involvement with psychoactive drugs. Although educational programs may be useful approaches, formal treatment programs are necessary for persons who are compulsive abusers or addicts.

One approach to drug education is to teach the pharmacology of psychoactive drugs, as is done in this text. Of course, this approach can be seen to provide directions for taking drugs. However, it can also be seen to provide accurate information for people to use in examining and modifying their own risk-taking behavior and thus making the informed decisions necessary to lead a healthy life in the community at large.

No program of drug education can guarantee to reduce the use of psychoactive drugs. A drug education program can, however, teach individuals the beneficial and harmful effects of a given drug (whether licit or illicit). Education may limit experimentation by some individuals. It will not dissuade those already involved in drugs, nor will it dissuade those who seek pharmacologic relief from their own psychiatric symptoms or disorder. In other words, it will not dissuade self-prescription for symptom relief. As stated in a White Paper from the U.S. Office of National Drug Abuse Policy (1992)[19]:

> Although [drug prevention] programs may not prevent someone from ever using drugs, they may well contribute toward a person ultimately leading a drug-free life. Furthermore, if a program can delay the onset of first use of a drug, while not the primary goal of prevention, it will decrease the likelihood of the user becoming addicted and a burden on society.

To alter the behavior of youths requires both education and examples set by teachers, peers, parents, and the whole community, including government officials. As stated by Goldstein (1994),[20] three steps are necessary:

1. Basic information has to be imparted—truthful information—to generate motivation for behavior change. Only honest, straightforward, and full information about the health risks of the addictive drugs will meet this requirement.

2. The means for behavior change have to be provided. Here many techniques have proven effective, especially teaching children how to resist peer pressure. It is important to promote a redefinition of drug-using peers as not "cool."

3. Methods for reinforcing the new behaviors have to be employed. This means, in short, that children need recognition, praise, and other rewards for not using drugs. Emphasis on how drugs detract from a healthy body and an attractive appearance, for example, appeals to adolescents' interest in athletics as well as to their developing sexuality and their striving for intimate peer relationships.

In essence, this approach is directed toward building one's self-esteem in a drug-free environment. While praiseworthy, this approach works best for those least likely to abuse drugs.[18]

Ultimately, prevention of drug abuse requires that adults be willing to set a consistent example by responsibly using or minimizing their use of psychoactive drugs. In addition, legislation must be consistent and in agreement with accepted, documented scientific evidence. Such action is particularly important regarding cigarettes and alcohol. The casualness with which we use these drugs and allow their promotion, distribution, and sale demonstrates both our ignorance and our hypocrisy about the use of addicting drugs.

Practical and Immediate Efforts to Stop Abuse

Perhaps the most important element of the public health approach is that there will be a single national policy for controlling the abuse of all the recreational mood-altering drugs. This policy will apply to each and every recreational mood-altering drug, whether it is currently legal or illegal. This policy will end the current OK/not-OK drug dichotomy.[16]

Such a policy must incorporate the following components:

- A scientifically based system for classifying recreational mood-altering drugs
- A broad definition of "responsible use" that takes into account age, drug, time, place, and other risk factors
- A rational price/tax structure for whatever drugs are legal
- Guidelines for prodrug advertising

Deterring the use of cigarettes and alcohol, which extract a multi-billion-dollar toll in lives, health, and productivity, should be the top priority in a drug abuse campaign. These substances should be the major focus of educational, regulatory, and enforcement efforts. In addition, we must be prepared to meet the challenge of the sudden and episodic emergence of fashionable, potent, and dangerous drugs, such as crack cocaine, methamphetamine, ICE methamphetamine, anabolic-androgenic steroids, and designer derivatives of psychedelics and narcotics.

Cigarettes. "There is no 'safe use' of cigarettes, and there is no such thing as responsible use of cigarettes."[16] "Cigarettes are the only product which, when used as directed, increase the risk of death and disease."[21] Such statements emphasize that cigarette smoking is the most widespread example of drug dependence, the most preventable cause of disease and disability, and the most unnecessary of modern epidemics in the world today. Forty-six million Americans still smoke, and cigarettes cause more illness and death than any other drug. The major problem is that most of the severe consequences of smoking have a delayed onset—often 20 years or more—at which time much of the damage is irreversible. Smoking and dependence develop early in life, usually during adolescence, when the feeling of personal invulnerability is maximal. As many as 3 million teenagers smoke, and up to 3,000 youngsters start smoking every day.

On August 28, 1996, the U.S. Food and Drug Administration (FDA) claimed jurisdiction over cigarettes and smokeless tobacco products, and President Clinton announced the first regulations for implementation of this jurisdiction. In a 1997 article, FDA Commissioner David Kessler and colleagues[22] explained the legal and scientific basis for this assertion of jurisdiction. In an accompanying article, Gostin and associates (1997)[23] offered a legal opinion and concluded that the FDA's claim was appropriate and that the courts should defend the FDA's historical and legislative mission to protect the public health. In brief, the FDA claims that the nicotine in cigarettes affects the "structure or any function of the body," and that, as a "drug delivery device," cigarettes are "intended" by the manufacturers to be used for pharmacological purposes and to sustain addiction. Accompanying this assertion was the release and publication of the "Children's Tobacco Rule,"[24] a comprehensive set of regulations that restrict the sale, distribution, promotion, and advertising of nicotine-containing cigarettes and smokeless tobacco to minors. Some of the promotion and advertising restrictions follow:

- Advertisements are restricted to black and white only, unless the ads cannot be viewed by minors. Ads must include a statement that the product is a nicotine delivery device for individuals aged 18 or more.

- No outdoor advertising within 1,000 feet of any school or playground.

- Restrictions on the sale, distribution, or offering of nontobacco products (hats, shirts, bags, and so on) displaying material linked to tobacco.

- Restriction on sponsorship of sporting events using brand name, logo, or other link to nicotine-containing products.

As might be expected, the tobacco industry is making legal challenges[22] that may or may not block the implementation of these FDA regulations. However, after 30 years of surgeon general's reports on the havoc caused by tobacco products, public sympathy seems to be swaying toward restrictions both on tobacco use by minors and on the depiction of cigarettes as being compatible with an active and healthy lifestyle. Although the government measures will not remove cigarettes from our culture, they might prepare adults who avoid becoming nicotine-dependent in teenage years to live cigarette-free in a society where cigarettes are readily available.

Alcohol. In addition to cigarettes, we should be equally concerned about the societal and medical effects of alcohol use. Alcohol is the direct cause of death for more than 31,000 Americans each year and an indirect cause of more than 37,000 deaths by accident or violence. Alcohol is a factor in 70 percent of homicides; 41 percent of the 40,676 traffic fatalities in 1994 (the latest year for available statistics) involved the drug; and two out of five people in the United States will be involved in an alcohol-related motor vehicle crash at some time during their lives.

Every year the average American consumes the equivalent of three gallons of pure alcohol. This amount of alcohol is equivalent to 591 twelve-ounce cans of beer, 115 fifths of table wine, or 35 fifths of 80 proof liquor. The total yearly cost of alcohol-related problems is about $150 billion, $45 billion of which are costs resulting from motor vehicle accidents. The remainder pays for the medical treatment of alcoholism; alcohol-related illness; fetal alcohol syndrome; loss of life, productivity, and property (including fire losses); crime; and social costs (for courts, jails, law enforcement, and so on). One out of four families is troubled by a family member who drinks alcohol. An estimated 10 million adults in the United States are alcoholics, and 7 million adults are problem drinkers. Alcohol-associated deaths account for at least 25 times more deaths than those caused by all the illegal drugs combined. Especially devastating are the injuries and fatalities among youths:

- More than 40 percent of teenage deaths result from automobile accidents, and more than half of them involve alcohol.
- Alcohol-related motor vehicle crashes are the number one public health problem among young people.
- Approximately 10 youths between 15 and 19 years of age die each day from alcohol-related traffic accidents.
- Youths between 15 and 24 years of age account for 37 percent of all alcohol-related traffic deaths.
- More than 30 percent of high school seniors report recent binge drinking. Junior and senior high school students consume 1.1 billion cans of beer each year, which translates into more than $200 million in revenues for the beer industry alone.[25]

In 1997 Liu and coworkers[26] surveyed more than 102,000 adults to determine how frequently adults in the United States drive while impaired by alcohol. Their results were "sobering" (see Table 14.1). Notably, the survey did not inquire about automobile accidents; it relied on a self-reported estimate of how many times respondents had driven in the last month "when you've had too much to drink." The data was then extrapolated to an average number of episodes of alcohol-impaired driving per responder per year, the total number of episodes per state per year, and the number of episodes per year per 1,000 population of each state. The average rate of alcohol-impaired driving per year per 1,000 adults was 655. The range was from 165 to 1,550. Overall, in the United States, there are more than 123 million episodes per year. The authors note, however, that this is a 20 percent decline from data obtained in 1986, a statistic that correlates with a 30 percent decline in alcohol-related traffic fatalities during the period 1982–1992. They conclude their report by recommending continued aggressive intervention to prevent alcohol-impaired driving. Effective policies include prompt license suspension for persons arrested for driving while impaired and lowering the legal blood alcohol level to, at most, 0.08 g% for adults and 0.02 g% for drivers younger than 21 years of age. . . . We also recommend strict enforcement of minimum drinking age laws and the passage of "zero tolerance" laws, which lower the legal alcohol concentration for drivers younger than 21 years of age.

A variety of counseling and educational recommendations were also listed. Hopefully,

through this combination of legal and medical [counseling] interventions, we can further reduce the unacceptable burden of injury and death from alcohol-related motor vehicle crashes and facilitate the early diagnosis and treatment of alcoholism.

Fleming and coworkers (1997)[27] tested a hypothesis that even brief interventional techniques in clinical settings might be effective in reducing alcohol consumption and binge drinking in problem drinkers who are not alcohol dependent. The study concluded that two 10- to 15-minute counseling interventions with men drinking more than 14 drinks per week and women drinking more than 11 drinks per week resulted, after 12 months, in a 14 percent reduction in alcohol use by men and a 31 percent reduction by women. Episodes of binge drinking and excessive drinking were reduced even more. The authors concluded that brief interventions can significantly decrease alcohol use and health resource utilization.

Youths and Drugs of Abuse

Use of drugs of abuse by adolescents shows little sign of decrease and, indeed, appears to have stabilized or slightly increased. Farrow and Schwartz (1992)[28] studied illicit drug use in adolescents (in Washington, D.C.) from urban (95 percent black) and suburban areas (89 percent white). In general, there were more similarities in patterns of use than there were differences. White suburban youths were heavier users of tobacco products, alcohol, and inhalants and experienced more difficulties with blackouts, family conflicts, school absence, suicidal ideation, and loss of peer relationships. Black urban youths experienced a higher peer use of marijuana.

Kandel and Davies[29] in 1996 studied 7,600 adolescents in New York State, classifying them into six mutually exclusive categories of drug use: nonusers, alcohol and/or cigarettes only, marijuana use only, users of illicit drugs other than marijuana but neither cocaine or crack,

TABLE 14.1 Estimated percentage, total episodes, and rate of alcohol-impaired driving among adults aged 18 years or older by state (Behavioral Risk Factor Surveillance System, 1993)

State	% of respondents[a]	Average no. of episodes of alcohol-impaired driving per respondent per year[b]	Total no. of episodes of alcohol-impaired driving per year[c]	No. of episodes of alcohol-impaired driving per 1,000 population
Alabama	1.8	23.2	1,274,664	422
Alaska	2.5	61.9	581,231	1,550
Arizona	1.8	22.2	1,162,574	409
Arkansas	1.6	37.3	1,038,343	593
California	2.5	23.2	12,959,400	569
Colorado	2.5	20.4	1,292,671	511
Connecticut	3.0	19.7	1,504,816	598
Delaware	2.3	25.9	311,212	604
District of Columbia	1.1	17.1	93,848	194
Florida	3.2	30.7	10,243,747	972
Georgia	1.5	19.7	1,414,240	288
Hawaii	2.0	34.8	539,921	683
Idaho	2.2	22.7	360,856	495
Illinois	2.2	25.1	4,671,622	545
Indiana	2.5	25.7	2,628,257	633
Iowa	2.9	24.9	1,484,651	718
Kansas	3.3	26.8	1,618,591	883
Kentucky	1.0	27.1	726,593	264
Louisiana	2.4	23.0	1,671,233	555
Maine	1.0	17.0	153,137	165
Maryland	0.8	27.6	839,759	226
Massachusetts	2.8	25.3	3,229,058	701
Michigan	4.6	23.2	7,429,420	1,074
Minnesota	3.2	16.9	1,779,735	546
Mississippi	1.8	35.0	1,147,705	625
Missouri	2.7	27.3	2,951,544	743

[a] Percentage of respondents who gave a response (not zero) to the question: "And during the past month, how many times have you driven when you've had perhaps too much to drink?"
[b] Includes only those persons who reported at least 1 episode of alcohol-impaired driving in the month prior to being surveyed.
[c] Calculated using population weighting factor for the state.

TABLE 14.1 Estimated percentage, total episodes, and rate of alcohol-impaired driving among adults aged 18 years or older by state *(continued)*

State	% of respondents[a]	Average no. of episodes of alcohol-impaired driving per respondent per year[b]	Total no. of episodes of alcohol-impaired driving per year[c]	No. of episodes of alcohol-impaired driving per 1,000 population
Montana	2.5	21.8	315,992	540
Nebraska	3.8	25.4	1,121,706	971
Nevada	4.5	32.5	1,312,035	1,459
New Hampshire	4.4	20.6	749,413	903
New Jersey	2.5	39.7	5,786,669	977
New Mexico	2.7	33.5	1,009,449	918
New York	2.1	28.0	8,219,729	596
North Carolina	1.5	28.1	2,144,462	417
North Dakota	4.3	23.4	463,484	1,009
Ohio	1.8	29.5	4,392,909	542
Oklahoma	0.9	23.2	468,879	200
Oregon	1.7	55.4	2,054,640	933
Pennsylvania	2.7	25.8	6,439,911	705
Rhode Island	3.2	28.2	702,598	900
South Carolina	1.7	25.2	1,134,258	433
South Dakota	3.1	22.9	350,987	698
Tennessee	0.8	40.0	1,223,373	328
Texas	3.6	26.6	12,065,625	964
Utah	1.5	24.7	432,377	379
Vermont	2.7	24.8	280,030	664
Virginia	2.3	23.5	2,575,968	537
Washington	2.0	17.9	1,335,253	354
West Virginia	1.4	54.5	1,045,364	772
Wisconsin	5.3	23.9	4,638,901	1,275
All respondents	2.5	26.3	123,272,837	655

Data from Liu, Siegel, Brewer, et al. (1997),[26] p.124.

cocaine but not crack users, and crack users.* The results clearly indicated that adolescents who use illicit drugs show deficits in school performance, quality of family relationships, and health and increased psychological symptoms, especially depression and deviance. The perception of drug use by peers and the participation in delinquent activities were the most important factors that differentiated users from nonusers. Lowered academic commitment and detachment from parents were also important determinants.

> Parental alcohol and cigarette use were important for initial experimentation with a legal drug; parental use of a medically prescribed tranquilizer is important for experimentation with illicit drugs. . . . The children . . . may use illicit drugs to handle their own feelings of psychological distress. . . . For some youngsters, the use of illicit drugs may represent a form of self-medication.[29]

How might drugs of abuse be self-administered to treat psychological distress? Perhaps some examples will help answer this question.

1. The nicotine in cigarettes can serve an antidepressant function (see Chapter 6), leading to nicotine dependence, leading to the long-term development of cigarette-induced toxicities.

2. Ethanol in alcohol exerts antianxiety, disinhibiting, and sedative actions and "dulls" input. This can, in the short term, ameliorate anxiety symptoms (see Chapter 3), allow one to "cope," and increase socialization. However, this can lead to alcohol dependency and eventually to alcohol-induced toxicities (alcoholism).

3. Cocaine and the amphetamines can exert a mood-elevating action and ameliorate feelings of worthlessness (at least in the short term); prolonged or repeated use can lead to dependency and all of the problems associated with these drugs (see Chapter 5).

4. Opioids are incredibly effective at dulling pain, be it physical or psychological (see Chapter 10). When all else becomes intolerable, opioids become the ultimate "coping" drug, allowing temporary toleration of an otherwise intolerable situation. Used for this purpose, the progression to dependency and addiction is predictable.

---

*Hatsukami and Fischman (1996)[30] note that, despite the classifications made by Kandel and Davies, there is little to pharmacologically differentiate crack cocaine from cocaine hydrochloride. The differences are mainly in the dose of drug and the pharmacokinetics of more rapid absorption when the drug is smoked.

5. Marijuana (see Chapter 11) appears to exert a sedative, calming, perhaps analgesic influence, together with an increased feeling of well-being. As a symptom reliever, it may be used to calm anxiety, depression, and social isolation.

Yamada and coworkers (1996)[31] confirmed the adverse effects of adolescent alcohol and marijuana use by tabulating the detrimental effects of these drugs on high school graduation. Results suggested that "marijuana use and frequent drinking are substitute activities" for each other.

Winnail and coworkers (1995)[32] demonstrated an inverse relationship between physical activity and the use of tobacco products and marijuana in a study of 4,800 adolescents. They postulate that increased physical activity might have a positive effect to decrease drug use. However:

> It seems more likely that higher levels of physical activity for white males, in combination with a host of other factors such as parental bonding, expectations for school performance, ability to resist peer pressure, self-esteem, and self-efficacy, contributed to the observed decrease in tobacco and marijuana use.

What then are some of the conclusions to be drawn about drug use in adolescents? I might summarize them as follows:

- Drug use in adolescents is similar across ethnic boundaries.
- Those who progress to greater degrees of substance abuse have different perceptions of drug use by their peers (than do nonusers), have greater participation in deviant activities, have lowered academic commitment, and have greater detachment from parents.
- Parental alcohol and drug use is associated with drug experimentation by their children.
- Some adolescent drug users may use drugs to self-medicate their own feelings of psychological distress.
- Illicit drug use is inversely related with academic achievement, parental bonding, ability to resist peer pressure, self-esteem, and self-efficacy.

How can these conclusions be addressed? Again, a few comments:

- The majority of adolescents are not more than occasional users of illicit drugs and their occasional use is restricted to alcohol, cigarettes, and marijuana. Thus, adolescents can be educated by peers (as in the ATLAS program; see Chapter 13) about the adverse and aversive effects of drugs.

- Peer efforts should be primarily directed toward nonusers and occasional users, setting peer standards for leading a drug-free, healthy, and active life.

- Education must involve parents in order to induce them to modify their own use of cigarettes, alcohol, and prescription drugs. If quitting is difficult, sharing this with adolescents may go a long way toward helping the child avoid escalations in drug use.

- An estimated 12 percent of children, 7.5 million young Americans, suffer from psychological disorders.[33] Many seek symptomatic relief through illicit drugs. Recognizing this fact and seeking professional help may "mainstream" youths and help guide them away from using an illicit drug for symptom amelioration. Hopefully, the underlying disorder can be treated before dependency is added as a comorbid diagnosis.

- Psychosocial interventions aimed at increasing self-image, reductions in peer influences, diagnosing and treating comorbid disorders,[5] reducing the parental use of drugs, and improving academic commitment will be successful and certainly cost effective.

- Crits-Christoph and Siqueland (1996)[3] review the effectiveness of various family therapy approaches for the treatment of adolescent drug abusers. Not only does the adolescent have a "drug problem," but the family system likely is similarly involved, each with a "drug problem" or other sort of psychological distress.

Treatment Issues

In past years, many people equated physical dependence with addiction. Indeed, in older views, the defining problem of addiction was physical dependence, implying that fear of withdrawal following drug removal was the "engine driving addictive substance use."[34] In such a view, detoxification was seen as the principle treatment for addiction. Free the addicted individual from the clutches of the drug by assisting him or her through withdrawal and the grip of the addiction was broken. Extending this concept to treatment, it is not surprising that treatment focused on detoxification, often in a clinical, residential, or hospital setting. Even today, detoxification is often still a primary goal of addiction treatment.

A more contemporary view of addiction treatment was necessitated by the observation that most individuals who go through detoxification eventually relapse to the reinstatement of drug use. As stated by DuPont and Gold (1995),[35] we must

> focus on reward rather than withdrawal as the engine of addiction. Clearly, the positive aspects of the drug experience support drug self-administration. . . . The reinforcing properties of drugs are powerful motivational forces that are preferred by the subjects to natural reinforcers.

Thus, drug reinforcement is the unifying feature of drug abuse and dependence.[35] We then can view *drug abstinence* as a behavioral and physical state induced by the absence of the drug of abuse to which the addict had adapted. It is behaviorally reinforcing to reverse the abstinence state by the readministration of a drug (i.e., relapse is behaviorally reinforcing). The state of abstinence is, therefore, not a return to "normal," as presumed by old models of addiction and withdrawal. Abstinence is characterized by a mental state of apathy, boredom, depression, malaise, anhedonia, and craving for relief. The individual "needs" the drug to feel "normal." Thus, relapse is driven both by the negative reinforcement of abstinence and the positive reinforcement of the drug.

These observations imply that the use of highly addicting drugs leads to permanent changes in brain chemistry, probably through alterations in the "synaptic plasticity" of receptors that underlie learning, memory, and reinforcement,[36,37] so that abstinence from a drug does not return one to normal but to an abnormal, anhedonistic state that requires the drug for chemical "normalization." One obvious implication is that addiction can best be prevented by establishing a zero-tolerance goal of primary prevention so that the drug-induced brain changes caused by addictive substance use do not occur.[35] Achieving such "harm reduction" will not be achieved through legalization of currently illegal drugs.[38]

Treatment Goals

The first goal of treatment of drug and alcohol addiction is to help the addicted person become and stay drug and alcohol free.[39] Long-term work is then needed to help individuals avoid relapse and improve the quality of their life, including dealing with their comorbid medical and psychiatric disorders.[35,40] There are three phases to the treatment of addiction[35,41]:

1. Getting started, the process of developing a willingness to enter treatment.

2. Stopping use. Medical treatment of both withdrawal and abstinence is important.

3. Staying clean and sober. Relapse-preventing pharmacotherapy (to reduce drug craving) is an important new area of interest and research, as are the traditional psychosocial interventions.[3]

In essence, this is a 12-step fellowship approach to developing "a new way of life and a complex relapse-prevention program for all drugs of abuse."[42]

To these, I add a fourth phase, which accompanies the third: Treatment of concurrent psychiatric illnesses, so that depression, anxiety, eating disorders, sleep disorders, bipolar illness, panic disorders, and so on are addressed and aggressively treated.[43]

Relapse-Prevention Psychopharmacology

In discussing the pharmacology of addiction treatment, we differentiate the use of drugs to ameliorate acute withdrawal from drugs that reduce the drive (craving) to addictive drug use that results from drug reward, recognizing that relapse can occur even after years of abstinence.

We have already discussed several drugs that have been used to ameliorate withdrawal symptoms and/or reduce the rate of relapse:

- *Naltrexone* (Trexan; see Chapter 10) is a long-acting, orally absorbed opioid antagonist that has made some relapsing alcoholics more amenable to positive behavioral change. As an opioid antagonist, it is also used to treat opioid dependency, negating any potentially positive effects of narcotic administration. As discussed in Chapter 3, it is also used to reduce the craving for alcohol.[43]

- *Disulfiram* (Antabuse; Chapter 3) is an aversive agent used in some alcoholics. The drug reduces the reward of drinking alcohol by the threat of painful symptoms if alcohol is consumed.

- *Clonidine* (Catapres) is used to ameliorate the signs and symptoms of withdrawal from abused agents, decreasing the peripheral manifestations of withdrawal. It is most commonly used to ameliorate the discomforts that accompany withdrawal from opioids.

Substitute drugs for the replacement of abused drugs include:

- *Nicotine patches* for nicotine dependency (Chapter 6)

- *Methadone* (Dolophine) for opioid dependency (Chapter 10)
- *Buprenorphine* (Buprenex) for opioid dependency (Chapter 10)

In addition to these drugs, there has recently been increasing interest in ibogaine (Endabuse) and acamprosate to reduce drug craving. *Ibogaine* is an alkaloid, with psychedelic properties, obtained from the West African shrub *Tabernanthe iboga*. For centuries the shrub has been used for initiation rites in a number of African societies; individuals believe that the drug enables them to contact ancestors in the spirit world. Properties assigned to ibogaine include those of a stimulant, a performance enhancer, a hallucinogen, and an aphrodisiac.[44]

Ibogaine was isolated in 1901. The structure (see Figure 14.5) closely resembles those of serotonin and harmine. In the late 1980s, it was noted that in animal experiments ibogaine reduced the self-administration of both cocaine and morphine and attenuated the symptoms of morphine withdrawal.[44] Claims have been made that ibogaine "interrupts the dependency syndrome, allowing patients to maintain a drug-free lifestyle for at least six months."[44] Side effects in animals consist of ataxia (staggering), tremor, psychedelic-like mannerisms, and (in rats) cell damage (to Purkinje cells) in the cerebellum. In man, ibogaine can cause visual and other hallucinations associated with severe anxiety, apprehension, and tremor.

Rezvani and coworkers (1995)[45] reported that ibogaine attenuated alcohol intake in three strains of alcohol-preferring rats (see Figure 14.5). The mechanisms underlying this putative anticraving effect are unclear, but they may result from drug-induced modulation of a serotinergic system that, in turn, regulates dopamine release.[46-48] This would not be unexpected because of the structural similarity of ibogaine to serotonin. There are several interactions of ibogaine with multiple receptor systems.[49-51] Popik and coworkers (1995)[51] conclude: "The claimed 'anti-addictive' properties of ibogaine require rigorous validation in humans, after careful assessment of its neurotoxic potential."

Acamprosate, available in many European countries, is the calcium salt of N-acetyl-homotaurinate,[52] and it attenuates alcohol craving in laboratory animals and in humans who have been weaned from alcohol dependencey. The drug apparently blocks the alcohol-deprivation drive to relapse to ethanol consumption. The drug reduces calcium ion flows through NMDA-medicated glutamate neurotransmission (see Appendix IV). Spanagel and Zieglgansberger (1997)[52] review the anticraving actions of bothe acamprosate and naltrexone.

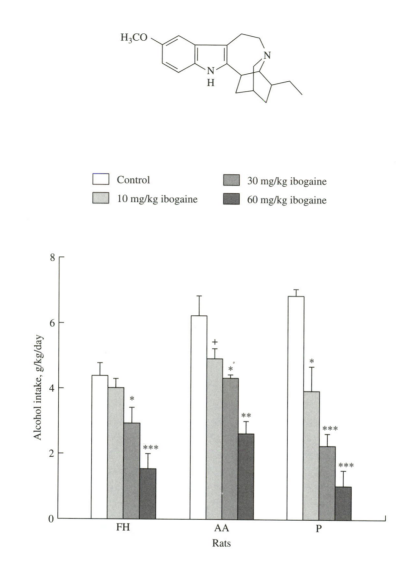

FIGURE 14.4 Ibogaine, structure (upper figure) and effects of three doses and control vehicle (clear bars, lower figure) on spontaneous intake of alcohol in three strains of alcohol-preferring rats (labeled FH, AA, and P). Data are means ± SEM. *p<0.05, **p<0.002, and ***p<0.001 compared with control. [Data from Rezvani, Overstreet, and Lee (1995),[45] p. 617.]

NOTES

1. D. L. Dunner, ed., "Psychopharmacology II," *Psychiatric Clinics of North America* 16, no. 4 (December 1993).

2. A. Goldstein, *Addiction: From Biology to Drug Policy* (New York: W. H. Freeman and Company, 1994), 9.

3. P. Crits-Christoph and L. Siqueland, "Psychosocial Treatment for Drug Abuse: Selected Review and Recommendations for National Health Care," *Archives of General Psychiatry* 53 (1996): 749–756.

4. D. R. Gerstein, H. J. Harwood, D. Fountain, N. Suter, and K. Malloy, "Evaluating Recovery Services: The California Drug and Alcohol Treatment Assessment General Report" (Sacramento, Calif.: California Department of Alcohol and Drug Programs, 1994).

5. B. R. Horner and K. E. Scheibe, "Prevalence and Implications of Attention-Deficit Hyperactivity Disorder Among Adolescents in Treatment for Substance Abuse," *Journal of the American Academy of Child and Adolescent Psychiatry* 36 (1997): 30–36.

6. R. C. Kessler, R. M. Crum, L. A. Warner, et al., "Lifetime Co-occurrence of DSM-III-R Alcohol Abuse and Dependency with Other Psychiatric Disorders in the National Comorbity Survey," *Archives of General Psychiatry* 54 (1997): 313–321.

7. E. L. Gardner, "Brain Reward Mechanisms," in J. H. Lowinson, P. Ruiz, R. B. Millman, and J. G. Langrod, eds., *Substance Abuse: A Comprehensive Textbook*, 2nd ed. (Baltimore: Williams & Wilkins, 1992), 70–99.

8. G. F. Koob, "Drugs of Abuse: Anatomy, Pharmacology, and Function of Reward Pathways," *Trends in Pharmacologic Sciences* 13 (1992): 177–182.

9. I. Stolerman, "Drugs of Abuse: Behavioral Principles, Methods, and Terms," *Trends in Pharmacological Sciences* 13 (1992): 170–176.

10. R. L. Bolster, "Pharmacological Effects of Cocaine Relevant to Its Abuse," in D. Clouet, K. Asqhar, and R. Brown, eds., *Mechanisms of Cocaine Abuse and Toxicity*, NIDA Research Monograph 88 (Rockville, Md.: National Institute on Drug Abuse, 1988), 1–13.

11. D. L. Simon, "Rapid Opioid Detoxification Using Opioid Antagonists: History, Theory, and the State of the Art," *Journal of Addictive Diseases* 16 (1997): 103–122.

12. N. S. Miller and M. S. Gold, "A Hypothesis for a Common Neurochemical Basis for Alcohol and Drug Disorders," *Psychiatric Clinics of North America* 16 (1993): 105–117.

13. K. Battig and H. Welzl, "Psychopharmacological Profile of Caffeine," in S. Garattini, ed., *Caffeine, Coffee, and Health* (New York: Raven Press, 1993), 213–253.

14. M. Herkenham, "Localization of Cannabinoid Receptors in Brain and Periphery," in R. G. Pertwee, ed., *Cannabinoid Receptors* (London: Academic Press, 1995), 150.

15. R. J. Cadoret, W. R. Yates, E. Troughton, G. Woodworth, and M. A. Stewart, "Adoption Study Demonstrating Two Genetic Pathways to Drug Abuse," *Archives of General Psychiatry* 52 (1995): 42–52.

16. S. Jonas, "Public Health Approach to the Prevention of Substance Abuse," in J. H. Lowinson, P. Ruiz, R. B. Millman, and J. G. Langrod, eds., *Substance Abuse: A Comprehensive Textbook,* 2nd ed. (Baltimore: Williams & Wilkins, 1992), 928–943.

17. R. Porter and M. Teich, eds., *Drugs and Narcotics in History* (New York: Cambridge University Press, 1995).

18. J. Shedler and J. Block, "Adolescent Drug Use and Psychological Health," *American Psychologist* 45 (1990): 612–630.

19. Office of National Drug Control Policy, Executive Office of the President, *Understanding Drug Prevention* (Washington, D.C.: U.S. Government Printing Office, 1992), 16.

20. A. Goldstein, *Addiction: From Biology to Drug Policy* (New York: W. H. Freeman and Company, 1994), 208–209.

21. A. C. Novello, "From the Surgeon General, U.S. Public Health Service," *Journal of the American Medical Association* 270 (1993): 806.

22. D. A. Kessler, P. S. Barnett, A. Witt, et al., "The Legal and Scientific Basis for FDA's Assertion of Jurisdiction Over Cigarettes and Smokeless Tobacco," *Journal of the American Medical Association* 277 (1997): 405–409.

23. L. O. Gostin, P. S. Arno and A. M. Brandt, "FDA Regulation of Tobacco Advertising and Youth Smoking: Historical, Social, and Constitutional Perspectives," *Journal of the American Medical Association* 277 (1997): 410–418.

24. U.S. Department of Health and Human Services, Food and Drug Administration, "Regulations Restricting Sale and Distribution of Cigarettes and Smokeless Tobacco to Protect Children and Adolescents," Final Rule, 21 CFR Part 801, et seq. (Aug. 28, 1996). Published in the *Federal Register* (Aug. 28, 1996) 61 *Federal Register* 44396.

25. J. F. Mosher, "Alcohol Advertising and Public Health: An Urgent Call for Action," *American Journal of Public Health* 84 (1994): 180–181.

26. S. Liu, P. Z. Siegel, R. D. Brewer, et al., "Prevalence of Alcohol-Impaired Driving: Results from a National Self-Reported Survey of Health Behaviors," *Journal of the American Medical Association* 277 (1997): 122–125.

27. M. F. Fleming, K. L. Barry, L. B. Manwell, et al., "Brief Physician Advice for Problem Alcohol Drinkers: A Randomized Controlled Trial in Community-Based Primary Care Practices," *Journal of the American Medical Association* 277 (1997): 1039–1045.

28. J. A. Farrow and R. H. Schwartz, "Adolescent Drug and Alcohol Usage: A Comparison of Urban and Suburban Pediatric Practices," *Journal of the National Medical Association* 84 (1992): 409–413.

29. D. B. Kandel and M. Davies, "High School Students Who Use Crack and Other Drugs," *Archives of General Psychiatry* 53 (1996): 71–80.

30. D. K. Hatsukami and M. W. Fischman, "Crack Cocaine and Cocaine Hydrochloride: Are the Differences Myth or Reality?" *Journal of the American Medical Association* 276 (1996): 1580–1588.

31. T. Yamada, M. Kendix, and T. Yamada, "The Impact of Alcohol Consumption and Marijuana Use on High School Graduation," *Health Economics* 5 (1996): 77–92.

32. S. D. Winnail, R. F. Valois, R. E. McKeown, R. P. Saunders, and R. R. Pate, "Relationship Between Physical Activity Level and Cigarette, Smokeless Tobacco, and Marijuana Use Among Public High School Adolescents," *Journal of School Health* 65 (1995): 438–442.

33. Members of the Committee for the Study of Research on Child and Adolescent Mental Disorders, "Report Card on the *National Plan for Research on Child and Adolescent Mental Disorders*," *Archives of General Psychiatry* 52 (1995): 715–723.

34. M. S. Gold and D. H. Eaton, "Drugs in History," *Journal of the American Medical Association* 275 (1996): 1364–1365.

35. R. L. DuPont and M. S. Gold, "Withdrawal and Reward: Implications for Detoxification and Relapse Prevention," *Psychiatric Annals* 25 (1995): 663–668.

36. G. Riedel, "Function of Metabotropic Glutamate Receptors in Learning and Memory," *Trends in Neuroscience* 19 (1996): 219–224.

37. W. S. Sossin, "Mechanisms for the Generation of Synapse Specificity in Long-Term Memory: The Implications of a Requirement for Transcription," *Trends in Neuroscience* 19 (1996): 215–218.

38. R. L. DuPont and E. A. Voth, "Drug Legalization, Harm Reduction, and Drug Policy," *Annals of Internal Medicine* 123 (1995): 461–465.

39. M. A. Schuckit, "Goals of Treatment," in M. Galanter and H. D. Kleber, eds., *The American Psychiatric Press Textbook of Substance Abuse Treatment* (Washington, D.C.: American Psychiatric Press, 1994), 3–10.

40. R. D. Weiss, "Inpatient Treatment," in M. Galanter and H. D. Kleber, eds., *The American Psychiatric Press Textbook of Substance Abuse Treatment* (Washington, D.C.: American Psychiatric Press, 1994), 359–368.

41. L. Grinspoon, ed., "Treatment of Drug Abuse and Addiction, Parts I, II, and III," *Harvard Mental Health Letter* 12, nos. 2,3, and 4 (August–October 1995).

42. M. S. Gold, "Neurobiology of Addiction and Recovery: The Brain, the Drive for the Drug, and the 12-Step Fellowship," *Journal of Substance Abuse Treatment* 11 (1994): 93–97.

43. R. M. Weinrieb and C. P. O'Brien, "Naltrexone in the Treatment of Alcoholism," *Annual Review of Medicine* 48 (1997): 477–487.

44. P. Popik, R. T. Layer, and P. Skolnick, "100 Years of Ibogaine: Neurochemical and Pharmacological Actions of a Putative Anti-Addictive Drug," *Pharmacological Reviews* 47 (1995): 235–253.

45. A. H. Rezvani, D. H. Overstreet, and Y.-W. Lee, "Attenuation of Alcohol Intake by Ibogaine in Three Strains of Alcohol-Preferring Rats," *Pharmacology, Biochemistry, and Behavior* 52 (1995): 615–620.

46. E. D. French, K. Dillon, and S. F. Ali, "Effects of Ibogaine, and Cocaine and Morphine After Ibogaine, on Ventral Tegmental Dopamine Neurons," *Life Sciences* 59 (1996): PL 199–205.

47. H. Sershen, A. Hashim, and A. Lajtha, "Effect of Ibogaine on Cocaine-Induced Efflux of [^{3}H]Dopamine and [^{3}H]Serotonin from Mouse Striatum," *Pharmacology, Biochemistry, and Behavior* 53 (1996): 863–869.

48. D. C. Mash, J. K. Staley, M. H. Baumann, R. B. Rothman, and W. L.

Hearn, "Identification of a Primary Metabolite of Ibogaine that Targets Serotonin Transporters and Elevates Serotonin," *Life Sciences* 57 (1995): PL 45–50.

49. E. E. Codd, "High Affinity Ibogaine Binding to a Mu Opioid Agonist Site," *Life Sciences* 57 (1995): PL 315–320.

50. H. Sershen, A. Hashim, and A. Lajtha, "Effect of Ibogaine on *Sigma*- and NMDA-Receptor-Mediated Release of [^{3}H]Dopamine," *Brain Research Bulletin* 40 (1996): 63–67.

51. P. Popik, R. T. Layer, L. H. Fossom, et al., "NMDA Antagonist Properties of the Putative Antiaddictive Drug, Ibogaine," *Journal of Pharmacology and Experimental Therapeutics* 275 (1995): 753–760.

52. L. B. Hough, S. M. Pearl, and S. D. Glick, "Tissue Distribution of Ibogaine After Intraperitoneal and Subcutaneous Administration," *Life Sciences* 58 (1996): PL 119–122.

53. R. Spangel and W. Zieglgansberger, "Anti-craving Compounds for Ethanol: New Pharmacological Tools to Study Addictive Processes," *Trends in Pharmacological Sciences* 18 (1997): 54–59.

Chapter 15

INTEGRATION OF DRUGS AND PSYCHOLOGICAL THERAPIES IN TREATING MENTAL AND BEHAVIOR DISORDERS

**Donald E. Lange and
Robert M. Julien**

Because no illness occurs in a vacuum, psychoactive medications should rarely be prescribed as the sole treatment; combinations of drug therapy plus psychological therapies provide more effective treatment than the use of either alone.[1,2] This chapter explores the interaction between pharmacotherapy and psychological therapies in the overall care of patients, a topic that is unavoidably intertwined with psychotherapy. In particular, this chapter

1. Describes the roles of medication and psychotherapy in the treatment of patients with mental disorders and the thorough assessment and accurate diagnosis vital to appropriate treatment

2. Provides an overview of the standard classification system used in mental health[3]

3. Discusses the major categories of mental disorders that require an integrated treatment approach

4. Discusses the practice standards that are being established for the treatment of major psychological disorders

Role of Medication

The use of psychoactive drugs in treating psychological illness is termed *psychopharmacotherapy*. The past 40 years have produced remarkable medicines that can ameliorate much of the symptomatology and suffering that accompanies both acute episodes and chronic persistence of such central nervous system (CNS) disorders as anxiety, depression, mania, psychosis, insomnia, epilepsy, parkinsonism, and pain. The limitations to drug therapy are many, however, and include

- Intolerance to or persistence of side effects
- Occasional severe toxicities
- Development of tolerance, dependence, and "addiction"
- Noncompliance
- Treatment resistance
- Amelioration of symptoms with failure to "cure" the underlying disease process

In addition to treating the symptomatology of mental disease, medication may serve a *prophylactic function*, altering brain chemistry in order to prevent the onset of a symptom complex (e.g., reducing the frequency of recurrence of symptomatology). Thus, drugs can be used both to ameliorate debilitating symptoms of acute or chronic conditions and to prevent the development of additional symptoms, allowing the introduction of nonpharmacological therapies. Illustrating this statement are the "new generation" of antipsychotic drugs (see Chapter 9), which can effectively ameliorate both the positive and the negative symptomatology of schizophrenia, permitting the use of psychosocial interventions that can assist with the integration of the patient into society and improve his or her functional level therein.

Therefore, it is rare that psychoactive drugs are the only answer to a psychological problem. Indeed, there may be little statistical difference between the effectiveness of antidepressant drugs and psychotherapeutic interventions when either treatment is used alone to treat depression. In combination, however, the two modalities provide a synergistic effect that significantly decreases the time to recovery.[4] Thus, judicious use of drugs, while important in the successful treatment of many mental disorders, is only part of an overall treatment strategy.

Role of Psychotherapy

In 1952 psychologist Hans Eysenck issued a challenge to mental health professionals by drawing their attention to a lack of reliable evidence that psychotherapy* was more helpful than doing nothing and waiting for the client to spontaneously recover. Over the next 45 years, this challenge was met; hundreds of studies have demonstrated that psychotherapy is better for a client than being placed on a waiting list.[5] Today, research is attempting to delineate which psychotherapeutic interventions are most effective for which psychiatric conditions, partly because of the current health care funding crisis, which demands closer accountability for funds spent. Out of this research some conclusions are becoming clear:

> Behavioral and cognitive behavioral therapies have more consistent and lasting effects than medications in the treatment of panic disorder, agoraphobia, simple phobias, and, to a lesser extent, social phobias. Medications and behavioral techniques are equally effective in obsessive-compulsive disorder, post-traumatic stress disorder, and generalized anxiety disorder. Behavioral therapies of the kind originally developed by Masters and Johnson are more effective than medications in the treatment of sexual dysfunction.[5]

Drugs provide only temporary relief in the treatment of insomnia, which is more effectively treated with behavioral therapy. In the treatment of major depression without psychotic features, behavioral, cognitive behavioral, and interpersonal psychotherapies are as effective as antidepressant drugs. Psychodynamically oriented therapies are less useful, more long term, and more costly but are better than no treatment. No psychological therapies are effective in the treatment of bipolar (manic-depressive) illness, but they are a useful adjunct to pharmacotherapy once the manic behavior is under control (see Chapter 8).

---

*As used in this chapter, the term *psychotherapy* covers a wide range of treatment modalities from education and supportive counseling to insight-oriented, dynamically based therapy.

Psychotherapy without medication is not an effective treatment for schizophrenia, but schizophrenic patients under pharmacologic control benefit from social skills training and related therapies (see Chapter 9). Almost all tested psychotherapies are short-term (under 15 or 20 sessions) and are best if carried out over about six months. Such short-term therapies provide more than temporary relief; they can lead to long-lasting behavioral changes. The efficacy and cost effectiveness of classical long-term psychoanalysis remains untested.[5]

Role of the Treatment Team

No single health-care provider is a sole caregiver. Usually a team of caregivers with members from several disciplines assists in the treatment of the patient. One team member is usually a clinician with prescription privileges (a physician or, increasingly, a nurse practitioner). Other clinicians, who do not prescribe medication, may have responsibility for psychotherapeutic interventions. Other caregivers may include nurses, pharmacists, counselors, vocational rehabilitation counselors, physical or occupational therapists, dieticians, spiritual counselors, family members, and psychiatric, occupational, or recreational assistants. Miller and Keitner (1996)[6] review the team approach, suggesting a "sequential" or "cascading" model when providing combined treatment. Various treatments (medication or psychotherapy) are administered in a sequential fashion based on the patient's response or lack of response to a previous treatment. If the patient responds to one treatment, no other may be needed; if there is no response, then a second treatment is added to the first. Continued nonresponse may lead to additional or substitute types of treatments.

Because the prescribing clinician has traditionally often acted alone, one might reasonably ask whether the treatment team concept is just idealistic, a "make-work" concept, and overly expensive or can deliver a higher quality of care with a better life for the patient at a manageable cost, the latter being increasingly important in this age of managed care and cost constraints. Several recent articles have addressed these concerns.

For example, several articles have addressed the issue of the costs associated with the treatment of patients with major depression. Henk and coworkers (1996)[7] conclude that, compared with nondepressed patients, depressed patients are greater utilizers of medical care, incurring $1,498 more per patient per year in medical costs. Meredith and coworkers (1996)[8] also discuss the economics of mental health delivery systems for treating depression. Katon and coworkers (1996)[9] discuss a multifaceted, multidisciplinary intervention program to improve treatment of depression in a more cost-effective manner. In essence, these researchers conclude that a treatment team relieves the prescribing physician of responsibility for handling psychological interventions, reduces hospitalizations, and provides longer, more intensive, more cost-effective case management. Katon and coworkers (1997),[10] addressing the collaborative management of patients with depression, noted that only 30 to 40 percent of primary care patients with major depression receive antidepressant medication and fewer than 10 percent receive specific psychotherapies known to be effective in treating depression. Therefore, they evaluated teamwork models to remedy the situation:

> In the psychiatrist/primary care model, a psychiatrist alternated visits with a primary care physician to assist in the education and pharmacologic treatment of the patient. In the psychiatrist/psychologist team model, the psychiatrist worked with a team of psychologists to improve adherence to and effectiveness of antidepressant treatment, with psychologists also providing brief behavioral treatment in the primary care clinic. It was found that the collaborative model was associated with improved adherence to treatment, increased patient satisfaction with depression care, and improved depression outcome compared with usual care by primary care physicians alone.[10]

The client's medications most certainly affect the delivery of and even the ability to deliver treatment. Each team member must continually evaluate changes in symptomatology caused by the medication. This assessment includes the interrelationships between drug effects, psychotherapeutic effects, and the patient's overall goals in treatment. Team members should assess how a particular drug affects the treatment strategy and, conversely, how psychotherapy affects the intended therapeutic effects of prescribed medications. Wells (1997)[11] documents the reductions in health-care costs and the improved patient well-being with this approach to care.

How might a treatment team function? Certainly, the nonprescribing clinicians must be thoroughly familiar with the pharmacology, uses, limitations, and side effects of the drugs being used by their clients. They must also know about alternative medications that may provide equal or superior effectiveness with a more reasonable spectrum of side effects for the particular client. These clinicians must be able to professionally converse with the prescribing physician, monitor drug therapy, and institute psychological therapies appropriate to the condition under treatment. All members of the treatment team need to know which drugs their clients are taking and which effects should be expected. All must monitor for both positive and negative effects and must be sensitive to the meaning that medications have to the clients. Indeed, effective psychotherapy depends on the ability of patients to comply with treatment requirements. Thus, patients must have at least a threshold level of concentration, cooperation, and motivation and be free of incapacitating symptomatology.

Psychotropic medication is frequently used to help achieve these prerequisite conditions. Although a drug is prescribed for its beneficial effects, some side effects may reduce the patient's mental activity, concentration, or cooperation, thus hindering his or her progress in psychotherapy. Similarly, inadequate doses of medication may decrease therapeutic effectiveness. Therefore, levels of the drug in the blood may be monitored, especially when there is either an inadequate response to the drug or when side effects become prominent.[12]

Regardless of their individual roles, all team members share certain basic functions. Most important is that of evaluation and assessment. For a clinical psychologist, this function may involve the administration of various psychometric instruments. A mental status examination frequently assists in establishing a tentative diagnosis. The purpose of assessment is to obtain a clear, objective report of the patient's signs and symptoms and, as much as possible, to relate these to possible causes. A psychological assessment may include a formal diagnosis, or it may be a description of the development of the patient's behavior. Either type of assessment should address both the strengths and the weaknesses of the patient. An assessment that also includes the etiology of the problem is most beneficial.

The clinician may list the possible explanations for the observed behaviors in a comprehensive format called the *differential diagnosis*, from which the causes may be determined. Frequently, further assessment is necessary to rule out some of the possible causes. Less plausible causes usually can be readily eliminated. The differential diagnosis then guides further assessment and treatment. Possible causal factors in the differential diagnosis often have markedly different treatments. Consequently, an accurate assessment and diagnosis of the causes of the patient's behavior must precede any treatment planning or therapeutic intervention. Evaluation by mental health professionals is often formalized into a standard diagnostic format. Most often used is the diagnostic system of the fourth edition of the *Diagnostic and Statistical Manual of Mental Disorders*, or DSM-IV.[3]

DSM-IV Classification of Mental Disorders

Diagnosis is the practice of distinguishing one disease from another. In clinical psychology, diagnosis is based on the signs and symptoms of a mental disorder, regardless of the morbid changes producing them. The DSM-IV classification provides a shorthand description of the patterns of behavior that can be expected with each disorder.

> DSM-IV is a categorical classification that divides mental disorders into types based on criteria sets with defining features. . . . In DSM-IV there is no assumption that each category of mental disorder is a complete discrete entity with absolute boundaries dividing it from other mental disorders or from no mental disorder. There is also no assumption that all individuals described as having the same mental disorder are alike in all important ways. This outlook allows more flexibility in the use of the system, encourages more specific attention to boundary cases, and emphasizes the need to capture additional clinical information that goes beyond diagnosis.[13]

Thus, the DSM-IV provides a set of guidelines for describing and characterizing clinical symptoms. Its categories also help in defining the etiology of the disorders. It also provides information about the context in which infrequently observed, abnormal behaviors occur as well as a description of the actions themselves.

In the DSM-IV classification system, each individual being diagnosed is not merely assigned a single diagnostic category (for example, bipolar disorder). Instead, he or she is characterized by clinically relevant factors that are grouped into five "axes":

- Axis I: primary classification (diagnosis) of the major problem requiring attention (for example, alcohol dependence)

- Axis II: mental retardation and personality disorders generally believed to begin in childhood or adolescence and persisting into adult life

- Axis III: any physical disorder that seems relevant to a case and that may have implications for present treatment (for example, asthma that is exacerbated by psychological factors)

- Axis IV: psychosocial and environmental problems that may affect the diagnosis, treatment, and prognosis of the mental disorders listed under Axes I and II (for example, illiteracy or unemployment)

- Axis V: global assessment of psychological functioning, social relationships, and occupational activities (including ratings of both the current level of functioning and the highest level of functioning during the past year)

In emergencies, a preliminary classification is made, even though much information is lacking. In such situations, any assessment is

TABLE 15.1 DSM-IV Axis I categories

Category	Examples
Disorders usually first diagnosed in infancy, childhood, or adolescence	Attention deficit and disruptive behavior disorders, learning disorders, certain eating disorders
Delirium, dementia, and amnestic and other cognitive disorders	Transient or permanent brain dysfunction attributable to such factors as aging, dementia due to head trauma or Alzheimer's, and amnestic disorders (memory loss)
Substance-related disorders	Disorders related to alcohol, all chemical withdrawal syndromes, and some disorders related to or caused by substances such as substance-induced psychotic disorders
Schizophrenia and other psychotic disorders	Chronic disorganized behavior and thought of psychotic proportions (delusions, hallucinations), incoherence, and social isolation; disorders that are well-organized systems of delusions without the incoherence, bizarreness, and other social isolation seen in schizophrenia
Mood disorders	Depression and bipolar disorder
Anxiety disorders	Anxiety, tension, and worry without psychotic features (delusions, hallucinations); post-traumatic (reactive, stress caused) disorders, whether brief or chronic
Somatoform disorders	Physical symptoms for which no medical causes can be found (symptoms apparently not under voluntary control and linked to psychological factors or conflicts)
Factitious disorders	Physical or behavioral symptoms that are voluntarily produced by the individual, apparently in order to play the role of patient and often involving chronic, blatant lying
Dissociative disorders	Sudden, temporary change in the normal functions of consciousness (for example, loss of memory, sleepwalking)
Sexual and gender identity disorders	Deviant sexual thoughts and behavior that are either personally anxiety provoking or socially maladaptive

TABLE 15.1 DSM-IV Axis I categories *(continued)*

Category	Examples
Eating disorders	Disorders of eating such as anorexia nervosa
Sleep disorders	Insomnia or difficulty in going to sleep or staying asleep, excessive daytime sleeping, complaints of sleep disturbance without objective evidence, impairment of respiration during sleep, disturbance of sleeping schedule, sleepwalking, sleep terrors
Impulse control disorders, not classified elsewhere	Maladaptations characterized by failure to resist impulses (for example, pathological gambling, chronic stealing of desired objects, habitual fire setting)
Adjustment disorders	Maladaptive reactions to identifiable life events or circumstances that are expected to lessen and cease when the stressor ceases; reactions may be dominated by depressed mood, anxiety, withdrawal, conduct disorder such as truancy, or a lessening in work or job performance
Mental disorders due to general medical condition, not classified elsewhere	Disorders that may be due to a medical condition, such as a psychotic disorder that emerges in response to renal failure
Other conditions that may be a focus of clinical attention	Includes such things as medication-induced movement disorders such as tardive dyskinesia or partner or parent/child relational problems

Abstracted from DSM-IV, pp. 13–24.

considered tentative and subject to revision as additional medical, psychological, and psychosocial assessments are made.

The first three axes constitute official diagnostic categories of the American Psychiatric Association. Axes IV and V are regarded as supplementary categories for use in clinical and research settings. It is common practice, however, to describe a case using all five axes. The major categories of Axis I classification are listed in Table 15.1. Here we consider 3 of the 16 Axis I categories—mood (or affective) disorders, schizophrenia, and anxiety disorders. These three were chosen because they are so prevalent,[14–16] and because they are the disorders most frequently treated with a combination of medication and psychotherapy.

TABLE 15.2 Prevalence of mental disorders in combined community and institutionalized population over 18 years of age

Disorder	1-year prevalence	No. of persons[a]
Any DIS ADM disorder	28.1 ± 0.5	44,679,000
Any DIS disorder except alcohol or drug	22.1 ± 0.4	35,139,000
Any mental disorder with comorbid substance use	3.3 ± 0.2	5,283,000
Any substance use disorder	9.5 ± 0.3	15,054,000
Any alcohol disorder	7.4 ± 0.3	11,766,000
Any drug disorder	3.1 ± 0.2	4,929,000
Schizophrenic/schizophreniform disorders	1.1 ± 0.1	1,749,000
Affective disorders	9.5 ± 0.3	15,143,000
Any bipolar	1.2 ± 0.1	1,908,000
Unipolar major depression	5.0 ± 0.2	7,950,000
Dysthymia	5.4 ± 0.2	8,586,000
Anxiety disorders	12.6 ± 0.3	20,034,000
Phobia	10.9 ± 0.3	17,331,000
Panic disorder	1.3 ± 0.1	2,067,000
Obsessive-compulsive disorder	2.1 ± 0.1	3,339,000
Somatization disorder	0.2 ± 0.0	365,000
Antisocial personality disorder	1.5 ± 0.1	2,385,000
Cognitive impairment (severe)	2.7 ± 0.1	4,293,000

Adapted from Regier and coworkers,[16] tab. 2, p. 88.
[a]The combined community and institutional civilian adult population was 159 million in 1980, 167 million in 1983, and 184 million persons in 1990. A 16.5 percent population increase from 1980 to 1990 is an adjustment factor that may be applied to these data to estimate the number of persons with disorders or service use in 1990. For example, the 44,679,000 persons with any mental or addictive disorder in 1980 would be increased to 52,051,000 in 1990.
   DIS, diagnostic interview schedule; ADM, alcohol, drug, and mental. Rates are standardized to the age, sex, and race distribution of the 1980 institutionalized and noninstitutionalized population of the United States aged 18 years and older. Data are mean ± standard error.

Forty-four million Americans are identified as having a psychological disorder (see Table 15.2). Of these, 1.7 million are identified as having schizophrenia, 15 million a mood disorder, and at least 20 million an anxiety disorder. Another 15 million are reported to have a substance abuse disorder (drugs or alcohol), which is often found in conjunction with one of the other three disorders. Patients with one of these four disorders are the most frequent users of the mental health delivery system. Several other widespread disorders of increasing recognition are not included in these numbers. Generalized anxiety disorder, dysthymia, and cyclothymia together add several million more individuals to the total. They are currently included in DSM-IV (they were excluded from the data in the early 1990s) because they are increasingly being treated with drugs; as drug treatment is instituted, patients responsive to the drugs become "labeled" with the diagnosis and the numbers can be tabulated.

Regier and coworkers (1993)[14–16] reported that only about half of the 44 million Americans with a mental health disorder received mental health services over their 12-month period of study; providers of these health services were equally split between specialists and general medical providers. The authors suggest that more individuals should be receiving treatment for their disorders. Only 64 percent of the individuals diagnosed with schizophrenia received treatment; the corresponding figures for individuals with a mood disorder or an anxiety disorder were 45 percent and 32 percent, respectively. Thus, many individuals diagnosed with mental and addictive disorders do not receive treatment, or, if they do receive treatment, it is not in a mental health setting.

Integrated Treatment of Major Mental and Behavioral Disorders

Mood Disorders

The term *mood* refers to a perceptual bias that alters how one views the world. Mood disorders may include major depressive, manic, or hypomanic episodes, dysthymia, or alternating recurrences of one or more such moods. All of us experience mood shifts, such as mild anxiety, depression, sadness, and grief, in response to difficult life events. These responses are natural and certainly do not constitute a mood disorder. The DSM-IV classification of mood disorders pertains to distinct, severe processes that interfere with daily activities. These dysfunctional processes are, however, amenable to treatment. General medical conditions may be a causal factor, as may drug use. A normal course of bereavement due to environmental factors (for example, death of a loved one) is not classified as a mood disorder, even though it may temporarily incapacitate the individual.

In general, mood disorders are subclassified by type and duration of the mood episode. For example, two weeks of severely depressed mood (as indicated by a specific set of four additionally related symptoms) is required for a diagnosis of a major depressive episode.[17] Two years of mildly depressed mood and the presence of two related symptoms is required for diagnosis of dysthymic disorder. The DSM-IV groups mood disorders into depressive disorders, bipolar disorders, substance-induced mood disorders, and mood disorders due to general medical conditions. The following features common to some mood disorders do not by themselves indicate any specific condition:

1. Pathological change in mood from despair to elation or vice versa
2. A change in interests or in the ability to obtain pleasure; greatly diminished or excessive involvement in pleasurable activities
3. Vegetative changes (changes in sleep, energy level, appetite, or libido)
4. Deviations in mannerisms that suggest changes in self-concept; such altered patterns may suggest worthlessness or a sense of great self-worth
5. Diminished ability to think, focus, concentrate, and/or make decisions
6. Recurrent suicidal ideation, suicidal plans, or suicide attempts

Assessment and Diagnosis. Careful assessment of psychological disorders is the initial step in effective treatment planning, whether the planned treatment is pharmacological, psychological, or a combination of both. Thorough assessment is helpful in distinguishing between functional and organic causes. In other words, not only do we need to develop a DSM-IV classification of symptom-based behavioral dysfunction, we also need to make a differential diagnosis of all possible causative factors for the observed behaviors.[18] This list is then narrowed to one or perhaps a few possibilities, so that the likely cause can be identified and more effectively treated.

Development of a differential diagnosis can be quite difficult. Consider a 19-year-old student who had been the "perfect" son. When initially seen, he was reporting delusions, had pressured speech, and was making psychotic verbalizations. It was established that he had been abusing alcohol, marijuana, and stimulant drugs. A differential diagnosis included both bipolar illness and polysubstance abuse. During a 1-week period of hospitalization, his symptoms remitted. He subsequently did well for 3 weeks, until his friends provided him with alcohol and drugs. He was arrested after a bar fight and began displaying his prior delusional symptoms and psychotic verbalizations. Two weeks later, during a second period of hospitalization, the symptoms again subsided. Recovery after discharge went well for about a month. Then he was arrested one evening when he was found directing traffic while naked. Hospitalized a third time, he strongly denied any drug or alcohol use. Finally, diagnosis of bipolar disorder was made after hypomanic symptoms returned in the absence of drug abuse. Without a valid differential diagnosis, effective treatment, which included the use of lithium carbamate (see Chapter 8), could not have been initiated.

A thorough assessment also includes an investigation of social and psychological factors that may contribute to pathology.[19] Other sociopsychological conditions may exacerbate existing physical or psychological problems. For example, cessation of cigarette smoking can be accompanied by the emergence or exacerbation of major depressive episodes,[20] a situation that not only requires treatment of the depression but is probably associated with repeated attempts to stop smoking, with repeated relapses to continued cigarette use.

Relieving symptoms through prescribed drugs fails to treat the root of the mood disorder, especially if the disorder results from a nonbiological, exogenous source. In such a case, long-term resolution of symptomatology can be achieved only through comprehensive psychosocial treatments.

Treatment. The biological, psychological, and social factors in mood disorders must be addressed in a comprehensive treatment plan.[8] Studies have shown that pharmacotherapy and psychotherapy effectively treat depression and are markedly superior to the usual office care supplied by a physician.[6,10,21] Also, combining medication and psychotherapy is more effective than either treatment alone.[2,22,23] Even reactive (exogenous) depression, adjustment mood disorders, and dysthymia[24] have biological components that require intervention with pharmacological agents along with psychotherapy.[25-27] Furthermore, with the most refractory mood disorders, a psychological or psychotherapeutic approach is made more effective with medication; both approaches work together to increase efficacy and prevent relapse. Medication often reduces symptoms arising from biochemical dysfunction to a level that allows the introduction of psychological interventions.[28]

An individual's basic perceptual beliefs, cognitive and intellectual processing, and experiences affect that person's interaction with the environment and with other individuals. Eventually a person develops a sense of how that self interacts with others. Individuals suffering from a mood disorder learn a pattern of behavior that may cause their problems to become worse and make the disorder resistant to treatment and intervention. Psychological therapies can change that pattern of behavior. There are many techniques, "from simple education to supportive counseling to insight-oriented dynamically based therapy."[29] Cognitive therapy, behavioral therapy, brief psychodynamic psychotherapy, group therapies, and others are frequently used and are effective interventions.

Miller, Norman, and Keitner (1989)[30] note that adding cognitive-behavioral therapy to standard antidepressant pharmacotherapy cuts the rate of relapse of depression by about one-half during the year following treatment termination. Schulberg and Rush (1994)[31] state: "It is thought that persons with more severe or chronic depression and partial responders to either treatment alone [psychotherapy or medication] may benefit from the combination."[31]

Children and adolescents are being increasingly diagnosed with mood disorders, including major depressive disorder and bipolar disorder.[32] Why there is an increase in the diagnosis of depression is unclear. As stated by Campbell and Cueva (1995)[33]:

> Systematic research is required to ascertain whether a marked increase of depression (or depressive symptomatology) in children and adolescents is an increase in rate of endogenous depression or a function of changing times and change in family structure. Nongenetic environmental factors may contribute up to 40 percent to 50 percent of the risk for depression.

In general, antidepressant medication is only slightly (or not at all) more effective than is placebo in treating depression in children and adolescents, with 35 to 50 percent responding positively to either placebo or active medication. Several children taking antidepressants have suddenly and unexpectedly died (see Chapter 7). This may not indicate a lack of efficacy of the drug but the powerful effect of the placebo.[33] Here, behavioral therapies and family interventions are perhaps more important than pharmacologic interventions. Fisher and Fisher (1996)[34] questioned the continued use of antidepressants in children despite their documented lack of effect. They concluded by questioning the ethical position of making "therapeutic decisions that are not anchored in existing scientific data."

Bipolar disorder in adolescents is not uncommon. Approximately 20 percent of all bipolar patients have their first episode during adolescence, 12 percent are hospitalized during this period of their life, and the peak age of onset is between 15 and 19 years of age. Lithium carbonate and valproic acid (see Chapter 8) are the mainstays of therapy.[35] In 1997 the American Academy of Child and Adolescent Psychiatry published practice parameters for the assessment and treatment of children and adolescents with bipolar disorder.[35] These parameters delineate both the pharmacologic and the psychosocial interventions. Practitioners working with children and adolescents are advised to be familiar with these practice parameters, as well as those published for use in treating adults (discussed later in this chapter).

Schizophrenia

The formal DSM-IV definition of schizophrenia is presented in Table 15.3. The symptoms of schizophrenia include hallucinations, delusions, disorganized speech, and bizarre behavior. These are often referred to as the "positive" symptoms of schizophrenia. "Negative" symptoms include impaired social interactions, impoverished and blunted affect, an absence of motivation, and significant social withdrawal (see Chapter 9). The disorder often begins in adolescence or young adulthood, frequently followed by a progressively deteriorating course, with few patients making a complete recovery.

Antipsychotic Medication. The use of the phenothiazines and other neuroleptic drugs to reduce the symptomatology of schizophrenia was discussed in Chapter 9. In the early 1990s it was stated:

> All of the symptoms associated with schizophrenia are affected to some degree by neuroleptics. Positive symptoms, including hallucinations, delusions, and disorganized thoughts, are more responsive to drug treatment than are negative symptoms, such as blunted affect, emotional withdrawal, and lack of social interest. . . . A substantial proportion of schizophrenic patients—about 10 to 20 percent—fail to demonstrate substantial improvement when they are treated with neuroleptics. This subgroup of treatment-refractory schizophrenic patients often requires long-term institutionalization in state hospitals and similar facilities. Clozapine and other atypical antipsychotic drugs may be particularly effective for these patients.[36]

Clozapine is the first of the "new generation" of antipsychotic drugs; others include risperidone, olanzapine (introduced in 1996), and mirtazapine (introduced in 1997). These newer agents are effective in at least 30 percent of patients who are severely disabled by negative symptoms. In addition, these new drugs are rapidly becoming accepted as first-line agents because of their effectiveness and their lack of extrapyramidal side effects. By relieving negative symptomatology, they make the patient "reachable" and more amenable to psychosocial interventions in efforts to improve their social functioning and their integration into society.

Psychotherapy and Rehabilitation. The development of the "new generation" of antipsychotic drugs increases the usefulness of psychotropic

---

TABLE 15.3 DSM-IV categories of schizophrenia and related disorders

---

Schizophrenia is a disturbance that lasts for at least 6 months and includes at least 1 month of active-phase symptoms (i.e., two [or more] of the following: delusions, hallucinations, disorganized speech, grossly disorganized or catatonic behavior, negative symptoms). Definitions for Schizophrenia subtypes (Paranoid, Disorganized, Catatonic, Undifferentiated, and Residual) are also included in this section.

Schizophreniform Disorder is characterized by a symptomatic presentation that is equivalent to Schizophrenia except for its duration (i.e., the disturbance lasts from 1 to 6 months) and the absence of a requirement that there be a decline in functioning.

Schizoaffective Disorder is a disturbance in which a mood episode and the active-phase symptoms of Schizophrenia occur together and were preceded or are followed by at least 2 weeks of delusions or hallucinations without prominent mood symptoms.

Delusional Disorder is characterized by at least 1 month of nonbizarre delusions without other active-phase symptoms of Schizophrenia.

Brief Psychotic Disorder is a psychotic disturbance that lasts more than 1 day and remits by 1 month.

Shared Psychotic Disorder is a disturbance that develops in an individual who is influenced by someone else who has an established delusion with similar content.

In **Psychotic Disorder Due to a General Medical Condition,** the psychotic symptoms are judged to be a direct physiological consequence of a general medical condition.

In **Substance-Induced Psychotic Disorder,** the psychotic symptoms are judged to be a direct physiological consequence of a drug of abuse, a medication, or toxin exposure.

Psychotic Disorder Not Otherwise Specified is included for classifying psychotic presentations that do not meet criteria for any of the specific Psychotic Disorders defined in this section or psychotic symptomatology about which there is inadequate or contradictory information.

Reproduced with permission from DSM-IV, pp. 273–274.

therapy in treating mental disorders. Similarly, the limits of medication demonstrate the need for concomitant psychotherapy and other rehabilitative procedures. While psychotropic medication frequently relieves symptomatology, the addition of psychotherapy can be important, particularly in an outpatient setting.

Having established the primary role of antipsychotics, there is evidence that psychosocial therapies, when administered with these agents, improve long-term prognosis. Because chronically psychotic patients have difficulties with social adjustment, reason dictates that they and their families could benefit from such interventions. Regardless of theoretical orientation, it is clear that practitioners should provide psychosocial therapy as part of a comprehensive treatment strategy.[38]

In general, most cost-benefit studies find that the addition of psychological therapies in an outpatient setting encourages drug compliance. Indeed, therapeutic interventions improve social skills and assist in the rehabilitation of cognitive functions. Psychological therapy in conjunction with drug therapy also extends relapse time and reduces the intensity of relapse episodes. Typically, the most beneficial strategy is a sociopsychological therapy emphasizing self-esteem, social skills, and cognitive rehabilitation. This emphasis addresses the interaction between the client's symptoms and their social and psychological consequences. These strategies develop and rehabilitate cognitive functions, resulting in a more positive self-image and more effective social and cognitive functioning. Medication addresses the biophysical component of the disorder. Social therapy, with structured or supported living, teaches and reinforces social skills. Psychological therapy addresses the intrapsychic and psychodynamic issues. Vocational rehabilitation is important in developing self-esteem and establishing financial independence.

Functions of the Treatment Team. The treatment team should teach the client the positive and negative effects of any prescribed drugs; it should also answer any questions and relieve any doubts that a patient has about any medication. Helping the client remain drug compliant is important in reducing the rate of relapse. Indeed, monitoring of drug levels in plasma can provide important information, improve drug effectiveness, and reduce unwanted side effects.[36] The client should also understand the limitations of his or her medication. A team member should help the client understand that motivation, medication, and psychological therapy are all important in stabilization and recovery.

Schizophrenia is relatively uncommon in children and adolescents.[33] Therefore, research in this area is lacking and individuals in this age group, if diagnosed with the disorder, are generally medicated with antipsychotics (haloperidol, clozapine, and others), as are adults.

Anxiety Disorders

Symptoms of anxiety are normal and serve as an early warning system that helps one avoid potentially dangerous situations. Excessive anxiety, however, may be a source of significant suffering and require intervention.[37] Because anxiety touches everyone, it becomes a disorder only when it is objectively uncomfortable or is perceived to be out of control. At such times, the usual feelings of anxiety increase and interfere with one's normal functioning. Severe symptoms of anxiety require assessment and treatment.

Understanding the underlying causes and formulating a differential diagnosis will help the clinician determine which drugs and which psychological interventions will be the most effective.[38] What we continue to discover is not only the subtlety of anxiety but also its pervasiveness. Indeed, anxiety accompanies almost every psychiatric disorder.

Regier and coworkers (1993)[16] (see Table 15.2) reported a one-year prevalence of all anxiety disorders in 12.6 percent of the U.S. adult population (20 million persons). Most of these individuals had a phobic disorder (10.9 percent or 17 million persons), while 1.3 percent had panic disorder and 2.1 percent had obsessive-compulsive disorder. Indeed, anxiety disorders had the highest prevalence rate of the major DSM-IV diagnostic groups.

Added to these 20 million persons are individuals who have generalized anxiety disorder (GAD), most of whom are undiagnosed. It is likely that mental health workers have not been aware of people with GAD because they perceive the symptoms, especially the worry, as part of their clients' daily lives. The exact incidence of GAD is unknown, although estimates run as high as 5 percent of the adult population. However, awareness is increasing, and more cases of GAD are reported every year. GAD is also becoming recognized as a condition responsive to medication (see the discussion of buspirone in Chapter 4) and to psychological intervention.

The chronicity of anxiety disorders is similar to that of mood disorders, more enduring than that of substance abuse disorders, but less deep-seated than that of the schizophrenias. Only about 30 percent of individuals with anxiety disorders receive treatment,[16] a percentage that is even lower if GAD is included. Thus, a high percentage of mental health and addictive disorders are actually anxiety disorders or have a high component of comorbid anxiety. Often, these disorders go untreated or are not treated by behavioral health specialists.

Characteristic of anxiety disorders are the symptoms of anxiety and avoidance behavior. Anxiety is a complex response that includes subjective feelings of dread, apprehension, fear, tension, and related psychomotor responses. The last may include motor tension, increases in autonomic responses (heart rate, blood pressure), vigilance, and scanning. The DSM-IV lists several subcategories of the anxiety disorders,[39] which are listed in Table 15.4.

Using drugs to treat anxiety disorders (in both adults and children) is controversial, with the controversy arising from diagnostic difficulties, from the chronic nature of many anxieties, and from the addictive potential associated with some of the drugs used in therapy. In the 1960s and 1970s, the benzodiazepine anxiolytics appeared to treat anxiety disorders quickly, effectively, and safely and replaced the barbiturate therapies of the 1950s. Over time, however, the potential addictiveness of benzodiazepine therapy became evident. Similarly, clinicians noted that anxiolytics, which reduced the outward symptoms of anxiety, could be counterproductive in some cases, producing depression and suppressing cognitive function. With the advent of the antidepressants and the observation that these drugs effectively treated many of the anxieties, sophistication in diagnosing and treating the anxieties similarly expanded:

> It is imperative for [both prescribing and nonprescribing] clinicians to become knowledgeable about the basic pharmacology of these drugs, along with their appropriate clinical indications, dosages, and duration of usage. Most importantly, their limitations must receive as much attention as their assets.[40]

Accurate assessment and diagnosis is especially vital in planning the appropriate treatment for anxiety disorders. Generally, more diffuse and severe anxiety symptoms require some initial pharmacological intervention. Less severe, more circumscribed symptoms of phobias may be more responsive to cognitive and behavioral therapy; in such cases, it is often unnecessary to resort to pharmacotherapy. Regarding combination therapy, Mavissakalian and Ryan (1997)[41] state:

> Although the integration of medication and behavior therapy for anxiety disorders is widely practiced clinically, there are not many controlled studies of the combined use of medication with behavioral techniques. . . . Medications alone are effective treatments of anxiety disorders, but they are more likely to require long-term maintenance treatments for indefinite periods of time. Although nearly equivalent in efficacy, benzodiazepines and antidepressants should not be considered equivalent when combined with behavioral treatments. Combined treatment, guided by some general principles . . . offers the best chance for relief and long-term recovery from anxiety disorders.

TABLE 15.4 DSM-IV categories of anxiety disorders

A **Panic Attack** is a discrete period in which there is the sudden onset of intense apprehension, fearfulness, or terror, often associated with feelings of impending doom. During these attacks symptoms such as shortness of breath, palpitations, chest pain or discomfort, choking or smothering sensations, and fear of "going crazy" or losing control are present.

Agoraphobia is anxiety about, or avoidance of, places or situations from which escape might be difficult (or embarrassing) or in which help may not be available in the event of having a Panic Attack or panic-like symptoms.

Panic Disorder without Agoraphobia is characterized by recurrent unexpected Panic Attacks about which there is persistent concern. **Panic Disorder with Agoraphobia** is characterized by both recurrent unexpected Panic Attacks and Agoraphobia.

Agoraphobia without History of Panic Disorder is characterized by the presence of Agoraphobia and panic-like symptoms without a history of unexpected Panic Attacks.

Specific Phobia is characterized by clinically significant anxiety provoked by exposure to a specific feared object or situation, often leading to avoidance behavior.

Social Phobia is characterized by clinically significant anxiety provoked by exposure to certain types of social or performance situations, often leading to avoidance behavior.

Obsessive-Compulsive Disorder is characterized by obsessions (which cause marked anxiety or distress) and/or by compulsions (which serve to neutralize anxiety).

Post-Traumatic Stress Disorder is characterized by the reexperiencing of an extremely traumatic event accompanied by symptoms of increased arousal and by avoidance of stimuli associated with the trauma.

Acute Stress Disorder is characterized by symptoms similar to those of Post-Traumatic Stress Disorder that occur immediately in the aftermath of an extremely traumatic event.

Generalized Anxiety Disorder is characterized by at least 6 months of persistent and excessive anxiety and worry.

Anxiety Disorder Due to a General Medical Condition is characterized by prominent symptoms of anxiety that are judged to be a direct physiological consequence of a general medical condition.

Substance-Induced Anxiety Disorder is characterized by prominent symptoms of anxiety that are judged to be a direct physiological consequence of a drug of abuse, a medication, or toxin exposure.

Anxiety Disorder Not Otherwise Specified is included for coding disorders with prominent anxiety or phobic avoidance that do not meet criteria for any of the specific Anxiety Disorders defined in this section (or anxiety symptoms about which there is inadequate or contradictory information).

Because Separation Anxiety Disorder (characterized by anxiety related to separation from parental figures) usually develops in childhood, it is included in the "Disorders Usually First Diagnosed in Infancy, Childhood, or Adolescence" section. Phobic avoidance that is limited to genital sexual contact with a sexual partner is classified as Sexual Aversion Disorder and is included in the "Sexual and Gender Identity Disorders" section.

Reproduced with permission from DSM-IV, pp. 393–394.

Panic Disorder. Panic disorder is one of the most common and most disabling anxiety disorders. A recent article[42] discusses Charles Darwin, describing how disabling this disorder was in his life. Indeed, panic disorder is considered a chronic condition that requires ongoing maintenance therapy[43,44] (pharmacologic[45,46] and psychological[47,48]). It is estimated[49,50] that the prevalence of panic disorder in the general community is about 1.6 percent to 3.2 percent in women and 0.4 percent to 1.7 percent in men. Between 8 percent and 13 percent of patients in primary care practices experience panic attacks. Further, patients with panic disorder account for more than 20 percent of emergency room visits and are 12 times more likely to visit the emergency room than the general population. Patients with panic attacks average 19 medical visits per year, a rate 7 times above normal; they also account for 15 percent of total medical visits. The use of medical services and the health care costs associated with these patients are therefore enormous. Added to those are disability costs and unemployment expenses (25 percent of these patients are fully unemployed). Certainly, appropriate treatment will reduce these disabilities and expenditures.

Comprehensive therapy reduces the severity of the course of panic disorder and enhances outcome. Pharmacologically, antidepressant drugs are now considered to be the pharmacological treatments of choice,[45] except for patients also experiencing severe agitation. For those patients, an anxiolytic, such as a benzodiazepine, is more effective on a short-term basis, until the anxiety and/or agitation resolves. Davidson (1997),[46] however, argues in favor of benzodiazepine therapy as primary treatment for panic disorder.

Of the antidepressants, the SSRIs (serotonin-specific reuptake inhibitors), such as fluvoxamine, fluoxetine, and clomipramine, appear to be superior to the traditional tricyclic antidepressants and to alternative agents such as maprotiline (see Chapter 8).[45] As Sheehan and Harnett-Sheehan (1996)[51] state:

> The emerging data suggest that serotonin uptake inhibitors are superior to placebo and better tolerated than most of the older alternatives. As a result they are now becoming first-choice treatments in panic disorder.

An estimated 50 percent of patients with panic disorder ultimately experience an episode of major depression,[52] an added impetus for the use of antidepressant medications over alternative agents. Psychological therapies must also address this comorbidity of panic disorder and depression.

Pollack (1997)[53] reviewed the psychopharmacology for panic disorder. He stated that, with the use of SSRIs, it is important to "start low" to minimize the increased anxiety associated with the initiation of treatment. Here, the benzodiazepines may be necessary. According to Pollack, buproprion and trazodone are "unique among antidepressants in their relative lack of efficacy in treating panic disorder and other anxiety conditions in contrast to most other antidepressants." Data for venlafaxine and nefazodone are not yet available. Pollack concludes by providing explicit dosage recommendations (see Table 15.5) to which the interested clinician is referred.[53]

Of the benzodiazepines, alprazolam (Xanax) is the most widely studied for treating panic disorder. Other benzodiazepines that have been studied include lorazepam (Ativan) and clonazepam (Clonopin). The benzodiazepines have a favorable profile of side effects, lacking the anticholinergic side effects of the TCAs and the increased anxiety of the SSRIs. Concomitant use (benzodiazepine plus SSRI) provides rapid anxiolysis and more comprehensive relief of panic and depressive symptoms.[53] In addition, the monoamine oxidase (MAO) inhibitors have been shown to be effective in treating panic disorder, particularly in patients who do not respond to more traditional antidepressant compounds.

For all antidepressant medications, treatment may need to be continued indefinitely, because there is a high rate of relapse with medication discontinuation. Clinically, cognitive-behavioral therapeutic (CBT) interventions are also indicated in the treatment of panic disorder. These interventions should target avoidance behaviors that patients have learned over time to reduce the frequency of panic attacks. One part of the CBT approach is teaching the patient specific relaxation and stress management techniques.

Otto (1997)[54] reviewed the "integrated treatment" of panic disorder. CBT techniques were more effective than drug therapy. CBT usually includes

> informational intervention; somatic management skills, including breathing retraining and relaxation skills, and of more importance, cognitive restructuring, which helps patients change their catastrophic responses and fears concerning the somatic sensations; interoceptive exposure (for example, exposing patients to rapid heartbeat, numbness and tingling, and showing them that these sensations do not have to drive them toward a panic attack); and situational exposure, to help agoraphobic patients overcome their fear of having panic attacks in certain situations or settings. . . . Interoceptive exposure . . . is the most important component.

TABLE 15.5 Pharmacology for panic disorder

Class	Agents	Starting and maintenance doses
SSRIs	Fluoxetine	5–10 mg/d; 20–80 mg/d
	Sertraline	25–50 mg/d; 50–200 mg/d
	Paroxetine	10 mg/d; 20–50 mg/d
	Fluvoxamine	25 mg/d; 50–300 mg/d
Tricyclic antidepressants	Imipramine	10 mg/d "test dose"
	Nortriptyline	Recommended dosage for all TCAs:
	Desipramine	2.25 mg/kg/d (imipramine equivalents)
	Amitriptyline	
	Doxepin	
Atypical antidepressants	Venlafaxine	18.75 mg b.i.d.
	Nefazodone	50 mg b.i.d.
MAOIs	Phenelzine	45–90 mg/d; 100–300 mg/d
	Tranylcypromine	30–60 mg/d; 300–500 mg/d
High potency benzodiazepines	Clonazepam	1–5 mg/d
	Alprazolam	2–10 mg/d

Reproduced with permission from Pollack (1997).[53]

Regarding combinations of CBT and medications, some studies report improvements, while others note that adding medications to CBT provides short-term gains but may reduce the long-term benefits of CBT. Certainly, CBT must be reinstituted at the time of medication discontinuation.[54] Spiegel and Bruce (1997)[55] review the combined use of CBT with benzodiazapine therapy for panic disorder.

Generalized Anxiety Disorder. Despite the considerable attention focused on anxiety disorder over the past decade, little attention has been devoted to the investigation of generalized anxiety disorder (GAD):

> The emerging picture is that GAD is a common and chronic disorder, affecting primarily women, and one that leads to significant distress and impairment. Subjects with GAD frequently utilize health care services and require medication treatment.[56]

Formerly called *anxiety neurosis*, GAD occurs at a rate that equals or exceeds the other anxiety disorders, such as panic disorder and social phobia. GAD is also comorbid with other psychological disorders, especially depression and dysthymia[57]:

> GAD is associated with disability, medically unexplained symptoms, and overutilization of medical resources. Two-thirds of individuals with current GAD had an additional current psychiatric diagnosis (usually major depression or dysthymia), and 98 percent of those with lifetime GAD had another lifetime psychiatric diagnosis. GAD may be a crucial factor in modifying the presentation, course, and outcome of major depression.

Patients with GAD have a moderate amount of disability and impairment in quality of life. GAD is especially common in the elderly.[58] Treatment of GAD is at an elementary stage. Certainly, one mainstay of the self-medication (or self-prescription) for GAD is alcohol, which effectively produces a short-term anxiolytic action (see Chapter 3). Acute drug therapy is well studied and appears to be highly effective in providing symptomatic relief, but relapse and recurrence are high.[59] Until recently benzodiazepines have been the prescribed agent of choice, but their use is associated with significant "emergent anxiety and/or withdrawal-related symptomatology"[60]:

> Twenty-five percent of patients treated with lorazepam showed rebound anxiety, and 40 percent of them utilized reserve medication because they found drug discontinuation to be intolerable.

More recently, buspirone (BuSpar) has been demonstrated to effectively reduce symptomatology with efficacy superior to placebo and equal to lorazepam.[61,62] Patients treated with buspirone show no rebound anxiety or benzodiazepine withdrawal syndrome.[62] As discussed in Chapter 3, buspirone is now considered to be the drug of first choice for GAD in situations where a slow onset of action is acceptable and the drug may be required for a prolonged time.[63] Hales and coworkers (1997)[64] present an algorithm for treating anxiety, emphasizing buspirone for persistent anxiety without panic attacks, the latter often requiring therapy with an SSRI-type antidepressant:

> Buspirone does not impair memory or motor coordination, is not associated with abuse or dependence, is not cross tolerant with alcohol, and does not produce a withdrawal reaction. In addition, buspirone has a progressive onset of action and produces few adverse drug reactions when combined with other agents. If the patient does not respond to buspirone, we encourage nefazodone, a 5-HT$_2$ antagonist, or one of the serotonin selective reuptake inhibitors.

Regarding formal psychotherapies, recent research is focusing on the efficacy of cognitive-behavioral interventions,[64] which teach clients to examine how their unrealistic thoughts and ruminations affect their behavioral functioning. Relaxation therapy, biofeedback, and stress management are used to teach patients how to relax even under stress. Many anxious people worry about being unable to cope. They fear losing control, "going crazy," or being publicly embarrassed. As a consequence, the fears increase the anxiety, causing a vicious circle. Anxious thoughts increase anxiety symptoms, which, in turn, generate even more anxious thoughts. Cognitive-behavioral techniques help patients break this circle by allowing them to deal appropriately with anxious thoughts and their related behavioral expressions.[63]

Because GAD is a chronic, relapsing, and debilitating disorder, both acute efficacy and long-term prevention of relapse must be considered when choosing both drug and psychotherapeutic interventions. Ideally, cognitive-behavioral therapies should accompany pharmacologic treatment.[65] Certainly, any psychotherapeutic intervention should begin before medication is discontinued in order to minimize the likelihood of relapse.

Specific Phobia and Social Phobia. The phobias are characterized by extreme anxiety about a specific object (specific phobia) or a generalized or discrete social situation (social phobia). Patients with social phobias are at high risk for developing mood or anxiety disorders and schizophrenia. According to learning theory, individuals select the behavior that moves them from a state of stress to a state in which the stress is reduced. Thus, if a conditioned stimulus is repeatedly presented in a manner that does not produce a conditioned emotional response, the original association is extinguished. The object of therapy based on this reasoning ("targeted exposure therapy") is to pair fear-evoking incidents with relaxation training in a sequence that finally leads to the presentation of the original fear-inducing or anxiety-arousing stimulus.

When the patient with a phobia displays severe anxiety symptoms, anxiolytics may be administered to treat acute symptoms. For longer-term pharmacological management, antidepressant agents are indicated, especially those with anxiolytic properties. Alprazolam (Xanax) can be quite effective, as are serotonin-specific antidepressants,[66] MAO inhibitors, and buspirone, either alone or in combination.[67]

Obsessive-Compulsive Disorder. Obsessive-compulsive disorder (OCD) is characterized by recurrent and disturbing thoughts (obsessions) and/or repetitive behaviors (compulsions) that the individual feels driven to perform but recognizes as irrational or excessive. Once thought to be a rare condition, it is now estimated to be present in about

2 percent of the general population, making it the fourth most common psychiatric disorder.[68]

> Although traditionally viewed as resistant to a variety of therapeutic interventions, recent advances have been made in the psychopharmacologic and behavioral therapy of OCD. In particular, the clear efficacy of serotonin reuptake inhibitors, such as clomipramine, fluvoxamine, fluoxetine, and sertraline, has been established in double-blind studies in patients with OCD. Consistent with these drug response data are the hypotheses that changes in serotonin function are critical to the treatment of OCD and perhaps involved in the pathophysiology of at least some patients with the disorder.[69]

SSRIs are commonly used for treating OCD, being effective in approximately 40 to 60 percent of OCD patients. Several recent papers explore the use of SSRIs in OCD.[70-72] Treatment guidelines for OCD were recently published [*Journal of Clinical Psychiatry* 58 (1997), Supplement 4.]

Dager (1993)[73] favors a combination of medication and behavioral therapy. He believes that in some cases behavioral conditioning can be useful as the primary intervention for compulsions, although the approach appears to be less effective for obsessional thinking. Systematic desensitization or cognitive-behavioral therapy is also used. A paradoxical behavioral approach known as exposure therapy is sometimes also used to treat OCD. In exposure treatment, the client is asked to experience the stimuli that produced the obsessional thinking or compulsive behavior. Although cognitive-behavioral therapies have been quite useful, other types have not. "Psychoanalysis and psychodynamically-oriented psychotherapy have been particularly unsuccessful in treating OCD."[73] Janicak, Davis, Preskorn, and Ayd (1993)[74] summarize:

> Because significant OCD symptoms often remain or recur, even when there is substantial improvement with a specific therapy, a combined complementary approach seems to be the optimal strategy for most patients.

March and Leonard (1996)[75] review OCD in children and adolescents, noting that 1 in 200 young persons suffer from the disorder.

> OCD-specific cognitive-behavioral psychotherapy and pharmacotherapy with a serotonin reuptake inhibitor define the psychotherapeutic and pharmacotherapeutic treatments of choice, respectively.[75]

Post-Traumatic Stress Disorder. It is generally accepted that transient and long-lasting neurological alterations may underlie acute and long-term neuronal responses to traumatic stress.[76] Comorbidity is frequent; individuals with post-traumatic stress disorder (PTSD) experience a high incidence of GAD, phobias, depression, and substance abuse.[76] Thus, the treatment of PTSD must be comprehensive and individualized, utilizing carefully balanced pharmacotherapeutic and psychotherapeutic interventions that address both the PTSD and any comorbid disorder. According to Vargas and Davidson (1993)[77]: "Symptom relief provided by pharmacotherapy enables the patient to participate more thoroughly in individual, behavioral, or group therapy."

Most drugs that are effective for PTSD are also useful for treating major depression and panic disorder. Thus, numerous drugs have been tried,[78] including TCAs,[79] MAO inhibitors,[80] trazodone,[81] the SSRIs,[82] and many other agents, including clonidine, guanfacin, brofaromine, valproate, carbamazepine, and benzodiazepines.[78] Obviously, no one drug or class of drugs is universally effective in treating the disorder, although some feel that "a serotonergic action is necessary for good clinical effect in PTSD, analogous to the situation in OCD."[77] Some clinicians advocate the use of hypnotic techniques to facilitate working through the traumatic events. This approach is based on the frequently observed interrelationship between dissociative reactions and physical trauma.

Eating Disorders. Only in recent years have eating disorders (bulimia nervosa and anorexia nervosa) been considered amenable to pharmacologic treatment. For bulimia, in particular, the role of medication has expanded with publication of double-blind, placebo-controlled studies demonstrating significant decrease in the frequency of binge-eating behavior in response to antidepressant medications (see Jimerson and coworkers [1996][83] for discussion). Among the antidepressant medications, TCAs, MAOIs, and SSRIs can all be used; the choice depends on the side effect profile that a given patient could tolerate. Similarly, short-term psychotherapies (e.g., CBT or interpersonal therapies) also reduce binge frequency equal to or exceeding the effects of medication treatment. Thus, it seems reasonable to expect that combination therapy would provide additive effects. This issue is addressed by Crow and Mitchell (1996),[84] who conclude that the literature is inconclusive. Combining medication and psychotherapy may improve the outcome in selected patients.

Most authors concur that to initiate treatment of bulimia, nonpharmacologic approaches should be attempted first and medication added for either the unresponsive patient or one in whom depression or an anxiety disorder is diagnosed as a comorbid disorder. Major depression is the most common comorbid disorder; others include anxiety disorders, substance abuse, and a past history of anorexia nervosa.[83]

Medication failure can result from poor compliance, from vomiting the medication, or from other causes. Blood level analysis may be necessary before concluding that the drug attempt was a failure. Numerous other agents have been tried, but none have been effective when subjected to carefully controlled trials. The course of bulimia may require long-term antidepressant therapy with careful monitoring of side effects and compliance.

In anorexia, pharmacologic treatment has a very limited role, with psychiatric therapy being more important. Here, psychotherapy, often with CBT components, group therapy, family therapy, nutrition counseling, and so on are all necessary. Drug therapy is primarily aimed at treating comorbid depression. However, double-blind studies of antidepressants (versus placebo) show little improvement in weight (weight gain), mood, or body perception. Certainly, however, a trial of antidepressant therapy is warranted in patients who do not respond to psychotherapeutic interventions.

The APA has published guidelines for the treatment of eating disorders, and D. M. Garner and P. E. Garfinkel have edited a textbook that addresses the integration of pharmacological and psycotherapeutic approaches to treating eating disorders (*Handbook of Treatment for Eating Disorders*, 2nd ed.; New York: Guilford, 1997).

Practice Standards

As the 1990s began, it became apparent that numerous psychopharmacologic interventions and psychotherapeutic treatments of various psychological disorders were being conducted with minimal evaluation for either therapeutic efficacy or cost effectiveness. Therefore, about 1991, several groups, including the American Psychiatric Association (APA), the federal government (through the Agency for Health Care Policy and Research, or AHCPR), and more recently, the American Academy of Child and Adolescent Psychiatry (AACAP), began developing and continue to publish "practice guidelines" that are, in essence, comprehensive reviews of patient care strategies to assist clinicians in making clinical decisions regarding the treatment of specific patients. The ultimate goal of these clinical practice guidelines is to improve the care of patients. The guidelines are not intended to serve as standards of care for medical, psychological, or legal purposes. They do, however, present a consensus of expert opinion regarding disorders, their diagnoses, and the efficacy of various treatments.

It is our opinion that all behavioral health professionals should be familiar with these practice guidelines, have them available for reference, and keep up with new guidelines as they are released. With the pharmacologic background presented in this text for reference, the practitioner should have little trouble integrating the material contained in the guidelines into his or her clinical practice.

In several instances there is an overlap between the guidelines developed by the APA and those developed by AHCPR. For example, in 1996 both groups published guidelines for the treatment of nicotine dependence. Despite the overlap, the general review, therapeutic principles, and conclusions are quite similar. Several of the guidelines have been referred to in earlier chapters, but because of their importance, all are listed here, hopefully to assist the reader in developing a personal library and to prepare the reader for forthcoming monographs.

APA Practice Guidelines

For many years, the APA has published its *Diagnostic and Statistical Manual of Mental Disorders* (DSM), now in its fourth edition (DSM-IV).[3] This manual is widely used, and it provides a diagnostics foundation for categorizing behavioral/mental disorders. In 1991 the APA embarked on a process of developing practice guidelines, which have been periodically published in its journal, the *American Journal of Psychiatry*. Commentaries to these guidelines are occasionally published in the *Journal of the American Medical Association*. Some of the commentaries are included here because they can assist readers in broadening their awareness of the issues involved.

In late 1996 the APA collected and published in book form the first five sets of guidelines[86]:

- "Psychiatric Evaluation of Adults"
- "Eating Disorders" (first published in February 1993 in the *American Journal of Psychiatry*)
- "Major Depressive Disorder in Adults" (first published in April 1993 in the *American Journal of Psychiatry*)
- "Treatment of Patients with Bipolar Disorder" (first published in December 1994 in the *American Journal of Psychiatry*)
- "Treatment of Patients with Substance Abuse Disorders: Alcohol, Cocaine, Opioids"

The sixth practice guideline published by the APA, "Practice Guideline for the Treatment of Patients with Nicotine Dependence,"[87] appeared as a supplement to the *American Journal of Psychiatry* in October 1996. It is also available in monograph form from the APA.[87] In April 1997 the APA published its seventh practice guideline, "Practice Guideline for the Treatment of Patients with Schizophrenia,"[88] followed the next month by its eighth guideline, "Practice Guideline for Treatment of Patients with Alzheimer's Disease and Other Dementias of Late Life." In addition to the seven sets of guidelines, the APA is in the process of developing practice guidelines for panic disorder and related anxiety disorders, geriatrics, and mental retardation.

As they are developed, the guidelines will be published as supplements in the *American Journal of Psychiatry*. Completed guidelines are scheduled for revision at three- to five-year intervals. All guidelines will probably be included in future editions of "Practice Guidelines."[86]

AHCPR Practice Guidelines

AHCPR was established by the federal government in December 1989 with the mission to enhance the quality and effectiveness of health care services and access to such services. AHCPR carries out this mission, in part, by publishing a wide variety of clinical practice guidelines intended for use by health care professionals, educators, medical review organizations, and consumers. The first set of guidelines was released on March 5, 1992, and was devoted to the management of acute pain following operative or medical procedures and trauma. This was followed by guidelines devoted to such medical topics as urinary incontinence, cataracts, sickle cell anemia, low back problems, heart failure, and many others. In the area of psychopharmacology and psychotherapeutics, the AHCPR guidelines include

- *Depression in Primary Care* (volume I, *Detection and Diagnosis*; volume II, *Treatment*), published in 1993[21, 22]
- *Diagnosis and Treatment of Anxiety and Panic Disorder in the Primary Care Setting*, published in 1994
- *Diagnosis and Treatment of Bipolar Disorder*, published in 1995
- *Smoking Cessation Clinical Practice Guidelines*, published in 1996[89]

The AHCPR reports can occasionally be difficult to locate due to limited printings, but they have been either republished or extensively discussed in other publications. The 1993 depression guidelines were discussed soon after their publication by Schulberg and Rush (1994)[90] and by Munoz and coworkers (1994)[91] and more recently by Persons and coworkers (1996)[2]. The 1996 guidelines on smoking cessation[89] were discussed in the *Journal of the American Medical Association* (April 24, 1996).[92]

The guidelines on smoking cessation were the eighteenth set of guidelines published by AHCPR. It was followed in late 1996 by the nineteenth, on the diagnosis and treatment of Alzheimer's disease. Unfortunately, additional guidelines will not be forthcoming, because in 1997 the AHCPR ceased this activity; in the future it will provide supportive services for other organizations developing practice guidelines. Copies of existing guidelines can be ordered through the AHCPR publications clearinghouse (1-800-358-9295).

AACAP Practice Parameters

In 1997 the Council of the AACAP published practice parameters for the assessment and treatment of children and adolescents with bipolar disorder.[93] A first for this population of patients, additional practice parameters for other neuropsychological disorders in children and adolescents will probably follow and will appear in the *Journal of the American Academy of Child and Adolescent Psychiatry*.

NOTES

1. P. G. Janicak, J. M. Davis, S. H. Preskorn, and F. J. Ayd, *Principles and Practice of Psychopharmacotherapy* (Baltimore: Williams & Wilkins, 1993), 268.
2. J. B. Persons, M. E. Thase and P. Crits-Christoph, "The Role of Psychotherapy in the Treatment of Depression," *Archives of General Psychiatry* 53 (1996): 283–290 (with four additional commentaries).
3. American Psychiatric Association, *Diagnostic and Statistical Manual of Mental Disorders*, 4th ed. (Washington, D.C.: American Psychiatric Association, 1994).
4. M. T. Shea et al., "Course of Depressive Symptoms over Follow-up: Findings from the National Institute of Mental Health Treatment of Depression Collaborative Research Program," *Archives of General Psychiatry* 49 (1992): 782–787.
5. S. J. Kingsbury, "Where Does Research on the Effectiveness of Psychotherapy Stand Today?," *The Harvard Mental Health Letter* (September 1995): 8.
6. I. W. Miller and G. I. Keitner, "Combined Medication and Psychotherapy in the Treatment of Chronic Mood Disorders," *Psychiatric Clinics of North America* 19 (1996): 151–170.
7. H. J. Henk, D. J. Katzelnick, K. A. Kobac, J. H. Griest, and J. W. Jefferson, "Medical Costs Attributed to Depression Among Patients With a History of High Medical Expenses in a Health Maintenance Organization," *Archives of General Psychiatry* 53 (1996): 899–904.

8. L. S. Meredith, K. B. Wells, S. H. Kaplan, and R. M. Mazel, "Counseling Typically Provided for Depression," *Archives of General Psychiatry* 53 (1996): 905–912.

9. W. Katon, P. Robinson, M. Von Korff, et al., "A Multifaceted Intervention to Improve Treatment of Depression in Primary Care," *Archives of General Psychiatry* 53 (1996): 924–932.

10. W. Katon, M. Von Korff, E. Lin, et al., "Collaborative Management to Achieve Treatment Depression Guidelines," *Journal of Clinical Psychiatry* 58, Suppl. 1(1997): 20–23.

11. K. B. Wells, "Caring for Depression in Primary Care: Defining and Illustrating the Policy Context," *Journal of Clinical Psychiatry* 58, Suppl. 1(1997): 24–27.

12. S. H. Preskorn, M. J. Burke, and G. A. Fast, "Therapeutic Drug Monitoring: Principles and Practice," *Psychiatric Clinics of North America* 16 (September 1993): 611–641.

13. American Psychiatric Association, *Diagnostic and Statistical Manual of Mental Disorders*, 4th ed. (Washington, D.C.: American Psychiatric Association, 1994), xxi–xxii.

14. R. W. Mandersheid, D. S. Rae, W. E. Narrow, B. Z. Locke, and D. A. Regier, "Congruence of Service Utilization Estimates from the Epidemiologic Catchment Area Project and Other Sources," *Archives of General Psychiatry* 50 (1993): 108–114.

15. W. E. Narrow, D. A. Regier, D. S. Rae, R. W. Mandersheid, and B. Z. Locke, "Use of Services by Persons with Mental and Addictive Disorders: Findings from the National Institute of Mental Health Epidemiologic Catchment Area Program," *Archives of General Psychiatry* 50 (1993): 95–107.

16. D. A. Regier, W. E. Narrow, D. S. Rae, et al., "The De Facto U.S. Mental and Addictive Disorders Service System: Epidemiologic Catchment Area Prospective One-Year Prevalence Rates of Disorders and Services," *Archives of General Psychiatry* 50 (1993): 85–94.

17. American Psychiatric Association, *Diagnostic and Statistical Manual of Mental Disorders*, 4th ed. (Washington, D.C.: American Psychiatric Association, 1994), 317–320.

18. P. G. Janicak, J. M. Davis, S. H. Preskorn, and F. J. Ayd, *Principles and Practice of Psychopharmacotherapy* (Baltimore: Williams & Wilkins, 1993), 187–201.

19. D. L. Dunner, "Diagnostic Assessment," *Psychiatric Clinics of North America* 16 (September 1993): 431–441.

20. K. B. Stage, A. H. Glassman, and L. S. Covey, "Depression After Smoking Cessation: Case Reports," *Journal of Clinical Psychiatry* 57 (1996): 467–469.

21. H. C. Schulberg, M. R. Block, M. J. Madonia, et al., "Treating Major Depression in Primary Care Practice: Eight-Month Clinical Outcomes," *Archives of General Psychiatry* 53 (1996): 913–919.

22. Depression Guideline Panel, *Depression in Primary Care*, vol. 1, *Diagnosis and Detection, Clinical Practice Guideline No. 5*, AHCPR Publication 93-0550 (Rockville, Md.: Department of Health and Human Services, Public Health Service, Agency for Health Care Policy and Research, 1993).

23. Depression Guideline Panel, *Depression in Primary Care*, vol. 2, *Treatment of Major Depression, Clinical Practice Guideline No. 5*, AHCPR Publication 93-0551 (Rockville, Md.: Department of Health and Human Services, Public Health Service, Agency for Health Care Policy and Research, 1993).

24. R. A. Friedman and J. H. Kocis, "Pharmacotherapy for Chronic Depression," *Psychiatric Clinics of North America* 19 (1996): 121–132.

25. American Psychiatric Association, "Practice Guideline for Major Depressive Disorder in Adults," *American Journal of Psychiatry* 150, Suppl. 4 (1993): 1–26.

26. E. Richelson, "Treatment of Acute Depression," *Psychiatric Clinics of North America* 16 (September 1993): 461–478.

27. J. H. Kocis, R. A. Friedman, J. C. Markowitz, et al., "Maintenance Therapy for Chronic Depression," *Archives of General Psychiatry* 53 (1996): 769–774.

28. M. E. Thase, M. Fava, U. Halbreich, et al., "A Placebo-Controlled, Randomized Clinical Trial Comparing Sertraline and Imipramine for the Treatment of Dysthymia," *Archives of General Psychiatry* 53 (1996): 777–784.

29. P. G. Janicak, J. M. Davis, S. H. Preskorn, and F.J. Ayd, *Principles and Practice of Psychopharmacotherapy* (Baltimore: Williams & Wilkins, 1993), 268.

30. I. Miller, W. Norman, and G. Keitner, "Cognitive-Behavioral Treatment of Depressed Inpatients: Six- and Twelve-Month Follow-up," *American Journal of Psychiatry* 146 (1989): 1274–1279.

31. H. C. Schulberg and A. J. Rush, "Clinical Practice Guidelines for Managing Major Depression in Primary Care Practice: Implications for Psychologists," *American Psychologist* 49 (1994): 34–41.

32. C. Z. Garrison, J. L. Waller, S. P. Cuffe, et al., "Incidence of Major Depressive Disorder and Dysthymia in Young Adolescents," *Journal of the American Academy of Child and Adolescent Psychiatry* 36 (1997): 458–465.

33. M. Campbell and J. Cueva, "Psychopharmacology in Child and Adolescent Psychiatry: A Review of the Past Seven Years. Part II," *Journal of the American Academy of Child and Adolescent Psychiatry* 34 (1995): 1262–1272.

34. R. L. Fisher and S. Fisher, "Antidepressants for Children: Is Scientific Support Necessary?," *Journal of Nervous and Mental Disease* 184 (1996): 99–102.

35. J. McClellan and J. Werry, principal authors, "Practice Parameters for the Assessment and Treatment of Children and Adolescents with Bipolar Disorder," *Journal of the American Academy of Child and Adolescent Psychiatry* 36 (1997): 138–157.

36. S. R. Marder, A. Ames, W. C. Wirshing, and T. Van Putten, "Schizophrenia," *Psychiatric Clinics of North America* 16 (1993): 567–588.

37. J. Zajecka, "Importance of Establishing the Diagnosis of Persistent Anxiety," *Journal of Clinical Psychiatry* 58, Suppl. 3 (1997): 9–13.

38. O. Brawman-Mintzer and R. B. Lydiard, "Biological Basis of Generalized Anxiety Disorder," *Journal of Clinical Psychiatry* 58, Suppl. 3 (1997): 16–25.

39. American Psychiatric Association, *Diagnostic and Statistical Manual of Mental Disorders*, 4th ed. (Washington, D.C.: American Psychiatric Association, 1994), 393–444.

40. P. G. Janicak, J. M. Davis, S. H. Preskorn, and F. J. Ayd, *Principles and Practice of Psychopharmacotherapy* (Baltimore: Williams & Wilkins, 1993), 405.

41. M. R. Mavissakalian and M. T. Ryan, "The Role of Medication," in W. T. Roth, ed., *Treating Anxiety Disorders* (San Francisco: Jossey-Bass, 1997), 175–203.

42. T. J. Barloon and R. Noyes, "Charles Darwin and Panic Disorder," *Journal of the American Medical Association* 277(1997): 138–141.

43. M. H. Pollack and M. W. Otto, "Long-Term Course and Outcome of Panic Disorder," *Journal of Clinical Psychiatry* 58, Suppl. 2 (1997): 57–60.

44. J. F. Rosenbaum, chairperson, "Panic Disorder: Making Clinical Sense of the Latest Research," *Journal of Clinical Psychiatry* 58 (1997): 127–134.

45. J. W. Jefferson, "Antidepressants in Panic Disorder," *Journal of Clinical Psychiatry* 58, Suppl. 2 (1997): 20–24.

46. J. R. T. Davidson, "Use of Benzodiazepines in Panic Disorder," *Journal of Clinical Psychiatry* 58, Suppl. 2 (1997): 26–28.

47. M. K. Shear and K. Weiner, "Psychotherapy for Panic Disorder," *Journal of Clinical Psychiatry* 58, Suppl. 2 (1997): 38–43.

48. D. H. Barlow, "Cognitive-Behavioral Therapy for Panic Disorder: Current Status," *Journal of Clinical Psychiatry* 58, Suppl. 2 (1997): 32–36.

49. W. Kayton, "Panic Disorder: Relationship to High Medical Utilization, Unexplained Physical Symptoms, and Medical Costs," *Journal of Clinical Psychiatry* 57, Suppl. 10 (1996): 11–18.

50. J. R. Marshall, "The Course and Impact of Panic Disorder," *Journal of Clinical Psychiatry* 58 (1997): 36–38.

51. D. V. Sheehan and K. Harnett-Sheehan, "The Role of SSRIs in Panic Disorder," *Journal of Clinical Psychiatry* 57, Suppl. 10 (1996): 51–58.

52. J. M. Gorman and J. D. Coplan, "Comorbidity of Depression and Panic Disorder," *Journal of Clinical Psychiatry* 57, Suppl. 10 (1996): 34–43.

53. M. H. Pollack, "Psychopharmacology Update," *Journal of Clinical Psychiatry* 58 (1997): 38–40.

54. M. W. Otto, "Integrated Treatment of Panic Disorder," *Journal of Clinical Psychiatry* 58 (1997): 40–42.

55. D. A. Spiegel and T. J. Bruce, "Benzodiazepines and Exposure-Based Cognitive Behavioral Therapies for Panic Disorder: Conclusions from Combined Treatment Trials," *American Journal of Psychiatry* 154 (1997): 773–781.

56. O. Brawman-Mintzer and R. B. Lydiard, "Generalized Anxiety Disorder: Issues in Epidemiology," *Journal of Clinical Psychiatry* 57, Suppl. 7 (1996): 3–8.

57. P. P. Roy-Byrns and W. Katon, "Generalized Anxiety Disorder in Primary Care: The Precursor/Modifier Pathway to Increased Health Care Utilization," *Journal of Clinical Psychiatry* 58, Suppl. 3 (1997): 34–38.

58. L. S. Schneider, "Overview of Generalized Anxiety Disorder in the Elderly," *Journal of Clinical Psychiatry* 57, Suppl. 7 (1996): 34–45.

59. E. Schweizer and K. Rickels, "The Long-Term Management of Generalized Anxiety Disorder: Issues and Dilemmas," *Journal of Clinical Psychiatry* 57, Suppl. 7 (1996): 9–12.

60. L. A. Mandos, K. Rickels, N. Cutler, et al., "Placebo-Controlled Comparison of the Clinical Effects of Rapid Discontinuation of Ipsapirone and Lorazepam After Eight Weeks of Treatment for Generalized Anxiety Disorder," *International Clinical Psychopharmacology* 10 (1995): 251–256.

61. J. J. Sramek, M. Tansman, A. Suri, et al., "Efficacy of Buspirone in Generalized Anxiety Disorder with Coexisting Mild Depressive Symptoms," *Journal of Clinical Psychiatry* 57 (1996): 287–291.

62. R. Delle Chiaie, P. Pancheri, M. Casacchia, et al., "Assessment of the Efficacy of Buspirone in Patients Affected by Generalized Anxiety Disorder, Shifting to Buspirone from Prior Treatment with Lorazepam: A Placebo-Controlled, Double-Blind Study," *Journal of Clinical Psychopharmacology* 15(1995): 12–19.

63. E. Schweizer and K. Rickels, "Strategies for Treatment of Generalized Anxiety in the Primary Care Setting," *Journal of Clinical Psychiatry* 58, Suppl. 3 (1997): 27–31.

64. R. E. Hales, D. A. Hilty, and M. G. Wise, "A Treatment Algorithm for the Management of Anxiety in Primary Care Practice," *Journal of Clinical Psychiatry* 58, Suppl. 3 (1997): 76–80.

65. A. G. Harvey and R. M. Rapee, "Cognitive-Behavioral Therapy for Generalized Anxiety Disorder," *Psychiatric Clinics of North America* 18 (1995): 859–870.

66. B. Black, T. W. Uhde, and M. E. Taylor, "Fluoxetine for the Treatment of Social Phobia," *Journal of Clinical Psychopharmacology* 12 (1992): 293–295.

67. D. J. Munjack, J. Brun, and P. L. Baltazar, "A Pilot Study of Buspirone in the Treatment of Social Phobia," *Journal of Anxiety Disorders* 5 (1991): 87–88.

68. R. Pary, S. Lippmann, and C. Tobias, "Obsessive-Compulsive Disorder," *Postgraduate Medicine* 96 (1994): 119–125.

69. Symposium, "New Frontiers on OCD Spectrum Research for Psychiatry and Primary Care," *Journal of Clinical Psychiatry* 57, Suppl. 8 (1996).

70. L. M. Koran, S. L. McElroy, J. R. Davidson, et al., "Fluvoxamine Versus Clomipramine for Obsessive-Compulsive Disorder: A Double-Blind Comparison," *Journal of Clinical Psychopharmacology* 16 (1996): 121–129.

71. T. A. Pigott, "OCD: Where the Serotonin Selectivity Story Begins," *Journal of Clinical Psychiatry* 57, Suppl. 6 (1996): 11–20.

72. O. T. Dolberg, I. Iancu, Y. Sasson, and J. Zohar, "The Pathogenesis and Treatment of Obsessive-Compulsive Disorder," *Clinical Neuropharmacology* 19 (1996): 129–147.

73. S. Dager, "Obsessive Compulsive Disorder," in *Psychopharmacology 1993* (Menlo Park, Ca.: Healthline, 1993), 2–4.

74. P. G. Janicak, J. M. Davis, S. H. Preskorn, and F.J. Ayd, *Principles and Practice of Psychopharmacotherapy* (Baltimore: Williams & Wilkins, 1993), 471.

75. J. S. March and H. L. Leonard, "Obsessive-Compulsive Disorder in Children and Adolescents: A Review of the Past 10 Years," *Journal of the American Academy of Child and Adolescent Psychiatry* 34 (1996): 1265–1273.

76. J. R. T. Davidson et al., "Posttraumatic Stress Disorder in the Community: An Epidemiological Study," *Psychological Medicine* 21 (1991): 713–721.

77. M. A. Vargas and J. Davidson, "Post-Traumatic Stress Disorder," *Psychiatric Clinics of North America* 16 (1993): 745.

78. L. Katz, W. Fleisher, K. Kjernisted, and P. Milanese, "A Review of the Psychobiology and Pharmacotherapy of Posttraumatic Stress Disorder," *Canadian Journal of Psychiatry* 41 (1996): 233–238.

79. S. M. Sutherland and J. R. Davidson, "Pharmacotherapy for Post-Traumatic Stress Disorder," *Psychiatric Clinics of North America* 17 (1994): 409–423.

80. R. DeMartino, R. F. Mollica, and V. Wilk, "Monoamine Oxidase Inhibitors in Posttraumatic Stress Disorder: Promise and Problems in Indochinese Survivors of Trauma," *Journal of Nervous and Mental Disease* 183 (1995): 510–515.

81. M. A. Hertzberg, M. E. Feldman, J. C. Beckham, and J. R. Davidson, "Trial of Trazodone for Posttraumatic Stress Disorder Using a Multiple Baseline Group Design," *Journal of Clinical Psychopharmacology* 16 (1996): 294–298.

82. C. R. Marmar, F. Schoenfeld, D. S. Weiss, et al., "Open Trail of Fluvoxamine Treatment for Combat-Related Posttraumatic Stress Disorder," *Journal of Clinical Psychiatry* 57, Suppl. 8 (1996): 66–70.

83. D. C. Jimerson, B. E. Wolfe, A. W. Brotman, and E. D. Metzger, "Medications in the Treatment of Eating Disorders," *Psychiatric Clinics of North America* 19 (1996): 739–754.

84. S. J. Crow and J. E. Mitchell, "Integrating Cognitive Therapy and Medications in Treating Bulimia Nervosa," *Psychiatric Clinics of North America* 19 (1996): 755–760.

85. J. Yager, guest ed., "Eating Disorders," *Psychiatric Clinics of North America* 19, no. 4 (December 1996).

86. American Psychiatric Association, *Practice Guidelines* (Washington D.C.: American Psychiatric Association, 1996).

87. American Psychiatric Association, "Practice Guidelines for the Treatment of Patients with Nicotine Dependence," *American Journal of Psychiatry* 153, no. 10, supplement (October 1996): 1–31. Also available from the APA, 1400 K Street, NW, Washington, D.C. 20005.

88. American Psychiatric Association, "Practice Guideline for the Treatment of Patients with Schizophrenia," *American Journal of Psychiatry* 154, no. 4, suppl. (April 1997): 1–63.

89. M. C. Fiore, D. W. Wetter, W. C. Bailey, et al., *Smoking Cessation Clinical Practice Guideline.* (Rockville, Md.: Agency for Health Care Policy and Research, Public Health Service, U.S. Department of Health and Human Services, 1996).

90. H. C. Schulberg and A. J. Rush, "Clinical Practice Guidelines for Managing Major Depression in Primary Care Practice: Implications for Psychologists," *American Psychologist* 49 (1994): 34–41.

91. R. F. Munoz, S. D. Hollon, E. McGrath, et al., "On the AHCPR *Depression in Primary Care* Guidelines: Further Considerations for Practitioners," *American Psychologist* 49 (1994): 42–61.

92. The Smoking Cessation Clinical Practice Guideline Panel and Staff, "The Agency for Health Care Policy and Research Smoking Cessation Clinical Practice Guideline," *Journal of the American Medical Association* 275 (1996): 1270–1280.
93. J. McClellan and J. Werry, principal authors, "Practice Parameters for the Assessment and Treatment of Children and Adolescents with Bipolar Disorder," *Journal of the American Academy of Child and Adolescent Psychiatry* 36 (1997): 138–157.

PHARMACOLOGICAL REGULATION OF FEMALE FERTILITY:

ORAL CONTRACEPTIVES AND RELATED DRUGS

Chapter 13 discusses the hormonal regulation of the male sex hormone *testosterone* and the problems associated with the use of anabolic-androgenic steroids. Normal testosterone levels are regulated by the hypothalamic release of a hormone called *gonadotropin-releasing factor* (GRF), which, in turn, induces the synthesis and release of two pituitary hormones, *follicle-stimulating hormone* (FSH) and *luteinizing hormone* (LH). A similar process occurs in the female, but the process is cyclical, resulting in the monthly cycle involving ovulation and menses (see Figure I.1).

It is pertinent here that contraceptive drugs (oral contraceptives, birth control pills) suppress the release of GRF from the hypothalamus and FSH and LH from the pituitary gland, inducing a state of "pseudopregnancy," suppressing fertility, and decreasing the possibility of pregnancy. Drugs that increase fertility perform in the opposite way.

Figure I.2 illustrates the principal organs of the human female reproductive system. These organs include the *ovaries, fallopian tubes, uterus,* and *vagina*. In the process of reproduction, ova (eggs) develop in the ovaries. Once developed, a single ovum is released and taken up

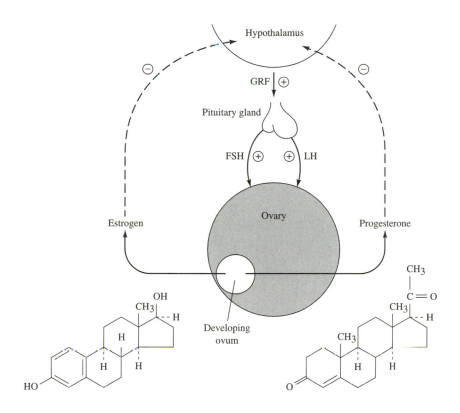

FIGURE I.1 Hormonal regulation of female fertility. The structures of naturally occurring estrogen (estradiol) and progesterone are also shown. GRF = gonadotropin-releasing factor; FSH = follicle-stimulating hormone; LH = luteinizing hormone; solid arrows = stimulation; dashed arrows = inhibition. See text for discussion.

(captured) by extensions of the fallopian tubes, called *fimbriae*, which gather the ovum into the fallopian tube. The ovum is then transported down the tube into the uterus. If the ovum becomes fertilized by a sperm (usually as the ovum passes down the fallopian tube), it implants itself on the inner wall of the uterus, where it develops into a fetus and placenta.

The Monthly Ovarian Cycle

After puberty and the development of ovarian function, a woman normally secretes various sex hormones in a rhythmic monthly pattern; as levels of these hormones change, corresponding changes occur in the activity of the female sexual organs. The duration of this cycle averages 28 days, but it may vary from 20 days to as long as 45 days.

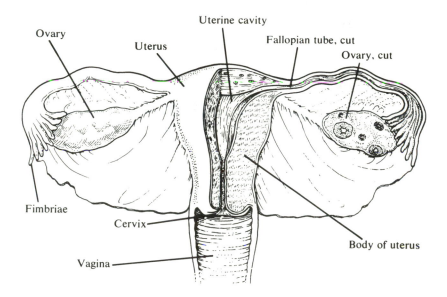

FIGURE I.2 Principal organs of the female reproductive system.

In order to accomplish the two most important aims of this cycle—the development and release of a single ovum and the proliferation of a uterine endometrium that is prepared for the implantation of a fertilized ovum—a coordinated sequence of hormonal events must occur. This sequence of events is illustrated in Figure I.3. At the beginning of the cycle, the levels of both estrogen and progesterone in the bloodstream are low, the endometrium that was built up during the preceding cycle begins to slough, and the woman menstruates for several days. Because the levels of estrogen and progesterone are low, the cells in the hypothalamus begin to release GRF. GRF is a 10-amino-acid peptide (a small protein), which on release is transported in the bloodstream from the hypothalamus to the pituitary gland, where it induces the release of FSH and LH. In response to increased FSH in the bloodstream, one or a few ovarian follicles (each one containing an ovum) begin to enlarge. Then, after 5 or 6 days, one of these ovarian follicles begins to develop more rapidly than the others, and begins to mature.

The maturing ovum then begins to release small quantities of estrogen into the circulating blood. The estrogen inhibits further secretion of GRF from the hypothalamus, therefore inhibiting further release of FSH from the pituitary gland. As a result of this inhibition, the other follicles that had also started to develop regress. The secretion of

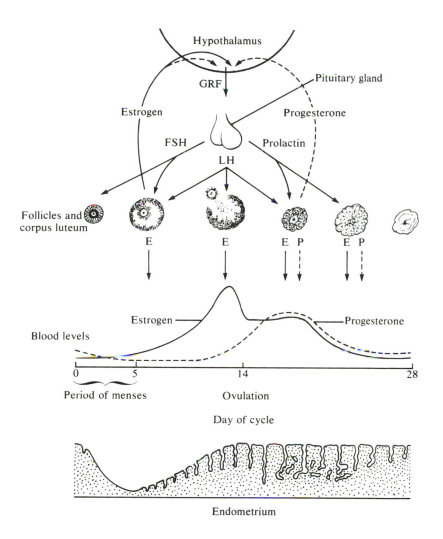

Figure I.3 Sequence of events in the brain, ovaries, and uterus during the monthly ovarian cycle in females. GRF = gonadotropin-releasing factor; FSH = follicle-stimulating hormone; LH = luteinizing hormone; E = estrogen; P = progesterone; solid arrows = stimulation; dashed arrows = inhibition.

estrogen by the one maturing ovum and the follicle in which it is contained reaches a peak just before midcycle (day 14). Near the end of this preovulatory phase, LH release peaks and prepares the ovarian follicle for ovulation by stimulating it to grow rapidly. The follicle swells until it eventually ruptures, and the developed ovum is released. This occurrence is referred to as the time of ovulation. Because LH is necessary for the final preovulatory development of the follicle and subsequent ovulation, the follicle will not rupture and ovulation will be inhibited if LH is not present (even with large quantities of FSH).

After ovulation, the ovum is gathered by the fimbriae into one of the fallopian tubes, where a sperm may fertilize it. Whether fertilized or not, the ovum then enters the uterus. The follicle from which the ovum was released changes to become a structure known as the corpus luteum, which secretes both estrogen and progesterone. These hormones released from the corpus luteum maintain the uterus in a state conducive to receiving a fertilized ovum. This state is established by the maintenance of a highly vascular endometrial lining (or endometrium) on the uterine wall. In addition, the estrogen and progesterone that are released from the corpus luteum act on the hypothalamus to inhibit the release of GRF. During the next 10 days, the corpus luteum regresses and, within about 12 days, ceases to function. At this point it no longer releases estrogen and progesterone, menstruation begins, and a new cycle follows if the ovum was not fertilized. If the ovum was fertilized and implanted, the endometrium begins to secrete large quantities of hormones that act to maintain pregnancy and prevent menstrual sloughing.

Oral Contraceptives

Oral contraceptives are the most effective pharmacological technique for preventing pregnancy. In 1996 about 17.5 million women in the United States were users of oral contraceptives. These products typically contain an orally absorbable estrogen derivative and/or progesterone derivative (called a progestin).* Available preparations can be classified according to their steroid content (see Table I.1 and Figure I.4):

1. Fixed combinations that contain constant amounts of an estrogen (usually ethinyl estradiol) and progestin (for example, norethindrone).

2. Multiphasic (biphasic or triphasic) combinations that usually contain constant amounts of estrogen and variable amounts of progestin; the dose of progestin changes from week to week, except for one product that has varying amounts of estrogen.

---

* Naturally occurring estrogen and progesterone cannot be utilized, because neither is absorbed following oral administration. Thus, synthetically produced derivatives that are effectively absorbed from the gastrointestinal tract are used. Two estrogen derivatives and six progestins are currently used in commercially marketed products (see Table I.1).

TABLE I.1 Oral contraceptives available in the United States

Trade name	Product type	Steroid composition			
		Progestin	mg	Estrogen	µg
Brevicon	Monophasic—low estrogen	Norethindrone	0.5	Ethinyl estradiol	35
Demulen 1/35	Monophasic—low estrogen	Ethynodiol	1.0	Ethinyl estradiol	35
Demulen 1/50	Monophasic—high estrogen	Ethynodiol	1.0	Ethinyl estradiol	50
Desogen	Monophasic—low estrogen	Desogestrel	0.15	Ethinyl estradiol	30
Estrostep	Tri-phasic	Norethindrone	1.0	Ethinyl estradiol	20, 30, 35
Jenest-28	Bi-phasic	Norethindrone	.5, 1.0	Ethinyl estradiol	35
Levlen	Monophasic—low estrogen	Levonorgestrel	0.15	Ethinyl estradiol	30
Lo/Ovral	Monophasic—low estrogen	Norgestrel	0.3	Ethinyl estradiol	30
Loestrin-1/20	Monophasic—very low estrogen	Norethindrone	1.0	Ethinyl estradiol	20
Loestrin-1.5/30	Monophasic—low estrogen	Norethindrone	1.5	Ethinyl estradiol	30
Micronor	Progestin—only	Norethindrone	0.35	—	
Modicon	Monophasic—low estrogen	Norethindrone	0.50	Ethinyl estradiol	35
Nelova 1/35	Monophasic—low estrogen	Norethindrone	1.0	Ethinyl estradiol	35
Nelova 10/11	Biphasic	Norethindrone	.5, 1.0	Ethinyl estradiol	35
Nor-Q.D.	Progestin—only	Norethindrone	0.35	—	
Nordette	Monophasic—low estrogen	Levonorgestrel	0.15	Ethinyl estradiol	30
Norethin 1/35	Monophasic—low estrogen	Norethindrone	1.0	Ethinyl estradiol	35

TABLE I.1 Oral contraceptives available in the United States *(continued)*

Trade name	Product type	Progestin	mg	Estrogen	μg
				Steroid composition	
Norethin 1/50	Monophasic—high estrogen	Norethindrone	1.0	Ethinyl estradiol	50
Norinyl 1 & 35	Monophasic—low estrogen	Norethindrone	1.0	Ethinyl estradiol	35
Norinyl 1 & 50	Monophasic—high estrogen	Norethindrone	1.0	Mestranol	50
Ortho-cept	Monophasic—low estrogen	Desogestrel	0.15	Ethinyl estradiol	30
Ortho-cyclen	Monophasic—low estrogen	Norgestimate	0.25	Ethinyl estradiol	35
Ortho-tricyclen[a]	Triphasic	Norgestimate	.18, .212, .25	Ethinyl estradiol	35
Ortho-Novum 1/35	Monophasic—low estrogen	Norethindrone	1.0	Ethinyl estradiol	35
Ortho-Novum 1/50	Monophasic—high estrogen	Norethindrone	1.0	Mestranol	50
Ortho-Novum 10/11	Bi-phasic	Norethindrone	0.5, 1.0	Ethinyl estradiol	35
Ortho-Novum 7/7/7	Triphasic	Norethindrone	0.5, 0.75, 1	Ethinyl estradiol	35
Ovcon-35	Monophasic—low estrogen	Norethindrone	0.4	Ethinyl estradiol	35
Ovcon-50	Monophasic—high estrogen	Norethindrone	1.0	Ethinyl estradiol	50
Ovral	Monophasic—high estrogen	Norgestrel	0.5	Ethinyl estradiol	50
Ovrette	Progestin—only	Norgestrel	0.075	—	
Tri-Levlen	Triphasic	Levonorgestrel	0.5, 0.075, 0.125	Ethinyl estradiol	30, 40, 30
Tri-Norinyl	Triphasic	Norethindrone	0.5, 1, 1.5	Ethinyl estradiol	35
Triphasil	Triphasic	Levonorgestrel	0.5, 0.075, 0.125	Ethinyl estradiol	30

[a] First oral contraceptive to receive FDA approval (March 1997) for use in the treatment of acne in women >14 years of age who have not responded to other acne treatments.

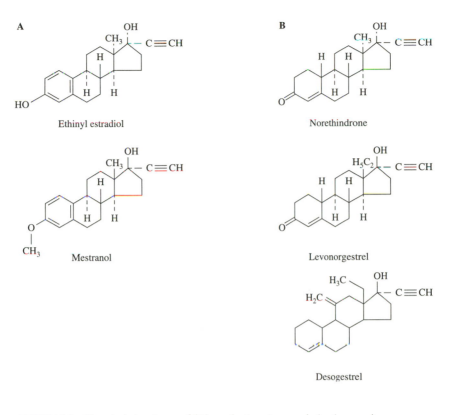

FIGURE I.4 Chemical structures of (**A**) synthetic estrogen derivatives and (**B**) synthetic progestins. Note the similarity in the structures.

3. "Minipills" (progestin-only pills) that contain constant amounts of progestin, with no estrogen at all.

Thirty-five years ago, the availability of orally absorbed estrogen and progestin fueled the technology to develop pharmacological control of ovulation as a means of preventing pregnancy. The problem was to find an appropriate combination of estrogen and progestin that would effectively suppress ovulation but limit the number and intensity of side effects. Excessive amounts of estrogen and progestin produce abnormal menstrual bleeding, whereas insufficient amounts do not completely inhibit the release of GRF, which could result in an unwanted pregnancy. Today, nearly four decades after the introduction of these agents, close to optimal balances have been achieved. Contemporary oral contraceptives are extremely safe and very effective at blocking conception. Indeed, we are probably at or near the lowest dose levels that can be achieved without sacrificing (pregnancy blocking) efficacy.

Combination Products

All but three of the oral contraceptive products that are currently available contain a combination of an estrogen and a progestin in very low, low, high, or variable doses. The low-dose combination pills contain 30 to 35 micrograms of ethinyl estradiol and afford a reasonable compromise between the toxicities that are produced by too much estrogen and the bothersome breakthrough bleeding that results from too little. The use of products that contain higher amounts of estrogen is diminishing rapidly in favor of the low-dose products, which appear to be equally effective in preventing pregnancy while causing only mild increases in breakthrough bleeding.

The variable-dose products are either *biphasic* or *triphasic*, depending on the number of variations in dosage during a given month's cycle. These products are designed to reduce the total hormone content that is administered to the body throughout the menstrual cycle while still providing contraception that is as effective as that obtained from products that contain higher doses. Advantages are more claimed than demonstrated.

The combination oral contraceptives are taken for 21 days of the menstrual cycle (usually days 5 to 24, counting the first day of menstruation as day 1). This is followed by one week without medication, toward the end of which withdrawal bleeding (menstruation) occurs.

By combining estrogen and progestin, combination pills block release of both FSH and LH by means of negative feedback effects on both the pituitary gland and the hypothalamus; ovarian follicles do not develop, and no ovulation occurs. The estrogen primarily inhibits the release of FSH. The progestin suppresses the release of LH and acts directly on the uterus to produce an endometrium that will not accept the implantation of a fertilized ovum. The progestin thickens the normal mucus discharge of the cervix so that sperm cannot gain access to the uterus and fallopian tubes, where fertilization occurs. In addition to suppressing the release of FSH, the estrogen also stabilizes the uterine lining (the endometrium) so that irregular shedding and unwanted breakthrough bleeding does not occur. The estrogen also potentiates the action of the progestin. All these actions minimize the likelihood of conception and implantation as long as the pills are taken faithfully.

Progestin-Only Contraceptives

During the early 1980s, there was concern that long-term use of the estrogen contained in the combination estrogen-progestin contraceptives

TABLE I.2 Pregnancies per 100 woman-years

Contraception method	Pregnancies
Oral contraceptive pills, combination	1
Oral contraceptive pills, progestin only	2–3
Intrauterine device (IUD)	1–6
Diaphragm with spermicidal cream or gel	2–20
Condom	3–36
Spermicidal aerosol foams	2–29
Spermicidal gels and creams	4–36
Periodic abstinence ("rhythm")	
All types	1–47
Calendar method	14–47
Temperature method	1–20
Mucus method	1–25
No contraception	60–80

might be harmful. These fears prompted the use of continuous progestational therapy without concomitant estrogen. (At that time, combination products contained much higher amounts of estrogen than they do today.)

A progestational agent given alone produces an endometrium that is not receptive to an ovum and a thick cervical mucus that is impervious to sperm transport, although an ovarian follicle still might mature. Thus, even if fertilization does occur, the progestin tends to prevent implantation of the fertilized ovum in the endometrium.

The administration of progestin alone (three such products are currently available), however, is not quite so reliable as the administration of a combination product; statistics indicate an approximately threefold increase in the incidence of unwanted pregnancies. Nevertheless, for women who experience significant side effects when using combination products, the administration of progestin-only products affords better contraceptive protection than do foams, creams, jellies, or the rhythm method, and it is certainly far better than no contraception at all. Table I.2 lists the pregnancy rates for various forms of contraception.

Undesirable Effects

The frequent, mild side effects that are induced by combination-type oral contraceptives resemble those that are experienced during early pregnancy and are generally attributed to the estrogen content. These effects include nausea, occasional vomiting, headache, dizziness, and breast discomfort. Because these side effects are usually related to the dose, products that have less estrogen generally have milder side effects. However, the incidence of breakthrough bleeding increases with decreasing doses of estrogen.

Other side effects are generally not too bothersome; they include weight gain and psychological changes that may result in depression in some women. These side effects are most frequently seen when progestin-only pills are taken.

When oral contraceptives are no longer taken, normal cyclic periods are usually resumed, but they are often not reestablished immediately. It may take several months or even longer, presumably because the hypothalamus, pituitary gland, and ovaries have been suppressed for a prolonged period of time. About 95 percent of women whose menstrual periods were normal before taking oral contraceptives resume normal periods within a few months after they stop taking the drug. In women who discontinue oral contraceptives to become pregnant, 50 percent conceive within three months; more important, after two years, only 7 to 15 percent fail to conceive. Thus, infertility does not seem to occur often, if at all, in women who discontinue the use of oral contraceptives.

Serious Side Effects

The possibility that oral contraceptives cause serious side effects has been a source of concern. These side effects include:

- Cardiovascular risks, such as arteriosclerosis, venous blood clots and emboli (thromboembolism), heart attacks, stroke, high blood pressure, and lipoprotein and cholesterol imbalance
- Cancer risks, especially uterine, cervical, liver, and breast cancer
- Diabetes mellitus (sugar diabetes)
- Adverse effects on a fetus if the drugs are taken during pregnancy

Few drugs have been subjected to more intense study than the oral contraceptives. All efforts were directed at maximizing the benefits of drug use while minimizing potential risks, especially those involving the cardiovascular system. Decreasing the amount of estrogen from 100 or 150 micrograms per tablet (levels in the pills of the 1960s) to 30 or 35 micrograms per tablet (levels of today) drastically reduced the cardiovascular risks. In healthy women who are not predisposed to

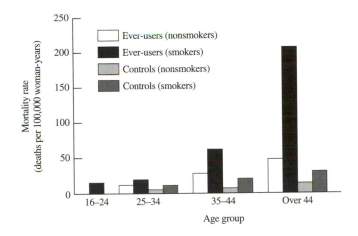

FIGURE I.5 Circulatory disease mortality rates by age, smoking status, and oral contraceptive use.

these conditions, the risks of blood clots, stroke, heart attack, hypertension, and atherosclerosis are minimal.[1–4] All reports state that women who use oral contraceptives can reduce their risk of cardiovascular disease by reducing or eliminating cigarette smoking.[4] Indeed, smoking increases all the potential risks in women who take oral contraceptives (see Figure I.5).[5] On the adverse side, the presence of hypertension (elevated blood pressure) is now generally considered to be a contraindication to the use of oral contraceptives.[4]

Data now demonstrate that concern over the risks of cancer is unwarranted. Such concern arose during the 1960s, when high-dose oral contraceptives were shown to be associated with a slightly increased risk of cervical cancer. Today, this risk is no longer considered significant. Indeed, the use of low-dose oral contraceptives does not increase the risk of breast or cervical cancer and may actually reduce a woman's risk of uterine and ovarian cancer by 40 to 50 percent,[6–8] as well as having a protective effect against pelvic inflammatory disease and heavy menstrual bleeding. Altered metabolism of glucose and insulin and the possible development of diabetes—other risks once thought to be associated with the use of oral contraceptives—are no longer major causes for concern.[8] Reproductive problems after use of oral contraception have not been substantiated; there is no increase in the occurrence of spontaneous abortions, pregnancy complications, or congenital malformations.

Conclusions and Contraindications

Stolley, Strom, and Sartwell (1989)[5] offer reasonable guidelines for the use of oral contraceptives:

- Women over 35 years of age should avoid the use of these products.
- Women who smoke cigarettes should avoid the use of these products and users should not smoke.
- The product that is effective at the lowest dose of estrogen that does not cause unacceptable breakthrough bleeding should be chosen.
- Women with high blood pressure or a tendency toward migraine headaches should be carefully educated and monitored.

Oral contraceptives are contraindicated in women with any of the following conditions:

- Venous thrombophlebitis, thromboembolic disorders, cerebral vascular disease, or coronary artery disease
- Impaired liver function or jaundice
- Known or suspected cancer of the breast or uterus
- Abnormal genital bleeding
- Known or suspected pregnancy
- Congenitally elevated blood cholesterol or lipid levels
- An addiction to cigarettes (for women over the age of 35 years)
- Hypertension

Additional information about oral contraceptives may be obtained from a physician or pharmacist. The insert that is packaged with oral contraceptives is written in layman's terms and expands on the information given here.

Alternatives to Oral Contraceptives

A few effective pharmacological alternatives do exist for women who want to avoid pregnancy but do not want to take a daily oral contraceptive tablet. Proven techniques and devices include the following:

- Diaphragms, condoms, intrauterine devices (IUDs), and contraceptive creams (vaginal spermicides)
- A long-acting, injected progestin (Depo-Provera)

- Implanted plastic tubes containing a long-acting, progestin-releasing contraceptive (Norplant)

Diaphragms, condoms, and IUDs are only approximately 90 to 95 percent effective. Even less effective are vaginal spermicides and the non-pharmacological strategies of the rhythm method, coitus interruptus, and douching. The most effective nonpharmacological technique for the temporary prevention of unwanted pregnancy is abstention. For permanent prevention, sterilization of men (vasectomy) and women (tubal ligation) are 100 percent effective but should not be considered reversible, even though surgical attempts at reversal can be successful.

Depo-Provera

Certain long-acting injectable products can be used as contraceptive agents. The most important is *medroxyprogesterone acetate*, marketed under the trade name *Depo-Provera*. This drug is a progestin that was approved for use in the United States in 1992 after being used for many years by millions of women worldwide as an effective contraceptive. A single dose of 150 milligrams is injected intramuscularly every 3 to 6 months. The advantages of this form of contraception include freedom from taking daily tablets, freedom from the side effects of estrogen, and the maintenance of normal FSH activity. Depo-Provera inhibits ovulation by blocking the midcycle surge of LH. It induces thickening of the cervical mucus and inhibits the development of the lush uterine endometrium that is necessary for the fertilized ovum to survive. Follicular development is not suppressed, because the normal estrogen cycle is maintained. The contraceptive protection that Depo-Provera provides is approximately equal to that afforded by the combination-type oral contraceptives. Disadvantages and side effects associated with Depo-Provera include breakthrough bleeding ("spotting"), weight gain, depression, headaches, and abdominal bloating.

As Figure I.6 illustrates, up to 8 months may be required for Depo-Provera to be totally eliminated from the body after injections are discontinued. Thus, regular menstrual periods take several months to a year to return, and fertility during that period is unpredictable.

Norplant

In 1992 a novel hormonal contraceptive device was introduced that delivers pregnancy-preventing progestin (*levonorgestrel*) for a maximum of 5 years following its surgical implantation under the skin of a woman's upper arm. The device consists of six flexible silicone rubber tubes, each containing 36 milligrams of levonorgestrel, which is re-

Provera blood level
ng/ml

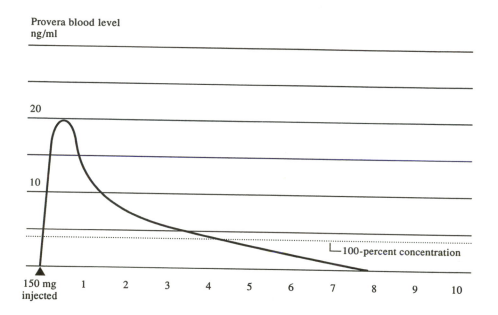

FIGURE I.6 Blood levels of Depo-Provera following a single intramuscular injection. [From Speroff, Glass, and Kase (1989),[8] 489.

leased at a low, constant rate over the 5-year period. Each tube is about the size of a matchstick. The tubes are inserted in a fanlike manner through a small skin incision. This implant has the advantage of being removable (with removal of the tubes). The gross cumulative pregnancy rate at 5 years is 2.6 pregnancies per 100 woman-years.

Side effects can lead to requests to have the tubes removed. The main complaints are bleeding (menstrual) irregularities and weight gain.[9] Total cumulative discontinuation rates after five years of Norplant use ranged from 36 to 60 per 100 women (35 to 60 percent).[10] Preinsertion counseling is of paramount importance to assist with the acceptance of side effects.[9,11] Unfortunately, follow-up (return visits by patients after device insertion) is poor, especially in adolescents.[12]

Postcoital Contraceptives

After unprotected intercourse, certain pharmacological measures may be used to prevent (or "terminate") an unwanted pregnancy. Older postcoital techniques included high doses of estrogen in preparations that were referred to as "morning after" pills. In one such regimen, large doses (e.g., 25 milligrams of diethylstilbestrol) were administered twice daily for 5 days. This pharmacological regimen apparently reduced the time required for a fertilized ovum to pass down the fallopian tube into the uterus, thus impairing the viability of the fertilized ovum in the uterus. More recently, high doses of either ethinyl estradiol (the oral contraceptive *Ovral*) or conjugated estrogens (Premarin) have been prescribed to accomplish much the same purpose.

On February 25, 1997, David A. Kessler, commissioner of the U.S. Food and Drug Administration (FDA), published a monograph in the *Federal Register*[13] proposing a campaign of education and promotion to advocate the use of oral contraceptives as emergency contraception after unprotected sex. This was an unusual action, because the FDA was formally advocating an "off-label" use of oral contraceptives, meaning that the drugs would be used for indications different from the ones for which they were approved. To date, the manufacturers of these drugs have displayed no interest in submitting requests for formal approval or an "indication" to market their products for such use (probably because of the fear of potential litigation or protest). Not only is the FDA action unusual, the social and political arguments are unique, with one side claiming victory for making an emergency contraceptive available, the other claiming that such action is abortion and removes the consequences of having unprotected sex. The FDA guidelines (see Table I.3) call for a strong dose of oral contraceptive within 72 hours of unprotected sex, followed by the same dose 12 hours later. Nausea and vomiting are common side effects because of the high dose of estrogen. Even though the FDA considers use of oral contraceptives after unprotected sex to be safe, using this technique as a method of routine contraception is probably unwise.

Mifepristone (RU-486)

In addition to the controversy about the FDA promotion of a "morning after" technique, their preliminary approval of the abortion-inducing drug mifepristone (formerly known as RU-486) is also controversial, but formal approval is expected in late 1997.

As discussed, progesterone is required to maintain the uterine lining (endometrium) in a state suitable for supporting a fertilized ovum. Pharmacological blockade of progesterone receptors in the uterus provokes endometrial necrosis and shedding (menstruation). Thus, if a woman is in the first trimester of pregnancy, the growing fetus will be aborted if she takes a progesterone antagonist.

Mifepristone is the first clinically available progesterone antagonist, and it is currently used in Europe (especially in France) and in the Far East. In actual use, the administration of mifepristone is followed

TABLE I.3 Morning-after pill[a]

Drug[b]	Dosage	Color
Ovral	Two up to 72 hours after sex; two 12 hours later	White
Nordette	Four up to 72 hours after sex; four 12 hours later	Light orange
Lo/Ovral	Four up to 72 hours after sex; four 12 hours later	White
Triphasil	Four up to 72 hours after sex; four 12 hours later	Yellow
Levlen	Four up to 72 hours after sex; four 12 hours later	Light orange
Tri-Levlen	Four up to 72 hours after sex; four 12 hours later	Yellow

[a] The Food and Drug Administration has published guidelines for "morning-after" contraception, in which high doses of birth-control pills are taken after unprotected sex.[13] The method prevents pregnancy 75 percent of the time.
[b] Drugs must be prescribed by a physician. The second dosage must be taken exactly 12 hours after the first.

Source: Food and Drug Administration, published in the *Federal Register* 62, no. 37 (Feb. 25, 1997), pp. 8609–8612.

in a couple of days by a dose of prostaglandin, which induces uterine contractions to ensure successful abortion. The clinical pharmacology of mifepristone has been reviewed by Robbins and Spitz (1996).[14]

In practice, a woman, in a doctor's office, takes three 200-milligram tablets of mifepristone. She returns 2 days later for two 200-milligram tablets of misoprostol (Cytotec, a prostaglandin), which induces uterine contractions. She remains under observation for 4 hours in order to monitor for adverse effects (nausea, cramping, excessive bleeding). If the chemical sequence is not effective in inducing abortion, a surgical abortion is performed, but this should be necessary in only about 5 to 10 percent of cases.

In a 1992 study of 800 women and female adolescents, Glasier and coworkers[15] compared the effectiveness of mifepristone as an abortifacient (without the prostaglandin) with the sequential administration of high doses of ethinyl estradiol and norgestrel. Administered within 72 hours after unprotected intercourse, none of the 402 females who received mifepristone became pregnant, while 4 of the 398 females who received ethinyl estradiol and norgestrel did. The authors concluded that the drug has the potential to avert unwanted and unplanned pregnancy.

Mifepristone has been the source of controversy since the initial reports demonstrated its efficacy as an abortifacient. In an editorial accompanying the Glasier report, Grimes and Cook (1992)[16] argue that mifepristone is actually not an abortifacient:

> Pregnancy begins when implantation [in the uterus of a fertilized ovum] is complete. Implantation begins five to six days after fertilization and is complete eight days later. When a woman's oocyte [egg] is fertilized in vitro, she cannot claim to be pregnant until the conceptus is implanted successfully [by artificial means] in her uterus. The same holds for fertilization in vivo. Since the postcoital contraceptive action of mifepristone occurs before implantation, it is not an abortifacient when used this way.

A letter to the editor in the same journal (followed by a rebuttal by Grimes and Cook) challenged the statement:

> Many people feel that a fertilized ovum constitutes a new human life and that preventing its implantation constitutes abortion. This is the central issue about mifepristone. . . . Redefining the meaning of contraception to include the prevention of implantation does not change the fact that preventing implantation is what many people find problematic with the drug.[17]

I leave conclusions to the reader. When after fertilization of the ovum is a woman pregnant? Is the nonimplanted ovum a living being? Is early pharmacological abortion the same as later surgical abortion of an implanted, fertilized ovum? The studies cited here do not answer these questions, but they do raise them.

The status of mifepristone as an abortifacient was reviewed by Murray and Muse[18] in 1996 in a volume that also reviews other, nonabortifacient uses of the drug both in gynecology[19–21] and as an anticancer agent in specific situations.[22] Cadepond, Ulmann, and Baulieu (1997)[23] also review the actions and uses of mifepristone.

Agents That Increase Fertility

Women who are having difficulty becoming pregnant may be candidates for drugs that can increase fertility. Infertility, as a medical diagnosis, may be caused by many factors, physical and psychological, in either the man or the woman. Certain types of infertility in women can be pharmacologically manipulated.

One such pharmacological approach is an extension of the sequence of events illustrated in Figure I.3. When estrogen acts on the hypothalamus, the release of GRF is inhibited, the release of FSH and LH by the pituitary gland is decreased, and follicular development is inhibited. If the action of estrogen on the hypothalamus is blocked, GRF is released, and this action, in turn, stimulates the release of FSH and LH from the pituitary gland. Subsequently, one or more ovarian follicles develop, and eventually at least one ovum is released. For a drug to block the inhibitory action of estrogen on the hypothalamus, it would have to attach to normal estrogen receptors (thus blocking the normal access of estrogen to the receptor) without causing any changes in cellular behavior (in pharmacological terms, it would have affinity for the receptors but be devoid of intrinsic activity).

Clomiphene

Clomiphene (Clomid), a compound that is frequently referred to as a "fertility pill," is a drug that has affinity for and binds to estrogen receptors in the hypothalamus but is devoid of intrinsic activity. Clomiphene has enabled many women who were previously unable to conceive to become pregnant. The drug has also been responsible for causing multiple births; sometimes four or five ova are released and fertilized in women who take the drug. However, the possibility of bearing more than one child is usually not considered a problem for couples who have not been able to conceive by other methods. Because clomiphene acts on the hypothalamus, the pituitary gland and ovaries must be functional if the drug is to improve a woman's chances of conception. Thus, the drug is ineffective if infertility is caused by a deficit in the man or when the woman's infertility is caused by pituitary or ovarian dysfunction.

Ordinarily the administration of clomiphene is started on day 5 of the menstrual period (day 1 being the first day of menses); it is then taken daily for 5 days. The drug is then stopped until the next menstrual cycle if the woman does not become pregnant. The procedure is then repeated, often with slowly increasing doses. Approximately 35 percent of formerly infertile women become pregnant when they take clomiphene. Side effects of clomiphene include ovarian cysts (14 percent), multiple pregnancies (8 percent), and birth defects (2.4 percent). The incidence of birth defects in nontreated women who conceive without the aid of clomiphene is approximately 1 percent.

Alternatives to Clomiphene

If a woman does not become pregnant after several trials on clomiphene, Pergonal (human postmenopausal hormone), Follutein (chorionic gonadotropin), or bromocriptine can be tried.

Pergonal is a commercial product that contains FSH and LH, which are extracted from the urine of postmenopausal women. *Follutein*, a hormone produced by the human placenta, is extracted from the urine of pregnant women and exerts actions that are virtually identical to those of pituitary LH. Thus, sequential injections of

Pergonal and then Follutein can, in anovulatory women, simulate the normal FSH and LH release found in fertile women. Pergonal is injected daily for 9 to 12 days, and then, after a day of rest, the woman is given a single injection of Follutein. Approximately 75 percent of women who are treated by this method ovulate, and approximately 25 percent of them become pregnant.

Bromocriptine is an agonist (stimulant) of dopamine receptors that inhibit the pituitary secretion of prolactin, restoring gonadotropin function and ovarian responsiveness. It seems to increase a woman's responsiveness to clomiphene.[10]

NOTES

1. M. Thorogood and M. P. Vessey, "An Epidemiologic Survey of Cardiovascular Disease in Women Taking Oral Contraceptives," *American Journal of Obstetrics and Gynecology* 163 (1990): 274–281.

2. G. Samsioe and L. A. Mattsson, "Some Aspects of the Relationship Between Oral Contraceptives, Lipid Abnormalities, and Cardiovascular Disease," *American Journal of Obstetrics and Gynecology* 163 (1990): 354–358.

3. E. P. Frohlich, "Vascular Complications in Women Using the Low Steroid Content Combined Oral Contraceptive Pills: Case Reports and Review of the Literature," *Obstetrical and Gynecological Survey* 45 (1990): 578–584.

4. D. B. Petitti, S. Sidney, A. Bernstein, et al., "Stroke in Users of Low-Dose Oral Contraceptives," *New England Journal of Medicine* 335 (1996): 8–15.

5. P. D. Stolley, B. L. Strom, and P. E. Sartwell, "Oral Contraceptives and Vascular Disease," *Epidemiologic Reviews* 11 (1989): 241–243.

6. K. Gast and T. Snyder, "Combination Oral Contraceptives and Cancer Risk," *Kansas Medicine* 91 (1990): 201–208.

7. D. R. Mishell, Jr., "Correcting Misconceptions About Oral Contraceptives," *American Journal of Obstetrics and Gynecology* 161 (1989): 1385–1389.

8. L. Speroff, R. H. Glass, and N. G. Kase, *Clinical Gynecologic Endocrinology and Infertility*, 4th ed. (Baltimore: Williams & Wilkins, 1989), 461.

9. S. L. Rosenthal, F. M. Biro, L. M. Kollar, et al., "Experience with Side Effects and Health Risks Associated with Norplant Implant Use in Adolescents," *Contraception* 52 (1995): 283–285.

10. R. W. Johnson Pharmaceutical Research Institute, "Pre-Introductory Clinical trials of Norplant Implants: A Comparison of Seventeen Countries' Experience," *Contraception* 52 (1995): 287–296.

11. C. Musham, E. G. Darr, and M. L. Strossner, "A Qualitative Study of the Perceptions of Dissatisfied Norplant Users," *Journal of Family Practice* 40 (1995): 465–470.

12. L. Dugoff, O. W. Jones, J. Allen-Davis, et al., "Assessing the Acceptability of Norplant Contraception in Four Patient Populations," *Contraception* 52 (1995): 45–49.

13. D. A. Kessler and the Food and Drug Administration, "Prescription Drug Products: Certain Combined Oral Contraceptives for Use as Postcoital Emergency Contraception," *Federal Register* 62, no. 37 (Feb. 25, 1997): 8609–8612.

14. A. Robbins and I. M. Spitz, "Mifepristone: Clinical Pharmacology," *Clinical Obstetrics and Gynecology* 39 (1996): 436–450.

15. A. Glasier, K. J. Thong, M. Dewar, et al., "Mifepristone (RU 486) Compared with High-Dose Estrogen and Progestin for Emergency Postcoital Contraception," *New England Journal of Medicine* 327 (1992): 1041–1044.

16. D. A. Grimes and R. J. Cook, "Mifepristone (RU 486)—An Abortifacient to Prevent Abortion?" *New England Journal of Medicine* 327 (1992): 1088–1089.

17. R. P. Hamel and M. T. Lysaught, letter to the editor of *New England Journal of Medicine* 328 (1993): 354–355.

18. S. Murray and K. Muse, "Mifepristone and First Trimester Abortion," *Clinical Obstetrics and Gynecology* 39 (1996): 474–485.

19. A. J. Morales, M. Kettel, and A. A. Murphy, "Mifepristone: Clinical Applications in General Gynecology," *Clinical Obstetrics and Gynecology* 39 (1996): 451–460.

20. O. Heikinheimo and D. F. Archer, "Mifepristone: A Potential Contraceptive," *Clinical Obstetrics and Gynecology* 39 (1996): 461–468.

21. M. S. Edwards, "Mifepristone: Cervical Ripening and Induction of Labor," *Clinical Obstetrics and Gynecology* 39 (1996): 469–473.

22. O. Sartor and W. D. Figg, "Mifepristone: Antineoplastic Studies," *Clinical Obstetrics and Gynecology* 39 (1996): 498–505.

23. F. Cadepond, A. Ulmann, and E.-E. Baulieu, "RU486 (Mifepristone): Mechanisms of Action and Clinical Uses, " *Annual Reviews of Medicine* 48 (1997): 129–156.

NONOPIOID ANALGESICS

There are two general classes of analgesic (pain-relieving) drugs. The first consists of the "centrally acting" analgesics, such as morphine and other opioids. These drugs act on specific opioid receptors both in the spinal cord and at higher levels of the central nervous system (CNS), reducing the intensity and central processing of afferent pain impulses. Opioids are discussed in Chapter 10. The second class of analgesic agents consists of "peripherally acting" drugs, such as aspirin and ibuprofen. Drugs in this class act at the local (peripheral) site of tissue injury to reduce pain and inflammation by interfering with the synthesis of prostaglandin hormones. These drugs are discussed here.

The nonopioid analgesics are a group of chemically unrelated drugs (see Figure II.1) that produce both analgesic and anti-inflammatory effects.[1-3] They block the generation of peripheral pain impulses by inhibiting the synthesis and release of prostaglandins.* These drugs do not bind to opioid receptors. Their effects include:

---

*Prostaglandins are body hormones that induce local inflammatory responses. Aspirin-like drugs inhibit the enzyme *cyclooxygenase (prostaglandin synthetase)*, which is responsible for the biosynthesis of certain prostaglandins.[1] In addition, studies suggest that the inhibition of prostaglandin synthesis is only part of aspirin's action;[3] the local anti-inflammatory action also results from aspirin's ability to disrupt white blood cell responsiveness to tissue injury, thus preventing the cellular release of tissue-disruptive enzymes.

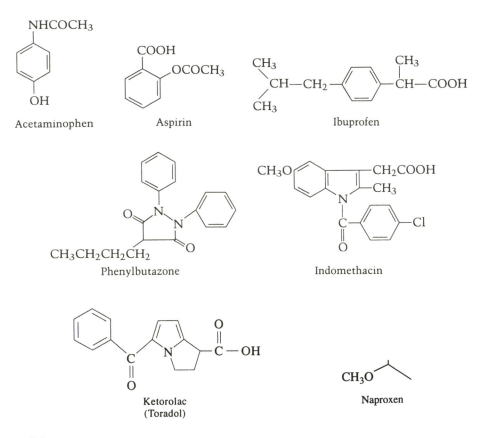

FIGURE II.1   Structural formulas of representative anti-inflammatory analgesics.

- Reduction of inflammation (anti-inflammatory effect)
- Reduction in body temperature when the patient has a fever (antipyretic effect)
- Reduction in pain without sedation (analgesic effect)
- Inhibition of platelet aggregation (anticoagulant effect)

Drugs classified as nonopioid analgesics include aspirin and other salicylates, ibuprofen, acetaminophen, indomethacin, phenylbutazone, ketorolac, ketoprofen, and naproxen. The prototype is aspirin; hence they can be referred to as aspirin-like drugs. They are also frequently called *nonsteroidal anti-inflammatory drugs*, or *NSAIDs*, although this term does not describe their full spectrum of effects (at least until one understands what that spectrum encompasses). These drugs are widely used (and are quite irreplaceable) to reduce both the inflammation and the pain associated with the various forms of arthritis. Gastric irritation tends to limit their long-term usefulness. Other uses and side effects are presented with discussion of individual agents.

Aspirin

In the United States, between 10,000 to 20,000 tons of *aspirin* are consumed each year.[1] It is our most popular and most effective analgesic, antipyretic, and anti-inflammatory drug. In daily low doses, it is also widely used to prevent blood clots in the coronary arteries, reducing the risks of having a heart attack.

As an analgesic, aspirin is most effective for low-intensity pain. The analgesic and anti-inflammatory effects follow peripheral inhibition of both prostaglandin synthesis and white blood cell responsiveness to injury. Its antipyretic effect follows the inhibition of prostaglandin synthesis in the hypothalamus, a structure in the brain that modulates body temperature. However, one caution is necessary regarding the use of aspirin to reduce fever in children. An association exists between the use of aspirin for the fever that accompanies varicella (chicken pox) or influenza and the subsequent development of Reye's syndrome, including severe liver and brain damage and even death.[4] Thus, in children, aspirin use is precluded for the treatment of virus-induced febrile illness.[1]

Aspirin increases oxygen consumption by the body, which increases the production of carbon dioxide, an effect that stimulates respiration. Therefore, an overdose with aspirin is often characterized by a marked increase in respiratory rate, which causes the overdosed person to appear to pant. This occurrence results in other severe metabolic consequences that are beyond this discussion.

Aspirin has important effects on blood coagulation.[3] For blood to coagulate, platelets* must first be able to aggregate, an action requiring the presence of prostaglandins. Aspirin can inhibit the aggregation of platelets and therefore reduce the formation of intravascular clots. Low doses of aspirin (for example, one-half tablet daily) are now widely used for preventing strokes and heart attacks, which can be caused by atherosclerosis, intravascular clotting, or the formation of emboli on either artificial or damaged heart valves.

---

* Platelets are small components of the blood that adhere to vascular membranes after injury to a vessel. They form an initial plug, over which a blood clot eventually forms to limit bleeding from a lacerated blood vessel.

Side effects of aspirin are common. Gastric upset occurs most frequently and can range from mild upset and heartburn to severe, destructive ulcerations of the stomach or upper intestine. In addition, poisoning due to aspirin overdosage is not infrequent and can be fatal. Mild intoxication can produce ringing in the ears, auditory and visual difficulties, mental confusion, thirst, and hyperventilation.

Acetaminophen

Acetaminophen (Tylenol) is an effective alternative to aspirin both as an analgesic and as an antipyretic agent. However, unlike aspirin, acetaminophen's anti-inflammatory effect is minor, and the drug is not clinically useful in treating either acute inflammation or chronic arthritis.[1] Also, because acetaminophen does not inhibit platelet aggregation, it is not useful for preventing vascular clotting or for prophylaxis against heart attacks or stroke. No reports have associated acetaminophen with Reye's syndrome; therefore, it has an improved margin of safety in children.

It should be noted that an acute overdose (either accidental or intentional) may produce severe or even fatal liver damage. Alcoholics appear to be especially susceptible to the hepatotoxic effects of even moderate doses of acetaminophen. Indeed, alcoholics should avoid acetaminophen while they persist in heavy consumption of alcohol.

Acetaminophen generally has fewer side effects than aspirin; the drug produces less gastric distress and less ringing in the ears. Acetaminophen has been proven to be a reasonable substitute for aspirin when analgesic or antipyretic effectiveness is desired, especially in children and in patients who cannot tolerate aspirin.

Ibuprofen and Related Drugs

Ibuprofen and several related drugs (see Table II.1) exert aspirin-like analgesic, antipyretic, and anti-inflammatory effects. These agents are often better tolerated than aspirin. Their effectiveness is comparable to or greater than that of acetaminophen, aspirin, codeine, aspirin with codeine, and propoxyphene.[2] Like other NSAIDs, their actions result from drug-induced inhibition of prostaglandin synthesis. The incidence and severity of side effects produced by these agents are somewhat lower than those of aspirin, but gastric distress and the formation of peptic ulcers have occasionally been reported. Like aspirin (but unlike acetaminophen), these compounds inhibit platelet aggregation and therefore interfere with the clotting process. These drugs should

TABLE II.1 Ibuprofen and related drugs: Available formulations and recommendations for anti-inflammatory therapy

Nonproprietary name	Trade name	Formulation	Usual anti-inflammatory dose
Ibuprofen	Motrin, Advil, Nuprin, Medipren	Tablets	400 mg, three to four times a day
Naproxen	Naprosyn, Aleve, Anaprox	Tablets, suspension	250–500 mg, twice a day
Fenoprofen	Nalfon	tablets, capsules	300–600 mg, three to four times a day
Ketoprofen	Orudis, Oravail	Capsules	150–300 mg, two to four times a day
Flurbiprofen	Ansaid, others	Tablets	50–75 mg, two to four times a day
Oxaprozin	Daypro	Tablets	600–1200mg, once daily

be used with caution in patients who suffer from peptic ulcer disease or bleeding abnormalities. At the present time, ibuprofen and related drugs are not recommended for use by pregnant women. They are not secreted in breast milk.

FDA-approved indications for ibuprofen and related drugs (e.g., ketoprofen [Oruvail]) include use as analgesics and use in the symptomatic treatment of various forms of arthritis, tendonitis, bursitis, and for dysmenorrhea (painful menstrual periods). The anti-inflammatory effect is comparable to that of aspirin. The generally lower level of gastrointestinal side effects must be measured against the generally greater expense of these drugs.

Phenylbutazone

Phenylbutazone (Butazolidin) is an older, effective anti-inflammatory agent (available since 1949) that was once widely used to relieve the inflammation associated with rheumatoid arthritis. However, significant, serious side effects have limited its long-term usefulness. Most patients who take phenylbutazone experience gastric distress and skin rashes.

More severe problems include ulcer formation, allergies, liver and renal dysfunction, and a variety of severe abnormalities in various types of blood cells.

Unlike most of the other anti-inflammatory drugs, the half-life of phenylbutazone is quite long (about 2 days). At present, phenylbutazone is considered to be a distant choice for clinical use.

Indomethacin, Sulindac, and Etodolac

Indomethacin (Indocin), available since 1963, is an effective anti-inflammatory drug that is used primarily for treating rheumatoid arthritis and similar disorders. Like phenylbutazone, its use is limited because of its toxicity. Indomethacin is an analgesic, antipyretic, and anti-inflammatory agent. Indeed, its clinical effects closely resemble those of aspirin. Side effects occur in about 50 percent of the patients who take indomethacin, with gastric dysfunction being most prominent. Paradoxically, drug-induced headache limits its use in about 50 percent of patients. Other side effects are rare but potentially serious.

Two newer NSAIDs structurally and pharmacologically related to indomethacin are *sulindac* (Clinoril) and *etodolac* (Lodine). Sulindac is itself inactive, but its metabolite (sulindac sulfide) is very active. Its efficacy is comparable to that of indomethacin, but perhaps with a lower level of gastrointestinal toxicities (less than indomethacin, but greater than many other NSAIDs). Etodolac is an effective analgesic and anti-inflammatory drug. Its side effects, which include skin rashes, headache, and gastrointestinal irritation and ulceration, appear to be fewer than those caused by many other NSAIDs.

Ketorolac

Ketorolac (Toradol) is a newer analgesic and anti-inflammatory agent; it is the first NSAID available in injectable form for use in the treatment of postsurgical pain. Administered either intramuscularly or intravenously, it is effective in the short-term treatment of moderate to severe pain.[5,6] Because it does not produce the accompanying "rush" or pleasure associated with intravenous opioid use, ketorolac is not considered to be a drug of abuse. Like the other NSAIDs, ketorolac indirectly inhibits prostaglandin synthesis. Its analgesic potency is comparable to that of low doses of morphine, and it offers an anti-inflammatory action not offered by morphine. Its concomitant use with morphine offers synergistic action, reducing the required analgesic dose of morphine by about 50 percent. The half-life of ketorolac is about 4 to 6 hours in most persons, but it is longer in the elderly. Ketorolac is not recommended for use in obstetrics, because it and all other inhibitors of prostaglandin synthesis can adversely affect uterine contraction and fetal circulation.[7]

Side effects of ketorolac include excessive bleeding (due to platelet inhibition) and renal failure; the latter is minimized by limiting the use of the drug to 24 to 48 hours after surgery. Available also in tablet form for oral use, analgesic efficacy differs little from other orally administered NSAIDs.

Miscellaneous NSAIDs

Other, more rarely used NSAIDs available in the United States include *mefenamic acid* (Ponstel), *meclofenamate sodium* (Meclomen), *tolmetin* (Tolectin), *diclofenac* (Voltaren), *piroxicam* (Feldene), and *nabumetone* (Relafen). These are primarily used in the treatment of arthritis.

Several other drugs are in various stages of clinical development. These agents are reviewed by Insel (1996),[1] who also provides references to in-depth discussion of individual agents.

NOTES

1. P. A. Insel, "Analgesic-Antipyretic and Anti-inflammatory Agents and Drugs Employed in the Treatment of Gout," in J. G. Hardman, L. E. Limbird, P. B. Molinoff, R. W. Ruddon, and A.G. Gilman, eds., *Goodman & Gilman's The Pharmacological Basis of Therapeutics*, 9th ed. (New York: McGraw-Hill, 1996), 617–657.
2. "Analgesics," in *Drug Evaluations Annual 1994* (Milwaukee: American Medical Association, 1993), 114–131.
3. G. Weissmann, "Aspirin," *Scientific American* 264 (1991): 84–90.
4. P. Pinsky, E. S. Hurwitz, L. B. Schonberger, and W. J. Gunn, "Reye's Syndrome and Aspirin. Evidence for a Dose-Response Effect," *Journal of the American Medical Association* 260 (1988): 657–661.
5. M. M.-T. Buckley and R. N. Brogden, "Ketorolac: Review of Its Pharmacodynamic and Pharmacokinetic Properties, and Therapeutic Potential," *Drugs* 39 (1990): 86–109.
6. J. C. Gillis and R. N. Brogden, "Ketorolac: A Reappraisal of Its Pharmacodynamic and Pharmacokinetic Properties and Therapeutic Use in Pain Management," *Drugs* 53 (1997): 139–188.
7. "Ketorolac Tromethamine," *The Medical Letter on Drugs and Therapeutics* 32 (1990): 79–81.

PHARMACOLOGIC TREATMENT OF PARKINSONISM

Chapter 9 discussed drugs used to treat schizophrenia. The most prominent side effects of those drugs (especially the classical neuroleptic agents) are disorders that resemble the movement disorders seen in idiopathic Parkinson's disease (parkinsonism). From a mechanistic point of view, these side effects result from blockade of dopamine$_2$ receptors. Parkinsonism is similarly associated with a loss of dopamine in the extrapyramidal motor areas of the basal ganglia (caudate and putamen),[1] and the symptomatology of parkinsonism resembles the side effects seen with use of neuroleptics. Thus, it should be little surprise that the drugs used to ameliorate neuroleptic side effects are used to treat parkinsonism.

Parkinson's disease is a neurodegenerative disease that occurs in about 1 percent of all adults over the age of 65. Although the cause of parkinsonism remains unknown, its symptoms clearly follow from a deficiency in the numbers and function of dopamine-secreting neurons located in the basal ganglia of the brain. The clinical disease emerges when dopamine is depleted to about 20 percent of normal. In other words, the disease results when about 80 to 90 percent of dopamine neurons are lost. (Recall from Chapter 9 that the antipsychotic efficacy of neuroleptic drugs occurs when about 80 percent of dopamine$_2$ receptors were blocked.)

494

The clinical syndrome of parkinsonism comprises four cardinal features[1]: bradykinesia (slowness and poverty of movement); muscle rigidity; resting tremor, which usually abates during voluntary movement; and an impairment of postural balance leading to disturbances of gait and falling. Older terms for parkinsonism include "shaking palsy" and "paralysis agitans."

The availability of effective treatments for the symptoms of parkinsonism has radically altered the prognosis of this disease. In most cases, good functional mobility can be maintained for many years and the life expectancy of an affected individual has been greatly expanded. Either replacement of the dopamine or administration of dopaminergic agonists can restore function and ameliorate much of the symptomatology. These two approaches (dopamine replacement or administration of a dopaminergic agonist) underlie the present-day treatment of the disease. Table III.1 lists the medications and the dosages used for the treatment of parkinsonism.

TABLE III.1 Drugs for Parkinson's disease

Agent	Trade name	Daily dose— useful range	Comments
Carbidopa/levodopa	Sinemet	200–1,200 mg levodopa	Half-life = 1–3 hours
Carbidopa/levodopa sustained release	Sinemet CR	200–1,200 mg levodopa	Bioavailability 75% of standard form
Pergolide	Permax	0.75–5.0 mg	Titrate slowly
Bromocriptine	Parlodel	3.75–40 mg	Titrate slowly
Selegiline	1-Deprenyl, Eldepryl	2.5–10 mg	
Amantadine	Symmetrel	200 mg	
Trihexyphenidyl	Artane	2–15 mg	Representative anticholinergic agent

Levodopa

Because a loss of dopamine is the primary problem in patients who have Parkinson's disease, replacement of the dopamine would be expected to ameliorate the symptoms of the disease. It does, but not by itself, because it does not cross the blood-brain barrier from plasma into the central nervous system (CNS). In an intuitive step, the precursor compound in the biosynthesis of dopamine from the amino acid tyramine, a substance called *dihydroxydopamine* or *DOPA* (see Figure III.1), crosses the blood-brain barrier and in the CNS is converted into dopamine, replacing that which is absent. Therefore, today, levodopa (the *levo* isomer being more active than the *dextro* isomer) is the most effective treatment for parkinsonian motor disability,

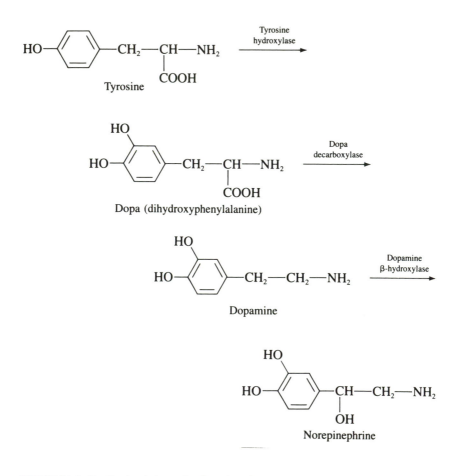

FIGURE III.1 Synthesis of dopamine from tyrosine.

and many practitioners consider an initial beneficial response an important diagnostic criterion for the diagnosis of parkinsonism.[2]

Mechanism of Action

Levodopa is itself largely inert; its therapeutic as well as its adverse effects result from its conversion to dopamine.[1] Administered orally, levodopa is rapidly absorbed into the bloodstream, where most of it (about 95 percent) is converted to dopamine in the plasma. Although only a small amount (about 5 percent) of levodopa crosses the blood-brain barrier and is converted to dopamine in the brain, it is enough to alleviate the symptoms of parkinsonism. Indeed, in the CNS, levodopa is converted to dopamine by "decarboxylation," primarily within the presynaptic terminals of dopaminergic neurons in the basal ganglia.[1]

One problem with this therapy, however, is that, when levodopa is administered by itself, large amounts are destroyed by enzymes located both in the intestine and in plasma, so that little drug is available to cross the blood-brain barrier. In addition, the levodopa in the peripheral circulation is converted to dopamine in the body, resulting in undesirable side effects, such as nausea.

Again, we return to basic pharmacology. A drug is needed to reduce the high levels of dopamine in the systemic circulation while maintaining sufficient quantities in the brain. To develop such a drug, the biosynthetic pathway that leads to dopamine (see Figure III.1) must be examined. Since the enzyme *dopa decarboxylase* is responsible for converting dopa to dopamine, by inhibiting this enzyme in the systemic circulation but not in the brain, systemic biotransformation of the drug should be reduced, with a concomitant reduction in blood levels of dopamine and therefore in side effects. The drug would need a unique characteristic: it would have to be active in the body but not cross the blood-brain barrier into the brain. Thus, the metabolic conversion would occur in the CNS but not in the periphery. An example of such a drug is *carbidopa*, which is available in combination with levodopa (the combination is known as Sinemet). By combining carbidopa with levodopa, the effective dose of levodopa is reduced by 75 percent, with a concomitant reduction in side effects and no loss of CNS therapeutic effect. The current treatment of parkinsonism relies heavily on the combination of levodopa and carbidopa (see Table III.1).

Limitations to Levodopa Therapy

While levodopa therapy has a dramatic effect on the symptoms of parkinsonism, as time goes on, the drug becomes less effective and the patient's symptoms fluctuate dramatically between doses. Eventually, this develops into what is called an "off-and-on" phenomenon, which is described in detail by Standaert and Young (1996)[1] and by Hughes (1997).[2] Part of the phenomenon is due to the short half-life of levodopa (1 to 3 hours) and can be minimized by increasing the dose and by decreasing the interval between doses. Here, however, one risks the development of levodopa-induced movement disorders (e.g., dyskinesias), which can be as uncomfortable and disabling as the rigidity and akinesia of parkinsonism.[1] A sustained-release preparation of levodopa/carbidopa (Sinemet CR) can be used to help provide a more stable blood level of the drug and hopefully reduce the dyskinesias.

Another unanswered question with levodopa therapy is whether or not this drug might theoretically accelerate the course of parkinsonism.[3] One theory of the disease is that the metabolism of dopamine produces free radicals that contribute to the death of the dopamine-releasing neurons. While unproven, it is a cause of concern that while we are ameliorating symptoms, we might be aggravating the disease. Thus, initiation of levodopa therapy is often delayed until the symptoms of parkinsonism actually cause an unacceptable degree of functional impairment.

Dopamine Receptor Agonists

Between one and five years after the start of levodopa therapy, most patients gradually become less responsive. This development may be related to a progressive inability of dopamine neurons to synthesize and store dopamine. To alleviate this problem, attempts have been made to identify drugs that will directly stimulate postsynaptic dopamine receptors in the basal ganglia. These drugs do not depend on the ability of existing dopaminergic neurons to enzymatically convert the drug to an active compound (i.e., levodopa to dopamine). In addition, if one accepts the free radical theory described in the previous paragraph, these drugs would avoid the biotransformation into potentially neurotoxic metabolites. These drugs might be effective in the late stages of parkinsonism, when dopamine neurons are largely absent or nonfunctional.

To date, two such dopamine receptor agonists are commercially available in the United States for the treatment of parkinsonism—bromocriptine (Parlodel) and pergolide (Permax). Both of these drugs are derived from the ergot alkaloid lysergic acid (see Chapter 12), and both have structures that closely resemble that of dopamine (see Figure III.2). A third lysergic acid derivative, lisuride, is being studied.

Bromocriptine is a potent agonist (stimulant) of dopamine$_2$ receptors and a partial agonist of dopamine$_1$ receptors. It is well absorbed

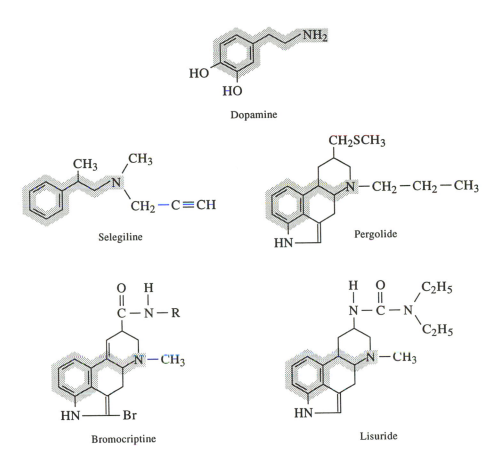

FIGURE III.2 Structures of dopamine and dopaminergic agonists that are used to treat parkinsonism. The shaded portions, which are shared by all these structures, resemble dopamine.

orally and has a half-life of about three to seven hours. Bromocriptine is used as an adjunct to levodopa in patients whose disease is not adequately controlled with levodopa; improving the patient's therapeutic response to a reduced dose of levodopa thus reduces the side effects of therapy. Because the efficacy of bromocriptine is often not sustained, its therapeutic usefulness is limited. Patient responsiveness also varies widely. Side effects include nausea, vomiting, hypotension, and mental disturbances. Recent studies, however, have pointed out the limited efficacy and significant adverse effects of bromocriptine and other dopamine agonists compared with levodopa as sole initial treatment.[2,4]

Pergolide closely resembles bromocriptine but is more potent and has a longer half-life (about 30 hours), although the clinical effect persists for only about 5.5 hours.[2] It is a potent agonist at both D_1 and D_2 receptors; how this related to any therapeutic difference from bromocriptine is unknown. Pergolide may be effective following a loss of responsiveness to bromocriptine. Thus, a patient's failure to respond to one dopaminergic agonist does not rule out a response to another.

Lisuride is a selective dopamine$_2$ receptor agonist whose use is limited by the occurrence of dyskinesias and neuropsychiatric toxicity. It probably will not become available in the United States.

Selegiline

Selegiline (l-Deprenyl, Eldepryl) effectively ameliorates the symptoms of parkinsonism through a unique mechanism. In Chapter 7, we discussed two types of the enzyme monoamine oxidase (MAO) and the emerging use of a selective MAO-A inhibitor (moclobemide) as a clinical antidepressant. In contrast to MAO-A (which is more closely involved with norepinephrine and serotonin nerve terminals), MAO-B has preferential affinity for dopamine neurons. MAO-B is selectively inhibited by selegiline. Selegiline also inhibits the local breakdown of dopamine, thus preserving the small amounts of dopamine that are present. Both actions enhance the therapeutic effect of levodopa. Selegiline is being used increasingly in the treatment of newly diagnosed, younger patients who have Parkinson's disease, because it appears to slow down the early progression of the disease and delays the need for initiating levodopa therapy.[5,6] Interestingly, selegiline is metabolized to several by-products, including amphetamine and methamphetamine. Thus, metabolism of this drug provides a third mechanism that may help to alleviate the dopamine deficiency. In summary, selegiline may contribute to therapy for parkinsonism through any of three mechanisms:

1. Inhibition of MAO-B

2. Inhibition of the breakdown of dopamine

3. Metabolism into the active intermediates amphetamine and methamphetamine (which augment dopamine neurotransmission; see Chapter 5)

There is one caution with selegiline. A report from the United Kingdom stated that, in combination with levodopa, selegiline may be associated with an increase in morbidity after five years of use.[7] The reason for this is unclear, and this observation has not been verified as yet by other researchers. Hughes (1997)[2] summarizes:

> The finding awaits confirmation and further clarification, and at this stage it is not possible to give clear prescribing guidelines for the use of selegiline, although many physicians are being cautious with its use at present.

Amantadine

Amantadine (Symmetrel) is an antiviral agent that, through an unknown mechanism, relieves the symptoms of parkinsonism. It is likely that amantadine releases dopamine from whatever dopamine neurons remain in the patient's basal ganglia. Amantadine also appears to potentiate the therapeutic effects of levodopa, although such potentiation is not consistent. Thus, amantadine is much less effective than levodopa for long-term relief of the symptoms of parkinsonism. Adverse effects include slurred speech, ataxia, gastric distress, hallucinations, confusion, and nightmares.

Muscarinic Receptor Antagonists

Although widely used before the introduction of levodopa, certain *anticholinergic agents* (muscarinic antagonists) are now used much less and are considered second-tier agents for the treatment of symptoms of parkinsonism. Their use was originally postulated to be on the basis of an unopposed cholinergic system after death of the dopaminergic neurons.

Occasionally, anticholinergic drugs are used as an adjunct to levodopa in patients with difficult-to-control tremors. Cognitive dysfunction limits their use, especially in the elderly. Representative agents include *trihexyphenidyl* (Artane), *procyclidine* (Kemadrin), *biperiden* (Akineton), *ethopropazine* (Parsidol), and *benzotropine* (Cogentin).

Nonpharmacologic Treatments for Parkinsonism

The drugs described have numerous limitations, not the least of which is reduced drug effect after about 10 years of treatment. Thus, alternatives to drug therapy are worth investigating. Alternatives include surgical transplantation of fetal "nigral" cells (dopamine-secreting cells from the substantia nigra)[8] and surgical implantation of stimulating electrodes in the basal ganglia. The indications for and the efficacy of such therapies are as yet unknown.

NOTES

1. D. G. Standaert and A. B. Young, "Treatment of Central Nervous System Degenerative Disorders," in J. G. Hardman, L. E. Limbird, P. B. Molinoff, R. W. Ruddon, and A. G. Gilman, eds., *Goodman & Gilman's The Pharmacological Basis of Therapeutics*, 9th ed. (New York: McGraw-Hill, 1996), 503–513.
2. A. J. Hughes, "Drug Treatment of Parkinson's Disease in the 1990s: Achievements and Future Possibilities," *Drugs* 53 (1997): 195–205.
3. P. Jenner, A. H. V. Schapira, C. Marsden, et al., "New Insights into the Cause of Parkinson's Disease," *Neurology* 42 (1992): 2241–2250.
4. M. A. Hely, J. G. L. Morris, W. C. J. Reid, et al., "The Sidney Multicentre Study of Parkinson's Disease: A Randomized, Prospective, Five Year Study Comparing Low Dose Bromocriptine with Low Dose Levodopa-Carbidopa," *Journal of Neurology, Neurosurgery, and Psychiatry* 57 (1994): 903–910.
5. C. Ward, "Does Selegiline Delay Progression of Parkinson's Disease? A Critical Re-evaluation of the DATATOP Study," *Journal of Neurology, Neurosurgery, and Psychiatry* 57 (1994): 217–220.
6. Parkinson Study Group, "Impact of Deprenyl and Tocopherol Treatment on Parkinson's Disease in DATATOP Subjects Not Requiring Levodopa," *Annals of Neurology* 39 (1996): 29–36.
7. A. J. Lees, "Comparison of Therapeutic Effects and Mortality Data of Levodopa and Levodopa Combined with Selegiline in Patients with Early, Mild Parkinson's Disease," *British Journal of Medicine* 313 (1995): 1602–1607.
8. C. W. Olanow, J. H. Kordower, and T. B. Freeman, "Fetal Nigral Transplantation as a Therapy for Parkinson's Disease," *Trends in Neuroscience* 19 (1996): 102–109.

THE BRAIN, NEURONS, SYNAPTIC TRANSMISSION, AND DRUG ACTION

Basic Anatomy of the Brain

The nervous system can be conveniently divided into two parts: the *central nervous system* (CNS) and the *peripheral nervous system*. The latter consists of the nerves that lie outside the brain and spinal cord and are both sensory from (afferent) and "motor" to (efferent) all the muscles and organs of the body. These nerves are considered peripheral even though their cell bodies might actually be located in the brain or spinal cord. For example, the cell bodies of the "motor neurons" that send efferent axons to our muscles are located in the ventral portions of the spinal cord. In this text, there is little focus on peripheral nerves, and they are referred to only as they may be involved in the side effects of psychoactive drugs. More complete information on the actions of drugs on the body and on the peripheral nervous system may be found in an earlier text by this author (1988).[1]

The human brain is thought to consist of perhaps 100 billion individual neurons located in the skull and the spinal canal. The *spinal cord* extends from the lower end of the medulla to the sacrum. It consists of neurons and fiber tracts involved in the following:

- Carrying sensory information from skin, muscles, joints, and internal body organs to the brain

- Organizing and modulating the motor outflow to the muscles (to produce coordinated muscle responses)
- Modulating sensory input (including pain-impulse input)
- Providing autonomic (involuntary) control of vital body functions

The lower part of the brain, attached to the upper part of the spinal cord, is the *brain stem* (see Figure IV.1). It is divided into three parts: the *medulla*, the *pons*, and the *midbrain*. All impulses that are conducted in either direction between the spinal cord and the brain pass through the brain stem, which is also important in the regulation of vital body functions, such as respiration, blood pressure, heart rate, gastrointestinal functioning, and the states of sleep and wakefulness. The brain stem is also involved in behavioral alerting, attention, and arousal responses. Depressant drugs, such as the barbiturates (see Chapter 2), depress the brain stem activating system; this action probably underlies much of their hypnotic action.

Behind the brain stem is a large bulbous structure—the *cerebellum*. The area immediately above the brain stem and covered by the cerebral hemispheres is the *diencephalon*. This area includes the hypothalamus, pituitary gland, various fiber tracts (bundles of axons that travel as a group from one area to another), subthalamus, and thalamus (see Figure IV.1). Almost completely covering the brain stem and the diencephalon are the left and right hemispheres of the *cerebrum*.

The cerebellum, a large, highly convoluted structure, is connected to the brain stem by large fiber tracts. The cerebellum is necessary for the proper integration of movement and posture. Some drugs exert noticeable effects on cerebellar activity. Drunkenness, which is characterized by ataxia (loss of coordination and balance, staggering, and other deficits), appears to be caused largely by an alcohol-induced depression of cerebellar function. Other drugs that can cause ataxia include the benzodiazepines and anticonvulsant-antimanic drugs, such as carbamazepine and valproic acid.

The *diencephalon* can be subdivided into several areas, but we discuss just three—the *subthalamus*, the *hypothalamus*, and the *limbic system*. The subthalamus is a small area underneath the thalamus and above the midbrain. It contains a variety of small structures that, together with the basal ganglia, constitute one of our motor systems, the *extrapyramidal system*. Patients who have Parkinson's disease (see Appendix III) have a deficiency of the neurotransmitter dopamine in the terminals of their nerve axons, which originate from cell bodies in the substantia nigra (one of the subthalamic structures).

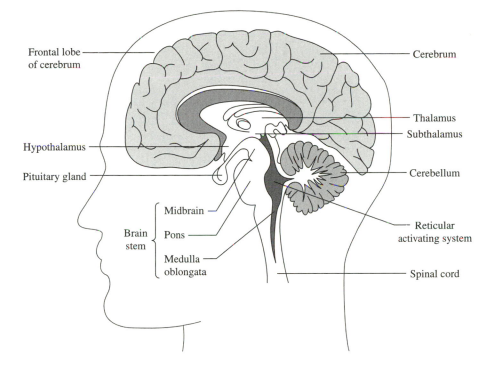

Frontal lobe of cerebrum

Hypothalamus

Pituitary gland

Brain stem
- Midbrain
- Pons
- Medulla oblongata

Cerebrum

Thalamus

Subthalamus

Cerebellum

Reticular activating system

Spinal cord

FIGURE IV.1   Midline section of the brain illustrating several structures lying below the cerebral cortex.

The hypothalamus is a collection of neurons in the lower portion of the brain near the junction of the midbrain and the thalamus. It is located near the base of the skull, just above the pituitary gland (the function of which it largely modulates). The hypothalamus is the principal center in the brain responsible for the integration of our entire autonomic (involuntary or vegetative) nervous system. Thus, it helps control such vegetative functions as eating, drinking, sleeping, regulation of body temperature, sexual behavior, blood pressure, emotion, and water balance. In addition, the hypothalamus closely controls hormonal output of the pituitary gland. Neurons in the hypothalamus produce substances called *releasing factors*, which travel to the nearby pituitary gland (see Chapter 13), ultimately inducing the production and secretion of hormones that regulate the menstrual cycle and ovulation in females and sperm formation in males. The hypothalamus is a site of action for many psychoactive drugs, either as a site for the primary action of the drug or as a site responsible for side effects associated with the use of a drug.

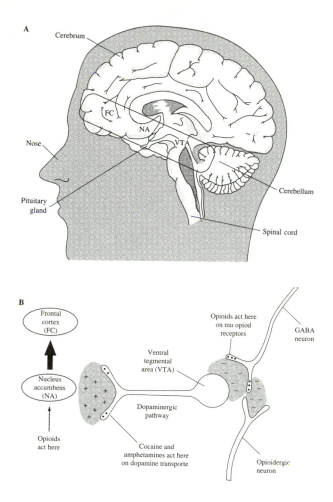

FIGURE IV.2 The limbic dopaminergic reward pathway. (**A**) Human brain sliced open lengthwise, showing the relevant midbrain and forebrain area, outlined by an oval, with ventral tegmental area (VTA), nucleus accumbens (NA), and frontal cortex (FC) labeled. (**B**) Diagram of the area outlined in (**A**). Heavy dots = stored neurotransmitter at nerve endings; + = excitatory neurotransmitter; – = inhibitory neurotransmitter.

Closely associated with the hypothalamus is the *limbic system,* the major components of which are the *amygdala* and the *hippocampus.* These structures exert primitive types of behavioral control; they integrate emotion, reward, and behavior with motor and autonomic functions. Because the limbic system and the hypothalamus interact to regulate emotion and emotional expression, these structures are logical sites for the study of psychoactive drugs that alter mood, affect, emotion, or responses to emotional experiences. The classical notion that the limbic system is important in learning and memory tasks has prompted investigations of both this structure and the hypothalamus as sites of action for compounds that affect these functions.

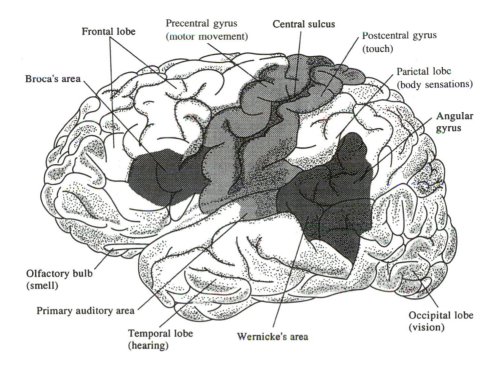

Frontal lobe

Precentral gyrus
(motor movement)

Central sulcus

Postcentral gyrus
(touch)

Broca's area

Parietal lobe
(body sensations)

Angular
gyrus

Olfactory bulb
(smell)

Primary auditory area

Temporal lobe
(hearing)

Wernicke's area

Occipital lobe
(vision)

FIGURE IV.3 Surface structure of the brain, showing major areas of the cerebral cortex.

The hypothalamic and limbic areas contain structures important in psychopharmacology and the abuse potential of drugs. Included here are the dopamine-rich reward centers (see Figure IV.2) that involve the ventral tegmental area, the median forebrain bundle, and the nucleus accumbens. The activity of these dopaminergic neurons is affected by opioid, GABAergic, and other neuronal influences. Throughout this text, this reward system is discussed as a site of the behavior-reinforcing action of psychoactive drugs that are subject to compulsive abuse.

In humans the *cerebrum* is the largest portion of the brain. It is separated into two distinct hemispheres, left and right, with numerous fiber tracts connecting the two. Because skull size is limited and the cerebrum is so large, the outer layer of the cerebrum, the *cerebral cortex*, is deeply convoluted and fissured. Like other portions of the brain, the cerebral cortex is divided by function; it contains centers for vision, hearing, speech, sensory perception, and emotion. The various regions of the cerebral cortex can be classified in several ways, one being by the type of function or sensation that is processed. Figure IV.3 illustrates some of this categorization.

The Neuron

The *neuron* is the basic component of the CNS, and each neuron shares common structural and functional characteristics (see Figure IV.4). A typical neuron consists of the *soma* (cell body), which contains the nucleus (within which is the genetic material of the cell). Extending from the soma in one direction are many short fibers, called *dendrites* (hundreds of widely branched extensions), that receive input from other neurons through *receptors* located on the dendritic membrane. Upon receipt of a "signal" from another cell, an electrical current is generated

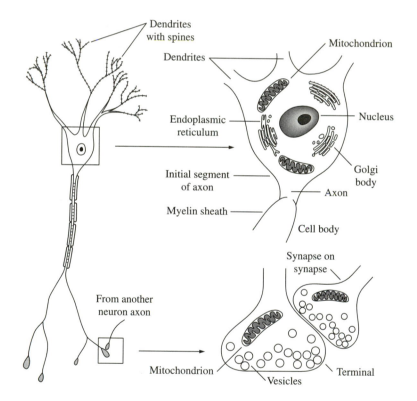

FIGURE IV.4   Major parts of a neuron. The genetic material (DNA) is contained in the nucleus, and several specialized organelles are present in the material of the cell outside the nucleus, the cytoplasm. The cell is covered by a thin wall, or membrane. Mitochondria are present in the cell body, the fibers, and the terminals. The terminals also contain small, round vesicles that contain neurotransmitter chemicals. Synaptic connections from the fibers of other neurons cover the cell body and dendrites. In many neurons the synapses on dendrites can be seen as little spines. The axon itself has no synapses on it except sometimes at its synaptic terminals, where other neuron axon terminals may form synapses on synapses. [From Thompson (1993),[2] p. 31.]

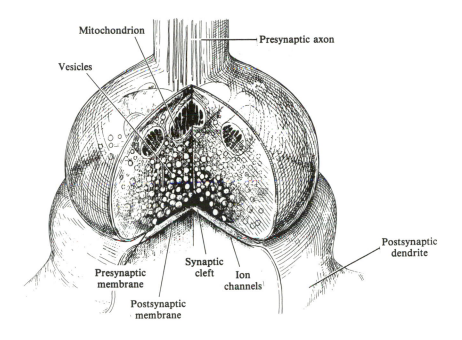

Mitochondrion

Vesicles

Presynaptic axon

Postsynaptic
dendrite

Synaptic
cleft

Presynaptic
membrane

Ion
channels

Postsynaptic
membrane

FIGURE IV.5 Three-dimensional drawing of a synapse. The axon terminal is the top knoblike structure, and the spine of the receiving neuron is the bottom one. Note that there is a space (synaptic cleft) between the presynaptic terminal membrane and the postsynaptic cell membrane.

and travels down the dendrite to the soma. Extending in another direction from the soma is a single elongated process called an *axon*, which varies in length from as short as a few millimeters to as long as a meter (meter-length examples are the axons that run from the motor neurons of the spinal cord out to the muscles that they innervate). The axon, in essence, transmits electrical activity (in the form of *action potentials*) from the soma to other neurons or to muscles, organs, or glands of the body. Normally, the axon conducts impulses in only one direction—from the soma, down the axon, to a specialized structure that, together with one or more dendrites from another neuron, forms a complex microspace called a *synapse* (see Figure IV.5). The axon also functions to transport proteins and other substances from the soma to nerve terminals.

A given neuron in the brain may receive several thousand synaptic connections from other neurons. Hence if the human brain has 10^{11} neurons, then it has at least 10^{14} synapses, or many trillions. The number of possible different combinations of synaptic connections among the neurons in a single human brain is larger than the total number of atomic particles that make up the known universe. Hence the diversity of the interconnections in a human brain seems almost without limit.[2]

It is interesting that our brains have the maximal number of neurons at birth; once a neuron dies, it is not replaced. What continues to develop during our lifetimes is the number and pattern of synaptic connections, which are shaped, synthesized, and "sculpted" by experience and appear to form the anatomical basis of memory.[3] In this text, we commonly refer to synapses as the major site of drug action and, therefore, further explore their anatomy and physiology.

The term *synapse* refers to the point of functional contact between an axon terminal and another cell (see Figure IV.5). As used here, a synapse consists of a minute space (the *synaptic cleft*) between the presynaptic membrane (which is the axon terminal) of one neuron and the postsynaptic membrane of the receiving neuron. The presynaptic terminal contains numerous structural elements, the most important of which (for our purposes) are the small synaptic vesicles, each of which contains several thousand molecules of neurotransmitter chemical. These vesicles store the transmitter, which is available for release (see Figure IV.6). Through a process called *exocytosis*, molecules of transmitter are released into the synaptic cleft. The transmitter substance diffuses across the synaptic cleft and attaches to receptors on the postsynaptic membrane (e.g., dendrites of the next neuron), thereby transmitting information chemically from one neuron to another. Because the neurons do not physically touch each other, synaptic transmission is a chemical rather than an electrical process.

When a chemical transmitter (e.g., serotonin, dopamine, acetylcholine) attaches to its postsynaptic "receptor," it is said to "occupy" its receptor; in fact, this is a dynamic process, with the transmitter reversibly binding and detaching for as long as the "neurotransmitter" persists in the synaptic cleft. Most psychoactive drugs act through various processes that either potentiate or oppose the actions of a neurotransmitter at its receptors. These receptors are, in fact, large proteins (chains of amino acids) that form various large macromolecular structures. Examples of such receptors are illustrated throughout this text; the GABA$_A$ receptor is illustrated in Figures IV.7 and IV.8. "Activation" of such receptors (by attachment of a neurotransmitter) often opens a "gate" or pore through which ions flow to alter postsynaptic cell functioning. In other cases, the receptor is coupled to intracellular ("G") proteins located within the postsynaptic neuron; activation of the receptor by transmitter induces release of the G-protein (which was

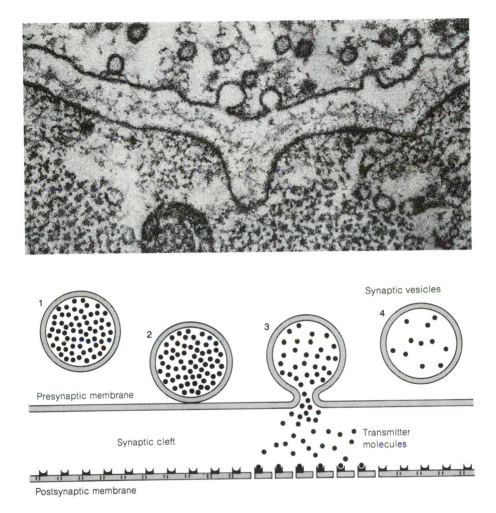

FIGURE IV.6 *Top:* Photomicrograph of a synapse in action taken with the electron microscope. Vesicles are releasing their transmitter chemical into the synaptic cleft. *Bottom:* Schematic of the process.

bound to the terminal chain of the receptor). In turn, the G-protein ultimately alters intracellular enzyme function.

It may sound as if this process of synaptic transmission takes a rather long time, but the process is remarkably fast and efficient, its length determined by multiple factors described by Clements (1996).[4] Indeed, the process may be as short as a fraction of a millisecond for transmitter release (from presynaptic vesicles), diffusion (across the

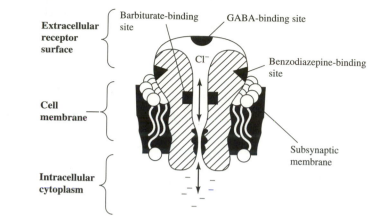

FIGURE IV.7 GABA_A receptor in a perpendicular section through the membrane. The localization of the various binding sites is purely hypothetical. [Reprinted with permission from W. E. Haefely, J. R. Martin, J. G. Richards, and P. Schoch, "The Multiplicity of Actions of Benzodiazepine Receptor Ligands," *Canadian Journal of Psychiatry* 38, Suppl. 4 (1993): 5102–5107.]

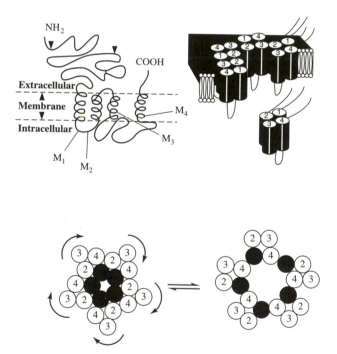

FIGURE IV.8 Presumed topology of the GABA_A receptor. *Top left:* Single subunit with its large extracellular terminal part, and the four transmembrane domains (M1 to M4) with their intracellular connecting stretches. *Top right:* Arrangement of the transmembrane domains of five subunits to form a central channel. *Bottom:* The transmembrane domains in a transverse section through the membrane when the channel is closed (*left*) and open (*right*). [Reprinted with permission from W. E. Haefely, J. R. Martin, J. G. Richards, and P. Schoch, "The Multiplicity of Actions of Benzodiazepine Receptor Ligands," *Canadian Journal of Psychiatry* 38, Suppl.4 (1993): 5102–5107.]

cleft), receptor interaction (on the postsynaptic membrane), and transmitter removal from the cleft (by either metabolic inactivation or by active reuptake by a "transporter protein" back into the presynaptic terminal).

We must address a point of possible confusion that is important as it relates to drug action. To discuss this point, we will use dopamine as a representative neurotransmitter. Following its synthesis, storage, and release, dopamine binds to the postsynaptic receptor to produce its characteristic effects. Its transmitter action is terminated by its "active reuptake" back into the presynaptic terminal and then into the storage granules, where it is protected from metabolic degradation and is stored for reuse. Dopamine therefore has "affinity" for (binds to) three structurally different protein "receptors": the postsynaptic receptor, the presynaptic transporter, and the transporter located on the surface of the storage granule.[5] The postsynaptic receptor is a protein of about 420 amino acids with 7 membrane-spanning regions, similar to the serotonin receptor; the two transporter receptors are 619 amino acid proteins with 12 membrane-spanning regions (see Chapter 5). Dopamine binds to all three, but drugs can be specific for one receptor. For example, cocaine binds to (and blocks the action of) the presynaptic transporter, augmenting the action of dopamine and resulting in its characteristic behavioral stimulant and behavioral reinforcing actions.

Similarly, the antihypertensive (blood pressure–lowering) drug reserpine blocks the storage granule transporter, making the transmitter available to destructive enzymes (e.g., MAO) that ultimately deplete the nerve terminal of transmitter, lowering blood pressure and inducing a state of depression. Conversely, chlorpromazine (see Chapter 9) binds to and blocks certain postsynaptic dopamine receptors, thus inhibiting the synaptic actions of dopamine, resulting in the amelioration of the positive symptomatology of schizophrenia and the production of extrapyramidal motor movements, actions that are essentially the opposite of that exerted by cocaine. Thus, drugs can have much more specific receptor effects than the endogenous transmitter for that receptor.

Before leaving the topic of the anatomy of the neuron, we briefly discuss the cell body of the neuron (the soma) as it influences neurotransmitter availability at the synapse. Like all cells of the body except red blood cells, the soma has a *nucleus* that contains the basic genetic material (DNA) for the cell (see Figure IV.4). Because the neuron is a specialized type of cell, its DNA expresses a subset of genes that encode the special structural and enzymatic proteins that endow the neuron with its size, shape, location, and other functional characteristics.[6]

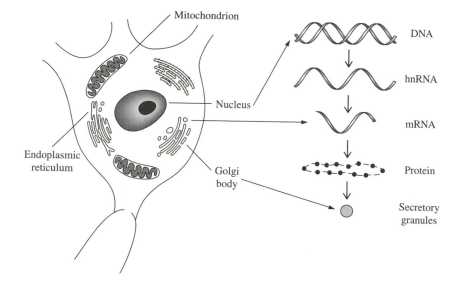

FIGURE IV.9 Formation of transmitter substances and "packaging" in vesicles from genetic material in the nucleus. DNA-encoded information is transcribed in the nucleus to a primary transcript form (hnRNA), which is edited and exported from the nucleus to the cytoplasm as messenger RNA (mRNA). This is then translated from the genetic nucleic acid code of RNA into the amino acid sequence of the protein that is to be expressed. Within the Golgi body portion of the endoplasmic reticulum, the transmitter is packaged into secretory organelles for transport down the axon to the neuron terminals.

Also located in the soma are the *mitochondria*, which provide the biological energy for the neuron. This energy, in the form of *adenosine triphosphate* (or ATP), is made available for all the various chemical reactions carried out in the cell (such as neurotransmitter synthesis, storage, release, and reuptake).

In response to stimuli, the DNA in the nucleus is transcribed into a second similar molecular form as strands of ribonucleic acid (RNA), which is then "edited" by several rapid steps and exported from the nucleus to the cytoplasm of the soma.[6] The edited RNA is called *messenger RNA*, and this nuclear material is then translated from the nucleic acid code of the RNA into the amino acid sequence of the protein that is to be expressed (see Figure IV.9). "Expression" or "translation" occurs on the endoplasmic reticulum, where the neurotransmitters are

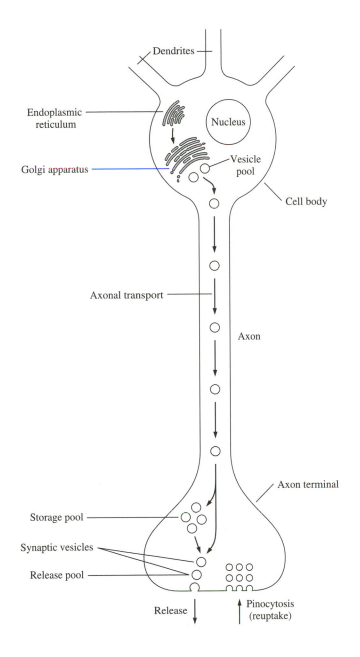

FIGURE IV.10 Axon transport. Chemicals are moved from the cell body to the terminals. It is believed that they move along the axon in microtubules that fill the axon.

synthesized and then "packaged" into vesicles that are then transported in specialized *microtubules* down the axon to the synaptic terminals, where they await release (see Figure IV.10). Indeed, even the presynaptic receptors (such as the dopamine transporter) are made in the soma and carried down the axon, where they embed themselves in the cell membrane and exert their receptor functions.

Receptors

In the human brain there are hundreds of different types of receptors, including multiple subtypes of receptors for such transmitter chemicals as norepinephrine, dopamine, GABA, glutamate, histamine, acetylcholine, opioids, and serotonin. This multitude of receptors can be divided into three classes. One class is the *"fast" receptors*, which are linked directly to an ion channel and which mediate millisecond responses when activated by a transmitter (one example is the $GABA_A$ receptor). Structurally, the proteins that make up this receptor contain four membrane-spanning elements (see Chapters 2 and 4).

A second class of receptors is referred to as *G-protein–coupled receptors*, which are somewhat slower in action and serve to modulate postsynaptic cellular function. These modulatory receptors in turn may be directly coupled to ion channels that are linked to intracellular "second messengers" (see Figure IV.11). These receptors all appear to be from a family of G-protein–binding proteins characterized by seven transmembrane-spanning segments with terminal chains inside the cell and in the synaptic cleft (see Figure IV.12).

The third class of transmitter receptors, termed *transporter proteins*, is located on presynaptic nerve terminals, the function of which is to reduce the amount of transmitter in the synaptic cleft. These proteins usually have 12 transmembrane spanning elements and are the site of action of antidepressant drugs and cocaine. The transporter protein receptor for dopamine (blocked by cocaine) is illustrated in Figure 5.5; the similar receptor for serotonin (blocked by certain antidepressants) is illustrated in Figure 7.3.

Specific Neurotransmitter Chemicals

Acetylcholine

Acetylcholine (ACh) was first identified as a transmitter chemical in the peripheral nervous system and in brain tissue, and deficiencies in acetylcholine-secreting neurons are associated with learning and memory dysfunctions, as seen in Alzheimer's disease. In addition, drugs

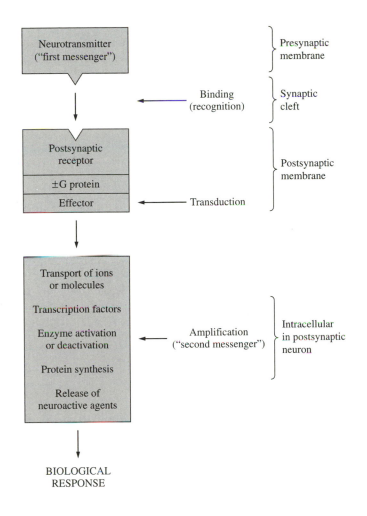

FIGURE IV.11   Schematic model of transmitter-receptor interaction.

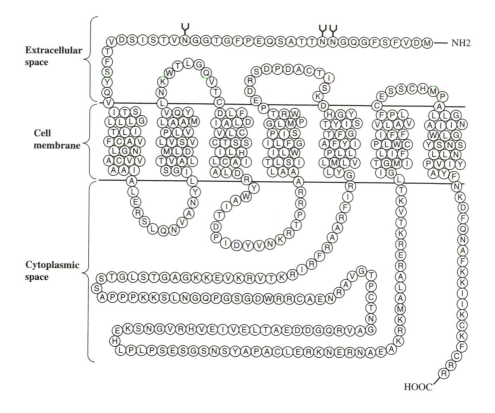

FIGURE IV.12 Schematic representation of the primary structure of the rat serotonin$_{1A}$ receptor.

such as scopolamine, which block central "cholinergic" receptors, are exceedingly effective amnestic agents (see Chapter 12). Thus, acetylcholine may be a critical neurotransmitter for normal intellectual functioning.

ACh is synthesized in a one-step reaction from two precursors and then stored within synaptic vesicles for release. This reaction and the dynamics of ACh release, metabolism, and resynthesis are shown in Figure IV.13. Like other neurotransmitters, ACh is released into the synaptic cleft, rapidly diffuses across the cleft, and reversibly binds to postsynaptic receptors.

Unlike most other neurotransmitters, once ACh has exerted its effect on the postsynaptic dendritic membrane, its action is terminated by the enzyme *acetylcholine esterase* (AChE). The enzymatic reaction that degrades ACh is important, because many drugs (referred to as

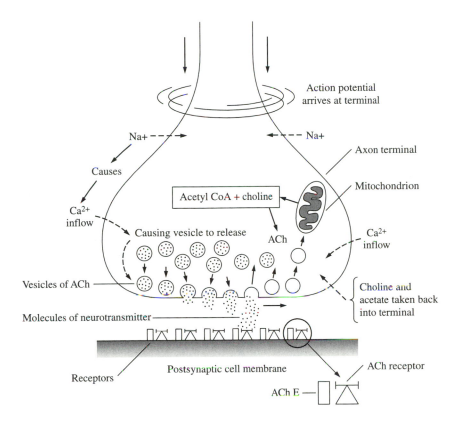

FIGURE IV.13 Chemical synapse. Acetylcholine (ACh) is used as the example. It is made in the axon terminal from acetyl coenzyme A (acetyl CoA) and choline, stored in vesicles, and released. When the action potential arrives at the terminal, closed calcium channels in the terminal are opened and Ca^{2+} rushes into the terminal, triggering vesicles to fuse with the membrane and release ACh molecules into the synaptic cleft. They attach to ACh receptors on the postsynaptic membrane and trigger the opening of Na^+ channels. ACh is immediately broken down at the receptors by acetylcholine-esterase (AChE) into choline and acetate, which are taken back up by the terminal and reused. [From Thompson (1993),[2] p. 77.]

AChE inhibitors) inhibit this enzyme. *Irreversible AChE inhibitors* (such as malathion) are potent toxins, exploited in agriculture as insecticides; other irreversible ACHE inhibitors (such as Sarin and Soman) are used in the military as lethal nerve gases. Less toxic, *reversible AChE inhibitors* can be used as cognitive enhancers, by increasing ACh

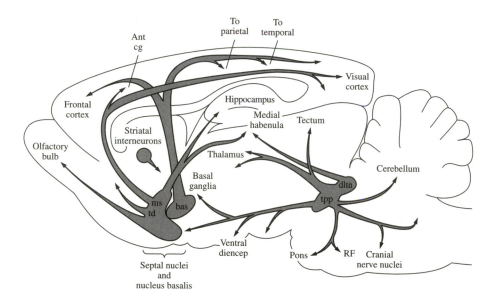

FIGURE IV.14 Schematic representation of the major cholinergic systems in the rat brain. As illustrated, central cholinergic neurons exhibit two basic organizational schemata: (1) local circuit cells (i.e., those that morphologically are arrayed wholly within the neural structure in which they are found) exemplified by the interneurons of the caudate-putamen nucleus (striatal interneurons); and (2) projection neurons (i.e., those that connect two or more different regions). Of the cholinergic projection neurons that interconnect central structures, two major subconstellations have been identified: (1) the basal forebrain cholinergic complex composed of neurons in the medial septal nucleus (ms) and nucleus basalis (bas) and projecting to the entire non-striatal telencephalon; and (2) the pontomesencephalotegmental cholinergic complex, composed of cells in the pendunculopontine (tpp) and laterodorsal (dltn) tegmental nuclei and projecting ascendingly to the thalamus and other diencephalic loci and descendingly to the pontine and medullary reticular formation (RF), cerebellum, and cranial nerve nuclei.

levels in the CNS, thereby delaying the decline in cognitive function and activities of daily living in patients with Alzheimer's disease. Donepezil (Aricept), which became available in 1997, is an example.

ACh is distributed widely in the brain (see Figure IV.14). Simply, the cell bodies of cholinergic neurons in the brain lie in two closely related regions. One involves the *septal nuclei* and the *nucleus basalis*. The axons of these neurons project to forebrain regions, particularly the hippocampus and cerebral cortex.[7] The second constellation of cholinergic neurons originates in the midbrain region and projects anteriorly to the thalamus, basal ganglia, and diencephalon and posteriorly to the reticular formation, pons, cerebellum, and cranial nerve nuclei. In addition to its generally agreed-on role in learning and memory, this diffuse network is consistent with suggestions that ACh may be involved in circuits that modulate pain and other sensory reception;[8] in mechanisms related to behavioral arousal, attention, energy conservation, and mood; and in REM activity during sleep.

Catecholamines: Dopamine and Norepinephrine

The term *catecholamine* refers to compounds that contain a "catechol" nucleus (a benzene ring with two attached hydroxyl groups) to which is attached an amine group (see Figure IV.15). In the CNS, the term usually refers to the transmitter *dopamine* (DA) and its metabolic product (in some neurons) *norepinephrine* (NE). A large number of psychoactive drugs exert their effects by altering the synaptic action of NE and DA.

The chemical synthesis of DA is illustrated in Figure IV.15. NE is produced by an additional step involving oxidation of the proximal carbon of the ethyl side chain. Biosynthesis of the catecholamines begins with the amino acid tyrosine and is an exceedingly complicated process involving genetic and enzymatic regulation.[9] Following synthesis, the transmitter is stored in vesicles for release into the synaptic space. Interestingly, such release is tightly controlled (modulated) by *presynaptic receptors* ("autoreceptors") that are activated not only by NE or DA but by such substances as ACh, prostaglandins, other amines, and possibly glutamate and/or endorphins. Such autoreceptors will probably become important targets of action for newly developed drugs, such as the recently introduced antidepressant mirtazapine (see Chapter 7). In addition, drugs such as the amphetamines (see Chapter 5) can induce the release of stored catecholamines.

Following release, NE and DA exert their characteristic postsynaptic effects. Inactivation in the synaptic cleft occurs primarily by active reuptake of the transmitter from the synaptic cleft back into the presynaptic nerve terminal. Within the nerve terminal,catecholamines can be inactivated by enzymes, such as monoamine oxidase (MAO). The products of inactivation are further metabolized and eliminated from the body through the urine. The class of antidepressants referred to as MAO-inhibitors (both irreversible and reversible; see Chapter 7) act by inhibiting MAO and thereby increasing the amounts of DA and NE available for synaptic release.

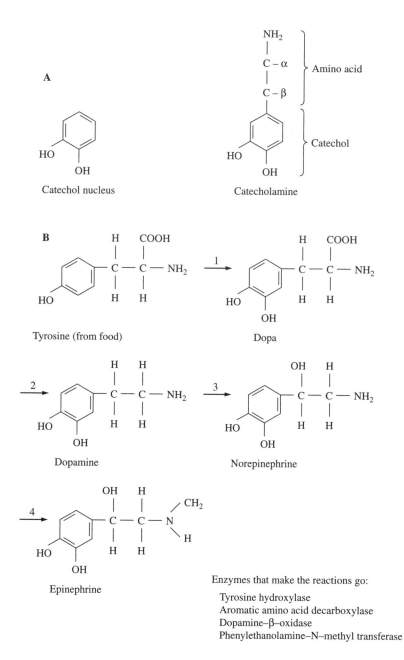

FIGURE IV.15 (**A**) Catechol and catecholamine structure. All catecholamines share the catechol nucleus, a benzene ring with two adjacent hydroxyl (OH) groups. (**B**) Structures and synthesis of the catecholamines. Tyrosine, an amino acid found in foods, is converted into dopa, then into dopamine, next into norepinephrine, and, finally (in the peripheral nervous system), into epinephrine, depending on which enzymes (1–4) are present in the cell.

Postsynaptic Action of Catecholamines. Unlike transmitters such as ACh and GABA (see Chapter 4), which affect ion channels, postsynaptic binding of DA or NE triggers a sequence of chemical events within the postsynaptic cell membrane (see Figure IV.11), ultimately affecting either ion channels or intracellular metabolic activity. It is likely that the antidepressant drugs exert their slow onset of action (several weeks to therapeutic effect) by ultimately reregulating as yet unidentified processes in postsynaptic neurons as a result of their blocking the presynaptic reuptake pump and making more transmitter available at the postsynaptic receptor, thus ultimately "desensitizing" postsynaptic intracellular function.

Norepinephrine Pathways. The cell bodies of NE neurons are located in the brain stem, mainly in the *locus ceruleus* (see Figure IV.16). From there, axons project widely throughout the brain, to nerve terminals in

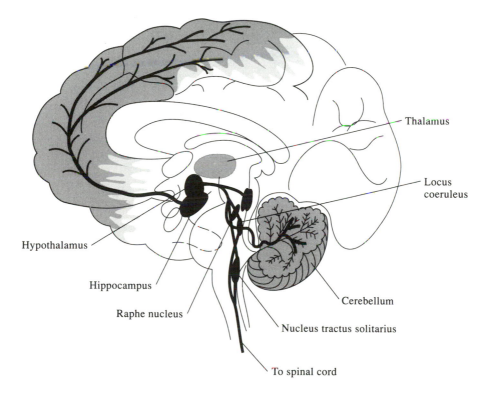

Thalamus

Locus coeruleus

Hypothalamus

Hippocampus

Raphe nucleus

Cerebellum

Nucleus tractus solitarius

To spinal cord

FIGURE IV.16 NE projection system in the human brain. The cell bodies are in the locus ceruleus and adjacent regions of the brain stem and project widely to the forebrain and cerebellum and to the brain stem and spinal cord.

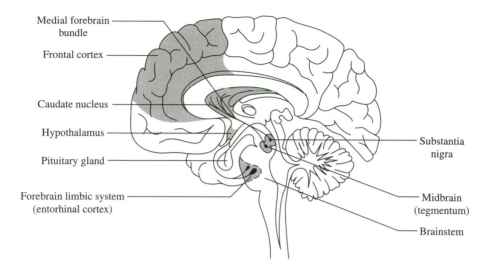

FIGURE IV.17 The three dopamine systems in the brain. One is a local circuit in the hypothalamus; another is the pathway from the substantia nigra to the caudate nucleus of the basal ganglia, which is involved in motor functions and Parkinson's disease; the third consists of cell bodies in the brain stem and midbrain (tegmentum) that project widely to the cerebral cortex and forebrain limbic system (entorhinal cortex). [From Thompson (1993),[2] p. 133.]

the cerebral cortex, the limbic system, the hypothalamus, and the cerebellum. Axonal projections also travel to the dorsal horns of the spinal cord, where they exert an analgesic action (as discussed in Chapter 10). The release of NE produces an alerting, focusing, orienting response, positive feelings of reward, and analgesia. NE release may also be involved in basic instinctual behaviors, such as hunger, thirst, emotion, and sex.

Dopamine Pathways. Dopamine pathways in the brain originate in the brain stem and are one-neuron pathways, sending axons both rostral to the brain and caudal to the spinal cord. Thompson (1993)[10] describes three dopamine circuits (see Figure IV.17). First, cell bodies in the hypothalamus send short axons to the pituitary gland. Such neurons are believed to function in the regulation of certain body hormones. Alterations in hormone function are commonly seen in schizophrenics taking phenothiazine antipsychotics, which block these dopamine receptors (see Chapter 9). Second, cell bodies in the brain stem structure called the substantia nigra project to the basal ganglia, playing a major role in the regulation of movement. Parkinsonism, its treatment with l-DOPA (see Appendix III), and antipsychotic-induced extrapyramidal side effects (Chapter 9) all involve this pathway. Third, cell bodies in the midbrain (ventral tegmentum), near the substantia nigra, project to higher brain regions including the cerebral cortex (especially the frontal cortex) and the limbic system, including the limbic cortex, nucleus accumbens, amygdaloid complex, and the entorhinal cortex, the latter being the major source of neurons projecting to the hippocampus. Alterations in the development of this pathway are thought to be involved in the pathogenesis of schizophrenia and its amelioration by neuroleptic drugs.[11]

Serotonin (5-Hydroxytryptamine, 5-HT)

Serotonin was first investigated as a CNS neurotransmitter when LSD was found to resemble serotonin structurally. At that time, it was hypothesized that drug-induced hallucinations might be caused by alterations in the functioning of serotonin neurons. (Today, we call LSD a *partial agonist* of serotonin receptors; see Chapter 12.) There is increasing interest in the role of serotonin in depression, sleep, sex, and the regulation of body temperature. Indeed, use of drugs that block the presynaptic reuptake of serotonin (the SSRIs; see Chapter 7) can be associated not only with alleviation of depression but with such side effects as insomnia, anxiety, loss of libido, and precipitation of a "serotonin syndrome."

Significant amounts of serotonin are found in the upper brain stem, with a large collection in the pons and the medulla (areas that are collectively called the *raphe nuclei*). Rostral projections from the brain stem terminate diffusely throughout the cerebral cortex, hippocampus, hypothalamus, and limbic system (see Figure IV.18). Serotonin projections largely parallel those of NE, although they are not as widespread. Serotonin seems to have an effect that is opposite to that of NE. Caudal projections of serotonin axons from the raphe nuclei to the spinal cord may be involved in the modulation of both pain (see Chapter 10) and spinal reflexes.

Glutamate (Glutamic Acid)

Glutamate appears to be the primary excitatory neurotransmitter in the brain, its receptors being found on the surface of virtually all neurons. Interestingly, glutamate is also the precursor for the major inhibitory neurotransmitter GABA, the latter being formed from glutamate under control of the enzyme *glutamic acid decarboxylase*. Glutamate neurotransmission plays a critical role in cortical and hippocampal cognitive

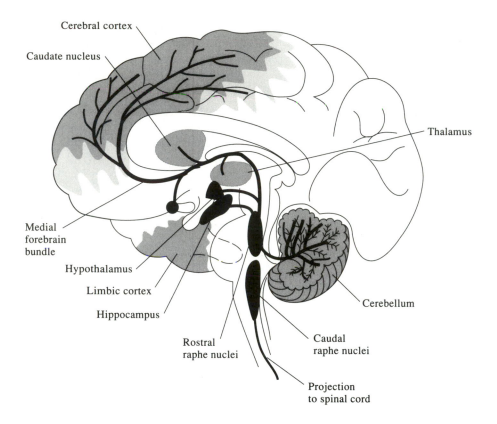

FIGURE IV.18 Serotonin pathways in the rat brain. Cell bodies and fiber tracts (axonal projections) are shown in black. Serotonergic terminals are represented by the shaded areas.

function, pyramidal and extrapyramidal motor function, cerebellar function, and sensory function.[12]

The glutamate receptor is schematically shown in Figure IV.19. Glutamate is obtained from foods and from metabolism and is stored in and released from nerve terminals. Postsynaptically, glutamate interacts with any of several different types of "glutamate receptors"; the transmitter then dissociates from the receptor and is inactivated by active reuptake into the presynaptic nerve terminal.

Glutamate acts not on a single receptor but on a "family" of receptors, with three distinct types. *AMPA* and *kainaic acid receptors* control the flow of sodium and potassium ions through a pore in the receptor, mediating rapid excitation of the postsynaptic neuron. Experimental

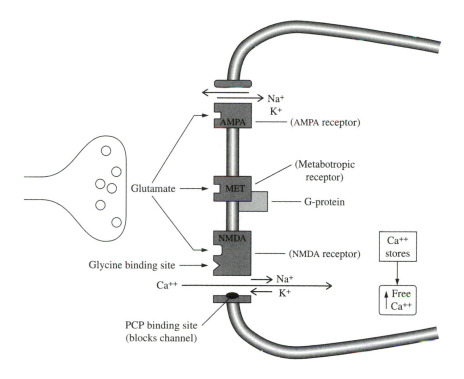

FIGURE IV.19 Glutamate receptor family. The AMPA receptor controls fast sodium and potassium channels; the NMDA receptor controls calcium channels; the metabotropic receptor controls a second-messenger system via a G-protein that acts on the intracellular machinery of the cell.

antianxiety drugs may act by blocking these receptors, reducing brain excitability. Lerma et al (1997)[13] discuss the possible roles of kainate-type glutamate receptors in hippocampal neurons.

Metabotropic receptors regulate ion channels and enzymes, producing second messengers coupled to G-proteins (like catecholamine and serotonin receptors described earlier).[14] Riedel (1996)[15] reviews the role of these receptors in learning and memory, via second messenger-induced alterations in synaptic plasticity that underlie memory formation. Conn and Pin (1997)[16] review the pharmacology of these receptors and their agonist and antagonist drugs, many of which have potential usefulness in treating a number of neurologic and psychologic disorders.

The *N-methyl-D-aspartate* (NMDA) *receptor* is a glutamate-activated ion channel, primarily for calcium ions, that is widely distributed in the brain and spinal cord, with particularly high receptor densities in the hippocampus and cerebral cortex. These receptors appear to also be involved in the developmental plasticity of the brain and in processes of learning and memory. They are rather selectively blocked by phencyclidine (PCP; see Chapter 12), a drug whose actions are characterized by analgesia, amnesia, and psychedelic effects. Overactivity of glutamate-NMDA receptors may be involved in neurotoxicity following ischemia (lack of oxygen) or other types of brain injury.[17] Here, excess inflow of calcium ions leads to greatly increased postsynaptic neuronal transcription of messenger RNA with a complex series of events that stimulate gene expression and protein synthesis involving cellular destructive enzymes. NMDA antagonists may aid in the protection of brain tissue following injury (such as after a stroke).

Gamma-Amino-Butyric Acid (GABA)

GABA is found in high concentrations in the brain and spinal cord and is a major inhibitory neurotransmitter. Indeed, benzodiazepine binding to its receptor site on GABA$_A$ receptors increases the flow of chloride ions through the membrane, an action associated with the anxiolytic effects of this class of drugs (see Chapter 4). *GABA$_A$ receptors* are found in high density in the cerebral cortex, hippocampus, and cerebellum. Likewise, activation of *GABA$_B$ receptors* in the amygdala is associated with the membrane-stabilizing, antiaggressive properties of valproic acid (see Chapter 8).

GABA$_A$ and *GABA$_B$ receptors* originate from two separate receptor families.[18] The GABA$_A$ receptor is a ligand-gated ion channel with multiple binding sites for drugs, such as barbiturates and benzodiazepines. Importantly for future pharmacologic research, about 10 different subtypes of the GABA$_A$ receptor occur,[18] certainly allowing for the development of agonists and antagonists of specific GABA$_A$ receptor subtypes. Such drugs might be novel antianxiety agents, anticonvulsants, cognitive enhancers, and so on.

GABA$_B$ receptors are G-protein–coupled receptors, a part of the superfamily of helical receptors similar to the serotonin$_{1A}$ and dopamine receptors discussed earlier.

Opioid Peptides

In 1967 it was proposed that chemicals exist in the brain that provide analgesia by acting on specific receptors and that the opioid narcotics might mimic these natural analgesic substances by binding to the same receptors. In 1973 opioid receptors were identified in localized areas of the brain. First, high concentrations of opioid receptors line the wall of the fourth ventricle in the brain stem. In that area, either morphine or electrical stimulation produces analgesia, which can be blocked by naloxone (Narcan, a pure opioid antagonist). The medial thalamus also has a high concentration of opioid receptors. This area of the brain appears to mediate deep pain that is poorly localized and emotionally influenced—the kind of pain most strongly affected by opioids. Opioid receptors are also found in areas of the spinal cord involved with the integration of incoming sensory information. Here, opioids reduce the intensity of painful stimuli. Receptors are also located in a nucleus of the brain stem that receives pain fibers from the face and the hands, as well as in those centers of the brain stem that are involved in the mediation of cough, nausea, and vomiting, maintenance of blood pressure, and control of stomach secretions.

The greatest concentration of opioid receptors in the CNS is located in the limbic system in the amygdala. Although opioids are not thought to exert analgesic actions through these limbic receptors, they probably exert influences through these receptors that affect emotional behavior (see Chapter 10). Very few opioid receptors are found in the cerebral cortex, and none have been found in the cerebellum.

In 1976 three types of opioid receptors were identified: *mu, kappa,* and *sigma receptors.* In 1981 a fourth type of receptor, the *delta receptor,* was added. More recently, subtypes of these receptors have been identified, and the existence of the opioid sigma receptor has been disputed.

Mu receptors are located primarily in the brain stem and medial thalamic areas. They appear to mediate morphine-induced analgesia and respiratory depression. Kappa receptors are located primarily in the spinal cord, where they mediate spinal analgesia. In the brain stem, kappa receptors mediate the sedation and miosis (pupil constriction) that are induced by opioids. Delta receptors are thought to be involved in alterations of affective behavior and euphoria. Delta receptors also appear to be specific target receptors for the enkephalin peptides.

The discovery of opioid receptors did not prove the existence of naturally occurring compounds in the brain that act on these receptors. In 1975, however, researchers isolated crude extracts from the brain that produced actions similar to those produced by morphine in a preparation of small intestines from guinea pigs. In particular, the brain extract inhibited normal intestinal contractions, an action that could be blocked by naloxone. Two proteins were isolated from this crude extract, each of which consisted of five amino acids. These two proteins were named met-enkephalin and leu-enkephalin. Later these proteins were isolated from pig brain, beef brain, human cerebral spinal fluid, and the pituitary gland of several species. Also isolated from the pituitary gland was a longer protein, called beta-lipotropin, within which was found met-enkephalin and other peptides that have opioid activity.

Several possible functions have been postulated for the endorphins, but their mechanism of analgesic action is not clear. A variety of evidence indicates that they are true neurotransmitters located in specific neuronal systems in the brain. They mediate the integration of sensory inputs related to pain, perception, and emotional behavior. This system probably is normally relatively inactive; otherwise, pure narcotic antagonists, such as naloxone, would displace them from their receptors and initiate pain (or at least produce an increased responsiveness) to a painful stimulus. The interesting possibility that endorphins may play a role in stress responses, in mental illness, and in drug craving has been raised. The opioid antagonist naloxone seems to ameliorate the hallucinogenic episodes experienced by chronic schizophrenic patients; in patients who experience chronic pain, naloxone alters endorphin levels; and in alcoholics, naloxone can reduce the craving for alcohol.[19] Certainly, these reported uses will stimulate additional attempts to clarify the role of endorphins in various emotional states.

NOTES

1. R. M. Julien, *Drugs and the Body* (New York: W. H. Freeman and Company, 1988).
2. R. F. Thompson, *The Brain: A Neuroscience Primer*, 2nd ed. (New York: W. H. Freeman and Company, 1993), 2–3.
3. W. S. Sossin, "Mechanisms for the Generation of Synapse Specificity in Long-term Memory: The Implications of a Requirement for Transcription," *Trends in Neurosciences* 19 (1996): 215–218.
4. J. D. Clements, "Transmitter Timecourse in the Synaptic Cleft: Its Role in Central Synaptic Function," *Trends in Neurosciences* 19 (1996): 163–171.
5. J. R. Cooper, F. E. Bloom, and R. H. Roth, *The Biochemical Basis of Neuropharmacology*, 7th ed. (New York: Oxford, 1996), 293–330.
6. Ibid., 51–54.
7. R. F. Thompson, *The Brain: A Neuroscience Primer*, 2nd ed. (New York: W. H. Freeman and Company, 1993), 122.
8. J. R. Cooper, F. E. Bloom, and R. H. Roth, *The Biochemical Basis of Neuropharmacology*, 7th ed. (New York: Oxford, 1996), 211.
9. Ibid., 226–244.

10. R. F. Thompson, *The Brain: A Neuroscience Primer*, 2nd ed. (New York: W. H. Freeman and Company, 1993), 133.
11. C. A. Ross and D. Pearlson, "Schizophrenia, the Heteromodal Association Neocortex and Development: Potential for a Neurogenetic Approach," *Trends in Neurosciences* 19 (1996): 171–176.
12. J. T. Greenamyre and R. H. Porter, "Anatomy and Physiology of Glutamate in the CNS," *Neurology* 44 (1994): S7–S13.
13. J. Lerma, M. Morales, M. A. Vicente, and O. Herreras, "Glutamate Receptors of the Kainate Type and Synaptic Transmission," *Trends in Neurosciences* 20 (1997): 9–12.
14. J.-P. Pin and R. DuVoisin, "The Metabotropic Glutamate Receptors: Structure and Functions," *Neuropharmacology* 34 (1995): 1–26.
15. G. Riedel, "Function of Metabotropic Glutamate Receptors in Learning and Memory," *Trends in Neurosciences* 19 (1996): 219–224.
16. P. J. Conn and J.-P. Pin, "Pharmacology and Functions of Metabotropic Glutamate Receptors," *Annual Review of Pharmacology and Toxicology* 37 (1997): 205–237.
17. J. K. Deshpande, "Ischemic Brain Injury: An Update on Mechanisms and Treatment," *American Journal of Anesthesiology* 23 (1996): 206–211.
18. R. M. McKernan and P. J. Whiting, "Which GABA$_A$-Receptor Subtypes Really Occur in the Brain?," *Trends in Neurosciences* 19 (1996): 139–143.
19. R. Spanagel and W. Zieglgansberger, "Anti-Craving Compounds for Ethanol: New Pharmacological Tools to Study Addictive Processes," *Trends in Pharmacological Sciences* 18 (1997): 54–59.

Abstinence syndrome. State of altered behavior that follows cessation of drug administration.

Acetylcholine. Neurotransmitter in the central and peripheral nervous systems.

Additive effect. Increased effect that occurs when two drugs that have similar biological actions are administered. The net effect is the sum of the independent effects exerted by the drugs.

Adenosine. Chemical neuromodulator in the CNS, primarily at inhibitory synapses.

Adenylate cyclase. Intracellular enzyme that catalyzes the conversion of cyclic AMP to adenosine monophosphate.

Affective disorder. Type of mental disorder characterized by recurrent episodes of mania, depression, or both.

Agonist. Drug that attaches to a receptor and produces actions that mimic or potentiate those of an endogenous transmitter.

Aldehyde dehydrogenase. Enzyme that carries out a specific step in alcohol metabolism: the metabolism of acetaldehyde to acetate. This enzyme may be blocked by the drug disulfiram (Antabuse).

Alzheimer's disease. Progressive neurological disease that occurs primarily in the elderly. It is characterized by a loss of short-term memory and intellectual functioning. It is associated with a loss of function of acetylcholine neurons.

Amphetamine. A behavioral stimulant.

Anabolic-androgenic steroid. Testosterone-like drug that acts to increase muscle mass and incurs other masculinizing effects.

Anandamide. Endogenous chemical compound that attaches to cannabinoid receptors in the CNS and to specific components of the lymphatic system.

Anandamide receptor. Receptor to which anandamide and tetrahydrocannabinol bind.

Anesthetic drugs. Sedative-hypnotic compounds used primarily in doses capable of inducing a state of general anesthesia that involves both loss of sensation and loss of consciousness.

Antagonist. Drug that attaches to a receptor and blocks the action of either an endogenous transmitter or an agonist drug.

Anticonvulsant. Drug that blocks or prevents epileptic convulsions. Some anticonvulsants (e.g., carbamazepine, valproic acid) are also used to treat certain nonepileptic psychiatric disorders.

Antidepressant. Drug that is useful in treating mental depression in depressed patients but does not produce stimulant effects in normal persons. Subdivided into seven classes or categories.

Antipsychotic drugs. Class of psychoactive drugs that have the ability to calm psychotic states and make the psychotic patient more manageable. Two classes are defined: classical and new generation.

Anxiolytic. Drug used to relieve the symptoms associated with anxiety and related disorders. Classically, refers to the benzodiazepines.

Attention deficit hyperactivity disorder (ADHD). Learning and behavioral disability characterized by reduced attention span and hyperactivity.

Autonomic nervous system. Portion of the peripheral nervous system that controls or regulates the visceral, or automatic, functions of the body (such as heart rate and blood pressure).

Barbiturates. Class of chemically related sedative-hypnotic compounds that share a characteristic six-membered ring structure.

Basal ganglia. Part of the brain that contains vast numbers of dopamine-containing synapses. Forms part of the extrapyramidal system. Parkinson's disease follows dopamine loss in this structure.

Benzodiazepines. Class of chemically related sedative-hypnotic agents of which chlordiazepoxide (Librium) and diazepam (Valium) are examples.

Beta-lipoprotein. 91-amino-acid protein containing amino acid sequences that have morphine-like activity.

Bipolar disorder. Affective disorder characterized by alternating bouts of mania and depression. Also referred to as *manic-depressive illness.*

Blackout. Period of time during which one may be awake but memory is not imprinted. It is common in people who have consumed excessive alcohol.

Brain syndrome, organic. Pattern of behavior induced when neurons are either reversibly depressed or irreversibly destroyed. Behavior is characterized by clouded sensorium, disorientation, shallow and labile affect, and impaired memory, intellectual function, insight, and judgment.

Brand name. Unique name licensed to one manufacturer of a drug. Contrasts with *generic name*, the name under which any manufacturer may sell a drug.

Caffeine. Behavioral and general cellular stimulant found in coffee, tea, cola drinks, and chocolate.

Caffeinism. Habitual use of large amounts of caffeine.

Cannabis sativa. Hemp plant; contains marijuana.

Carbidopa. Drug that inhibits the enzyme dopa decarboxylase, allowing increased availability of dopa within the brain. Contained in Sinemet.

Central nervous system (CNS). Brain and spinal cord.

Cirrhosis. Serious, usually irreversible liver disease. Usually associated with chronic excessive alcohol consumption.

Clonidine (Catapres). Antihypertensive useful in ameliorating the symptoms of narcotic withdrawal.

Cocaine. A behavioral stimulant.

Codeine. Sedative and pain-relieving agent found in opium. Structurally related to morphine but less potent; constitutes approximately 0.5 percent of the opium extract.

Comorbid disorder. Psychiatric disorder that coexists with a second psychiatric disorder (e.g., multisubstance abuse in a patient with a major depressive disorder).

Convulsant. Drug that produces convulsions by blocking inhibitory neurotransmission.

Crack. Street name for a smokable form of potent, concentrated cocaine.

Cross dependence. Condition in which one drug can prevent the withdrawal symptoms associated with physical dependence on a different drug.

Cross tolerance. Condition in which tolerance of one drug results in a lessened response to another drug.

Delirium tremens (DTs, "rum fits"). Syndrome of tremulousness with hallucinations, psychomotor agitation, confusion and disorientation, sleep disorders, and other associated discomforts, lasting several days after alcohol withdrawal.

Dementia. General designation for nonspecific mental deterioration.

Depo-Provera. Long-acting, injectable preparation of progesterone, useful as a long-acting female contraceptive.

Detoxification. Process of allowing time for the body to metabolize and/or excrete accumulations of drug. Usually a first step in drug abuse evaluation and treatment.

Diethylstilbestrol. Synthetically produced estrogen occasionally used in high doses as a postcoital contraceptive.

Differential diagnosis. Listing of all possible causes that might explain a given set of symptoms.

Dimethyltryptamine (DMT). Psychedelic drug found in many South American snuffs.

Disinhibition. Physiological state of the central nervous system characterized by decreased activity of inhibitory synapses, which results in a net excess of excitatory activity.

Dopamine transporter. Presynaptic protein that binds synaptic dopamine and transports the neurotransmitter back into the presynaptic nerve terminal.

Dose–response relation. Relation between drug doses and the response elicited at each dose level.

Drug. Chemical substance used for its effects on bodily processes.

Drug absorption. Mechanism by which a drug reaches the bloodstream from the skin, lungs, stomach, intestinal tract, or muscle.

Drug administration. Procedures through which a drug enters the body (oral administration of tablets or liquids, inhalation of powders, injection of sterile liquids, and so on).

Drug dependence. State in which the use of a drug is necessary for either physical or psychological well-being.

Drug interaction. Modification of the action of one drug by the concurrent or prior administration of another drug.

Drug misuse. Use of any drug (legal or illegal) for a medical or recreational purpose when other alternatives are available, practical, or warranted, or when drug use endangers either the user or others with whom he or she may interact.

Drug receptor. Specific molecular substance in the body with which a given drug interacts to produce its effect.

Drug tolerance. State of progressively decreasing responsiveness to a drug.

DSM-IV. *Diagnostic and Statistical Manual of Mental Disorders*, Fourth Edition (1994), a publication of the American Psychiatric Association.

Electroconvulsive therapy (ECT). Nonpharmacological treatment used for major depression.

Endorphin. Naturally occurring protein that causes endogenous morphine-like activity.

Enkephalin. Naturally occurring protein that causes morphine-like activity.

Enzyme. Large organic molecule that mediates a specific biochemical reaction in the body.

Enzyme induction. Increased production of drug-metabolizing enzymes in the liver, stimulated by certain drugs that increase the rate at which the body can metabolize them. It is one mechanism by which pharmacological tolerance is produced.

Epilepsy. Neurological disorder characterized by an occasional, sudden, and uncontrolled discharge of neurons.

Estrogen. Body hormone secreted primarily from the ovaries of females in response to stimulation by follicle-stimulating hormone (FSH) from the pituitary gland.

Fetal alcohol syndrome. Symptom complex of congenital anomalies, seen in newborns of women who ingested high doses of alcohol during critical periods of pregnancy.

G-protein. Specific intraneuronal protein.

Gamma-aminobutyric acid (GABA). Inhibitory amino acid neurotransmitter in the brain.

Generic name. Name that identifies a specific chemical entity (without specifically describing the chemical). Often marketed under different brand names by multiple manufacturers.

Hallucinogen. Psychedelic drug that produces profound distortions in perception.

Harmine. Psychedelic agent obtained from the seeds of *Peganum harmala*.

Hashish. Extract of the hemp plant (*Cannabis sativa*) that has a higher concentration of THC than does marijuana.

Heroin. Semisynthetic opiate produced by a chemical modification of morphine.

Hypothalamus. Structure located at the base of the brain, above the pituitary gland.

Hypoxia. State of relative lack of oxygen in the tissues of the body and the brain.

ICE. Street name for a smokable, free-based form of potent, concentrated methamphetamine.

Levodopa. Precursor substance to the transmitter dopamine, useful in ameliorating the symptoms of Parkinson's disease.

Limbic system. Group of brain structures involved in emotional responses and emotional expression.

Lithium. Alkali metal effective in the treatment of mania and depression.

Lysergic acid diethylamide (LSD). Semisynthetic psychedelic drug.

Major tranquilizer. Drug used in the treatment of psychotic states.

Mania. Mental disorder characterized by an expansive emotional state, elation, hyperirritability, excessive talkativeness, flights of ideas, and increased behavioral activity.

MAO inhibitor (MAOI). Drug that inhibits the activity of the enzyme monoamine oxidase.

Marijuana. Mixture of the crushed leaves, flowers, and small branches of both the male and female hemp plant (*Cannabis sativa*).

Mescaline. Psychedelic drug extracted from the peyote cactus.

Minor tranquilizer. Sedative-hypnotic drug promoted primarily for use in the treatment of anxiety.

Mixed agonist–antagonist. Drug that attaches to a receptor, producing weak agonist effects but displacing more potent agonists, precipitating withdrawal in drug-dependent persons.

Monoamine oxidase (MAO). Enzyme capable of metabolizing norepinephrine, dopamine, and serotonin to inactive products.

Monoamine oxidase inhibitor (MAOI). See **MAO inhibitor**.

Morphine. Major sedative and pain-relieving drug found in opium, comprising approximately 10 percent of the crude opium exudate.

Muscarine. Drug extracted from the mushroom *Amanita muscaria* that directly stimulates acetylcholine receptors.

Myristin. Psychedelic agent obtained from nutmeg and mace.

Neurotransmitter. Endogenous chemical released by one neuron that alters the electrical activity of another neuron.

Nicotine. Behavioral stimulant found in tobacco.

Ololiuqui. Psychedelic drug obtained from the seeds of the morning glory plant.

Opioid. Natural or synthetic drug that exerts actions on the body similar to those induced by morphine, the major pain-relieving agent obtained from the opium poppy (*Papaver somniferum*).

Opium. Crude resinous exudate from the opium poppy.

Parkinson's disease. Disorder of the motor system characterized by involuntary movements, tremor, and weakness.

Peptide. Chemical composed of a chain-link sequence of amino acids.

Pergonal. Preparation of follicle-stimulating hormone extracted from the urine of postmenopausal females.

Peyote. Cactus that contains mescaline.

Pharmacodynamics. Study of the interactions of a drug and the receptors responsible for the action of the drug in the body.

Pharmacokinetics. Study of the factors that influence the absorption, distribution, metabolism, and excretion of a drug.

Pharmacology. Branch of science that deals with the study of drugs and their actions on living systems.

Phencyclidine (Sernyl, PCP). Psychedelic surgical anesthetic. Acts by binding to and inhibiting ion transport through the NMDA-glutamate receptors.

Phenothiazine. Class of chemically related compounds useful in the treatment of psychosis.

Physical dependence. State in which the use of a drug is required for a person to function normally. Such a state is revealed by withdrawing the drug and noting the occurrence of withdrawal symptoms (abstinence syndrome). Characteristically, withdrawal symptoms can be terminated by readministration of the drug.

Placebo. Pharmacologically inert substance that may elicit a significant reaction largely because of the mental "set" of the patient or the physical setting in which the drug is taken.

Potency. Measure of drug activity expressed in terms of the amount required to produce an effect of given intensity. Potency varies inversely with the amount of drug required to produce this effect—the more potent the drug, the lower the amount required to produce the effect.

Progesterone. Hormone secreted from the ovaries in response to stimulation by luteinizing hormone (LH) from the pituitary gland.

Progestins. Group of synthetically produced progesterones; most frequently found in oral contraceptive tablets.

Psilocybin. Psychedelic drug obtained from the mushroom Psilocybe mexicana.

Psychedelic drug. Drug that can alter sensory perception.

Psychoactive drug. Chemical substance that alters mood or behavior as a result of alterations in the functioning of the brain.

Psychological dependence. Compulsion to use a drug for its pleasurable effects. Such dependence may lead to a compulsion to misuse a drug.

Psychopharmacotherapy. Clinical treatment of psychiatric disorders with drugs.

Psychotherapy. Nonpharmacological treatment of psychiatric disorders utilizing a wide range of modalities, from simple education and supportive counseling to insight-oriented, dynamically based therapy.

Receptor. Location in the nervous system at which a neurotransmitter or drug binds to exert its characteristic effect.

Reye's syndrome. Rare CNS disorder that occurs in children; associated with aspirin ingestion.

Risk-to-benefit ratio. Arbitrary assessment of the risks and benefits that may accrue from administration of a drug.

Scopolamine. Anticholinergic drug that crosses the blood-brain barrier to produce sedation and amnesia.

Second messenger. Intraneuronal protein that, when activated by an excitatory G-protein, initiates the neuronal response to the initial neurotransmitter attachment to an extracellular receptor.

Sedative-hypnotic drugs. Chemical substances that exert a nonselective general depressant action on the nervous system.

Serotonin (5-hydroxytryptamine, 5-HT). Synaptic transmitter in both the brain and the peripheral nervous system.

Serotonin-specific reuptake inhibitor (SSRI). Second-generation antidepressant drug.

Side effect. Drug-induced effect that accompanies the primary effect for which the drug is administered.

Tardive dyskinesia. Movement disorder that appears after months or years of treatment with neuroleptic (antipsychotic) drugs. It usually worsens with drug discontinuation. Symptoms are often masked by the drugs that cause the disorder.

Teratogen. Chemical substance that induces abnormalities of fetal development.

Testosterone. Hormone secreted from the testes that is responsible for the distinguishing characteristics of the male.

Tetrahydrocannabinol (THC). Major psychoactive agent in marijuana, hashish, and other preparations of hemp (*Cannabis sativa*).

Therapeutic drug monitoring (TDM). Process of correlating the plasma level of drugs with therapeutic response.

Toxic effect. Drug-induced effect either temporarily or permanently deleterious to any organ or system of an animal or person. Drug toxicity includes both the relatively minor side effects that invariably accompany drug administration and the more serious and unexpected manifestations that occur in only a small percentage of patients who take a drug.

INDEX